Entry Level

# RESPIRATORY
# THERAPIST *Exam Guide*

# Entry Level
# RESPIRATORY THERAPIST *Exam Guide*

## fourth edition

**JAMES R. SILLS, MEd, CPFT, RRT**
Director, Respiratory Care Program
Rock Valley College
Rockford, Illinois

*Original illustrations by*
Sandra Hogan, Rock Valley College, Rockford, Illinois

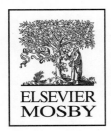

ELSEVIER
MOSBY

**ELSEVIER**
**MOSBY**

11830 Westline Industrial Drive
St. Louis, Missouri 63146

ENTRY LEVEL RESPIRATORY THERAPIST EXAM GUIDE, FOURTH EDITION

---

**Notice**

Pharmacology is an ever-changing field. Standard safety precautions must be followed, but as new research and clinical experience broaden our knowledge, changes in treatment and drug therapy may become necessary or appropriate. Readers are advised to check the most current product information provided by the manufacturer of each drug to be administered to verify the recommended dose, the method and duration of administration, and contraindications. It is the responsibility of the licensed prescriber, relying on experience and knowledge of the patient, to determine dosages and the best treatment for each individual patient. Neither the publisher nor the author assumes any liability for any injury and/or damage to persons or property arising from this publication.

---

Previous editions copyrighted 2000, 1994, 1991 by Mosby, Inc.

ISBN-13: 978-0-323-02824-0
ISBN-10: 0-323-02824-1

*Managing Editor:* Mindy Hutchinson
*Senior Developmental Editor:* Melissa K. Boyle
*Publishing Services Manager:* Pat Joiner
*Senior Project Manager:* Karen M. Rehwinkel
*Design Manager:* Bill Drone

Printed in the United States of America

Last digit is the print number:   9   8   7   6   5   4

*This book is dedicated to my wife*
***Deb***
*and our children*
***Rachael*** *and* ***David,***
*who make my life full and complete;*
*the memory of our first dog* ***Amber,***
*our new dog* ***Abby****, who takes me for long walks;*
*my* ***Mom*** *and the memory of my* ***Dad****;*
*and*
***Carl Hammond****,*
*who taught me respiratory care.*

*Words to live by:*
*The journey of 1000 miles begins with a single step.*
*Lao Tzu*
*Hope for the best but plan for the worst.*

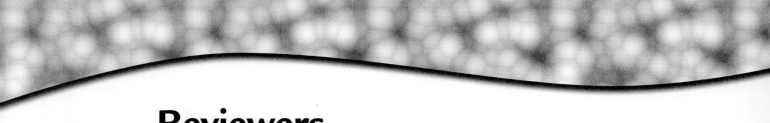

# Reviewers

**REGINA CLARK, MEd, RRT**
Program Director
Northwest Mississippi Community College
Southern, Mississippi

**SINDEE KALMINSON KARPEL, MPA, RRT, AE-C**
Clinical Coordinator
Cardiovascular Technology and Respiratory Care
  Programs
Edison Community College
Fort Myers, Florida

**STEPHEN MICKLES, EdS, RRT**
Program Director
Respiratory Care Program
St. Petersburg College
Pinellas Park, Florida

**DENNIS WISSING, PhD, RRT, CPFT**
Professor and Program Coordinator
Department of Cardiopulmonary Science
Louisiana State University Health Sciences Center
Shreveport, Louisiana

# Foreword

The fourth edition of Jim Sills' *Entry Level Respiratory Therapist Exam Guide* clearly demonstrates that good work will stand the test of time. Again, the profession of respiratory therapy will have the opportunity to harvest the many benefits from the author's unique ability to provide a straightforward and clear-cut presentation of the essential knowledge, skills, and professional attributes currently required by the National Board of Respiratory Care (NBRC) to successfully pass the Certified Respiratory Therapist (CRT) examination.

The fourth edition now provides the reader with an added discussion of all the new test items listed by the NBRC. No other work provides the respiratory practitioner with this resource. Items no longer tested by the NBRC have been eliminated. In addition, all of the pre-test and post-test questions provided in each chapter have

been updated to mirror the revised content of the NBRC exam. Finally, both the pre-test and the post-test examinations are now available on a CD-ROM, giving the reader two computer-based exam experiences.

For the reader preparing for the NBRC Entry Level examination, the *Entry Level Respiratory Therapist Exam Guide* is a "go-to-first" resource. As we prepare to meet the increased respiratory demands that will undoubtedly be thrust upon us by the "baby-boomers" heading toward the hospital industry, both the future respiratory practitioner and respiratory patient will surely reap the fruits of this important and valuable respiratory therapy contribution.

**Terry Des Jardins**
**Parkland College**
**Champaign, Illinois**

# Preface

This text is designed to discuss the current content examined on the Certification Examination for Entry Level Respiratory Therapists. In addition, it includes many suggestions on how to prepare for the examination and hints on frequently tested topics. Each chapter ends with self-assessment questions. To help the test-taker better prepare for the real examination, two practice tests modeled on the real National Board for Respiratory Care (NBRC) examination are included. New to this edition, both the pre-test and post-test are on the included CD-ROM. Both have been revised as needed to stay within the scope of testable material listed by the NBRC for the entry level respiratory therapist. It is suggested that the pretest be taken before using this book and studying for the actual exam. Study the results of the pre-test to help determine your strengths and weaknesses. This will help to focus your studying. Then take the post-test. Its results will help you to further refine your studying. It is my sincere hope that using this text will help every graduate to earn the Certified Respiratory Therapist (CRT) credential.

**James R. Sills, MEd, CPFT, RRT**

# Introduction

## INTRODUCTION AND RECOMMENDATIONS FOR EXAMINATION SUCCESS

Every item listed on the National Board for Respiratory Care (NBRC) Certification Examination for Entry Level Respiratory Therapists (CRT) Content Outline, released in August 2003, is discussed in this text. A program graduate preparing for the examination can use this text to help focus on what needs to be studied. "Exam Hints" within the chapters point out commonly tested items, and self-assessment questions are included at the end of each chapter. The pre-test and post-test on the enclosed CD-ROM will help you to analyze your strengths and weaknesses. It is recommended that the pre-test be taken and analyzed before beginning the text and studying. After studying, take the post-test. Both tests are designed to follow the real examination in format, question styles, difficulty levels, and relative weight of tested areas.

The text includes bold headings followed by two codes. The first (in parentheses) is the NBRC code for that subject found in the above-listed August 2003 examination detailed content outline. My choice of words is a paraphrasing of theirs. Occasionally a heading appears without an NBRC code after it. These headings are added because they help you understand what the NBRC is testing. Discussion of pathologic processes is included in the general discussion of each section as they relate to the treatment or procedure that the respiratory therapist would perform. It is recommended that you study the major types of adult and infant disease states and abnormal conditions.

The second code [in brackets] is the NBRC code for the difficulty level of the questions used to test your understanding of the material. R stands for Recall, Ap stands for Application, and An stands for Analysis. The NBRC asks questions at these three different levels of difficulty.

## ENTRY LEVEL EXAMINATION

The entry level examination consists of 140 actual questions. (The NBRC also includes 20 extra questions being pre-tested for future versions of the examination. These questions are not scored as part of your examination. Since it is not possible to tell the actual from the pretested questions, take each question seriously.) The examination is offered in a computer-based testing format. Make sure that you follow all commands listed on the computer screens so that you do not make any mistakes. You have 3 hours to complete the examination. Do not leave any questions unanswered. A passing score is listed as 75% or greater (at least 105 correct questions). However, you could get fewer than 105 correct and still pass because the Application and Analysis questions are weighted more heavily than the Recall ones (see below). Those passing the examination are awarded the Certified Respiratory Therapist (CRT) credential by the NBRC. The actual content of a given examination is a closely guarded secret. Several examinations are usually maintained at a given time by the NBRC, with others in production. Old examinations are retired. Not everyone takes the same examination even at the same test site. The best way to prepare is to know the types of things that may be tested and how the test is constructed. There are three difficulty levels to the questions:

## Recall [R]

*Recall* refers to remembering previously learned factual information. "Identify" is a commonly used action verb in these types of questions. You may be asked to identify specific facts, terms, methods, procedures, principles, or concepts. Prepare for these types of questions by studying the full range of factual information, equations, etc., seen in respiratory care practice. These types of questions are on the lowest order of difficulty. You either know the answer or you do not; there is little to ponder more deeply. It is very important to have a solid understanding of the factual basis of respiratory care to do well in this and the next two categories of questions.

## Application [Ap]

*Application* refers to being able to use factual type of information in real clinical situations that may be new to you. "Apply," "classify," and "calculate" are commonly used action verbs in these types of questions. You may be asked to apply laws, theories, concepts, or principles to new, practical clinical situations. Calculations may have to be performed. Charts and graphs, such as those seen in pulmonary function testing, may need to be used. These types of questions are on a higher order of difficulty than the Recall types. Critical thinking must be applied to the factual information to answer these questions.

## Analysis [An]

*Analysis* refers to being able to separate a patient care problem into its component parts or elements to evaluate the relationship of the parts or elements to the whole problem. "Evaluate," "compare," "contrast," "revise," or "select" are commonly used action verbs in these types of questions. You may be questioned about revising a patient care plan or evaluating therapy. These types of questions necessitate the highest level of critical thinking. You may have to recall previously learned information, apply it to a patient care situation, and make a judgment on the best way to care for the patient.

You will find that the NBRC uses two different types of questions on the examination in these three ways:

## One Best Answer

This type of question has a stem (the question) followed by four possible answers (A, B, C, and D). You must select the *best* answer from among those presented. Only one is clearly best even though other possible answers may be good. Carefully read the stem to make sure that you do not misunderstand the clear intent of the question. Controversial issues may be questioned. The use of "should" in the stem indicates the need to select the answer that would be selected by the majority of practitioners.

Some questions may be worded in such a way that the *false* answer must be excluded. In other words, three answers are correct and one is incorrect. The use of "except" indicates this type of question. Other phrases to pay attention to include "What would be the *first* thing . . . ," "What would be the *most* important thing . . . ," or "What would be the *least* important thing. . . ."

## Multiple True-False

This type of question has a stem (the question) followed by four or five possible answers coded with Roman numerals (I, II, III, IV, and V) and then four combinations of the answers coded by letters (A, B, C, and D). The stem may ask you to include all true statements or all false statements in the final answer. You must select the letter that represents the correct combination of answers.

No controversial answers should be offered. They are all either clearly correct or incorrect, and this is the key to selecting the best answer. Read each possible answer as separate from the others, and mark each possible answer as true or false. Even if you are not sure of every option, you should be able to determine the best answer. After finding an option that you know is false, cross off any of the answers that contain it. After finding an option that you know to be true, cross off any answers that do not contain it. Through the process of elimination the best answer will be the remaining one.

## Situational Sets

Situational sets involve the use of a patient care scenario that may include such information as the patient's history, vital signs, blood gas values, or pulmonary func-

tion results. Three to five questions follow that ask you about patient or equipment management. These questions are the "one best answer" or "multiple true-false" types as discussed above. However, because of the amount of information offered and the critical thinking required, these questions are categorized as being at the Application or Analysis level of difficulty. It is important to carefully read the scenario to fully understand the information. Then, after reading a related question, refer back to the scenario for information that can help you pick the best answer. Do this for each question and also refer to the prior questions for information that may help you with the current one.

## GENERAL SUGGESTIONS FOR EXAMINATION PREPARATION

1. Take the pre-test on the CD-ROM. Analyze the results to determine your strengths and weaknesses.
2. Begin studying about 2 months before the examination. Pace yourself so that everything can be covered in the time that you have. Avoid "cramming" a few days before the examination; this test demands more than the simple recall of facts.
3. Study the most important and heavily tested areas first. Work down to the less important areas. See the table at the end of this section.
4. Spend extra time on any weak areas that are heavily tested.
5. Take the post-test on the CD-ROM. Analyze the results to determine your strengths and continued weaknesses. Spend additional time studying the remaining weak areas.
6. The NBRC has established certain H & R Block offices as testing centers. Schedule yourself to take the examination at a date and time you know you can make. Get clear directions to the office, plan your route and time needed, and add more for unexpected traffic.
7. Eat a good meal before the examination. Avoid alcohol, even if you are nervous, so you have a clear head.
8. Do not "cram" just before the examination. If you are not prepared by now, a few more hours will not really help. If necessary, brush up on a few test areas.
9. Get a good night's sleep before the examination. Avoid sleeping pills.
10. Attempt to relax before the examination with the self-confidence that comes from knowing that you are well prepared.

## RELATIVE WEIGHTS OF THE VARIOUS TESTED AREAS ON THE ENTRY-LEVEL EXAMINATION

I have analyzed the content of each of the 140 questions on the available entry-level examinations covering the 1998 and 2003 examination content outlines. Each question has been matched to one of the chapters in the table on the next page. The numbers of questions and percentages are averages and may not be followed exactly

| Examination Content Found in Each Chapter | | |
|---|:---:|:---:|
| **Chapter** | **Number of Questions** | **Examination Percentage** |
| 1  Patient Assessment | 9 | 7% |
| 2  Infection Control | 4 | 3% |
| 3  Blood Gas Analysis and Monitoring | 10 | 7% |
| 4  Pulmonary Function Testing | 7 | 5% |
| 5  Advanced Cardiopulmonary Monitoring | 2 | 1% |
| 6  Oxygen Therapy | 12 | 9% |
| 7  Hyperinflation Therapy | 2 | 1% |
| 8  Humidity and Aerosol Therapy | 7 | 5% |
| 9  Pharmacology | 11 | 8% |
| 10  Bronchopulmonary Hygiene Therapy | 3 | 2% |
| 11  Cardiac Monitoring and Cardiopulmonary Resuscitation | 6 | 4% |
| 12  Airway Management | 9 | 7% |
| 13  Suctioning the Airway | 4 | 3% |
| 14  Intermittent Positive-Pressure Breathing | 3 | 2% |
| 15  Mechanical Ventilation | 43 | 31% |
| 16  Home Care and Pulmonary Rehabilitation | 3 | 2% |
| 17  Special Procedures | 3 | 2% |
| Miscellaneous pulmonary conditions or diseases | 2 | 1% |
| TOTAL | 140 | 100% |

on other versions of the entry-level examination. However, the relative weights can offer solid guidance as to what content is relatively more important or less important. Study time can be spent accordingly.

I recommend that the content of Chapters 1, 3, 4, and 5 be thoroughly understood. This information is questioned directly and also incorporated into questions covering other chapters. Examples: (1) Blood gas values are incorporated into the oxygen therapy questions. (2) Bedside spirometry values are incorporated into pharmacology questions dealing with the effectiveness of bronchodilator therapy. (3) Blood gas values and bedside spirometry values are incorporated into mechanical ventilation questions. The content in Chapter 15 (Mechanical Ventilation) is the most heavily questioned of all. You must understand mechanical ventilation to do well on the examination.

**James R. Sills, MEd, CPFT, RRT**

## Important Addresses and Phone Numbers

For information on the examination process, taking a practice exam, getting a copy of the exam detailed content outline, and to schedule taking an exam, contact:

**National Board for Respiratory Care**
8310 Nieman Road, Lenexa, Kansas 66214-1579
(913) 599-4200
Fax: (913) 541-0156
E-mail: nbrc-info@nbrc.org
Internet address: http://www.nbrc.org

For information on purchasing self-assessment examinations, contact:

**Applied Measurement Professionals**
8310 Nieman Road, Lenexa, Kansas 66214-1579
(913) 541-0400
Fax: (913) 541-0156
Internet address: http://www.goAMP.com

For information on accredited respiratory care educational programs, contact:

**Committee on Accreditation for Respiratory Care**
1248 Harwood Road, Bedford, Texas 76021-4244
(817) 283-2835
Fax: (817) 354-8519
Internet address: http://www.coarc.com

For information on state credentialing requirements, contact:

**American Association for Respiratory Care**
9425 N. MacArthur Boulevard, Suite 100, Irving TX 75063-4706
(972) 243-AARC (2272)
Fax: (972) 484-2720
E-mail: info@aarc.org
Internet address: http://www.aarc.org

# Contents

**CD-ROM Contents**

Pre-test: Practice Entry Level Examination

Pre-test: Practice Entry Level Examination Answer Key

CRT Self-Examination

CRT Self-Examination Answer Key

**Entry Level**

# RESPIRATORY
# THERAPIST *Exam Guide*

# 1 Patient Assessment

A review of the most recent Entry Level Examinations has shown an average of 9 questions (7% of the exam) that cover patient assessment issues.

## MODULE A

### Review the patient's chart and recommend diagnostic procedures based on the current information

Notes: (1) This discussion involves noninvasive bedside activities that apply to adults in most respiratory care settings. Some assessment items have been placed in later chapters because they are procedure specific. (2) Remember the NBRC code for question difficulty: R = Recall, Ap = Application, An = Analysis.

1. **Review the patient's history: present illness, admission notes, diagnosis, do not resuscitate (DNR) orders, respiratory care orders, and progress notes** (National Board for Respiratory Care [NBRC] code: IA1) **[Difficulty: R]**

   **a. Patient history**

Review the complete initial patient history and admission notes, and identify the following:
   1. Date of history taking
   2. Patient data (name, age, sex, race, and occupation)
   3. Primary complaints
   4. Secondary complaints
   5. History and symptoms of present illness
   6. Family history
   7. Medical history of cardiopulmonary disease

The chart should also contain the physician's written initial diagnosis for the patient. After the medical history has been completed and the diagnosis determined, the patient should be placed into one of the following four patient illness categories. Refer to Table 1-1 for examples of each category.
   1. Crisis/acute onset of illness
   2. Intermittent but repeated illness
   3. Progressive worsening
   4. Mixed patterns/multiple problems

It is important that the clinician obtain a *brief* history before beginning therapeutic procedures. Determine how the patient has been doing since the last treatment (e.g., has there been a change in dyspnea, cough and secretions, or chest pain?). This helps to guide therapy as effectively as possible.

   **b. Do not resuscitate (DNR) status**

The physician and patient and family should determine the patient's cardiopulmonary resuscitation status. A patient with a terminal condition, such as end-stage chronic obstructive lung disease, will often choose not to be resuscitated. If it has been determined that the patient does not want to be resuscitated, his/her DNR status should be clearly posted on the chart and in the patient's room. All members of the health care team should be aware of the patient's decision.

   **c. Current respiratory care orders**

Physician orders, including verbal orders to the nurse or respiratory therapist, must include the patient's name, the date and time, complete and proper orders for each therapeutic procedure, and the physician's signature. Incomplete, improper, or questionable orders must be confirmed by a call to the physician for clarification or correction.

   **d. Progress notes**

Review any patient progress notes from the physician, nurse, and respiratory therapist before you see the patient and begin the therapeutic procedure. Look for any cardiopulmonary or other organ system changes that may have an impact on the patient's ability to tolerate the treatment. This may necessitate revising the therapy, getting different equipment, or seeking help. Check for new patient care orders if the physician notes a change in the patient's care plan.

2. **Review the results of the patient's physical examination and vital signs** (NBRC code: IA2) **[Difficulty: R, Ap]**

Review the results of the physical examinations performed by the physician(s), nurse(s), and respiratory therapist(s). Review the following organ systems:
   • Pulmonary
   • Cardiovascular
   • Neuromuscular
   • Renal

| TABLE 1-1 | Patient Illness Categories |
|-----------|---------------------------|
| **Category** | **Examples** |
| Crisis/acute onset of illness | Trauma, heart attack, allergic reaction, aspiration of a foreign body, pneumothorax, pulmonary embolism, and some pneumonias |
| Intermittent but repeated illness | Asthma, chronic bronchitis, congestive heart failure, angina pectoris, myasthenia gravis, and some pneumonias |
| Progressive worsening | Congestive heart failure, chronic bronchitis, emphysema, and upper respiratory tract infection leading to bronchitis or pneumonia |
| Mixed patterns/ multiple problems | Chronic obstructive pulmonary disease and cystic fibrosis complicated by multiple problems, mucus plugging, or infection; mixes of congestive heart failure and chronic lung disease; mixes of neuromuscular and lung disease; mixes of renal failure and congestive heart failure with chronic lung disease |

| TABLE 1-2 | Normal Resting Respiratory Rates | |
|-----------|------|--------|
| **Age (years)** | **Male** | **Female** |
| 0–1 | $31 \pm 8$ | $30 \pm 6$ |
| 1–2 | $26 \pm 4$ | $27 \pm 4$ |
| 2–3 | $25 \pm 4$ | $25 \pm 3$ |
| 5–6 | $22 \pm 2$ | $21 \pm 2$ |
| 9–10 | $19 \pm 2$ | $19 \pm 2$ |
| 13–14 | $19 \pm 2$ | $18 \pm 2$ |
| 15–16 | $17 \pm 3$ | $18 \pm 3$ |
| 17–18 | $16 \pm 3$ | $17 \pm 3$ |
| Older than 18 | $16 \pm 3$ | $17 \pm 3$ |

From Eubanks DH, Bone RC: Comprehensive respiratory care, ed 2, St. Louis, 1990, Mosby.

### a. Current vital signs

Review current vital signs in the patient's chart. Compare admission vital signs with what you currently observe in the patient. Look for a change in pattern that would suggest a worsening or an improvement in the patient.

### b. Temperature

The textbook "normal" oral body temperature is 37° C (98.6° F), but a range from 35.8° to 37.4° C (96.5° to 99.5° F) is normal. Make sure the patient has not eaten any hot or cold foods recently, and that he or she has not been smoking just before the temperature is taken.

A rectal or core temperature is commonly taken in extremely sick patients because it is more accurate and reliable than an oral temperature. Normal rectal temperature is 36.4° to 38° C (97.5° to 100.4° F). Some variance, although less than in oral temperature, is normal. Axillary temperatures are used as a last resort in stable patients; they run almost 1° C (1° F) lower than oral temperatures and are less accurate and reliable.

The variations in temperature noted previously depend on the time of day, the activity level, and, in women, the menstrual cycle. For example, a lower body temperature is normal when a person is in a deep sleep. An oral temperature higher than 37.4° C (99.4° F) in a patient with a history of respiratory disease indicates a fever, which is typically caused by atelectasis or pulmonary or systemic

infection. Patients are commonly treated to keep the fever below 39° C (103° F) if possible. In general, a rectal temperature below 36° C (97° F) is considered hypothermic. Some procedures, such as open heart surgery, involve lowering a patient's temperature to reduce metabolism and oxygen ($O_2$) needs. Rectal temperature must be kept above 90° F (32° C) to prevent the occurrence of cardiac arrhythmias that result from the cold.

### c. Respiratory rate

The respiratory rate ($f$ for frequency) is the number of breaths the patient takes per minute. The clinician can count this number by looking at or feeling the chest or abdomen for movement. Normal rate varies with age (Table 1-2). When respiratory rate is determined, the patient is assumed to be resting but awake with a normal temperature and metabolic rate. A respiratory rate above or below normal is a cause for concern.

Hyperthermia (fever), acidemia, hypoxemia, fear, anxiety, and pain cause a patient to breathe more rapidly. Hypothermia, alkalemia, hyperoxia in the patient breathing on hypoxic drive, sedation, and coma cause a patient to breathe more slowly.

Even in healthy people, considerable variation is noted in the respiratory rate. The respiratory rate should be considered along with the patient's tidal volume ($V_T$) and minute volume for a more complete impression of how the patient is breathing. The respiratory rate should be carefully measured in any patient with cardiopulmonary disease or with a respiratory rate outside of the normal range. This rate should be checked as needed to follow up on the patient's condition.

### d. Blood pressure

Blood pressure (BP) is determined by the pumping ability of the left ventricle (made up of the heart rate [HR] and stroke volume), arterial resistance, and blood volume. Normal BP results when all three factors are in balance with each other. If one factor is abnormal, the other two have some ability to compensate. For example, if the patient has lost a lot of blood, the body attempts to maintain BP by increasing arterial resistance and HR.

### Normal blood pressures
Adult: Lower than 120/80 mm Hg
Infant to child younger than 10 years old: 60–100/ 20–70 mm Hg

As with other vital signs, some variation in BP exists among individuals. The patient's normal BP must be known before a comparison can be made with the current value. Carefully measure the BP in any patient with cardiopulmonary disease or a history of hypotension or hypertension.

Hypotension in the adult is seen as a systolic BP of less than 80 mm Hg. Recommend a BP measurement for any patient who has a history of hypotension, appears to be in shock, has lost considerable blood, has a weak pulse, shows mental confusion, is unconscious, or has low urine output.

Hypertension in the adult is noted as a systolic BP of 140 mm Hg or greater, or a diastolic BP of 90 mm Hg or greater. Carefully measure the BP of patients with hypertension, bounding pulse, or symptoms of stroke (e.g., mental confusion, headache, and sudden weakness or partial paralysis). Fear, anxiety, and pain also cause the patient's BP to rise temporarily.

### e. Heart/pulse rate

The HR, which is the number of heartbeats per minute, can be counted by listening to heart tones with a stethoscope, or by feeling any of the common sites at which an artery is easy to locate. Table 1-3 shows normal pulse rates based on age. The patient is assumed to be alert but resting when the pulse is counted. Carefully measure the HR of any patient with cardiopulmonary disease or with any of the aforementioned conditions to assess for hypotension or hypertension.

| TABLE 1-3 | Normal Pulse Rates According to Age |
|---|---|
| **Age** | **Beats/min** |
| Birth | 70–170 |
| Neonate | 120–140 |
| 1 year | 80–140 |
| 2 year | 80–130 |
| 3 year | 80–120 |
| 4 year | 70–115 |
| Adult | 60–100 |

From Eubanks DH, Bone RC: Comprehensive respiratory care, ed 2, St. Louis, 1990, Mosby.

## MODULE B
### Radiographic imaging

### 1. Review the patient's imaging findings (NBRC code: IA5 and IIIE1) [Difficulty: R]

Look for the results of radiographs (x-rays) of the chest or upper airway, computed tomography (CT) scans, positron emission tomography (PET) studies, ventilation/perfusion (V/Q) scans, angiograms, and magnetic resonance imaging (MRI) studies. If possible, review these results to gain a better understanding of the patient's condition.

### 2. Review the patient's chest radiograph film to evaluate and monitor the patient's response to respiratory care procedures (NBRC code: IIIE1) [Difficulty: R, Ap]

A chest x-ray examination is needed whenever a significant change is noted in the patient's cardiopulmonary condition, or whenever an invasive thoracic procedure (e.g., chest tube insertion, endotracheal intubation, or pulmonary artery catheter placement) is performed.

Chest x-ray examination should be recommended in the following situations:

a. After an endotracheal or tracheostomy tube has been placed or repositioned
b. After the jugular or subclavian route has been used to insert a central venous pressure (CVP) or pulmonary artery (Swan-Ganz) catheter
c. After a chest tube has been placed in the pleural space to remove air or fluids
d. If hemoptysis (bloody sputum) appears
e. When a sudden deleterious change occurs in the patient's cardiopulmonary condition
f. When the balloon on the pulmonary artery catheter has been left inflated for a prolonged period and a pulmonary infarct is suspected
g. When a pneumothorax is suspected

An upper airway x-ray (anterior and/or lateral) examination should be recommended for a patient who has symptoms of upper airway obstruction. These could include the following:

a. Aspirated foreign body
b. Laryngeal edema
c. Laryngeal tumor
d. Epiglottitis

A CT scan provides a more detailed image than is seen on a conventional x-ray film. It enables identification of abnormalities of the lungs and mediastinum. Indications include, but are not limited to, the following:

a. Tumor
b. Hematoma
c. Abscess and cyst
d. Pleural effusion
e. Aortic or other vascular abnormalities (after intravenous contrast material is given)

**Exam Hint**

**T**he National Board for Respiratory Care (NBRC) may use the term *radiograph* in examination questions rather than *x-ray*.

### 3. Look for the presence of, or any changes in, the pneumothorax, or for subcutaneous emphysema or any other extrapulmonary air (NBRC code: IB6b) [Difficulty: R, Ap]

Free air that leaks into the interstitial spaces of the lung or body cavities is abnormal in any patient. Causes for an air leak include barotrauma/volutrauma (alveolar rupture related to the use of excessive pressure and/or volume from a mechanical ventilator); ruptured bleb (congenital or acquired blister on the visceral pleura); puncture wound through the chest wall; and needle puncture through the pleural space during insertion of a CVP or pulmonary artery catheter through the subclavian or jugular vein. Once air under pressure is forced through a bronchial or alveolar tear into the interstitial tissues, it tends to follow the path of least resistance. This may result in the finding of air in any of the following areas, either singly or in combination.

*Pneumothorax* is air in the pleural space. The lung tends to collapse toward the hilum. A pneumothorax is identified on the chest radiograph as an area of black (indicating air) that surrounds the collapsed lung. No lung markings are visible in the air-filled space, and the edge of the lung can be seen (Fig. 1-1). If the air is under sufficient pressure to shift the lung and mediastinal structures to the opposite side, the condition is called *tension pneumothorax*. This is a serious condition and can lead to death if not quickly identified and treated. A pleural chest tube should be placed into the affected side to remove the air and reexpand the lung.

*Subcutaneous emphysema* is air found in the soft tissues such as the skin, axilla, shoulder, neck, or breast of the affected side. In extreme cases, the air forces its way into skin and soft tissues throughout the body. The chest x-ray appearance is one of scattered dark areas (air pockets) that are seen within the various soft tissues (Fig. 1-2).

Free air can be found pathologically in other areas. *Pneumomediastinum* is air in the mediastinal space (see Fig. 1-2). *Pneumopericardium* is air in the pericardial space (Fig. 1-3). Both of these conditions can be very serious. A cardiac tamponade is created if the pressure around the heart is great enough to interfere with its function. *Pneumoperitoneum* is air in the peritoneal space. This condition can be dangerous in an infant if such a volume of air limits the movement of the diaphragm. Pulmonary interstitial emphysema (PIE) is air disseminated throughout the

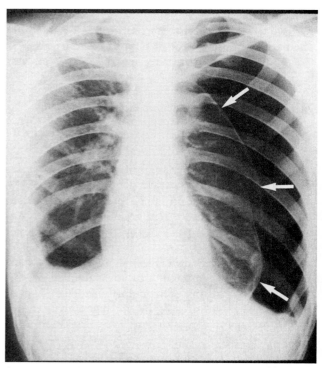

**Fig. 1-1** Frontal x-ray film of an adult male with a left-sided tension pneumothorax. Arrows indicate the edge of the collapsed lung. Note how the mediastinum is shifted to the right, the right lung is compressed, and the left hemidiaphragm is depressed. *(From Des Jardins TR, Burton GG: Clinical manifestations and assessment of respiratory disease, ed 3, St. Louis, 1995, Mosby.)*

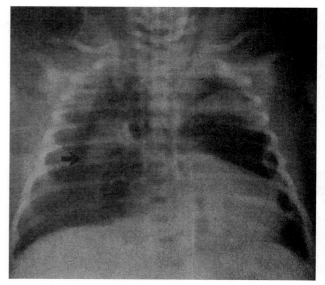

**Fig. 1-2** Frontal x-ray film of a neonate showing subcutaneous emphysema in the shoulders and neck area. Other abnormal air in the patient's chest includes a pneumomediastinum, which outlines the right lobe of the thymus gland *(arrow)* and a left anterior pneumothorax. *(From Carlo WA, Chatburn RL, editors: Neonatal respiratory care, Chicago, 1988, Mosby.)*

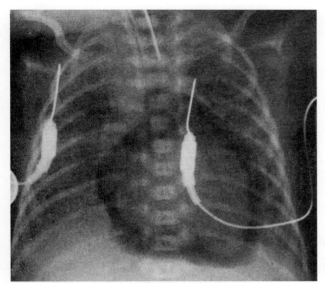

**Fig. 1-3** Frontal x-ray film of a neonate showing a pneumopericardium that resulted from pulmonary interstitial emphysema. Note the dark outline of air around the heart. Chest tubes have been placed to remove air from around the heart and the right pleural space from an earlier pneumothorax. An endotracheal tube is also seen. *(From Koff PB, Eitzman DV, Neu J: Neonatal and pediatric respiratory care, ed 2, St. Louis, 1993, Mosby.)*

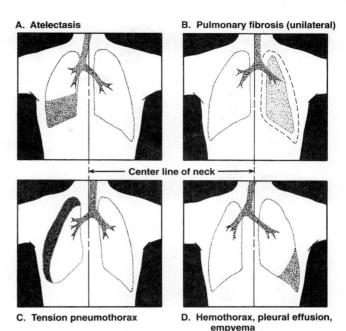

**Fig. 1-4** Conditions causing tracheal deviation and mediastinal shift (simulated chest x-ray findings). **A,** Unilateral atelectasis with tracheal deviation *toward* the affected lung. **B,** Unilateral pulmonary fibrosis with tracheal deviation *toward* the affected lung. **C,** Tension pneumothorax with tracheal deviation *away* from the affected lung. **D,** Pleural fluid with tracheal deviation *away* from the affected lung. The normal lung expands farther than the abnormal lung during inspiration.

interstitial spaces of the injured lung(s). The lungs appear cystic or "bubbly" on the chest x-ray image (see Fig. 1-3). The air may further leak into any of the locations previously discussed. PIE is most commonly seen in infants with infant respiratory distress syndrome (RDS) who require mechanical ventilation.

---

### Exam Hint

**Q**uestions pertaining to recommending a chest x-ray examination to rule out or confirm a pneumothorax have regularly appeared on the entry level examination. Signs and symptoms that the patient may have a pneumothorax include sudden chest pain with increased dyspnea and shortness of breath (SOB), absent breath sounds over a lung field, tracheal deviation, asymmetrical chest movement, a sudden increase in peak pressure or plateau pressure on the patient's ventilator, and air in the soft tissues.

---

### 4. Look for the presence of, or any changes in, mediastinal shift (NBRC code: IB6d) [Difficulty: R, Ap]

The mediastinum is the area between the lungs that contains the heart and great vessels, trachea, hilar structures, and esophagus. In the neonate, the heart and other mediastinal structures should be located approximately in the center of the chest, with the left ventricle to the left of center. In the adult, most of the heart and mediastinal structures should be detected left of center in the chest. Any shift of the mediastinum (and heart) is abnormal, as is shown by several conditions in Fig. 1-4. Either atelectasis or pulmonary fibrosis, if unilateral and great enough, results in a shift *toward* the problem area. Tension pneumothorax results in a shift *away* from the problem area. Fluid in the pleural space, if great enough, results in a shift *away* from the problem area.

### 5. Look for the presence of, or any changes in, pulmonary infiltrates or consolidation (NBRC code: IB6b) [Difficulty: R, Ap]

Pulmonary infiltration occurs when blood plasma (water) passes from the pulmonary vascular bed into the lung tissues. Usually, this fluid moves into the lung because the alveolar capillary membrane is damaged. On a chest x-ray film, an infiltrate often appears as a faint, white blurring of the lung and associated structures.

Consolidation is the filling of the alveoli with fluid from an infiltrate, aspirated vomitus, blood, or water. It is often segmental or lobar. Consolidation is noticed on the chest x-ray film as a dense, white shadow because fluid has

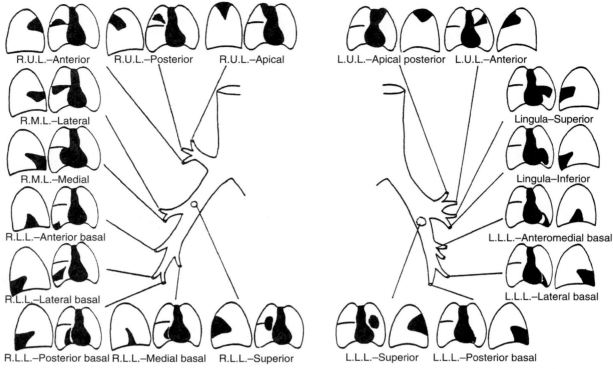

R.U.L.–Anterior    R.U.L.–Posterior    R.U.L.–Apical

L.U.L.–Apical posterior    L.U.L.–Anterior

R.M.L.–Lateral

Lingula–Superior

R.M.L.–Medial

Lingula–Inferior

R.L.L.–Anterior basal

L.L.L.–Anteromedial basal

R.L.L.–Lateral basal

L.L.L.–Lateral basal

R.L.L.–Posterior basal  R.L.L.–Medial basal    R.L.L.–Superior

L.L.L.–Superior    L.L.L.–Posterior basal

**Fig. 1-5** Simulated frontal and lateral x-ray findings for consolidation in the various segments of both lungs. *LLL,* Left lower lobe; *LUL,* left upper lobe; *RLL,* right lower lobe; *RML,* right middle lobe; *RUL,* right upper lobe. *(From Cherniack RM: Respiration in health and disease, ed 3, Philadelphia, 1983, WB Saunders.)*

replaced all of the air. The mediastinum and heart are seen in their normal locations. Fig. 1-5 shows both the posteroanterior (P-A) and the lateral chest x-ray appearance of consolidation in each of the segments of both lungs. Air bronchograms may also be noticed on an x-ray film that reveals consolidation.

### 6. Look for the presence of, or any changes in, atelectasis (NBRC code: IB6b) [Difficulty: R, Ap]

Atelectasis is the collapse of alveoli; no air is found within them. This problem is commonly seen postoperatively in the lower lobes of patients who have had abdominal or thoracic surgery who do not breathe deeply because of the pain. The x-ray appearance of atelectasis reveals an increase in lung markings and a decrease in lung volumes. If atelectasis is one sided, the mediastinum may shift toward the affected side (see Fig. 1-4, **A**). If atelectasis is bilateral, the mediastinum can remain properly located. If atelectasis is severe enough, the lungs have a uniform white appearance (Fig. 1-6).

### 7. Look for the positions of, or any changes in, the hemidiaphragms (NBRC code: IB6d) [Difficulty: R, Ap]

In infants and adults, anteroposterior (A-P) or P-A chest x-ray and lateral chest x-ray films normally reveal a domed

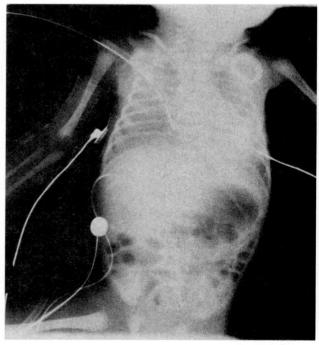

**Fig. 1-6** Frontal x-ray film of a neonate with severe atelectasis from infant respiratory distress syndrome. Also note the right pleural chest tube and wires to various monitoring systems. *(From Des Jardins TR, Burton GG: Clinical manifestations and assessment of respiratory disease, ed 3, St. Louis, 1995, Mosby.)*

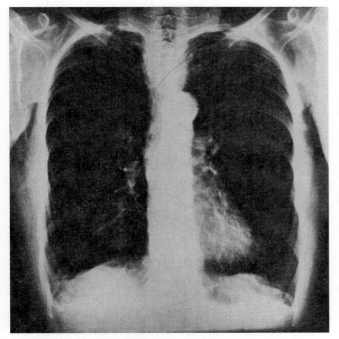

**Fig. 1-7** Frontal x-ray film of an adult with advanced chronic obstructive pulmonary disease. Both lungs are overinflated and hyperlucent. The ribs are spread more widely than normal. Often, these patients have a cardiothoracic ratio that is smaller than normal because the heart is elongated and the lateral chest diameter is increased. *(From Sheldon RL: Clinical application of the chest radiograph. In Wilkins RL, Krider SJ, Sheldon RL: Clinical assessment in respiratory care, ed 3, St. Louis, 1995, Mosby.)*

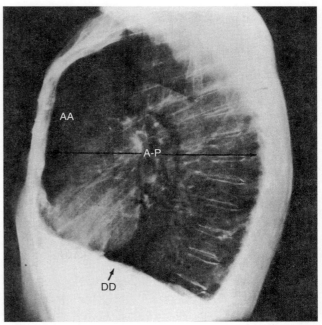

**Fig. 1-8** Lateral x-ray study of an adult with advanced chronic obstructive pulmonary disease. Note the characteristic shape of a "barrel chest" from the overinflated lungs. The anteroposterior *(A-P)* diameter of the chest is increased. *AA* marks an increased anterior airspace between the heart and sternum. The angle of the manubrium and body of the sternum is more obtuse than normal. *DD* marks depressed hemidiaphragms that are flattened. *(From Sheldon RL: Clinical application of the chest radiograph. In Wilkins RL, Krider SJ, Sheldon RL: Clinical assessment in respiratory care, ed 3, St. Louis, 1995, Mosby.)*

shape of the hemidiaphragms, with the edges turning down to acute costophrenic angles. The edges of the hemidiaphragms should be smooth, with no unusual dips or peaks. Conditions that result in an abnormal position of one hemidiaphragm include unilateral atelectasis, pleural fluid, tension pneumothorax, and check-valve bronchial obstruction (see Figs. 1-1 and 1-4). Asthma and chronic obstructive pulmonary disease result in the depression of both hemidiaphragms (Figs. 1-7 and 1-8). Improvement in the patient's condition should result in a return of the hemidiaphragm(s) to a close-to-normal position.

### 8. Look for the presence of, or any changes in, hyperinflation (NBRC code: IB6d) [Difficulty: R, Ap]

Hyperinflation is defined as an excessive amount of air in one or both lungs. To some degree, specific chest x-ray findings vary with the underlying condition that causes the hyperinflation. Unilateral hyperinflation is caused by a check-valve obstruction from a foreign body or airway tumor. At first glance, a tension pneumothorax appears as unilateral lung hyperinflation. Remember that with this condition, the chest wall can be pushed out while the lung is collapsed (see Fig. 1-1).

The adult with asthma, bronchitis, and emphysema (chronic obstructive pulmonary disease [COPD]) and the newborn with meconium aspiration show both lungs overinflated and both hemidiaphragms depressed (see Figs. 1-7 and 1-8). Other x-ray findings include widened intercostal spaces, hyperlucent lung fields, small vertical heart, small cardiothoracic diameter, and decreased vascularity of peripheral areas of the lungs with enlarged hilar vessels. In addition, lateral chest x-ray findings in the patient with COPD are the same and include anterior bowing of the sternum, increased retrosternal air space, and kyphosis.

### 9. Look for the presence of, or any changes in, pleural fluid (NBRC code: IB6d) [Difficulty: R, Ap]

Pleural fluid is typically seen on a P-A or A-P film as obscuring the costophrenic angle because gravity tends to draw the fluid to the lowest level (Fig. 1-9). Small amounts of fluid can sometimes be better visualized by means of a lateral decubitus x-ray. If the fluid can move freely within the pleural space, it will shift within a few minutes to the down side (Fig. 1-10). An empyema loculated (fixed) by adhesions does not move when the patient lies on his or

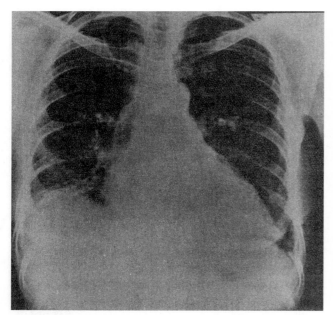

**Fig. 1-9** Frontal x-ray image of an adult showing a small pleural effusion in the right side of the chest. Note how the costophrenic angle and hemidiaphragm are obscured by the white shadow of fluid. *(From Sheldon RL: Clinical application of the chest radiograph. In Wilkins RL, Krider SJ, Sheldon RL: Clinical assessment in respiratory care, ed 3, St. Louis, 1995, Mosby.)*

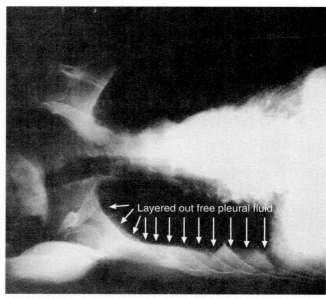

**Fig. 1-10** Lateral decubitus x-ray image of an adult showing the shift of a small pleural effusion to the now-dependent part of the pleural space. Arrows mark the layer of fluid. *(From Sheldon RL: Clinical application of the chest radiograph. In Wilkins RL, Krider SJ, Sheldon RL: Clinical assessment in respiratory care, ed 3, St. Louis, 1995, Mosby.)*

her side. If large amounts of fluid are removed by a thoracentesis procedure, a chest x-ray should be taken to confirm removal of fluid, reexpansion of the lung, and lack of pneumothorax.

### 10. Look for the presence of, or any changes in, pulmonary edema (NBRC code: IB6d) [Difficulty: R, Ap]

Pulmonary edema is watery fluid (plasma) that has leaked out of the pulmonary capillary bed into the interstitial spaces and alveoli. It is most commonly caused by left ventricular failure (congestive heart failure) but can also result from fluid overload, pulmonary capillary damage, or decreased osmotic pressure in the blood that results from a low level of protein.

Pulmonary edema appears on a P-A or A-P chest x-ray film as fluffy, white infiltrates in one or both lung fields. These tend to be more extensive in the lower lobes because of gravity that pulls the fluid to the basilar vessels from which it leaks. If the root cause is left ventricular failure, vessels in the hila are engorged and the left ventricle is enlarged (Fig. 1-11). A worsening problem causes more fluid to leak into the lungs and a greater quantity of white infiltrates to appear on succeeding chest x-ray examinations. Once the problem has been corrected, the lungs return to normal as the fluid is reabsorbed and removed.

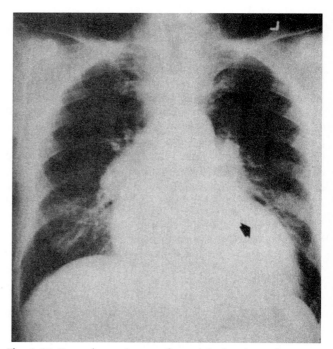

**Fig. 1-11** Frontal x-ray image of an adult showing pulmonary edema, increased pulmonary vascular markings, and enlarged left ventricle. Cardiothoracic diameter is increased, with the arrow showing where the border of the left ventricle should normally be seen. *(From Des Jardins TR: Clinical manifestations of respiratory disease, ed 2, Chicago, 1990, Mosby.)*

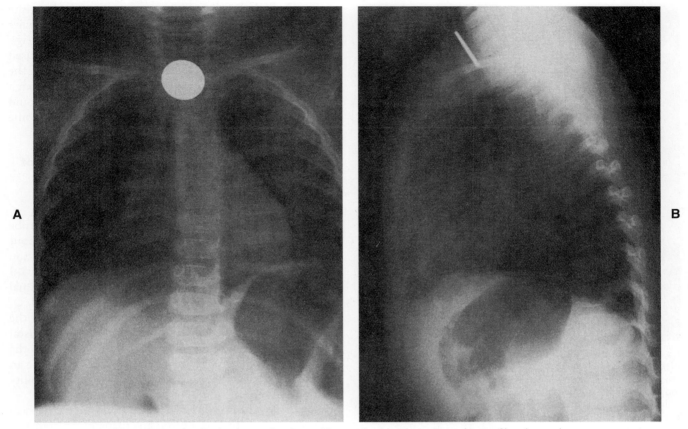

**Fig. 1-12** Foreign body obstruction in an 18-month-old girl. **A,** Frontal x-ray film shows the solid white disk of a coin, clearly seen in the hypopharynx. **B,** Lateral view of the chest shows the edge of the coin as a solid white line. *(From Hunter TB, Bragg DG: Radiologic guide to medical devices and foreign bodies, St. Louis, 1994, Mosby.)*

### 11. Look for the presence and position of any foreign bodies (NBRC code: IB6c) [Difficulty: R, Ap]

A foreign body is anything not naturally found in the chest. Metallic objects (e.g., bullets or swallowed or aspirated coins or metal buttons) are easily noticed because they completely block any x-ray penetration through the chest and are clearly outlined on the film as solid, white shadows (Fig. 1-12). Nonmetallic foreign objects (such as plastic pieces from toys and foods such as peanuts) are much more difficult to identify because they have about the same densities as normal body tissues. Determining the exact location of a foreign body may require P-A, lateral, and oblique chest x-ray studies. Lung volumes can be compared on inspiratory and expiratory films. A CT scan may prove more successful than an x-ray in revealing a nonmetallic foreign body.

All medical devices placed inside the body are made of radiopaque material and can be seen on a chest x-ray film as a white object or line. Chest tubes are placed to remove any abnormal collection of air or fluid from the thoracic cavity so that the function of the heart or lungs returns to normal. A pleural chest tube is placed to remove air or fluid from the pleural space (see Fig. 1-3). The insertion site and depth of tube insertion vary with the patient's disorder. (See Chapter 17 for further discussion of the placement of pleural chest tubes.)

A mediastinal or pericardial chest tube is placed to remove air or fluid from either of these spaces (see Fig. 1-3; Fig. 1-13). Cardiac tamponade can occur when air or fluid compresses the heart. After open heart surgery, most patients have one or more mediastinal chest tubes in place for several days to remove blood from around the heart. The insertion site lies below the sternum, and the tube is placed posterior to the heart in the pericardial or mediastinal space.

On chest x-ray film, a nasogastric tube is seen as a white line that extends from the patient's nose or mouth through the esophagus and into the stomach (on the left side below the diaphragm). A feeding tube may be placed as a nasogastric tube, or it may be surgically placed through the abdominal wall and into the stomach or small intestine.

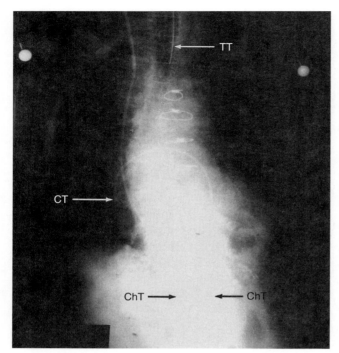

**Fig. 1-13** Frontal x-ray film of an adult patient with several medically necessary devices after open heart surgery. A properly placed pulmonary artery (Swan-Ganz) catheter is noted to loop through the right side of the heart and out into the right pulmonary artery. The catheter tip is marked by *CT*. Other devices include a properly placed endotracheal tube marked at *TT*, sternal wire sutures, ECG chest leads on each shoulder, and pericardial chest tubes (marked by *ChT*). *(From Sheldon RL: Clinical application of the chest radiograph. In Wilkins RL, Krider SJ, Sheldon RL: Clinical assessment in respiratory care, ed 3, St. Louis, 1995, Mosby.)*

A cardiac pacemaker is placed in one of two ways. An external pacemaker is recognizable on chest x-ray image by the long electrode leads that run through a vein in the right arm, through the superior vena cava, and into the right ventricle. The battery and control unit of an internal pacemaker are placed under the skin below a clavicle. The electrode leads run through the superior vena cava into the right ventricle.

Various venous catheters (pulmonary artery catheter, CVP catheter, umbilical artery catheter [UAC], and umbilical vein catheter [UVC]) should be seen on chest radiograph films in their entirety, that is, from their insertion points to their end points. Figs. 1-13 and 1-14 show the placement of several catheters.

## 12. Check the chest x-ray for size and patency of the patient's major airways (NBRC code: IB6d) [Difficulty: R, Ap]

On a properly taken chest x-ray film, the trachea and the right and left mainstem bronchi should be seen as straight, dark air columns that contrast with the white shadows of the various surrounding tissues. A white shadow within the airway could indicate a foreign body or tumor. Airway narrowing could also be caused by a tumor. This can be seen within the lumen of the airway or as a growth from outside the trachea or from a bronchus. A tumor that occurs outside the airway could press upon it, causing the airway to narrow or become occluded.

## 13. Check the chest x-ray for the position of the patient's endotracheal or tracheostomy tube (NBRC code: IB6a) [Difficulty: R, Ap]

The distal end of the endotracheal or tracheostomy tube should be seen within the lumen of the trachea and about midway between the larynx and the tracheal bifurcation to the right and left mainstem bronchi (see Figs. 1-3 and 1-13 for endotracheal tube placement). The proximal end of the tracheostomy tube (or a transtracheal $O_2$ catheter) can be seen on x-ray film as it comes out of the surgical insertion site in the suprasternal notch. The distal end should be centered within the trachea above the carina (see Fig. 1-13). These tubes are made of, or have an embedded line of, radiopaque material for easy visibility on x-ray film.

Care must be taken to avoid pushing the endotracheal tube more deeply into a bronchus (usually the right) or pulling it out. The tracheostomy tube and the transtracheal $O_2$ catheter are less likely to be displaced if they are properly handled. Take another x-ray to check the position of any of these tubes if clinical evidence shows that its position may have changed.

A properly inflated cuff fills the space between the tube and the patient's trachea and forms an airtight seal. An overinflated cuff puts excessive pressure on the trachea, which could cause it to dilate and be seen as a wider dark area than the rest of the tracheal air column. If this is noticed, cuff pressure should be measured. Excessive pressure should be reduced to a safer level.

---

### Exam Hint

**T**he NBRC will often have a question about how to identify the location of an endotracheal tube on chest x-ray. It should be seen in the middle of the trachea. If it is placed too deeply, the endotracheal tube will enter the right mainstem bronchus.

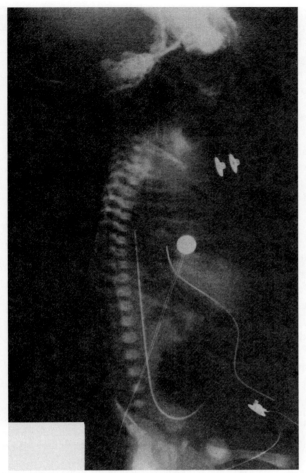
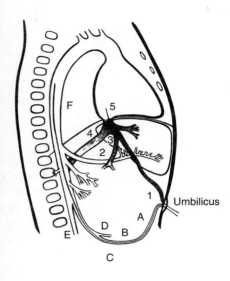

**Fig. 1-14** Lateral x-ray and drawing of the internal vascular structures of an infant with an umbilical artery catheter (UAC) and umbilical vein catheter (UVC) in place. The UAC passes through the umbilicus, umbilical artery *(A)*, hypogastric artery *(B)*, internal iliac artery *(C)*, common iliac artery *(D)*, and abdominal aorta *(E)* to the thoracic aorta *(F)*. The UVC passes through the umbilicus, umbilical vein *(1)*, portal vein *(2)*, ductus venosus *(3)*, and inferior vena cava *(4)* to the right atrium *(5)*. Other medical devices include an endotracheal tube and electrocardiogram leads. *(From Deming DD: Respiratory assessment of neonatal and pediatric patients. In Wilkins RL, Krider SJ, Sheldon RL: Clinical assessment in respiratory care, ed 3, St. Louis, 1995, Mosby.)*

## MODULE C

### Explain planned therapy and goals to the patient in understandable (nonmedical) terms to achieve the best results from the treatment or procedure (NBRC code: IIIA5) [Difficulty: R, Ap]

1. Avoid using technical and medical terms unless the patient has a medical background or asks you about the specifics of what you are doing. Generally, it is best to describe the procedure in layman's terms that do not demean the intelligence of the patient.

2. Describe the procedure in steps rather than as a whole process from beginning to end. Demonstrate each step for the patient. Ask the patient for any questions, and answer these or re-demonstrate. Coach the patient to perform each step and to correct any problems. Describe and demonstrate the next step and the next, until the procedure has been completed.

## MODULE D

### Interview the patient

### 1. What is the patient's level of consciousness/sedation? (NBRC code: IB4a) [Difficulty: R, Ap]

One common way of evaluating a patient's level of consciousness is to categorize him or her as alert, stuporous, semicomatose, or comatose.

### a. Alert

In the normal mental state, the patient is conscious or can be fully awakened from sleep by someone who calls his or her name. The patient can voluntarily ask and answer questions logically, and the conversation is relevant to the topic under discussion. The patient's movements and actions are willful and purposeful.

### b. Stuporous/very lethargic

The stuporous or very lethargic patient is sleepy or seems to be in a trance. He or she can be aroused to respond with willful, purposeful movements and actions, but the response may be slow. The patient may not respond to questions in a totally appropriate way.

### c. Semicomatose

The semicomatose patient does not perform requested movements or actions or answer questions appropriately. He or she responds defensively to pain. For example, if the right arm is pinched, the patient will withdraw it. Posturing of semicomatose patients includes the following:

1. Decerebrate: Legs are extended; arms are extended and rotated either inward or outward.
2. Decorticate: Legs are extended; arms are flexed, and the forearms may be rotated either inward or outward.
3. Opisthotonic: Legs, arms, and neck are extended, and the body is arched forward.

### d. Comatose/coma

The comatose patient has no spontaneous, oriented responses to the environment; pain causes no defensive movement, but heart and respiratory rates may increase.

Another common method by which the clinician can evaluate a patient's level of consciousness is the Glasgow Coma Scale, which uses a range from 3 to 15. The larger the total score that is reported, the more normal is the patient. A score of 15 is given to a patient who is normally awake and alert, whereas a score of 3 is given to an unresponsive patient (Table 1-4).

### 2. Is the patient oriented to time, place, and person? (NBRC code: IB4a) [Difficulty: R, Ap]

*Time* refers to the patient's knowing the date, day of the week, or time. Ask the patient, "Do you know what day of the week it is? Do you know what the date is?" (The patient must be able to see a calendar.) "Do you know what time it is?" (The patient must be able to see a clock.) If the patient can answer these questions, he or she is oriented to time. If not, inform and show him or her. Tell the patient that you will return at a certain time. Ask the same questions when you return.

*Place* refers to the patient's knowing where he or she is located (e.g., hospital and nursing care unit, extended care

| TABLE 1-4   Glasgow Coma Scale | | |
|---|---|---|
| **Test Parameter** | **Response** | **Score*** |
| **EYES** | | |
| Open | Spontaneously | 4 |
| | To verbal command | 3 |
| | To pain | 2 |
| | No response | 1 |
| **BEST MOTOR RESPONSE** | | |
| To verbal command | Obeys command | 6 |
| Moves arms to | Localizes pain | 5 |
| painful stimulus | Flexion—withdrawal | 4 |
| of knuckles | Flexion—abnormal | 3 |
| against sternum | movement (decorticate rigidity) | |
| | Extension—abnormal movement (decerebrate rigidity) | 2 |
| | No response | 1 |
| **BEST VERBAL RESPONSE (MAY AROUSE BY PAINFUL STIMULUS IF NECESSARY)** | | |
| | Oriented and converses | 5 |
| | Disoriented and converses | 4 |
| | Inappropriate words used | 3 |
| | Incomprehensible sounds | 2 |
| | No response | 1 |

From Apache II: a severity of disease classification system, ICU Research Unit, Washington, DC; product information from Upjohn, Kalamazoo, Mich.
*The total is obtained by adding the scores in all three areas. The range is 3 to 15.

facility, home). Ask the patient, "Do you know where you are?" If the patient knows, he or she is oriented to place. If not, inform the patient of his or her location. Tell the patient that you will return at a certain time. Ask the same question when you return.

*Person* refers to the patient's knowing his or her own name, address, and phone number. The patient should also know the names of obviously important people. Ask the patient, "Do you know who the president (or the physician) is?" If not, inform the patient. Tell the patient who you are and what your job is. When you return for your next treatment, ask the patient if he or she remembers who you are and what you do. If the patient remembers who the president (or the physician) is, and your name or job, he or she is oriented to person.

Orienting the stuporous or very lethargic patient to person, place, and time may improve cooperation in his or her care. Pain-relieving and sedative drugs, stroke, injury to or edema of the brain, and other illnesses may cause disorientation to person, place, or time.

| TABLE 1-5 | Teaching–Learning Process in Adaptation to Chronic Illness | | |
|---|---|---|---|
| **Stages of Adaptation** | **Patient's Behavior** | **Nurse's Behavior** | **Nurse's Facilitation of the Teaching-Learning Process** |
| Disbelief | Denies threatening condition to protect self and conserve energy; refuses to accept diagnosis; may claim to have something else; may behave so as to avoid the issue; may seem to accept diagnosis but avoids feelings about it | Allows patient to deny illness as he needs to; functions as noncritical listener; accepts patient's statements about how he feels; helps clarify patient's statements; does not point out reality | Orients all teaching to the present, not to tomorrow or next week; teaches as she does other nursing activities; assesses patient's level of anxiety; assures patient that he is safe and is being observed carefully; explains all procedures and activities to the patient; gives clear, concise explanations; coordinates activities to include rest periods |
| Developing awareness | Uses anger as a defense against being dependent and against feeling guilty about being sick | Listens to patient's expressions of anger and recognizes them for what they are; explores own feelings about illness and helplessness; does not argue with patient; gives dependable care with an attitude that it is necessary | Does not give anxious patient long lists of facts; continues development of trust and rapport through good physical care; orients teaching to present; explains symptoms, care, and treatment in terms of the fact that they are necessary now; does not mention long-range care needs |
| Reorganization | Accepts increased dependence and reorganizes relationships with significant others; members of patient's family may also use denial while they adapt to what patient's illness means to them | Establishes climate in which family and friends can express feelings about patient's illness; does not solve patient's problems but helps build communication so that patient and family can work together to solve problems | Assures family that patient is alright and safe; uses clear, concise explanations; does not argue about need for care |
| Resolution | Acknowledges changes seen in self; identifies with others with same problem | Encourages expression of feelings, including crying; understands own feelings of loss | Brings groups of patients with same illness together for group discussions; has a recovered person visit patient; teaches patient what he wants to learn (or perceives he needs to learn) first |
| Identity change | Defines self as an individual who has undergone change and is now different; "There are limits to my life because I have a disease" | Understands own feelings about patient becoming independent again | Realizes that as patient's own perceived needs are met, more mature (more progressive) needs will surface; is prepared to answer patient's questions as they arise |
| Successful adaptation | Can live comfortably or resignedly with himself as a person who has a specific condition | Initiates closure of nurse–patient relationship | Has helped develop a relationship with the patient in which the nurse is a guide with whom the patient can consult when he wishes |

From Kenner CV, Guzzetta CE, Dossey BM: Critical care nursing: body–mind–spirit, Boston, 1981, Little, Brown.

### 3. What is the patient's emotional state? (NBRC code: IB4a) [Difficulty: R, Ap]

Acute illness or injury with great pain may cause some patients to feel fear, anxiety, or panic. Therefore, the patient may be unable to concentrate on what you are saying, which could result in directions not being understood or followed. It is important to tell the patient that you are there to help and that you need the patient to calm down so you *can* help.

Authors have discussed chronic illness from various points of view. Table 1-5 presents a patient's reactions to chronic illness. Substitute "respiratory therapist" for "nurse" as you read.

A patient's statements and actions that indicate the *disbelief* stage of adaptation include the following:

  a. "I don't have (fill in the name of the disease or condition)"
  b. "There is nothing really wrong with me"
  c. "The laboratory test results are wrong"
  d. "The equipment is faulty"
  e. "The doctor/nurse/therapist is incompetent"
  f. The patient may refuse to take medications or follow treatments or other physician orders

A patient's statements and actions that indicate the *developing awareness* state of adaptation include the following:

  a. "The doctor/nurse/therapist doesn't know what he/she is doing"
  b. "It's all their fault"
  c. "Why is this happening to me?"
  d. The patient is angry about his or her illness
  e. The patient may strike out verbally or physically at staff members
  f. Some patients who do not get angry withdraw into a depression and wish to be left alone

A patient's statements and actions that indicate that he or she is progressing from the *reorganization* to the *successful adaptation* stage include the following:

  a. "I'll never be able to do (fill in type of activity) again"
  b. "I have to get on with my life"
  c. "At least I'm still alive and can do this for myself"
  d. The patient may be sad and cry often
  e. The patient may invent a nickname for his or her defect or diseased body part
  f. The patient accepts the disability and focuses on his or her abilities
  g. The patient works with family and others in planning for the future

### 4. Interview the patient to determine any advance directives. (NBRC code: IB4d) [Difficulty: R]

An advance directive is an advance declaration by a patient who is hopelessly and terminally ill that he/she does not wish to be connected to life support equipment. This statement could preclude the use of a mechanical ventilator, kidney dialysis equipment, cardiac pacemaker, or other means of artificially prolonging life. The advance directive can also declare if the patient does not want to be resuscitated if cardiac arrest should occur. This is commonly called a "do not resuscitate" (DNR) order and should be clearly noted in the patient's chart. The advance directive legal document should be part of the patient's medical record. The document may also be known as a "Living Will" in some states. A related legal document is the Durable Power of Attorney for Health Care. This document assigns another person, such as a relative or close friend, the right to make medical decisions when the patient is unable to do so. This can include

the stopping or withdrawal of medical treatment and the DNR order.

Always be sensitive to a patient's feelings about such a personal and difficult decision. The patient's emotional state (previous discussion) may very well determine readiness for an advance directive. A related issue is the patient's ability to cooperate (see below) based on his/her emotional and physical condition.

### 5. What is the patient's level of pain? (NBRC code: IB4a) [Difficulty: R, Ap]

It has been shown that unmanaged pain can slow down a patient's recovery from trauma or surgery. Because pain is a subjective feeling of the patient, only the patient can determine how severe the pain is. Some patients will have a low pain threshold and will report pain sooner and at a higher level than those with a high pain threshold. Therefore, the acceptable way to determine pain level is to have the patient rate it. Commonly, the patient is told to self-rate a pain level of "0" when there is no pain and to assign a number up to a pain level of "10" for the most severe pain possible. Additionally, the patient should be asked to point with one finger to the area with the greatest pain. After the patient is given a pain medication, and it has had time to take effect, the patient is again asked to rate the pain on the 0 to 10 scale. If the patient can tolerate the new pain level, it may not be necessary to give more medication. However, if the pain is still too great, additional medication may be given, if allowed within the physician's orders for pain management.

### 6. What is the patient's ability to cooperate? (NBRC code: IB4a) [Difficulty: R, Ap]

The patient's ability to cooperate can be judged on the basis of his or her responses to questions on level of consciousness, orientation to time, place, and person, pain level, and emotional state. An alert patient should be able to understand and follow directions and to allow an effective treatment or cooperate in a procedure. On the other hand, if the patient truly refuses the treatment or procedure, it should not be forced. Contact the patient's nurse or physician about the refusal; the physician must then decide what to do.

An alert but panicked, fearful, or anxious patient may be unable to cooperate fully until he or she is calmed by a clear explanation of who you are, what you will do, and why the treatment or procedure is important. Try to reassure the patient to improve cooperation.

If the patient appears alert but does not understand the questions, check whether he or she is deaf or does not speak English. Writing materials, a picture board, or a sign language interpreter is needed with a deaf patient. A native language translator is needed with a patient who does not speak English.

| TABLE 1-6 | Severity of Dyspnea in Evaluating Permanent Impairment | | | |
|---|---|---|---|---|
| **Class I** | **Class II** | **Class III** | **Class IV** | **Class V** |
| Dyspnea only on severe exertion ("appropriate" dyspnea) | Can keep pace with person of same age and body build on the level without breathlessness but not on hills or stairs | Can walk a mile at own pace without dyspnea but cannot keep pace on the level with a normal person | Dyspnea present after walking about 100 yd on the level or on climbing one flight of stairs | Dyspnea on even less activity or at rest |

From Burton GG: Practical physical diagnosis in respiratory care. In Burton GG, Hodgkin JE, editors: Respiratory care: a guide to clinical practice, ed 2, Philadelphia, 1984, Lippincott.

The stuporous or very lethargic patient may be aroused by a loud voice or gentle shaking. He or she may not be able to cooperate fully, so the practitioner may have to modify the treatment plan or its method of delivery to compensate for the patient's lack of cooperation.

Pain relievers and sedatives may make an alert patient seem stuporous. If the stuporous patient has not been medicated, ask the nurse or physician what may have recently changed in the patient's condition.

A semicomatose patient may present the greatest problems to the clinician who is attempting to provide treatment or perform a procedure. These patients do not cooperate in any way. In addition, some of their involuntary body posturings make correct positioning impossible. A comatose patient does not cooperate in any procedure or treatment. For either type of patient, equipment or procedures must be modified because of his or her inability to cooperate.

### 7. Does the patient complain of dyspnea or orthopnea? (NBRC code: IB4b) [Difficulty: R, Ap]

Dyspnea is the patient's subjective feeling of shortness of breath (SOB) or labored breathing. Dyspnea is normal after vigorous exercise but abnormal in a resting patient. Orthopnea is the condition in which a patient must sit erect or stand to breathe comfortably. In a patient with orthopnea, lying flat causes dyspnea.

Table 1-6 classifies the degrees of dyspnea, and Table 1-7 lists different kinds of dyspnea, including orthopnea. Only Class I is normal dyspnea (on severe exertion). Classes II to V are progressively severe and limiting for the patient. Any orthopnea is abnormal, and the more often the patient must sit up to breathe, the more limited his or her activity will be.

Following are examples of questions that the clinician should ask in evaluating dyspnea:

a. "How far can you walk before you feel SOB?"
b. "How many flights of stairs can you climb before you feel SOB?"

| TABLE 1-7 | Causes of Dyspnea Related to Preferred Body Position |
|---|---|
| **Kind of Dyspnea** | **Clinical Correlations** |
| Orthopnea (must sit up to breathe; often occurs at night as paroxysmal nocturnal dyspnea) | Congestive heart failure |
| Obstructive sleep apnea (periodically stops breathing, particularly when lying on back) | Obesity; obstructive sleep apnea syndromes |
| Emphysematous habitus | COPD |
| Platypnea | Pleural effusion; dyspnea associated with various body positions |
| Orthodeoxia | Pulmonary fibrosis; dyspnea improved when patient is lying flat |

*COPD,* Chronic obstructive pulmonary disease.
From Burton GG: Patient assessment procedures. In Barnes TA, editor: Respiratory care practice, Chicago, 1990, Mosby.

c. "How far can you go when you are walking as fast as your spouse?"
d. "Is there anything you do that makes the SOB *worse*?"
e. "Is there anything you do that makes the SOB *better*?"
f. "How long does the SOB last after you stop to rest?"
g. "Is the SOB worse at any particular time of the *day*?"
h. "Is the SOB worse at any particular time of the *year*?"

Following are examples of questions that the clinician should ask in evaluating orthopnea:

a. "Do you wake up at night with SOB?"
b. "Does your nighttime SOB get better after you sit up on the side of your bed or in a chair?"
c. "Do you get SOB when you are lying down to take a nap?"

d. "Do you use extra pillows behind your head and back to prevent SOB at night or during a nap?"

e. "How many pillows do you need to prevent SOB at night or during a nap?"

## 8. What is the patient's sputum production like? (NBRC code: IB4b) [Difficulty: R, Ap]

### a. Time of maximal and minimal expectoration

Interview the patient to determine the following:

1. Time of maximal expectoration: Ask the patient, "When do you cough up the most (in the morning, after eating spicy foods, after a breathing treatment, after smoking, work, exposure to dusts, etc.)?"

2. Time of minimal expectoration: Ask the patient, "When do you cough up the least (during certain nonallergic seasons, after a breathing treatment, after consuming milk or milk products, etc.)?"

### b. Quantity

Some practitioners prefer to know a specific amount, such as teaspoons, tablespoons, or milliliters. Others prefer to use subjective measures such as "a little" or "a lot." Interview the patient to determine the following:

1. How the quantity of sputum relates to the times of maximal and minimal expectoration and the patient's lifestyle: Ask the patient, "Is there anything you do that increases or decreases the amount you cough out?" For example, the patient states that he coughs up 20 mL after breathing treatments but can cough up nothing after eating a bowl of ice cream.

2. Whether the amount coughed up changes in a cyclical way: Ask the patient, "Do you cough up the most in the mornings or at night? Is there a work or lifestyle habit that changes how much you cough up? Is there a seasonal allergic condition that influences your asthma and sputum production?"

### c. Adhesiveness of the sputum

Interview the patient to determine the following:

1. "Are there times or things you do during the day that seem to result in your secretions' becoming thicker or thinner?"

2. "Do your medications (such as acetylcysteine [Mucomyst]) make the secretions easier to cough out?"

3. "Do certain foods make your secretions easier to cough out?"

## 9. What is the patient's work of breathing? (NBRC code: IB4b) [Difficulty: R, Ap]

Work of breathing (WOB) refers to the patient's subjective feeling about his or her breathing ability. A person at rest should feel no difficulty in breathing. During vigorous exercise, a person should be aware that he or she is working harder than normal to breathe, which is expected. After the patient recovers from exercise, the WOB should again be easy.

Patients with acute or chronic lung disease feel that they breathe with some difficulty. Because this is a subjective feeling of the patient, it is helpful to have the patient quantify it. Ask the patient to rate his or her WOB on a 1-to-10 scale with 1 being "easy breathing" and 10 being "extremely difficult breathing."

If bronchospasm or secretions have increased, the patient should feel that his or her WOB has worsened. If medications such as bronchodilators or mucolytics are effective, the patient should feel that his or her breathing is easier.

## 10. What are the patient's learning needs? (NBRC code: IB5) [Difficulty: R, Ap]

Based on previously gathered information, the respiratory therapist should be able to determine what the patient understands of his or her condition and what needs to be taught. Assess the following, and provide the appropriate information:

### a. Age-appropriate teaching

The patient is taught on the basis of his or her age and ability to understand. This is especially important with small children because they commonly have the following fears when hospitalized:

1. Fear of abandonment (separation anxiety). Small children are afraid of being abandoned in the hospital by their parents.

2. Fear of the unknown. Equipment and procedures must be explained so the child is not left to rely on his or her imagination.

3. Fear of punishment. Children may imagine that their illness is a punishment because they have done something wrong.

4. Fear of bodily harm. Procedures should be explained so the child understands what is going to happen.

5. Fear of death. Children who are sick but are expected to recover need to understand that they will get better. Children may feel afraid, and talking about these feelings or about fear of death should be encouraged.

### b. Language-appropriate teaching

Use nonmedical terms whenever possible. The patient's native language must be used so that he or she understands the situation. A translator may be needed.

### c. Education level

The way patients are taught and the level of difficulty presented should match their educational level and knowledge of the medical condition.

#### d. Previous disease knowledge

Patients should be taught as needed about their condition.

#### e. Medication knowledge

Patients should be taught as needed about their medication(s), including how medications are to be taken (e.g., metered-dose inhaler with spacer).

### MODULE E

**Use *observation* to determine the patient's complete respiratory condition**

#### 1. Evaluate the patient's general appearance (NBRC code: IB1a) [Difficulty: R, Ap]

Start by quickly inspecting the patient from head to toe, including how he or she is dressed and is functioning in the room, without the patient's knowing that he or she is being observed. The patient who is not suffering from cardiopulmonary disease should be able to lie flat in bed or on either side with no breathing difficulty. The patient with a one-sided lung condition, such as lobar pneumonia, pleurisy, or broken ribs, may prefer to lie with the good side down. The patient with severe airway obstruction, such as asthma, bronchitis, or emphysema, tends to sit up in a chair or on the edge of the bed and use locked arms and shoulders for support. This enables the patient to use accessory muscles (Fig. 1-15). The patient with orthopnea does not want to lie flat because of the resulting SOB. Orthopnea is commonly seen in patients with congestive heart failure and pulmonary edema.

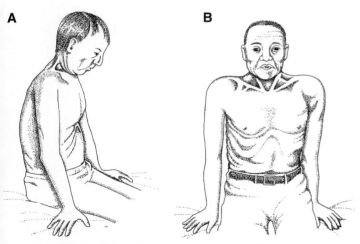

**Fig. 1-15** Typical posture seen in patients using accessory muscles of respiration. The shoulders are locked for more effective use of the accessory muscles. (*A, From Burton GG: Practical physical diagnosis in respiratory care. In Burton GG, Hodgkin JE, editors: Respiratory care, ed 2, Philadelphia, 1984, Lippincott. B, From Barriascout JR: Chest physical therapy and related procedures. In Burton GG, Hodgkin JE, editors: Respiratory care, ed 2, Philadelphia, 1984, Lippincott.)*

#### 2. Determine whether the patient is cyanotic (NBRC code: IB1a) [Difficulty: R, Ap]

Cyanosis is an abnormal blue or ashen-gray coloration of the skin and mucous membranes. It is most easily seen in white patients at the lips and nail beds, and in darker-pigmented people at the inner portion of the lip or lower eyelid or nail beds. Cyanosis is commonly caused by hypoxemia; the more bluish a patient's color appears, the more hypoxemic he or she is. Despite this, cyanosis is not an accurate measure of a patient's oxygenation. A patient with cyanosis should have an arterial blood gas (ABG) sample drawn for arterial oxygen pressure ($PaO_2$) measurement, or pulse oximetry should be performed for oxygen saturation ($SpO_2$) measurement so that oxygenation can be evaluated.

#### 3. Determine whether the patient is diaphoretic (NBRC code: IB1a) [Difficulty: R, Ap]

Diaphoresis is profuse sweating that is normally seen after vigorous exercise. A patient is expected to sweat after a stress test or even an $O_2$-assisted walk, but diaphoresis in a patient who is resting in bed should be investigated. The body releases adrenaline into the bloodstream when it is severely stressed, and diaphoresis is one of many bodily effects caused by the release of adrenaline. Similar sweating may be seen if a large dose of the drug epinephrine is given.

Diaphoresis in a patient is a nonspecific sign of serious cardiopulmonary difficulties. It may be seen any time the patient is in shock or is hypoxemic. Patients who are suffering from a myocardial infarct are commonly diaphoretic. The practitioner should promptly evaluate the diaphoretic patient's pulse, respiratory rate, BP, and ABGs.

#### 4. Determine whether the patient has nasal flaring (NBRC code: IB1a) [Difficulty: R, Ap]

Nasal flaring is a dilation of the nares on inspiration. A person who is breathing comfortably should have little or no nasal flaring, whereas a person who is exercising vigorously may have some. Nasal flaring seen in a patient who is resting in bed is a sign of increased WOB. The patient is attempting to reduce airway resistance by dilating the nares. Patients of any age have nasal flaring when they are experiencing increased WOB, but it is most commonly seen in the premature newborn (Fig. 1-16).

Nasal flaring, which is not specific to any disease or condition, can be seen in idiopathic respiratory distress syndrome (IRDS), acute respiratory distress syndrome (ARDS), or any condition in which pulmonary compliance is decreased or airway resistance is increased.

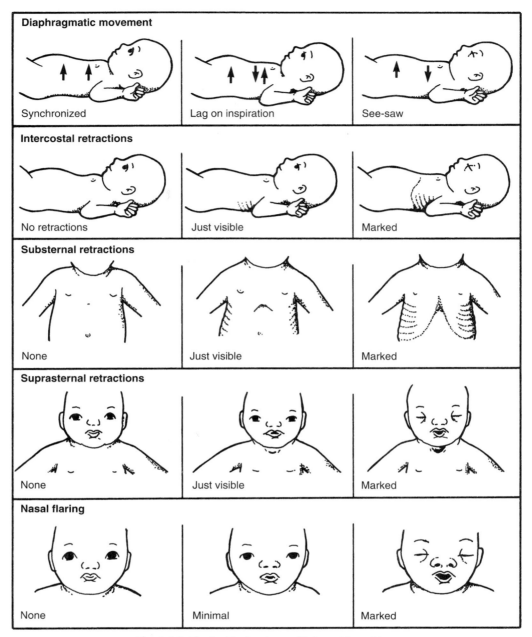

**Diaphragmatic movement**

| Synchronized | Lag on inspiration | See-saw |

**Intercostal retractions**

| No retractions | Just visible | Marked |

**Substernal retractions**

| None | Just visible | Marked |

**Suprasternal retractions**

| None | Just visible | Marked |

**Nasal flaring**

| None | Minimal | Marked |

**Fig. 1-16** Physical indications of labored breathing.

### 5. Determine whether the patient has clubbing of the fingers (NBRC code: IB1a) [Difficulty: R, Ap]

Clubbing of the fingers (digital clubbing) is an abnormal thickening of the ends of the fingers. (It can also occur in the toes.) The key finding is an angle greater than 160 degrees between the top of the finger and the nail when seen from the side. Clinically, a lateral and A-P thickening of the ends of the fingers is noticeable. Fig. 1-17 compares normal and clubbed fingers. The fingernail and toenail beds may be cyanotic.

The underlying cause is not completely understood, but it seems to be related to chronic hypoxemia, at least in part. This results in arteriovenous anastomosis with thickening of the tissues. Clubbing is seen in patients with COPD, bronchogenic carcinoma, bronchiectasis, sarcoidosis, and infective endocarditis.

### 6. Determine whether the patient has peripheral edema (NBRC code: IB1a) [Difficulty: R, Ap]

Peripheral edema occurs when fluid leaks from the capillary bed into the tissues. It is most commonly seen in the

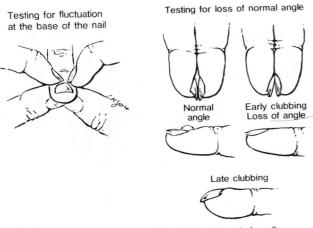

Testing for fluctuation at the base of the nail

Testing for loss of normal angle

Normal angle

Early clubbing Loss of angle

Late clubbing

**Fig. 1-17** Signs of and test for clubbing. *(From Lehrer S: Understanding lung sounds, Philadelphia, 1984, WB Saunders.)*

ankles and feet or along the back when the patient is lying supine. The clinician can measure the extent of edema by pressing a finger into the tissues. Normal skin springs back, whereas edematous skin remains pitted or depressed. Pitting edema is graded as 1+ for less than ¼-inch (mild) indentation, 2+ for ¼- to ½-inch (moderate) indentation, and 3+ for ½- to 1-inch (severe) indentation. Obviously, the deeper the pitting is, the greater is the extent of peripheral edema in the patient.

Peripheral edema is most commonly seen in patients with congestive heart failure or those who are overloaded with fluid. Patients with septicemia often have peripheral edema because the bloodborne pathogen (usually *Staphylococcus*) causes abnormal capillary leakage.

7. **Determine the shape (configuration) of the patient's chest** (NBRC code: IB1a) **[Difficulty: R, Ap]**

The patient should be sitting up straight or standing erect when he or she is being examined for chest configuration. Look at the patient from the front, back, and both sides to see the symmetry. Fig. 1-18 shows the appearance of the chest in a normal infant and a normal adult, as well as the appearance of barrel chest, funnel chest, pigeon chest, and thoracic kyphoscoliosis. Several variations on curvature of the spine exist. *Kyphosis* is an exaggerated A-P curvature of the upper portion of the spine. *Lordosis* is an exaggerated A-P curvature of the lower portion of the spine. *Scoliosis* is either right or left lateral curvature of the spine. *Kyphoscoliosis* is either right or left lateral curvature combined with A-P curvature of the spine.

8. **Determine whether the patient has asymmetrical chest movement when breathing** (NBRC code: IB1a) **[Difficulty: R, Ap]**

Infants and adults normally have symmetrical chest movement when breathing at rest or during exercise. All breath-

ing efforts are best observed when the patient is shirtless. In females, it may be necessary to observe only the uncovered back to judge chest movement. Any kind of asymmetrical chest movement is abnormal and may be due to an abnormality of the chest wall or abdomen or a pulmonary disorder.

a. **Thoracic scoliosis or kyphoscoliosis**

(Refer to Fig. 1-18 for the back view of a patient with thoracic scoliosis or kyphoscoliosis.) The scoliosis patient in Fig. 1-18 would tend to have greater chest movement on the right side than on the left because of right spinal curvature. The left side of the chest and left lung would inflate more fully than the right if the spine curved to the left. These same findings are found in a patient with kyphoscoliosis.

b. **Flail chest**

The flail segment moves in the opposite direction from the rest of the chest (paradoxical movement). That is, with inspiration, the flail segment moves inward and the rest of the chest moves outward; during expiration, the flail segment moves outward as the rest of the chest moves inward. As the ribs heal, the segment stabilizes and moves with the rest of the chest.

c. **Pneumothorax**

The side with the collapsed lung does not move as much as the chest wall over the normal lung does (see Fig. 1-1).

d. **Atelectasis/pneumonia**

The side with atelectasis or pneumonia does not move as much as the chest wall over the normal lung does (see Fig. 1-4).

9. **Determine whether the patient has intercostal or sternal retractions when breathing** (NBRC code: IB1a) **[Difficulty: R, Ap]**

Intercostal retractions are noticed when the soft tissues between the ribs are drawn inward during inspiration as the chest wall moves outward. Suprasternal retractions are noticed when the soft tissues *above* the sternum are drawn inward during inspiration as the chest wall moves outward. Substernal retractions are noticed when the soft tissues *below* the sternum are drawn inward during inspiration as the chest wall moves outward (see Fig. 1-16).

A person who is breathing at rest should not have any retractions, although that same person may have some minor retractions during vigorous exercise. Retractions are commonly seen in conditions in which airway resistance is increased, or lung compliance is decreased. Both increase a patient's WOB. The patient must generate a more negative intrathoracic pressure to breathe, and as

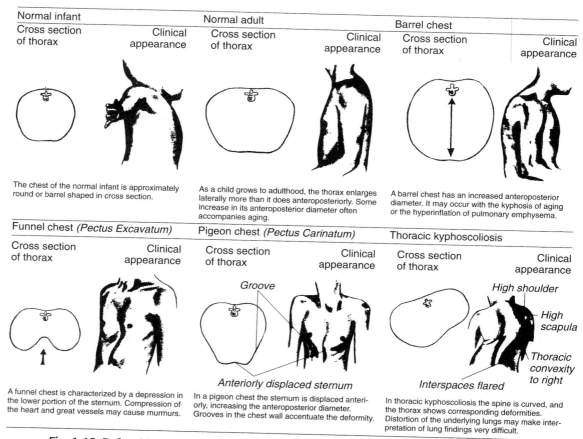

| Normal infant | | Normal adult | | Barrel chest | |
|---|---|---|---|---|---|
| Cross section of thorax | Clinical appearance | Cross section of thorax | Clinical appearance | Cross section of thorax | Clinical appearance |
| The chest of the normal infant is approximately round or barrel shaped in cross section. | | As a child grows to adulthood, the thorax enlarges laterally more than it does anteroposteriorly. Some increase in its anteroposterior diameter often accompanies aging. | | A barrel chest has an increased anteroposterior diameter. It may occur with the kyphosis of aging or the hyperinflation of pulmonary emphysema. | |
| Funnel chest (Pectus Excavatum) | | Pigeon chest (Pectus Carinatum) | | Thoracic kyphoscoliosis | |
| Cross section of thorax | Clinical appearance | Cross section of thorax | Clinical appearance | Cross section of thorax | Clinical appearance |
| A funnel chest is characterized by a depression in the lower portion of the sternum. Compression of the heart and great vessels may cause murmurs. | | In a pigeon chest the sternum is displaced anteriorly, increasing the anteroposterior diameter. Grooves in the chest wall accentuate the deformity. | | In thoracic kyphoscoliosis the spine is curved, and the thorax shows corresponding deformities. Distortion of the underlying lungs may make interpretation of lung findings very difficult. | |

**Fig. 1-18** Deformities of the thorax. *(From Bates B: A guide to physical examination and history taking, ed 4, Philadelphia, 1987, Lippincott.)*

result, various soft tissues are drawn inward during inspiration. This occurs in patients with IRDS, ARDS, pulmonary edema, pneumonia, asthma, bronchitis, and emphysema.

## 10. Determine whether the patient uses accessory muscles when breathing (NBRC code: IB1a) [Difficulty: R, Ap]

Accessory muscles of respiration should not be needed during passive resting breathing but may be used with vigorous breathing during exercise. Dyspneic patients typically use them even when they are resting. Abdominal muscles are used during active expiration, whereas the accessory muscles of inspiration are the intercostal, scalene, sternocleidomastoid, trapezius, and rhomboid. The accessory muscles of inspiration that are easiest for the clinician to observe in action are the sternocleidomastoids from the front and side of the patient and the trapezius from the back (Fig. 1-19).

Accessory muscle use in a resting patient demonstrates a greatly increased WOB. This finding is not specific for any one condition but is commonly seen in patients with emphysema (see Fig. 1-15).

## 11. Determine whether the patient has diaphragmatic movement when breathing (NBRC code: IB1a) [Difficulty: R, Ap]

Normally, an adult's diaphragm moves downward several centimeters toward the abdomen during inspiration as the chest wall moves outward. This is seen when the abdomen protrudes as its contents are forced forward. The chest and abdomen should rise and fall together during quiet and vigorous breathing efforts.

Two conditions exist in which this normal chest and abdominal movement does not occur. First, patients with emphysema, severe air trapping, and a barrel chest have a diaphragm that is depressed and flat rather than domed because of the air trapped in the lungs. On inspiration, the diaphragm continues to contract but is unable to displace the abdominal contents downward to permit air to be drawn into the lungs. These patients do not demonstrate the expected abdominal movement during inspiration. Of necessity, they use the accessory muscles of inspiration to assist breathing.

The second condition involves patients in whom airway resistance is increased or lung compliance is decreased. The greater negative intrathoracic pressure

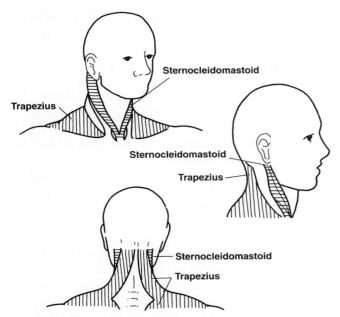

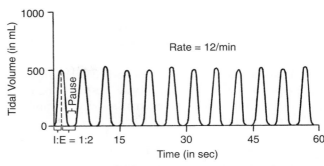

Fig. 1-20 Eupnea. *I*, Inspiratory time; *E*, expiratory time. Pause is time from the end of exhalation to the beginning of inspiration.

Fig. 1-19 The sternocleidomastoid and trapezius accessory muscles of respiration.

needed to draw the $V_T$ into the lungs can cause the chest wall to collapse inward as abdominal contents are displaced outward. The result is a kind of "see-saw" or paradoxical movement between the chest wall and the abdomen. Patients with IRDS typically demonstrate this because the premature neonate's rib cage is relatively compliant compared with the stiff lungs (see Fig. 1-16).

## 12. Determine the patient's breathing pattern (NBRC code: IB1a) [Difficulty: R, Ap]

Various respiratory patterns can be identified by characteristic respiratory rates, respiratory cycles, and $V_T$.

### a. Eupnea (normal breathing) (Fig. 1-20)

1. Normal respiratory rate for the age of the patient (see Table 1-2)
2. Normal respiratory cycle: When the flow of air into and out of the lungs is timed, the inspiratory/expiratory (I:E) ratio is 1:1.5 to 1:2. A pause of variable duration follows exhalation of the $V_T$, which changes the true I:E ratio to 1:2 to 1:4
3. Normal $V_T$ for the size of the patient (Fig. 1-20 refers to an average adult, but the following abnormal breathing patterns can be compared with it). Inspiration is achieved without the use of accessory muscles of inspiration, and exhalation is passive.

### b. Hypopnea (shallow breathing)

1. Respiratory rate is usually somewhat slower than normal

2. Normal respiratory cycle
3. $V_T$ decreased for the size of the patient
4. Possible causes: Deep sleep, sedation, coma, hypothermia, alkalemia, or restrictive lung disease
5. May be combined with bradypnea

### c. Hyperpnea (deep breathing)

1. Respiratory rate may be normal or somewhat faster
2. Normal respiratory cycle
3. $V_T$ increased for the size of the patient
4. Possible causes: Acidemia, fever, pain, fear, anxiety, or increased intracranial pressure
5. May be combined with tachypnea

### d. Bradypnea (slow breathing)

1. Respiratory rate is slower than normal
2. Expiration may be longer than normal as a result of a longer pause
3. $V_T$ may be decreased for the size of the patient
4. Possible causes: Deep sleep, sedation, coma, hypothermia, or alkalemia
5. May be combined with hypopnea

### e. Tachypnea (rapid breathing)

1. Respiratory rate is faster than normal
2. Inspiration may be faster than normal with the help of inspiratory accessory muscles. Expiration may be shorter than normal, and expiratory accessory muscles may be used to force out the air faster. The pause seen in eupnea is gone. The I:E ratio may be 1:2 or less
3. $V_T$ may be increased for the size of the patient
4. Possible causes: Acidemia, fever, pain, anxiety, or increased intracranial pressure
5. May be combined with hyperpnea

### f. Obstructed inspiration

1. Respiratory rate is slower than normal
2. Inspiratory time is equal to or longer than expiratory time. Inspiration is aided by use of the inspiratory accessory muscles; expiration is passive

3. $V_T$ may be normal or larger or smaller than normal depending on how the patient adapts to the increased WOB. A slower rate with a larger $V_T$ is most common
4. Possible causes: Croup, epiglottitis, foreign body aspiration with partial airway obstruction, post-extubation laryngeal edema, airway tumor, or airway trauma

### g. Obstructed expiration
1. Respiratory rate is slower than normal
2. Expiratory time is longer than normal; accessory muscles of inspiration and expiration may be used
3. $V_T$ may be normal or decreased for the size of the patient
4. Possible causes: Asthma, emphysema, bronchitis, cystic fibrosis, bronchiectasis, airway tumor, or airway trauma

### h. Kussmaul's respiration (rapid, large breaths)
1. Respiratory rate is faster than normal
2. I:E ratio approaches 1:1; both inspiratory and expiratory accessory muscles may be used
3. $V_T$ is increased for the size of the patient
4. Probable cause is acidemia (pH, 7.2 to 6.95) from diabetic ketoacidosis

### i. Cheyne-Stokes respiration (waxing and waning tidal volumes) (Fig. 1-21)
1. Respiratory rate varies from normal to faster and may include short periods of apnea
2. Respiratory cycle is normal or approximates normal unless the patient has periods of apnea
3. $V_T$'s increase and decrease over a variable time cycle; a 20-sec cycle is fairly common. Periods of apnea may occur between decreased $V_T$'s
4. Possible causes: Head injury, stroke, increased intracranial pressure, or congestive heart failure

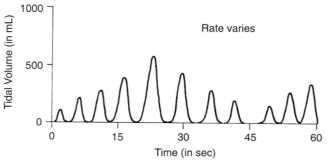

**Fig. 1-21** Cheyne-Stokes breathing pattern.

### j. Biot's respiration (unpredictably variable)
1. Respiratory rate varies from rapid to short periods of apnea
2. Respiratory cycle varies considerably
3. $V_T$ varies from shallow to large
4. Possible causes: Head injury, brain tumor, or increased intracranial pressure

### k. Apnea (cessation of breathing at the end of exhalation)
1. Apnea that lasts long enough to result in hypoxemia, bradycardia, and hypotension must be treated aggressively. Artificial respiration, with or without supplemental $O_2$, must be started immediately
2. The patient's previous breathing pattern must be evaluated if the cause of apnea is to be determined. Consider causes of heart attack, stroke, or upper airway obstruction in cases of normal breathing followed by apnea. Consider cause(s) of the original abnormal breathing in cases of an abnormal breathing pattern followed by apnea
3. Evaluate the previous $V_T$ variation for the reasons just listed
4. Possible causes: Airway obstruction, heart attack, stroke, or head injury

13. **Determine which type of cough the patient has** (NBRC code: IB1b) [Difficulty: R, Ap]
### a. Normal cough
A normal cough has four parts:
1. Person takes a deep breath.
2. Epiglottis and vocal cords close to trap the air within the lungs.
3. Abdominal and other expiratory muscles contract to increase the air pressure in the lungs.
4. Epiglottis and vocal cords open to allow the compressed air to escape explosively and remove any mucus or foreign matter.

All components must work individually and in a coordinated manner for the patient to have an effective cough. Serial, midinspiratory, huff, and assisted coughs are variations used by patients who, for some reason, cannot cough normally.

### b. Serial cough
All actions of a normal cough take place in a serial cough, except that the patient performs a series of smaller coughs rather than a single large one. This method of coughing may be used by postoperative patients who have such severe abdominal or thoracic pain that they cannot cough normally. As the pain lessens, the patient should be able to cough normally.

### c. Midinspiratory cough

All actions of a normal cough take place, except that the patient does not take as deep a breath. Patients with emphysema and chronic bronchitis (COPD) may use this to help prevent airway collapse when they cough.

### d. Huff cough

Patients with artificial airways may perform huff coughs. They cannot close the epiglottis and vocal cords, so they can only take a large breath and blow out with as much force as possible. This cough is still an effective way to remove watery secretions.

### e. Assisted cough

A patient with assisted cough needs direct help from the therapist, who gives the patient a deep breath with an intermittent positive-pressure breathing machine or manual ventilator. The therapist then helps the patient blow out the air quickly by pushing on the abdominal area to move the diaphragm up. This procedure is limited to conscious patients with neuromuscular defects who cannot cough effectively on their own.

## 14. Determine the quantity and characteristics of the patient's sputum
   (NBRC code: IB1b) [Difficulty: R, Ap]
### a. Quantity

Normally, a person is not aware of mucus production. The mucociliary escalator moves mucus toward the throat, where it is unconsciously swallowed. Normally, mucus is uninfected and is clear or white.

Infections that cause bronchitis or pneumonia typically result in the production of large amounts of mucus. The patient will report coughing and spitting up. Any increase in mucus or sputum production, to the extent that the patient is aware of it, is abnormal.

As has been mentioned previously, some practitioners prefer to use subjective measurements of sputum production such as "a little," "medium," or "copious." Objective or marked measurements, such as teaspoons, tablespoons, or milliliters, are preferred for quantifying production.

Note any changes in the amount of sputum the patient is producing in a timed manner, such as production per hour or per shift. Correlating sputum production with breathing treatments or other procedures that may increase or decrease its production or clearance is also wise.

### b. Characteristics

Homogeneity is best determined by letting a sputum sample stand in a test tube for several hours to allow stratification. This test is important in the patient with a pulmonary infection. Normal sputum separates into a relatively thin, white surface layer of gel that floats on a clear lower layer of water (sol). The patient with a pulmonary infection has more viscous sputum because it contains dead bacterial cells, dead white blood cells (WBCs), and cellular debris from infected lung tissues. These cells settle over time to the bottom of a sputum sample and create a third layer of sediment.

Fig. 1-22 shows how the layering would look in the sputum from a patient with a pulmonary infection that eventually clears up. Table 1-8 explains other details on sputum characteristics.

## 15. Determine whether the patient has excessive venous distension
   (NBRC code: IB1a) [Difficulty: R, Ap]

The internal and external or anterior jugular veins are observed by having the patient lie supine with the head elevated 30 degrees. The crest of the vein column should be seen just above the border of the midclavicle. A rough measure of the intravascular volume and CVP is taken by pressing on the veins at the base of the neck. The returning blood should fill the veins and make them distend (Fig. 1-23). When the pressure is released, the veins should return to their previous level of distension just above the level of the midclavicle. Increased venous distension is noted when the veins stand out at a level above the clavicle. This is seen in patients with right-sided heart failure (cor pulmonale), cardiac tamponade, fluid overload, or COPD, and when high airway pressures and positive end-expiratory pressure (PEEP) are needed for mechanical ventilation. The higher the veins are distended, the more the patient is compromised.

The veins should not collapse below the clavicle when the obstructing finger is removed. If this happens, the patient should lay his or her head flat. Normally, when flat, the external jugular vein should be partially distended. If the vein collapses on inspiration, low venous pressure is confirmed and the patient is probably hypovolemic. This is commonly seen with dehydration, hemorrhage, or increased urine output after the use of diuretics.

## 16. Determine the patient's capillary refill
   (NBRC code: IB1a) [Difficulty: R, Ap]

Capillary refill is the time needed for blood to refill the capillary bed after it has been forced out. The procedure is to pinch the fingernail or toenail until it blanches. After pressure is released, the pink color of the nail bed should return within 3 sec. A delay in the return to pink color indicates reduced blood flow to the extremities. Cyanotic nail beds also show reduced blood flow. Conditions that would result in a decreased capillary refill include decreased cardiac output, low BP from any cause, and the use of vasopressor medications.

**Infection**    **Improvement**    **Normal**

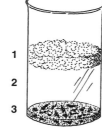 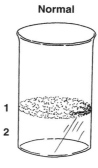

1. Gel layer:
   thicker than normal

2. Sol layer: thinner
   in ratio to gel
   layer than normal

3. Cellular debris:
   dead bacteria, WBCs,
   other cells

NOTE: The total volume of
sputum is greatly increased

1. Gel layer:
   reducing toward
   normal

2. Sol layer: returning
   to normal ratio with
   gel layer

3. Cellular debris:
   thinning out as fewer
   dead cells are being
   coughed out

1. Gel layer:
   normal volume

2. Sol layer: normal
   volume and ratio
   with the gel layer

NOTE: The total volume
of sputum is reduced
to normal; also, there
is no third layer of
cellular debris

**Fig. 1-22** Evaluation of the homogeneity of sputum in the infected patient. *WBCs,* White blood cells.

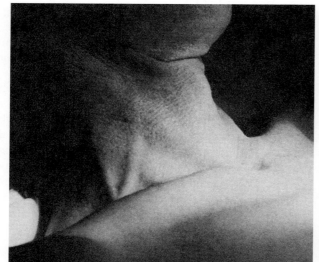 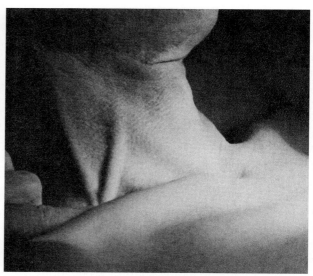

A                                         B

**Fig. 1-23** Evaluating distension of the external jugular vein. These photographs show a patient with right-sided heart failure. **A,** External jugular vein is distended above the level of the clavicle. **B,** Pressing a finger over the external jugular vein results in greater filling with blood and increased distension. When the pressure is released in a normal person, the vein should collapse to just above the superior border of the midclavicle. *(From Daily EK, Schroeder JS: Techniques in bedside hemodynamic monitoring, ed 4, St. Louis, 1989, Mosby.)*

| TABLE 1-8 | Sputum Characteristics | | | |
|---|---|---|---|---|
| **Sputum Type** | **Color** | **Contents** | **Illnesses** | **Odor** |
| Bloody (hemoptysis) | Red | Blood | Bronchogenic carcinoma; pulmonary hemorrhage; lung abscess; tuberculosis; pulmonary infarction | Typically none |
| Frothy or bubbly | Clear or pink | Water; plasma proteins; red blood cells | Pulmonary edema | Typically none |
| Mucoid | Clear or white | Water; complex sugars; glycoproteins; some cellular debris | Asthma; chronic bronchitis | Typically none |
| Mucopurulent | Light to medium yellow | Decreased water and complex sugars; increased cellular debris and causative organisms (if applicable); organisms are usually aerobes | Chronic and acute bronchitis | Typically none, but may exist depending on organism |
| Purulent | Dark yellow or green | Decreased water; greatly increased cellular debris and causative organisms that are usually aerobes; complex sugars | Bronchiectasis; lung abscess; pneumonia | Depending on organism, along with clearance of mucus; also may be foul tasting to the patient; odor usually not offensive |
| Purulent (fetid) | Dark yellow or green | Decreased water; may contain some blood; greatly exaggerated cellular debris and causative organisms that frequently are anaerobes; complex sugars | Bronchiectasis; lung abscess; cystic fibrosis | Offensive odor |

From DiPietro JS: Clinical guide for respiratory care and cardiopulmonary disease, Acton, Mass., 1998, Copley Custom Publishing.

## 17. Determine whether the patient has muscle wasting (NBRC code: IB1a) [Difficulty: R, Ap]

Muscle wasting is an abnormal condition of decreased muscle mass. The muscle wasting can be generalized or localized, depending on the underlying cause. Examples of conditions in which muscle wasting is seen include those discussed in the following paragraphs.

### a. COPD

COPD (emphysema and bronchitis) often results in muscle wasting because the patient is consuming an unusually large number of calories through the act of breathing. In addition, these patients often do not eat well because a full stomach restricts the movement of the diaphragm and worsens their WOB and SOB. These patients are frequently malnourished or undernourished. Their arms and legs may be thin, the joints in their shoulders, elbows, and knees may be prominent, and their ribs may be clearly outlined by deep intercostal spaces.

### b. Lung cancer

Lung cancer or other cancers usually result in a loss of muscle mass because the growing tumor consumes many calories. As a result, normal body tissues are not properly fed. These patients usually have thin arms and legs with prominent joints during advanced disease.

### c. Neurologic injuries

Neurologic injuries, such as transection of the spinal cord, result in atrophy of the affected muscles. Atrophy of the muscles, a decrease in their size from lack of use, is an unavoidable consequence of the permanent loss of nerve input to the affected muscles. For example, transection of the spinal cord at the first lumbar vertebra (L1) results in loss of nerve input to the legs. The patient is a paraplegic.

In time, the muscles of the legs atrophy; however, the arms retain their normal muscle mass if they are exercised. If the patient has a spinal transection that results in the loss of nerve input to both the arms and legs (quadriplegia), all of the limbs atrophy.

## MODULE F

**Use *palpation* to determine the patient's complete respiratory condition**

### 1. Determine the patient's heart rate, rhythm, and force (NBRC code: IB2a) [Difficulty: R, Ap]

The HR is most commonly counted by palpating the carotid, femoral, radial, and brachial arteries and the apical pulse of the heart. The apical pulse, or point of maximal impulse, is normally located in the area of the left midclavicular line in the fifth intercostal space (Fig. 1-24). This location indicates the apex of the heart (left ventricle). Other arterial sites, such as the temporal, dorsalis pedis, and posterior tibial, can be used but are more difficult to find. The pulse should be counted for a minimum of 30 sec, with 1 min providing the most accurate result. The rhythm is felt and mentally timed as the pulse rate is counted.

Palpating a pulse at any of the aforementioned sites reveals the timing between heartbeats. Normally, this rhythm is regular in people at rest or who are exercising

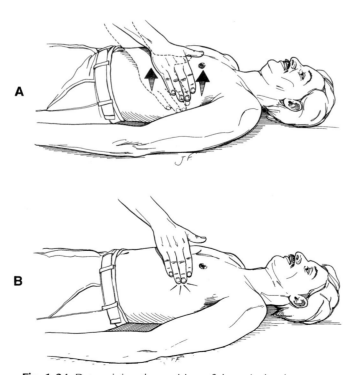

**Fig. 1-24** Determining the position of the apical pulse. **A,** Technique for locating the apical pulse by palpation. **B,** Location of the apical pulse. *(From Eubanks DH, Bone RC: Comprehensive respiratory care, ed 2, St. Louis, 1990, Mosby.)*

at a steady level. The time between beats should be about the same.

Respiratory effort may have some influence on heart rhythm. A heart rhythm that increases on inspiration and decreases on expiration is fairly common in children and occasionally is found in adults. This sinus arrhythmia, which is not really abnormal, occurs when the negative intrathoracic pressure during inspiration draws blood more quickly into the thorax and heart than during exhalation. The opposite may be true during mechanical ventilation with a high peak pressure or mean airway pressure. Then, the heart rhythm and rate may slow down during inspiration and speed up during expiration. In any other case, an irregular rhythm would indicate some sort of cardiac problem. An electrocardiogram (ECG) would be needed to help determine the specific cause.

The force of the pulse indicates the strength of the heart's contraction and BP. Normally, each heartbeat is felt with the same amount of force. A "thready" or variable force that is felt with each heartbeat is usually a sign of heart disease. Atrial fibrillation is an example of an irregular heart rhythm that results in an irregular force. The irregular rate and rhythm cause variable volumes of blood to be pumped with each contraction. A large volume of blood is felt as a strong pulse; a small volume of blood is felt as a weak pulse.

A "bounding" or greater-than-normal force felt with each beat is usually a sign of hypertension. For safety's sake, BP should be measured and compared with the patient's previous BP to detect possible change.

### 2. Determine whether the patient has asymmetrical chest movements during breathing (NBRC code: IB2b) [Difficulty: R, Ap]

Normally, the lungs and chest move in symmetry throughout the respiratory cycle. Asymmetrical chest wall movement during an inspiration indicates a lung or chest wall problem. If the patient does not have an abnormal chest wall configuration, the problem lies with the lungs. Less air is getting into the affected lung area(s), so the chest wall does not move out as far as it would over the normal lung. This nonspecific finding of lung disease can be seen in pneumonia, bronchial or lung tumor, and pneumothorax.

The therapist's hands should be placed over the chest for assessment of asymmetrical chest movement (Fig. 1-25). The thumbs should touch at the end of expiration. The patient is then instructed to breathe in deeply as asymmetrical movement is looked for and felt. In Fig. 1-25, parts *A* and *B* show the movement of the anterior apical lobes, *C* and *D* demonstrate the movement of the anterior middle and lower lobes, *E* and *F* show movement in the posterior lower lobes, and *G* and *H* reveal the movement of the costal margins.

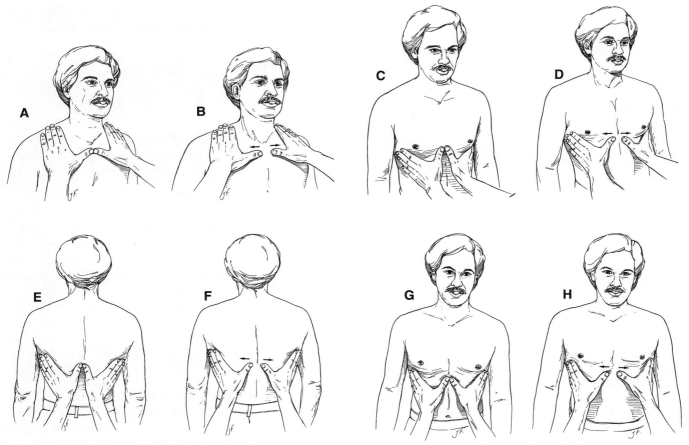

**Fig. 1-25** Palpation to assess symmetrical chest movements. **A,** Hand position over the apical lobes during expiration. **B,** Apical movement during inspiration. **C,** Hand position over middle and lower lobes during expiration. **D,** Middle and lower lobe movement during inspiration. **E,** Hand position over the posterior middle lobes during expiration. **F,** Movement of the posterior middle lobes during inspiration. **G,** Hand position to check for movement of the costal margins during expiration. **H,** Costal movement during inspiration. *(From Eubanks DH, Bone RC: Comprehensive respiratory care, ed 2, St. Louis, 1990, Mosby.)*

## 3. **Determine whether the patient has tactile fremitus** (NBRC code: IB2b) [Difficulty: R, Ap]

Tactile fremitus is a vibration that is felt through the chest wall when the patient speaks. Normally, when a sound is created in the larynx, its vibration is carried throughout the tracheobronchial tree to the lung parenchyma and the chest wall. The intensity or absence of the vibration gives the practitioner important information about the patient's condition.

Fig. 1-26 shows different methods of detecting tactile fremitus. Some practitioners prefer to use their fingertips, as shown in *A* and *B*, whereas others prefer the ulnar edge of the open or closed hand, as shown in *C* and *D*. All areas of the patient's chest must be assessed for tactile fremitus to detect any variations; this should be done over both lung fields to compare their symmetry and anterior and posterior differences (Fig. 1-26, *E* and *F*). Fig. 1-27 shows the posterior and anterior locations for evaluating tactile fremitus. Start with the supraclavicular fossae, and proceed to alternate intercostal spaces. An attempt must be made to preserve the adult female patient's modesty when anterior locations are evaluated. The patient may be asked to lift the breast to palpate beneath it.

When tactile fremitus is evaluated, the patient should say "99" in a normal voice as the practitioner's fingers or hand move from location to location. This procedure is also called *palpation for bronchophony.* The "99" should be spoken at least once for each location so that any variations can be determined. Having the patient speak more loudly or deeply should increase the intensity of the vibrations, which directly relates to the density of the underlying lung and chest cavity. Conditions that increase density result in more intense vibrations, and those that decrease density result in less intense vibrations. Vibrations are also reduced when they are blocked from penetration through

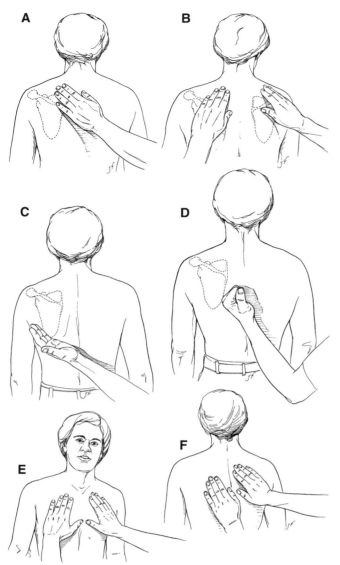

**Fig. 1-26** **A** to **D,** Techniques for feeling tactile fremitus. **E** and **F,** Anterior and posterior placement of the hands to detect tactile fremitus. *(From Eubanks DH, Bone RC: Comprehensive respiratory care, ed 2, St. Louis, 1990, Mosby.)*

| TABLE 1-9 | Abnormal Tactile Fremitus | |
|---|---|
| **Increased** | **Decreased** |
| **UNILATERAL** | **UNILATERAL** |
| Pneumonia | Pneumothorax |
| Atelectasis | Pleural effusion |
| Consolidation | Bronchial obstruction |
| **BILATERAL** | **BILATERAL** |
| Pulmonary edema | Thick chest wall (fat or muscle) |
| Acute respiratory distress syndrome | Chronic obstructive pulmonary disease |

to the surface. Table 1-9 gives conditions that alter tactile fremitus.

### 4. Determine whether the patient has secretions in the airway (NBRC code: IB2b) [Difficulty: R, Ap]

Rhonchial fremitus (or palpable rhonchi) is a type of tactile fremitus that is noticed when vibrations from airway secretions are felt through the chest wall as the patient breathes. These vibrations are abnormal and indicate that the patient has a significant secretion problem. Palpable rhonchi are not detected in a patient with clear airways. Having the patient cough or suctioning the

airway to remove secretions reduces or eliminates palpable rhonchi. Remember: An airway that is completely occluded by a mucus plug or foreign body does *not* reveal palpable rhonchi because no airflow exists. Breath sounds would also be absent in this area.

Different methods of detecting palpable rhonchi exist. Some therapists prefer to use their fingertips, whereas others prefer using the edge of the open or closed hand. All areas of the patient's chest must be assessed so that the exact location(s) of the secretions can be determined.

### 5. Determine whether the patient has crepitus (NBRC code: IB2b) [Difficulty: R, Ap]

Crepitus (or crepitation) is the sound heard when an area with subcutaneous emphysema is gently pressed. The dry crackling-like sound resembles that of Rice Krispies in milk. A stethoscope can help pinpoint the location of the sound. In extreme instances, the unaided ear can detect the sound. As the fingers of one hand are sequentially pressed into the affected area, the subcutaneous air moves away from the pressure points.

Subcutaneous emphysema is air under the skin that has leaked from a damaged lung. The skin appears puffy or edematous, characteristics that are most commonly seen in the tissues on the side of the leaking lung. Pressurized air dissects through the tissues by following the path of least resistance and most likely arrives at the skin in the axilla, neck, chest wall, and breast. In extreme cases, air is found under the skin throughout the body.

Crepitus, although not dangerous, is a serious finding because it indicates that the patient has a pulmonary air leak. Crepitus may be accompanied by pneumothorax, pneumomediastinum, or PIE. A chest x-ray examination should be performed immediately if the crepitation is a new finding.

### 6. Determine whether the patient has any tracheal deviation (NBRC code: IB2b) [Difficulty: R, Ap]

Normally, the trachea is located in a midline position within the neck and thorax. The clinician can find the

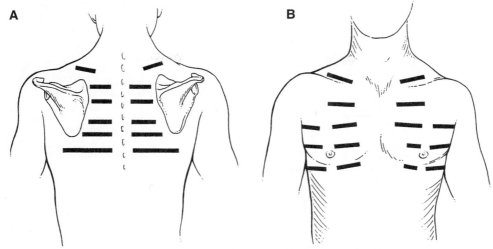

**A**    **B**

**Fig. 1-27** Locations on the posterior **(A)** and anterior **(B)** chest for feeling tactile fremitus and performing percussion. *(From Swartz MH: Textbook of physical diagnosis, Philadelphia, 1989, WB Saunders.)*

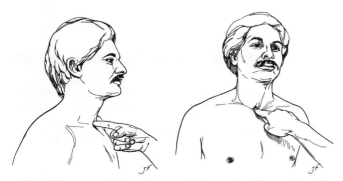

**Fig. 1-28** Detecting the position of the trachea by pressing the index finger into the suprasternal notch. *(From Eubanks DH, Bone RC: Comprehensive respiratory care, ed 2, St. Louis, 1990, Mosby.)*

trachea by having the upright or supine patient look straight ahead and gently inserting the index finger into the suprasternal notch (Fig. 1-28). The trachea should be detected in midline with soft tissues on both sides. A trachea that has shifted to one side is abnormal and can be caused by the following (see Fig. 1-4):

a. Atelectasis, which causes the trachea to be pulled *toward* the affected side
b. Pulmonary fibrosis, which causes the trachea to be pulled *toward* the most affected side
c. Tension pneumothorax, which causes the trachea to be pushed *away* from the affected side
d. Hemothorax, pleural effusion, and empyema, which push the trachea *away* from the affected side

Correction of the underlying pulmonary problem causes the trachea to return to its normal midline position.

## 7. Determine whether the patient has any tenderness (NBRC code: IB2b) [Difficulty: R, Ap]

Tenderness is an increased local sensation of pain when the chest is gently hit with the ulnar area of the fist. This tapping is done in a symmetrical pattern over the posterior and anterior lung areas and normally should not cause any pain. Intercostal tenderness is felt at the site of an inflamed pleura. Local tenderness and a history of trauma to some area of the chest lead to the conclusion of musculoskeletal pain. Chest x-ray examination might be indicated to reveal whether any ribs have been fractured. The absence of chest wall tenderness should lead to further investigation of the cause of the chest pain, such as angina pectoris (hypoxic heart pain).

## MODULE G

**Use *auscultation* to determine the patient's complete respiratory condition**

### 1. Breath sounds

**a. Determine if the patient has bilaterally normal breath sounds (NBRC code: IB3a) [Difficulty: R, Ap]**

Normal breath sounds can be classified into three different types (Fig. 1-29):

1. *Normal* breath sounds are also called *vesicular*. Normal breath sounds are heard over all areas of normally ventilated lungs. They have been variously described as "leaves rustling" or "like a gentle breeze." These faint sounds are heard as air is moved through the small airways of the lungs during the breathing cycle. The I:E ratio is about 3:1. The inspiratory sound is louder than the expiratory

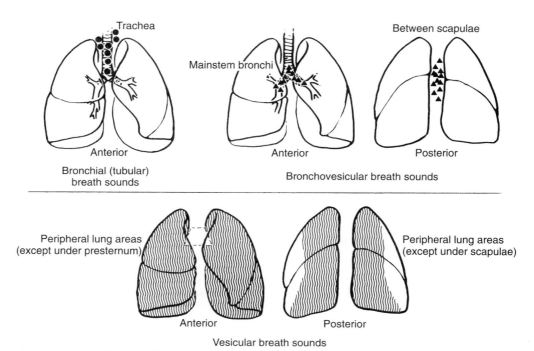

**Fig. 1-29** Breath sounds heard over the normal chest. *(From Lehrer S: Understanding lung sounds, Philadelphia, 1984, WB Saunders.)*

sound, and no pause can be noted between inspiration and expiration.

2. *Bronchial* breath sounds are also called *tracheal*. These breath sounds are heard over the trachea and main bronchi. Bronchial breath sounds have been described as louder, harsher, and higher pitched than normal breath sounds. They have a fairly uniform pitch on inspiration and expiration with a distinct pause in the transition of flow. The I:E ratio is about 1:1.5.

3. *Bronchovesicular* sounds are a cross between bronchial and vesicular sounds. The sound is more muffled than that of bronchial sounds but louder than vesicular sounds, and these sounds have the same pitch throughout inspiration and expiration. The I:E ratio is about 1:1.

Bronchial and bronchovesicular breath sounds are abnormal if they are heard in any areas other than those mentioned here. These sounds, when heard over areas that normally should be vesicular, indicate consolidation or atelectasis with a patent airway.

**b. Determine if the patient has abnormal breath sounds: increased, decreased, absent, or unequal breath sounds (NBRC code: IB3a) [Difficulty: R, Ap]**

This discussion is limited to variations in normal vesicular breath sounds. The abnormal appearance of bronchial and bronchovesicular breath sounds has been described previously.

**1. Increased normal vesicular breath sounds**

a. Found most often in children and in debilitated adults because their thinner chest walls transmit sounds better

b. Increased breath sounds are commonly described as harsh

**2. Decreased normal vesicular breath sounds**

a. Most commonly caused by pleural effusion, hemothorax, or empyema because of fluid between the lung and the stethoscope (see Fig. 1-4, *D*)

b. Pulmonary fibrosis because of decreased airflow (see Fig. 1-4, *B*)

c. Emphysema because of decreased airflow

d. Pleural thickening because of dampening from the thicker pleural tissues

**3. Absent normal vesicular breath sounds**

a. Pneumothorax because the lung is forced away from the chest wall (see Fig. 1-4, *C*)

b. Atelectasis because no air moves into the collapsed area (see Fig. 1-4, *A*)

c. Endotracheal tube placed into a bronchus instead of the trachea. In this case, the right bronchus is most commonly intubated, and breath sounds are absent over the left lung

d. Large pleural effusion

e. Obese patient

### 4. Unequal normal vesicular breath sounds

a. Pneumonia, consolidation, or atelectasis that decreases airflow into a segment or lobe

b. Foreign body or tumor in a bronchus that decreases airflow to the distal lung

c. Spinal or thoracic deformity that reduces airflow to the underlying lung

### c. Determine if the patient has abnormal breath sounds: wheezing (rhonchi) or crackles (rales) (NBRC code: IB3a) [Difficulty: R, Ap]

The term *adventitious* is used to collectively describe all types of abnormal breath sounds.

#### 1. Wheezing

Wheezing (also known as wheeze and rhonchi) has the following features or characteristics:

a. It is a continuous sound

b. It is more commonly heard on expiration than inspiration

c. Low-pitched, polyphonic expiratory wheezing is commonly associated with secretions in the airways. Coughing or tracheal suctioning often causes these sounds to be modified or eliminated. Common pulmonary conditions include bronchitis, pneumonia, or any other secretion-causing problem. A common term for these sounds is *rhonchi*

d. High-pitched, *monophonic* expiratory sounds are commonly associated with closure of one large airway (commonly found with an airway tumor)

e. High-pitched, *polyphonic* expiratory sounds are commonly associated with closure of many small airways, which is commonly found with bronchospasm in an asthmatic patient

f. Coughing or tracheal suctioning is unlikely to eliminate these high-pitched sounds

#### 2. Crackles (rales)

Crackles have the following features or characteristics:

a. They are discontinuous sounds

b. They are more commonly heard on inspiration than expiration

c. They may be caused by the sudden opening of collapsed airways. Early inspiratory crackles are heard in patients with obstructive lung diseases such as chronic bronchitis, bronchiectasis, asthma, and emphysema. Late inspiratory crackles are heard in patients with atelectasis, pneumonia, pulmonary edema, or fibrosis

d. They may be caused by air passing through secretions and are heard as a repeated sound during the same phase of the respiratory cycle

### d. Determine if the patient has abnormal breath sounds: stridor (NBRC code: IB3a) [Difficulty: R, Ap]

Stridor is heard as a harsh, monophonic, high-pitched, inspiratory sound over the larynx. (It is not the normal tracheal sound.) Stridor has these features or characteristics:

a. It can often be heard without a stethoscope

b. Common pediatric conditions include acute epiglottitis, laryngotracheobronchitis (LTB, or croup), and laryngomalacia (congenital stridor)

c. Common adult conditions include post-extubation laryngeal edema and laryngeal tumor

d. Stridor heard on inspiration and expiration is commonly caused by an aspirated foreign body, tracheal stenosis, or laryngeal tumor

### e. Determine if the patient has abnormal breath sounds: friction rub (NBRC code: IB3a) [Difficulty: R, Ap]

A friction rub (pleural friction rub) is the sound caused by the rubbing together of inflamed and adherent visceral and parietal pleurae, as seen in pleurisy. It is heard through a stethoscope and can be described as loud and grating, clicking, or the creaking of old leather. The inspiratory sound frequently is reversed from the expiratory sound as the pleural tissues rub against each other in the opposite direction.

A friction rub is heard most commonly over the lower lung areas when the patient complains of pleural pain on breathing. Coughing and suctioning do not affect it. Causes include pulmonary infarct or any pneumonia that leads to an abscess or empyema.

## 2. Heart sounds

### a. Determine if the patient has normal heart sounds (NBRC code: IB3b) [Difficulty: R, Ap]

The clinician can easily determine the patient's HR and rhythm by listening at the point of the apical pulse (see Fig. 1-24). Heart sounds are caused by the closing of the four heart valves during a cardiac cycle. The first heart sound, $S_1$, is heard as a "lub" sound when the mitral (bicuspid) and tricuspid valves close after the ventricles contract during systole. The second heart sound, $S_2$, is heard as a "dup" or "dub" sound when the pulmonary semilunar and aortic valves close after the ventricles relax during diastole. Obviously, if a heart sound cannot be detected, the patient should be assessed for cardiac arrest. Begin cardiopulmonary resuscitation if needed.

### b. Determine if the patient has arrhythmias (NBRC code: IB3b) [Difficulty: R, Ap]

A steady rhythm has approximately equal amounts of time between ventricular contractions. A slight increase in the HR and faster rhythm during inspiration than during expiration are considered normal because of the increased blood brought into the chest during inspiration when intrathoracic pressure is more negative. The opposite pattern might be found when a patient is mechanically ventilated with high peak airway pressures, which would indicate that venous return to the heart is decreased during a mechanically delivered inspiration.

Any sudden variations in rate and rhythm not related to the respiratory cycle are abnormal. Occasionally, a third ($S_3$) or fourth ($S_4$) heart sound is heard. A patient with these extra sounds is described as having a "gallop" rhythm. This pathologic finding is usually noted in patients with congestive heart failure.

The origin of most arrhythmias is difficult to determine solely on the basis of their sound patterns; an ECG is indicated. A premature ventricular contraction (PVC) is noted by two rhythmic characteristics: The heartbeat is premature, and a complete compensatory pause is noted between the PVC and the following normal beat. A complete compensatory pause is the time interval of two normal heartbeats. (See the representative rhythm strip in Chapter 11 [Fig. 11-22]).

### c. Determine the presence of abnormal heart sounds: murmurs (NBRC code: IB3b) [Difficulty: R, Ap]

A murmur is an abnormal fluttering or humming sound heard during the cardiac cycle. The murmur indicates that blood is flowing through one or more heart valves when it should not. The valve(s) could be either incompetent (not closing properly and causing blood to leak) or stenotic (narrowed and preventing normal blood flow). Fig. 1-30 shows the areas where a stethoscope should be

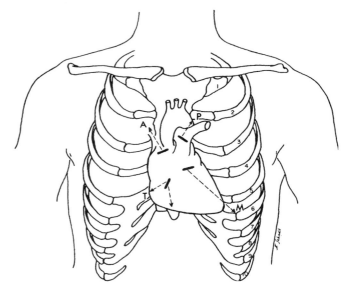

**Fig. 1-30** Areas for listening for heart murmurs. Solid bars show the approximate location of the valves within the heart (*A*, aortic valve; *P*, pulmonary semilunar valve; *M*, mitral valve; *T*, tricuspid valve). Arrows indicate where each valve sound is best heard. *(From Prior JA, Silberstein JS: Physical diagnosis: the history and examination of the patient, ed 6, St. Louis, 1982, Mosby.)*

placed to listen for a murmur from each of the four valves. The bell should be held lightly on the chest to hear low-frequency sounds and firmly on the chest to hear high-frequency sounds. Listening may be enhanced when the patient lies on his or her left side. A systolic murmur would be heard after the $S_1$ sound but before the $S_2$ sound. The sound sequence would be "lub-murmur-dup, lub-murmur-dup." A diastolic murmur would be heard after the $S_2$ sound but before the $S_1$ sound. The sound sequence would be "lub-dup-murmur, lub-dup-murmur." It is beyond the scope of this text to fully describe all of the possible types and causes of murmurs. However, one must understand that the presence of a murmur indicates a defective cardiac valve.

### d. Determine the patient's blood pressure (NBRC code: IB3c) [Difficulty: R, Ap]

Measure blood pressure (BP) on any patient to establish a baseline normal value, and when you think the BP may significantly increase or decrease. The BP should be the same on any arm or leg, although an arm is typically used. Place the proper cuff around the arm, and inflate the cuff pressure to above the patient's normal value. Place the diaphragm of the stethoscope over the brachial artery, and slowly let the air out of the cuff. The first distinct sound heard as the blood flows through the artery is the systolic pressure, and the last distinct sound is the diastolic pressure. Clinical practice is needed for accurate determination of BP.

## MODULE H
### Evaluate and monitor patient objective and subjective responses to respiratory care

### 1. Auscultate the patient's breath sounds and interpret any changes (NBRC code: IIIE11) [Difficulty: R, Ap]

Breath sounds should be evaluated after any treatment or procedure that could result in a change. These would include aerosolized bronchodilator therapy, suctioning, and bronchopulmonary hygiene therapy. Effective treatment should result in improved breath sounds.

### 2. Recommend and review a chest radiograph (NBRC code: IIIE1) [Difficulty: R, Ap]

A chest x-ray should be taken to reveal a pulmonary or cardiac condition with viewable bone or organ problems. This could include pneumothorax, foreign body in the airway or lung, broken ribs, or pleural effusion.

### 3. Look for changes in the patient's sputum characteristics (NBRC code: IIIE5) [Difficulty: R, Ap]

Sputum characteristics should be evaluated after any treatment or procedure that could result in a change. These would include aerosolized mucolytic therapy, suctioning, and bronchopulmonary hygiene therapy. Effective treatment should result in improved breath sounds.

### 4. Stop the treatment or procedure if the patient has an adverse reaction to it (NBRC code: IIIF1) [Difficulty: R, Ap, An]

Patient safety should always be an important consideration during a treatment or procedure. The respiratory therapist should know the complications and hazards of any patient care activity that is performed. These complications and hazards are discussed in the following chapters. Be prepared to stop the treatment or procedure if the patient has an adverse reaction to it. Additionally, be prepared to recommend to the physician that the treatment or procedure should be terminated if it is likely to result in additional adverse reactions.

## MODULE I
### Respiratory care plan

### 1. Analyze available information to determine the patient's pathophysiologic state (NBRC code: IIIH1) [Difficulty: R, Ap, An]

The limitations of this text prevent in-depth discussion of the various cardiopulmonary conditions and disorders that befall patients who are cared for by respiratory therapists. However, some discussion of cardiopulmonary conditions is included in the following chapters as the respiratory therapies are presented.

### Exam Hint

The NBRC is known to ask questions about cardiopulmonary pathologies. Take time to study at least the most common disorders, such as asthma, emphysema and chronic bronchitis (COPD), bacterial pneumonia, tension pneumothorax, and heart failure with pulmonary edema.

### 2. Determine the appropriateness of the prescribed respiratory care plan, and recommend modifications when indicated

a. Review the interdisciplinary patient and family care plan (NBRC code: IIIH2b) [Difficulty: R, Ap]

b. Review the planned therapy to establish the therapeutic plan (NBRC code: IIIH2a) [Difficulty: R, Ap]

c. Determine the appropriateness of the prescribed therapy and goals for the patient's pathophysiologic state (NBRC code: IIIH3) [Difficulty: R, Ap, An]

d. Recommend changes in the therapeutic plan if supportive data exist (NBRC code: IIIH4) [Difficulty: R, Ap]

e. Conduct patient and family education and disease management programs (NBRC code: IIIK2) [Difficulty: R, Ap]

If the patient is to receive the best care possible, the respiratory therapist must know the indications, contraindications, complications, and hazards of the respiratory care procedures that the patient will receive. The patient must be assessed before, during, and after the treatment or procedure for determination of its effectiveness. The key goal of an appropriate care plan is that the patient's condition is treated in the best way possible. Modifications to the care plan must be made, as needed, as the patient's condition changes.

The respiratory therapist should be a member of the patient care team that includes physician, nurse, and others who decide how best to care for the patient. The following steps are necessary in developing the respiratory care plan for any patient:

1. Determine an expected outcome or goal(s)
2. Develop a plan to achieve success
3. Decide how to measure goal achievement
4. Plan a timeline for measuring the patient's progress
5. Document the patient's response to care and the final outcome

**f. Discontinue treatment based on the patient's response** (NBRC code: IIIG1f) [Difficulty: R, Ap]

Typically, three events can result in discontinuation of a patient's treatment. First, the patient has recovered and no longer needs the treatment or procedure. It is expensive and wasteful to perform unnecessary treatments. Second, the patient has had an adverse reaction and is likely to have an adverse reaction every time the treatment or procedure is repeated. For example, the patient's blood pressure goes too high whenever he is placed into a head-down position for postural drainage. Third, the patient's condition is terminal, and the patient or responsible family member wants all treatment to be stopped.

> **Exam Hint**
>
> **B**e prepared to use information from the respiratory care plan to help you make decisions about patient care. Expect questions that relate to what would be the best recommendations for care.

### MODULE J
#### Respiratory care protocols

1. **Develop the outcomes of respiratory care protocols** (NBRC code: IIIH6b) [Difficulty: R, Ap]
2. **Apply respiratory care protocols to patient care situations** (NBRC code: IIIH8) [Difficulty: R]
3. **Monitor the outcomes of respiratory care protocols** (NBRC code: IIIH7b) [Difficulty: R, Ap]

Respiratory care protocols are set treatment plans that are designed to be used for management of certain patient care conditions. They have been developed to improve the quality of patient care by ensuring that the necessary treatment(s) or procedure(s) are delivered as quickly as possible. Common respiratory care protocols include oxygen therapy, aerosolized bronchodilator therapy, hyperinflation therapy (incentive spirometry vs. intermittent positive pressure ventilation), and aspects of mechanical ventilation and weaning.

The goal of all protocols is to restore the patient's condition to as close to normal as possible. When it is not possible to restore normal conditions, acceptable conditions must be listed as the target for care. The patient must be evaluated before, during, and after a protocol is used to determine if improvement has occurred. On the basis of the results of the patient assessment, the care can be upregulated (increased) or downregulated (decreased). Protocol information is listed as indicated in later chapters of this text.

### MODULE K
#### Quality assurance and quality control

1. **Develop outcomes of quality improvement programs** (NBRC code: IIIH6a) [Difficulty: R, Ap]
2. **Perform respiratory care quality assurance** (NBRC code: IIIH5) [Difficulty: R]
3. **Monitor outcomes of quality assurance programs** (NBRC code: IIIH5) [Difficulty: R]
4. **Perform quality control procedures for blood gas analyzers, co-oximeters, blood gas sampling devices, oxygen analyzers, mechanical ventilators, and flowmeters** (NBRC code: IIC1,2,3,4) [Difficulty: R]

Quality improvement (QI) refers to the processes used to identify areas of needed improvement in patient care services. Quality assurance (QA) refers to any evaluation of services provided and the results achieved as compared with accepted standards. These standards are developed through a process called *benchmarking*, wherein agreement is reached on fair and reasonable patient care criteria and outcomes. The later chapters of this text provide information on quality control procedures in the NBRC areas listed previously.

### MODULE L
#### Record any performed treatment(s) or procedure(s) on the patient's chart, and communicate with other members of the health care team.

1. **Record in conventional terminology any treatment(s) or procedure(s) performed, including the date, time, frequency of therapy, medication, and ventilatory data** (NBRC code: IIIA1a) [Difficulty: R, Ap]
2. **Apply computer technology to document patient management** (NBRC code: IIIA3a) [Difficulty: R]
3. **Apply computer technology to monitor workload assignments** (NBRC code: IIIA3b) [Difficulty: R]
4. **Record and evaluate the patient's response to treatment(s) or procedure(s), including the following:**
   a. **Record and interpret the following: heart rate and rhythm, respiratory rate, blood pressure, body temperature, and pain level** (NBRC code: IIIA1b3, IIIA1b4) [Difficulty: R, Ap]
   b. **Record and interpret the patient's breath sounds** (NBRC code: IIIAb2) [Difficulty: R, Ap]
   c. **Record and interpret the type of cough the patient has and the nature of the**

**sputum** (NBRC code: IIIAb2) [Difficulty: R, Ap]

d. **Record and evaluate any effects of therapy or adverse reactions the patient has had to treatment(s) or procedure(s)** (NBRC code: IIIA1b1) [Difficulty: R, Ap, An]

e. **Record and evaluate the patient's subjective and attitudinal responses to therapy** (NBRC code: IIIA1b1) [Difficulty: R, Ap, An]

5. **Recheck any math work and make note of incorrect data** (NBRC code: IIIA1c) [Difficulty: R, Ap]

Errors made in charting must be corrected by drawing a single mark through the error and writing in the correct information. Some prefer that the error be further clarified by writing in "error" next to it and adding initials. *Never* erase or use any covering material over an error.

> **Exam Hint**
>
> **O**ne question is often asked about the proper way to document patient care or how to document a charting error. Remember that a charting error should never be hidden or covered up. Typically, the error is identified, the correct information is written, and the charting therapist signs his or her name.

6. **Communicate with other members of the health care team about significant clinical information regarding the patient** (NBRC code: IIIA2a) [Difficulty: R, Ap]

Inform the patient's nurse or physician and the supervising therapist if any serious question or problem occurs with the patient. Routine communication should occur as needed between these people and any other caregiver.

7. **Communicate information relevant to coordinating patient care and discharge planning [e.g., scheduling, avoiding conflicts, and sequencing therapies]** (NBRC code: IIIA2b) [Difficulty: R, Ap]

Common scheduling problems include eating times and times when the patient must go to another department such as radiology or physical therapy. Some procedures, such as giving aerosolized medications and performing chest physiotherapy, should be performed before eating.

Typically, the discharge plan would include the following:

1. Patient evaluation that determines the patient is ready for discharge. The patient needs to have recovered sufficiently before leaving the hospital

2. Determination of the best place for the patient to go for further recovery and the necessary patient care resources. It needs to be determined if the patient can go home or should go to an extended care facility. If the patient is to go home, it needs to be determined if the family can provide the necessary care. If not, arrangements for home care respiratory therapists and nurses will be needed

3. Determination that the patient's financial resources are adequate. If not, social services will need to be contacted to work with the patient's insurance company or other financial support agencies

**BIBLIOGRAPHY**

American Association for Respiratory Care: Clinical Practice Guideline: Discharge planning for the respiratory care patient, *Respir Care* 40:1308, 1995.

Barkauskas VH, Stoltenberg-Allen K, Baumann LC, Darling-Fisher C: *Health & physical assessment*, St. Louis, 1994, Mosby.

Barnes TA, editor: *Core textbook of respiratory care practice*, ed 2, St. Louis, 1994, Mosby.

Burton GC, Hodgkin JE, Ward JJ, editors: *Respiratory care: a guide to clinical practice*, ed 4, Philadelphia, 1997, Lippincott.

Cherniack RM, Cherniack L: *Respiration in health and disease*, ed 3, Philadelphia, 1983, WB Saunders.

Clochesy JM, Breu C, Cardin S, et al, editors: *Critical care nursing*, ed 2, Philadelphia, 1996, WB Saunders.

Des Jardins TR, Burton GG: *Clinical manifestations of respiratory disease*, ed 4, Chicago, 2000, Mosby.

DiPietro JS, Mustard MN: *Clinical guide for respiratory care practitioners*, Norwalk, Conn, 1987, Appleton-Century-Crofts.

Erickson B: *Heart sounds and murmurs—a practical guide*, ed 3, St. Louis, 1997, Mosby.

Eubanks DH, Bone RC: *Comprehensive respiratory care*, St. Louis, 1985, Mosby.

Fink JB, Hunt GE, editors: *Clinical practice in respiratory care*, Philadelphia, 1999, Lippincott Williams & Wilkins.

Hess DR, MacIntyre NR, Mishoe SC, et al, editors: *Respiratory care principles & practice*, Philadelphia, 2002, WB Saunders.

Kacmarek RM, Dimas S, Mack CW: *The essentials of respiratory therapy*, ed 3, Chicago, 1990, Mosby.

Kenner CV, Guzzetta CE, Dossey BM: *Critical care nursing: body-mind-spirit*, Boston, 1981, Little, Brown.

Lehrer S: *Understanding lung sounds*, Philadelphia, 1984, WB Saunders.

Levitsky MG, Cairo JM, Hall SM: *Introduction to respiratory care*, Philadelphia, 1990, WB Saunders.

Pagana KD, Pagana TJ: *Manual of diagnostic and laboratory tests*, St. Louis, 1998, Mosby.

Peters RM: Chest trauma. In Moser KM, Spragg RG, editors: *Respiratory emergencies*, ed 2, St. Louis, 1982, Mosby.

Rau JL, Pearce DJ: *Understanding chest radiographs*, Denver, 1984, Multi-Media Publishing.

Shapiro BA, Kacmarek RM, Cane RD, et al, editors: *Clinical application of respiratory care*, ed 4, St. Louis, 1991, Mosby.

Stillwell SB, McCarter RE: *Pocket guide to cardiovascular care*, ed 2, St. Louis, 1994, Mosby.

Tilkian AG, Boudreau Conover M: *Understanding heart sounds and murmurs*, ed 2, Philadelphia, 1984, WB Saunders.

Wilkins RL, Hodgkin JE, Lopez B: *Lung sounds, a practical guide*, St. Louis, 1988, Mosby.

Wilkins RL, Krider SJ, Sheldon RL: *Clinical assessment in respiratory care*, ed 4, St. Louis, 2000, Mosby.

Wilkins RL, Stoller JK, Scanlan CL, editors: *Egan's fundamentals of respiratory care*, ed 8, St. Louis, 2003, Mosby.

## SELF-STUDY QUESTIONS

1. You have finished charting on your patient when you notice that an error was made. You should do which of the following?
   A. Tell the nurse so that she will tell the physician.
   B. Tell the nurse so that she will chart the correct information.
   C. Place a line through the error, initial it, and write in the correct information.
   D. Have your supervisor chart the correct information.

2. In listening to a patient's lungs, you notice bronchial breath sounds in her right lower lobe. These would indicate which of the following?
   A. Normal lungs
   B. Pneumothorax
   C. Consolidation in her right lower lobe
   D. Pleural effusion in her right lower lobe

3. You are called to start a new aerosolized medication treatment. After reading the physician's order, you notice that the drug dosage is outside the normal department guidelines. You should do which of the following?
   A. Give the treatment as ordered.
   B. Contact the physician to confirm that the order is indeed correct.
   C. Give the treatment as ordered, and leave a note in the chart asking for clarification for the next treatment.
   D. Have the nurse rewrite the order.

4. You are called to the Emergency Department to help care for a patient who was in a car accident and has chest injuries, including broken ribs. While palpating her neck, you feel a crepitation. What is the most likely cause of this?
   A. She has a laryngeal tumor.
   B. Blood is in the back of her throat.
   C. She has aspirated a tooth.
   D. She has an air leak from her lung.

5. You are called to help in the evaluation of a 55-year-old male patient. You notice the following signs and symptoms: oral temperature of 40° C (104.5° F), diaphoresis, respiratory rate of 22, the use of accessory muscles of respiration, and palpable rhonchi in the right lower lobe. You would suspect the following diagnosis:
   A. Bacterial pneumonia
   B. Heart attack
   C. Pneumothorax
   D. Viral pneumonia

6. A patient, since being told of the diagnosis of cancer, has become argumentative about his care and threatens to hit the nurse and therapist. He should be evaluated for
   A. Language barrier problems
   B. Hypercarbia
   C. Emotional state
   D. Hypoxemia

7. To help determine your patient's level of consciousness, you should ask the following questions:
   I. "Do you know what day this is?"
   II. "Can I see your identification wristband?"
   III. "Do you know where you are?"
   IV. "How are you feeling today?"
   V. "Do you know who the president is?"
   A. II and IV only
   B. III only
   C. V only
   D. I and III only

8. To help you determine whether your patient has orthopnea, you would ask the following:
   A. "How many flights of stairs can you climb before you become short of breath?"
   B. "Do you know who the governor is?"
   C. "Do you need to use extra pillows behind your head and back to keep from getting short of breath when you sleep?"
   D. "Do any particular foods seem to make it harder for you to cough up your secretions?"

9. In observing an infant's chest configuration, you notice that it is the same size in both the A-P and lateral dimensions. This would indicate that the patient has
   A. A normal chest
   B. Funnel chest/pectus excavatum
   C. Pulmonary emphysema with air trapping
   D. Lordosis

10. In examining your patient, you notice that she has diminished breath sounds in her right lower lobe, and her trachea is shifted to the right. These signs indicate which condition?
    A. Right-sided pneumothorax
    B. Right-sided atelectasis
    C. Left-sided pneumothorax
    D. Left-sided pneumonia

11. In palpating your patient for symmetrical chest movements, you notice that his left side does not move as much as his right side. This indicates that he has which condition(s)?
    I. Emphysema
    II. Congestive heart failure
    III. Left-sided pneumonia
    IV. Left-sided pneumothorax
    V. Right-sided pneumonia
    A. I and II only
    B. III and IV only
    C. IV and V only
    D. II only

12. You are called to the Emergency Department to help evaluate a pediatric patient. On entering the room, you observe the patient's breathing effort and can hear a harsh, high-pitched sound on inspiration. Which of the following is true?
    A. Sounds are tracheal and normal.
    B. Sounds are bronchovesicular and not normal.
    C. Sounds are stridorous and indicate a respiratory emergency.
    D. Sounds are bronchial and indicate a respiratory emergency.

13. You are called to evaluate a patient's breathing pattern. You notice that the patient's tidal volumes go from small to large to small and then stop for 10 sec before starting up again. The pattern repeats itself. This patient's breathing pattern would best be called
    A. Eupnea
    B. Obstructed expiration
    C. Kussmaul's respiration
    D. Cheyne-Stokes respiration

14. A tension pneumothorax is identified by the following:
    I. Chest x-ray film shows a shift of the mediastinum toward the affected lung.
    II. Chest x-ray film shows an elevation of the hemidiaphragm on the affected side.
    III. The patient's vital signs suddenly deteriorate.
    IV. Chest x-ray film shows a depression of the hemidiaphragm on the affected side.
    V. Chest x-ray film shows a shift of the mediastinum away from the affected lung.
    VI. Vital signs are essentially unchanged.
    A. I, II, and VI only
    B. III, IV, and V only
    C. I, II, and III only
    D. I, III, and IV only

15. Your patient is complaining of localized pain over the lower right area of the chest while breathing. When auscultating her chest, you hear a rasping noise at her point of pain on both inspiration and expiration. This is most likely
    A. Pleural friction rub
    B. Normal breath sounds
    C. Wheeze
    D. Rhonchi

16. Your patient has distended external jugular veins, even though her head and body are raised 45 degrees above her legs. This would indicate that she
    A. Is hypertensive
    B. Is fluid overloaded
    C. Has emphysema
    D. Is dehydrated

17. Tactile fremitus would be decreased in all of the following conditions EXCEPT
    A. Pneumothorax
    B. COPD
    C. Pulmonary edema
    D. Pleural effusion

18. A frail, thin patient known to have lung cancer is admitted to the hospital. His family members are also present. What should be asked of them to make sure that the proper level of care is delivered?
    A. The last time that he ate
    B. The last time that he had a bowel movement
    C. Whether any advance directives have been documented
    D. Whether he has brought his home care medications with him

19. It is most important to ask a patient with broken legs from a recent car crash about the following:
    A. Level of pain
    B. Level of consciousness
    C. Work of breathing
    D. Emotional state

20. All of the following could result in a mediastinal shift on a chest x-ray film EXCEPT
    A.  Right hemothorax
    B.  Bilateral lower lobe pneumonia
    C.  Left tension pneumothorax
    D.  Right lower lobe atelectasis

21. A patient who is suffering respiratory distress would exhibit all of the following EXCEPT
    A.  Normal respiratory rate
    B.  Nasal flaring
    C.  Intercostal retractions
    D.  Use of accessory muscles of inspiration

## ANSWER KEY AND RATIONALE

1.  **C.** From a legal point of view, a charting error should never be obliterated. Simply correct and initial the correct information. Only the person making the error should correct it.

2.  **C.** Bronchial breath sounds are not normal in the right lower lobe and indicate consolidation of the alveoli. Neither pneumothorax nor pleural effusion can be identified by bronchial breath sounds.

3.  **B.** Never give an overdose of a medication. Personally contact the physician to clarify the error. (Rarely, a larger-than-usual dose of medication is given under special circumstances. The physician must make it clear that he or she is aware of the large dose and wants it delivered.)

4.  **D.** The patient's history of injury and crepitus indicates air under the skin. The air under her skin would have to come from a lung tear.

5.  **A.** All of the patient's symptoms point to a bacterial pneumonia problem. The other options may have some but not all of the noted symptoms.

6.  **C.** The patient is reacting with anger to his diagnosis of cancer. He should be evaluated for emotional state. The other problems should not cause anger.

7.  **A.** The correct two questions relate to the patient's level of consciousness and understanding. The first question relates to the patient's understanding of *time*. The third question relates to the patient's understanding of *place*. The fifth question relates to the patient's understanding of *person*.

8.  **C.** Orthopnea relates to the patient's inability to lie down and breathe comfortably. Extra pillows are needed to raise the head and body. The other questions relate to other areas of assessment.

9.  **A.** An infant's chest is basically round in dimension. See Fig. 1-18.

10. **B.** Diminished breath sounds mean that less air than normal is entering an area. A tracheal shift to the side of the diminished breath sound indicates less air in the lung. Both of these point to atelectasis.

11. **B.** Left-sided pneumonia and pneumothorax both result in decreased movement on that side. Emphysema and congestive heart failure would not cause a one-sided change in movement. Right-sided pneumonia would result in less movement on the right side.

12. **C.** Inspiratory stridor is the only listed breath sound that can be heard with the unaided ear. It is a respiratory emergency.

13. **D.** Only Cheyne-Stokes respiration fits the description. See Fig. 1-21.

14. **B.** The high air pressure found with a tension pneumothorax causes the mediastinal contents to be shifted to the opposite side and the diaphragm on the affected side to be depressed. These drastic changes can cause the patient's vital signs to rapidly deteriorate.

15. **A.** A pleural friction rub is identified as a localized area of abnormal grating breath sound; it is often localized to an area of pain on breathing.

16. **B.** Fluid overload causes the jugular veins to be distended. Dehydration may result in the jugular veins being flat. Emphysema and hypertension should not have any effect on the jugular veins.

17. **C.** Tactile fremitus would be decreased in pneumothorax and COPD because the lung is overinflated. A pleural effusion would block and decrease the sounds coming from the lung. See Table 1-19.

18. **C.** It is appropriate to ask about advance directives such as a "do not resuscitate" order in a patient with a fatal illness. Eating and bowel habits are not essential to know at this time. He will be given new orders for medications during his stay in the hospital, so it does not matter if he brought his medications with him.

19. **A.** It is important to assess the patient's level of pain from the broken legs. Severe pain should be managed with increased medication. The other issues are less important to assess unless there is an apparent problem.

20. **B.** All listed items except bilateral lower lobe pneumonia would shift the mediastinum. Because bilateral lower lobe pneumonia affects both lungs, the mediastinum would stay centered properly.

21. **A.** A patient with respiratory distress should have an *increased* respiratory rate.

# 2 Infection Control

A review of the most recent Entry Level Examinations shows an average of 4 questions (3% of the exam) that cover infection control issues.

## MODULE A

### Follow established infection control policies and procedures (e.g., Standard Precautions) (NBRC code: IIID8) [Difficulty: R]

#### 1. Hand washing or cleansing

Hand washing or cleansing is probably the single most important procedure for reducing the spread of infection. Washing with plain soap and warm tap water is acceptable in most cases. Antimicrobial soap should be used if called for in the infection control protocol. In many institutions, an isopropyl alcohol and skin softener/cleansing agent is used unless the hands are obviously contaminated. When contaminated with body fluids, the hands should be washed. In any case, respiratory therapists should wash or cleanse their hands before and between each patient contact. The following times are recommended:

  a. When coming on duty
  b. When hands are obviously soiled or after contamination by blood or other patient body fluids
  c. Before contact with the face and mouth of patients, especially if the patient has an artificial airway
  d. Before setting up equipment or pouring medicines
  e. When leaving an isolation area or handling contaminated articles from an isolation area
  f. After handling soiled dressings, sputum containers, urinals, bedpans, catheters, etc.
  g. After removing patient care gloves
  h. After personal use of the toilet
  i. After using hands to cover a cough and after blowing or wiping the nose
  j. Before eating or serving food
  k. Upon completion of duty

The most common bacterial organisms spread by personal contact are *Staphylococcus aureus*, *Escherichia coli*, and *Streptococcus* species. Suspect personal contact and poor hand cleansing whenever a patient gets one of these infections.

#### 2. Standard precautions

Standard (formerly called *universal*) precautions are designed for care of all patients regardless of their diagnosis or presumed infection status. Barriers such as gloves, masks, and other items are used to prevent contact with body fluids. This approach to patient care has been adopted because of the concern of health care workers and the public that the human immunodeficiency virus (HIV), hepatitis B, or other deadly pathogens can be spread unknowingly by contact. Box 2-1 includes specific standard precaution guidelines established by the Centers for Disease Control and Prevention (CDC) and the Occupational Safety and Health Administration (OSHA).

#### 3. Respiratory care equipment and procedures

The following guidelines are recommended to minimize the spread of infection by equipment and procedures. Follow the manufacturer's specific guidelines when applicable.

  a. Each patient should have his or her own equipment.
  b. Disposable equipment should be discarded after use.
  c. Reusable equipment should undergo high-level disinfection or should be sterilized between patients.
  d. Equipment such as $O_2$ masks, large-volume nebulizers, and aerosol tubing should be changed every 24 hr.
  e. Ventilator breathing circuits should not be changed more often than every 48 hr and may be used for up to 5 days if a heat-moisture exchanger is used for humidification.

## BOX 2-1   Standard Precautions to Prevent the Spread of Infection

**EXCLUSION FROM PATIENT CONTACT**

Any health care worker with exudative skin lesions should not work in the direct care of patients

**BARRIERS**

1. Gloves should be worn under these conditions: During direct contact with blood, body fluids, secretions, mucous membranes, and wounds; when handling all items or surfaces contaminated by blood or body fluids; when performing venipuncture; or when handling intravenous catheters or monitoring devices.
2. Gloves must be changed between patients or if the gloves become torn or punctured, as with a needle-stick injury.
3. Hands should be washed immediately after the gloves are removed; the hands or any other body areas must be washed immediately if contaminated by blood or other body fluid.
4. Masks, eye goggles, or face shields, as well as gowns or aprons, should be worn when a procedure is performed that may lead to the splashing or splattering of blood, secretions, or body fluids.
5. Contaminated masks, goggles, face shields, gowns, and aprons should be removed and disposed of properly.
6. Contaminated worker uniforms should be left at the hospital for cleaning.

**NEEDLE AND INSTRUMENT PRECAUTIONS**

1. Care should be taken when needles and sharp instruments are handled.
2. Used needles and sharp instruments should be placed into puncture-resistant containers for proper disposal; reusable needles should be placed into a puncture-resistant container for transport.
3. No attempt should be made to manually recap arterial blood gas or other needles, remove them from the syringe, or bend or cut them (needle-covering systems or methods of pushing the needle into a rubber cube are widely used; these require the use of only one hand with no touching of the needle).

**PATIENT SPECIMENS**

1. Blood and body fluids should be placed into leak-proof, sturdy plastic bags for transportation to the laboratory.
2. The laboratory requisition form should be placed on the outside of this bag.

**CARDIOPULMONARY RESUSCITATION**

1. Mouth-to-mouth breathing should be avoided even though no evidence exists that saliva transmits human immunodeficiency virus infection.
2. Mouth-to-valve mask resuscitators and manual resuscitators (bag-valve) should be readily available for use in ventilating patients.

---

f. Sterile water should be used for procedures, and the unused portion should be discarded after 24 hr.
g. Add water to reservoir systems immediately before use.
h. Discard any unused water in a reservoir system before refilling.
i. Drain and discard any water collected in tubing; do *not* drain water back into the reservoir.
j. Medications should be stored under the conditions set by the manufacturer, should be discarded if they appear abnormal, and should be discarded on the expiration date.
k. Unused portions of medications should be discarded after 24 hr.
l. Sterile syringes should be used when medications are measured.
m. Sterile suction catheters should be used and sterile gloves worn whenever the patient's airway is suctioned.

### Exam Hint

**P**ast examinations have questioned the types of routine procedures that should be performed to control the spread of infection through respiratory care equipment.

### 4. Transmission-based precautions

Transmission-based precautions are used for patients known or suspected to be infected or colonized with epidemiologically significant pathogens, which are spread through airborne or droplet transmission or by contact with dry skin or contaminated surfaces. These precautions are used with standard precautions. The following are general guidelines and specific diseases or conditions established by the CDC for the three identified types of patient isolation categories. Hospitals may establish extra standards and post them at the door to the patient's room.

### a. Airborne precautions

Airborne precautions are used in addition to standard precautions for patients with known or suspected illness transmitted by airborne droplet nuclei, including pulmonary tuberculosis (TB), varicella (chicken pox), and rubeola (measles).

#### 1. Room placement

Patients under airborne precautions must be placed in a room with negative airflow and ultraviolet (UV) light capabilities.

#### 2. Gloves and hand washing

Use standard precautions.

#### 3. Respiratory protection

a. If a patient is known or suspected of having TB, a National Institute for Occupational Safety and Health (NIOSH)–approved respirator mask must be worn by all caregivers who enter the room.
b. If a patient is known or suspected of having varicella or rubeola, a NIOSH-approved respirator mask must be worn by all *susceptible* caregivers who enter the room.

#### 4. Patient transport

a. Transport personnel must wear a NIOSH-approved respirator mask, as discussed previously.
b. The patient must wear an isolation mask when out of his or her room.

#### 5. Patient equipment

Use standard precautions.

### b. Droplet precautions

Droplet precautions are used in addition to standard precautions for patients known or suspected of having serious illness transmitted by large-particle droplets such as influenza, invasive *Haemophilus influenzae* (type b), *Neisseria meningitidis* disease (including meningococcal bacteremia and meningitis), *Mycoplasma pneumoniae*, and *Bordetella pertussis*.

#### 1. Room placement

A private room is preferred, but patients with the same infection may be placed in the same room.

#### 2. Gloves and hand washing

Use standard precautions.

#### 3. Gown

Use standard precautions.

#### 4. Respiratory protection

a. Use standard precautions.
b. Caregivers must wear an isolation mask if working within 3 ft of the patient.

#### 5. Patient transport

a. Transport personnel must wear an isolation mask if working within 3 ft of the patient.
b. The patient must wear an isolation mask when out of his or her room.

#### 6. Patient equipment

Use standard precautions.

### c. Contact precautions

Contact precautions are used in addition to standard precautions for patients known or suspected of having epidemiologically important organisms that can be transmitted by direct contact with environmental surfaces, such as patients with diarrhea, inadequately contained wound infections, or localized herpes zoster (shingles).

#### 1. Room placement

A private room is preferred, but patients with the same infection may be placed in the same room.

#### 2. Gloves and hand washing

a. Wear gloves when you enter the patient's room.
b. Change gloves after contact with any contaminated item.
c. Remove gloves and wash hands before you leave the patient's room.

#### 3. Gown

a. Wear a gown when you enter the patient's room if you anticipate substantial contact with the patient, environmental surfaces, or patient items.
b. Remove the gown and wash hands before you leave the room.

#### 4. Respiratory protection

Use standard precautions.

#### 5. Patient transport

a. Limit transportation of the patient from the room.
b. If transportation is required, caregivers must wear a gown and gloves.

#### 6. Patient equipment

a. Each patient should have his or her own dedicated noncritical equipment (e.g., thermometer, commode, blood pressure cuff, sphygmomanometer, and stethoscope).

b. Clean and disinfect all patient care equipment after the patient has been discharged.

## MODULE B
### Decontaminate respiratory care equipment

Decontamination is the process of disassembling, washing (to remove debris), rinsing, and disinfecting or sterilizing used patient care equipment. As a result of the process, the equipment is free of any pathogens so that it can be used with another patient. Obviously, once disinfected, the equipment must be aseptically reassembled and stored for future use.

### 1. Choose the appropriate agent and method for disinfection and sterilization (NBRC code: IIB1) [Difficulty: R]
#### a. Disinfection

Disinfection is a procedure that significantly reduces the microbial contamination of the equipment that has been processed. All disinfection processes destroy the vegetative form (the cell) of pathogenic organisms, including the vast majority of respiratory system pathogens. However, a few *Bacillus*-type bacteria are difficult to kill because they have a particularly tough cell wall, or they have spores for reproduction. Spores are analogous to seeds in that they grow into bacteria under the right conditions and are resistant to drying, heat, and many chemicals that kill the bacterial cell. Therefore, a spore-forming organism may be able to reproduce itself after the cells have been killed. Obviously, disinfection can be used only on equipment that is *not* contaminated by spore-forming bacteria. Knowledge of what pathogen has infected the patient, if possible, can help the clinician to determine the appropriate disinfection (or sterilization) method that should be used on contaminated equipment. Various disinfecting agents kill different types of organisms, depending on the length of exposure time.

Another consideration in selection of the appropriate disinfection method is how the equipment will be used in patient care. Equipment or instruments that do not directly touch the patient are classified as *noncritical* (low risk of spreading infection) and can undergo low-level disinfection (e.g., an electrocardiograph machine). Low-level disinfectants are agents capable of killing some vegetative bacteria, fungi, and lipophilic viruses. Equipment or instruments that touch surface mucous membranes and the skin but do not penetrate them are listed as *semicritical* and must undergo high-level disinfection (e.g., laryngoscope blades and a bronchoscope). Agents that kill all microorganisms except bacterial spores are classified as *high-level* disinfectants.

A third consideration in selection of the best disinfection method is the type of equipment that needs to be decontaminated. Certain processes and agents can be used only on certain types of equipment. Table 2-1 lists various ways of disinfecting reusable patient care equipment that has become decontaminated in the hospital.

The fourth consideration in choice of disinfection method is the setting in which the patient is receiving care. The previous discussion relates to patients in the hospital or in a long-term care facility. Home care patients typically do not use hospital or long-term care facility methods of disinfection because their costs are high. Instead, the plastics used in such equipment as home care medication nebulizers are usually cleaned as follows:

a. Disassemble as needed.

b. Run hot water from the tap to eliminate as many organisms as possible. Clean the sink.

c. Use hot water to wash the equipment in a detergent solution.

d. Place the equipment into an acetic acid (white vinegar) solution for disinfection. It should soak for 60 minutes. (Grocery store–purchased white vinegar contains 5% acetic acid. However, it may be diluted with three parts of water to yield a 1.25% solution.) After use, the acetic acid must be thrown away because it will no longer be effective.

e. After it has been soaked, the equipment should be rinsed in hot water and placed on a clean towel to air dry.

A 1.25% or higher solution is classified as a low-level disinfectant and will kill most vegetative bacteria (including *Pseudomonas aeruginosa*) and some fungi and viruses. However, *Mycobacterium tuberculosis*, nonlipid viruses, and spores will not be killed.

---

**Exam Hint**

**E**xpect to see one question about the use of white vinegar or acetic acid to disinfect equipment in the home. The percentage of acetic acid that is used should not matter.

---

#### b. Sterilization

Sterilization is a procedure that destroys all living microbial organisms and renders them unable to reproduce. All sterilization procedures destroy the vegetative forms and spores of all microscopic organisms. Examples of spore-forming bacteria include *Bacillus anthracis* (anthrax), *Clostridium botulinum* (botulism), *Clostridium tetani* (tetanus), and *Clostridium perfringens* (gas gangrene). Any equipment or instruments that penetrate body tissue are listed as "critical" (i.e., they carry a high risk of spreading infection) and must be sterilized before use on another patient (e.g., a surgical scalpel). As has been discussed previously, the method of sterilization that should be used depends on the type of equipment under consideration. Table 2-2 lists various methods of sterilization for

| TABLE 2-1 | Methods of Disinfection Used in the Hospital Setting | | | | | | |
|-----------|------------------------|---------|----|--------|--------|-------|----------|
| | | Microbes effective against | | | | | |
| Method | Conditions | Bacteria | TB | Spores | Viruses | Fungi | Comments |
| **LOW AND INTERMEDIATE DISINFECTION** | | | | | | | |
| Pasteurization | Complete immersion in water heated to 70°C (170°F) for 30 min | Yes | Yes | No | Yes | Yes | Used with rubber and many plastics used in respiratory care, especially those that are sensitive to a high temperature **Avoid use** with any item that cannot be immersed or will be damaged at this temperature |
| Alcohols (70% ethyl or 90% isopropyl) | Complete immersion for several minutes or pooling of the alcohol on the equipment | Yes | Yes | No | Lipophilic only | Yes | Used with metallic or plastic surfaces of large pieces of equipment that cannot be disinfected by any other means. May also be used with most plastics **Avoid use** with any item that cannot be immersed or will absorb or be damaged by the alcohol |
| Iodines (iodine or iodophor with 70% ethyl alcohol) | Complete immersion for several minutes or pooling of the solution on the equipment | Yes | Yes | No | Yes | Yes | Used with metallic or plastic surfaces of large pieces of equipment that cannot be disinfected by any other means. May also be used with most plastics **Avoid use** with any item that cannot be immersed or will absorb or be damaged by the alcohol |
| **HIGH LEVEL DISINFECTION: GLUTARALDEHYDE SOLUTIONS** | | | | | | | |
| Alkaline glutaraldehyde (Cidex, Cidex 7, Sporicidin) | Complete immersion for 10 min | Yes | Yes | No | Yes | Yes | Used with rubber and many plastics used in respiratory care, especially those that are heat sensitive. Care must be taken to thoroughly rinse items after disinfection **Avoid use** with any item that cannot be immersed or will absorb the solution |
| Acid glutaraldehyde (Sonacide) | Complete immersion for 20 min | Yes | Yes | No | Yes | Yes | Used with rubber and many plastics used in respiratory care, especially those that are heat sensitive. Care must be taken to thoroughly rinse items after they have been disinfected **Avoid use** with any item that cannot be immersed or will absorb the solution |

*TB*, Tuberculosis.

| TABLE 2-2 Methods of Sterilization | | |
|---|---|---|
| **Method** | **Conditions** | **Comments** |
| Steam autoclave | Autoclave chamber with an internal steam pressure of 15 lb per sq in, 121°C (250°F), 15 min | Used with glass, cloth, bandages, unsharpened stainless steel instruments<br>**Avoid use** with many plastics used in respiratory care, rubber, dextrose solutions, sharpened stainless steel instruments, electrical devices, or machines |
| Dry heat | Autoclave chamber at 160°-180°C (320°-356°F), 2 hr use | Used with glass or sharpened stainless steel instruments<br>**Avoid use** with many plastics used in respiratory care, rubber, dextrose solutions, electric devices, or machines |
| Ethylene oxide gas | Specific guidelines vary depending on the manufacturer of the chamber and the supplies or equipment being sterilized. In general, a gas concentration of 800-1000 mg/L must be kept for 3-4 hr at 50%-100% relative humidity and 49°-57°C (120°-135°F). Great care must be taken to pre-dry all items before gassing and to properly aerate them after sterilization | Used with heat-sensitive and moisture-sensitive items as are many plastics used in respiratory care<br>**Avoid use** with supply pouches or plastic films, such as aluminum foil, nylon, thermoplastic resin (Saran), Mylar, cellophane polyamide, polyester, or other films that are not penetrated by the gas, or with PVC that has been previously sterilized by the manufacturer with gamma radiation |
| **GLUTARALDEHYDE SOLUTIONS** | | |
| Alkaline glutaraldehyde (Cidex, Cidex 7, Sporicidin) | Complete immersion. Cidex products for 10 hr; Sporicidin for 6 hr and 45 min | Used with rubber and many plastics in respiratory care, especially those that are heat sensitive; care must be taken to thoroughly rinse items after they have been cleaned<br>**Avoid use** with any item that cannot be immersed or that will absorb the solution |
| Acid glutaraldehyde (Sonacide) | Complete immersion for 1 hr at 60°C (140°F) | Used with rubber and many plastics used in respiratory care, especially those that are heat sensitive; care must be taken to thoroughly rinse items after they have been cleaned<br>**Avoid use** with any item that cannot be immersed or will absorb the solution |

*PVC*, Polyvinyl chloride.

reusable supplies and patient care equipment that become decontaminated in the hospital.

## 2. Disinfect or sterilize respiratory care equipment (NBRC code: IIB1) [Difficulty: R]

As has been discussed, the choice of whether to disinfect or sterilize equipment depends on how it is used clinically, what type of pathogen is involved, and from what material the equipment is made. Most respiratory pathogens are not spore-formers, so low-level or high-level disinfection is acceptable. Either a glutaraldehyde solution or pasteurization is used in most departments for disinfecting plastic masks, hoses, and so forth.

Any department that processes its own equipment must have adequate facilities. A "dirty" area must exist where contaminated equipment is brought for disassembly, scrubbing of secretions or blood, and rinsing. Equipment is then placed into either the glutaraldehyde solution or a pasteurizing machine. After that, equipment is taken to a "clean" area to be rinsed, dried, reassembled, and placed into plastic bags for storage. Care must be taken not to recontaminate the equipment during this procedure. Items that must be sterilized are usually processed through the "dirty" area before being sent to the central supply department, where the equipment is sterilized based on the criteria defined in Table 2-2.

## 3. Monitor the sterilization process to ensure its effectiveness (NBRC code: IIB1) [Difficulty: R]

The term *surveillance* describes the monitoring of equipment to ensure that the disinfection or sterilization process has been successful and that in-use equipment is not a source of patient contamination. Processing (chemical) indicators are used to ensure that disinfection or sterilization has been done correctly. Examples include special tapes used to hold the wrapping around packages of equipment being autoclaved or placed into ethylene oxide. These tapes change color when the autoclave has reached the proper temperature or the correct concentration of ethylene oxide has been reached. The color change shows the user that the package has been processed correctly; therefore, the package's contents are sterile.

Another example is a biologic indicator placed into the wrapped package before sterilization. These biologic indicators are bacterial spores that are killed only if the required conditions are met. After the equipment and spores have been sent through the sterilization process, the spores are placed into conditions favorable for growth. If no growth occurs, they are dead; therefore, no other living organisms have survived.

Equipment that is held in storage or used in patient care is also randomly sampled for contamination. There are three different ways to take a sample for culturing of possible organisms. The first involves wiping a sterile swab onto an equipment surface, then rubbing it over a plate of growth medium or placing it into a tube of liquid broth. The second is used to check inside lengths of tubing, which necessitates pouring a liquid broth through the tube and into a sterile container. The third involves sampling the aerosol that a nebulizer produces. A hose is usually attached to the outlet of the nebulizer. The other end of the hose is connected to a funnel, which is attached to a culture plate where the droplets impact. In all three examples, the growth of any organism in the growth medium indicates a form of contamination. Laboratory tests then determine whether the organism is pathogenic. If so, measurements must be taken to improve the disinfection or sterilization process.

## MODULE C
### Biohazardous materials

## 1. Make sure that biohazardous materials are properly handled (NBRC code: IIB2) [Difficulty: R]

A respiratory therapist is most likely to come into contact with biohazardous materials in the form of infectious waste, body fluids, or needles and syringes. All must be handled and disposed of properly to keep the practitioner and patient safe. Although hospital policies vary, infectious waste and body fluids are usually placed into a red bag. The bag is removed from the patient care area and is incinerated to ensure that all pathogens are killed.

Needles, syringes, or any sharp objects are placed into a sharps container, which is also red and usually marked with a biohazard symbol. Every patient room should have a sharps container in place so that used needles and syringes can be easily disposed of. If at all possible, the needle should not be recapped after use. Instead, the used needle and syringe should simply be dropped into the slot in the container. Nothing should ever be forced into the container, and fingers should never be pushed into it. When full, the sharps container should be sealed closed and removed for proper disposal.

## BIBLIOGRAPHY

American Association for Respiratory Care: Guidelines for the prevention of nosocomial infections, *AARTimes*, Dallas, September 1983.

American Respiratory Care Foundation: Guidelines for disinfection of respiratory care equipment used in the home, *Resp Care* 33:801, 1988.

Carter C, Stone MK: Respiratory microbiology, infection, and infection control. In Hess DR, MacIntyre NR, et al, editors: *Respiratory care principles & practice*, Philadelphia, 2002, WB Saunders.

Chatburn RL, Kallstrom TJ, Bajaksouzian S: A comparison of acetic acid with a quaternary ammonium compound for disinfection of hand-held nebulizers. *Respir Care* 33(3):179, 1988.

Cidexplus, 28-day solution, Product Insert, Johnson & Johnson Medical, Arlington, Tex.

Eubanks DH, Bone RC: *Comprehensive respiratory care*, ed 2, St Louis, 1990, Mosby.

Fink JB: Infection control and safety. In Fink JB, Hunt GE, editors: *Clinical practice in respiratory care*, Philadelphia, 1999, Lippincott Williams & Wilkins.

*Infection control precautions*, OSF Saint Anthony Medical Center, Rockford, Ill, 1998.

Meyer R, Scanlan CL: Principles of infection control. In Wilkins RL, Stoller JK, Scanlan CL, editors: *Egan's fundamentals of respiratory care*, ed 8, St Louis, 2003, Mosby.

Pagana KD, Pagana TJ: *Mosby's manual of diagnostic and laboratory tests*, St Louis, 1998, Mosby.

Washington JA: Infectious disease aspects of respiratory therapy. In Burton GG, Hodgkin JE, Ward JJ, editors: *Respiratory care*, ed 4, Philadelphia, 1997, Lippincott-Raven.

## SELF-STUDY QUESTIONS

1. Hand washing should be performed
   I. When coming on duty
   II. After obtaining a sputum sample
   III. After using the toilet
   IV. Before eating
   A. I only
   B. III only
   C. II and III only
   D. All of the above

2. You are about to refill a patient's nebulizer for an aerosol mask when you notice that the water bottle is dated as having been opened 2 days ago. You would proceed to
   A. Refill the nebulizer
   B. Throw away the water
   C. Refill the nebulizer but throw away any remaining water
   D. Call your supervisor for advice

3. Which of the following pertains to the care of a patient with droplet precautions?
   I. A private room must be assigned.
   II. Gowns must be worn by all persons who enter the room.
   III. Gowns are not necessary for routine procedures such as checking equipment.
   IV. The patient must wear an isolation mask if he or she is leaving the room.
   V. Masks must be worn by all persons who are in close personal contact with the patient.
   A. I, III, IV, and V only
   B. I, II, and IV only
   C. V only
   D. I and IV only

4. The patient with new, major burns is placed into the following type of isolation:
   A. Airborne precautions
   B. Contact precautions
   C. Droplet precautions
   D. Enteric precautions

5. The respiratory care department often reuses plastic $O_2$ masks and tubing between patients. What is the best way to disinfect them?
   A. Pasteurization
   B. Steam autoclave
   C. Ethylene oxide
   D. Dry heat

6. The best method of sterilizing a contaminated Bird Mark 7 IPPB unit is
   A. 10-hour soak in Cidex 7
   B. Steam autoclave
   C. Ethylene oxide
   D. 20-minute soak in Sonacide

7. You suspect that several large-volume jet nebulizers are the cause of an outbreak of pneumonia in the recovery room. To determine if the in-use nebulizers are contaminated, which method of surveillance would you recommend?
   A. Check if the ethylene oxide tape changed color after the units were sterilized.
   B. Swab the air intake ports on the nebulizers.
   C. Check for bacterial growth in the aerosol droplets from each nebulizer.
   D. Check the Cidex in which they were soaked for contamination.

8. A patient you are caring for has been diagnosed with pulmonary TB. What precautions should you take to prevent infection?
   A. Have a tuberculin skin test performed.
   B. Wear a NIOSH-approved respirator when you care for the patient.
   C. Have the patient wear an isolation mask when you are in his room.
   D. Have the patient wear a NIOSH-approved respirator when you are in his room.

9. Two patients with tracheostomy tubes who are on the same patient floor have been found to have *S. aureus* infection of their tracheostomy sites. What would be the most likely source of the organism?
   A. Infected tracheostomy tubes from the manufacturer
   B. Hand contact from a caregiver
   C. Infected suction catheters from the manufacturer
   D. Infected saline solution or water that was put into the patients' nebulizers

10. An asthmatic patient who is receiving public assistance needs to be able to effectively clean her small-volume medication nebulizer. What would you recommend that she do?
    A. Wash it once a week with a bar of soap.
    B. Rinse it daily with tap water, and dry with a dish towel.
    C. Wash it once a week with her dish soap, and dry with a dish towel.
    D. Soak it in white vinegar after her last treatment each day.

## ANSWER KEY AND RATIONALE

1. **D.** All of the items are indications to wash hands to protect either the patient or the respiratory therapist.
2. **B.** Water bottles should be dated and the unused water thrown away after 24 hr.
3. **A.** A private room is indicated to prevent the spread of infection to a roommate. A gown is not needed because the infection is not spread by contact. A mask on the patient prevents the spread of droplets by coughing. Anyone within 3 ft of the patient must wear a mask to prevent the inhalation of droplets from the patient.
4. **B.** Contact precautions should help to prevent the spread of infection from a caregiver to the patient's burned areas.
5. **A.** Pasteurization is the simplest way to disinfect most plastic items used in respiratory care. The other three methods are used for sterilization of equipment. Many plastic items melt if subjected to the high temperatures that are reached in steam autoclave and dry heat systems.
6. **C.** Ethylene oxide gas is the only method of sterilization that can be used on this piece of equipment without damaging it. Cidex and Sonacide are both liquid solutions that would get into internal components of the unit and could not be removed. The heat of steam autoclaving would melt and destroy the plastic body of the unit.
7. **C.** The best way to find out if the *nebulizers* are the source of contamination is to have aerosol droplets from each one sprayed onto a growth medium, then determine if bacteria grow out. The ethylene oxide and Cidex sterilization procedures may or may not be a problem and could be checked separately for contamination. An uncontaminated air intake port does not prevent the output of contaminated aerosol if the nebulizer is the source.

8. **B.** A NIOSH-approved respirator protects the wearer from inhaling droplet nuclei that may contain TB. Having the patient wear a mask does not protect the caregiver from inhaling suspended droplet nuclei. A TB skin test does not protect against inhalation of suspended droplet nuclei.
9. **B.** The *S. aureus* organism is commonly found on unwashed hands. A caregiver who did not wash properly is the most likely cause of both infections. Separate tracheostomy tubes, suction catheters, or sterile water or saline bottles are unlikely sources of the same infectious organism in two patients.
10. **D.** A white vinegar (acetic acid) soak is the only effective way listed to kill commonly encountered bacteria. A bar of hand soap will help to remove common bacteria from the hands. However, it is not as effective as white vinegar at killing bacteria. Tap water will not effectively kill bacteria. Although washing the equipment with dish soap may be beneficial, it is not going to kill as many bacteria as will be killed by acetic acid.

# 3 Blood Gas Analysis and Monitoring

A review of the most recent Entry Level Examinations shows an average of 10 questions (7% of the exam) that cover blood gas analysis and monitoring. In addition, arterial blood gas results are often included in questions related to oxygen therapy and mechanical ventilation.

## MODULE A

### Make a recommendation to obtain a blood sample for blood gas analysis (NBRC code: IB9) [Difficulty: R, Ap]

Blood can be sampled from a systemic artery, a pulmonary artery, or an "arterialized" capillary for determination of a patient's pressures of oxygen ($O_2$), carbon dioxide ($CO_2$), acid-base status (pH), and related values. A pulmonary artery sample is taken to assess a patient's mixed venous values, and an "arterialized" capillary sample is taken from a neonate when an arterial sample cannot be obtained. The term *arterial blood gas* (ABG) is commonly used when the discussion involves drawing a sample of blood from a patient's systemic artery.

Three broad, general indications for this recommendation follow:
   a. To check a patient's oxygenation status ($PaO_2$)
   b. To check a patient's pH
   c. To check a patient's ventilation status ($PaCO_2$)
Some specific indications follow.

### 1. Cardiac failure
   a. Congenital heart defect
   b. Heart attack (myocardial infarction)
   c. Congestive heart failure with or without pulmonary edema

### 2. Chronic obstructive pulmonary disease (COPD)
   a. Asthma
   b. Emphysema
   c. Bronchitis
   d. Bronchiectasis
   e. Cystic fibrosis

### 3. Pneumonia that causes hypoxemia
### 4. Trauma
   a. Broken ribs
   b. Flail chest
   c. Pneumothorax
   d. Hemothorax
   e. Upper airway trauma

### 5. Ventilatory failure
   a. Overdosage of sedatives or pain relievers
   b. Stroke or head (brain) injury
   c. Spinal cord injury
   d. Neuromuscular diseases, such as myasthenia gravis or Guillain-Barré syndrome

### 6. Airway obstruction
   a. Foreign body aspiration
   b. Laryngotracheobronchitis (croup)
   c. Epiglottitis

### 7. Miscellaneous
   a. Smoke inhalation
   b. Carbon monoxide (CO) poisoning
   c. Near-drowning
   d. Infant respiratory distress syndrome/hyaline membrane disease
   e. Acute respiratory distress syndrome (ARDS)
   f. No indwelling arterial line in the patient
   g. A shunt percentage calculation or alveolar-arterial $O_2$ pressure difference [$P(A - a)O_2$] calculation must be made
   h. Cardiopulmonary resuscitation

> ### Exam Hint
>
> **E**xpect at least one question in which the respiratory therapist is expected to recommend that either an arterial blood gas sample or a pulse oximeter reading be performed.

## MODULE B
### Obtain an arterial blood gas sample

### 1. Perform quality control procedures for a blood gas sampling device (NBRC code: IIC1) [Difficulty: R, Ap]

A properly assembled sampling device should not create problems with obtaining the blood sample. Following are quality control (QC) procedures for an arterial sampling device and steps that can be taken to correct a problem.

#### a. Properly assemble the blood gas syringe and needle

To assemble a blood gas syringe, use sterile technique to screw the selected needle onto the syringe. Add heparin (if the syringe does not already contain it) by aspirating liquid heparin through the needle into the syringe. Coat the inside of the syringe with liquid heparin by tipping the needle up, pulling the plunger back, and pushing the plunger forward to squirt the excess heparin out the needle. This ensures that the needle and dead space of the needle are filled with heparin and that the inside of the syringe is coated.

The plunger should easily slide within the barrel of the syringe; a blood clot or debris within the needle would plug it and prevent this. Replace and safely dispose of an obstructed needle, or get a new syringe and needle. The needle should have an automatic capping device to reduce the chance of an accidental puncture of the therapist.

#### b. Make sure no air bubbles are in the syringe

An air bubble results in a mixing of room air gas conditions with the patient's arterial blood gas conditions. This usually results in an $O_2$ reading that is too high, a $CO_2$ level that is too low, and a pH that is too high. If an air bubble is found within the syringe, tilt it so that the needle is up. The bubble rises by itself or may be raised by tapping of the syringe. Push the plunger into the syringe to eject the air bubble. Cap off the hub of the syringe or needle to prevent air from entering the syringe.

#### c. Use the proper amount of heparin

This is a matter of concern only when liquid heparin is added to a needle and syringe. Aspirate about 1 mL of 10 mg/mL or 1000 units/mL sodium heparin through the needle into the syringe. Pull the plunger back to coat the inside of the syringe. Push the plunger forward to squirt the excess heparin out through the needle. A 2- to 4-mL blood sample should not be affected by this concentration. Remember that inadequate heparin could result in clotting of the blood sample. Excessive heparin can alter the blood gas values by lowering the pH and $CO_2$ levels and raising the $O_2$ level.

#### d. Promptly cool down the blood gas sample

If the sample cannot be analyzed within 10 min of the time it is drawn, it should be placed into an ice water bath. Failure to do so causes the living blood to consume the available $O_2$ and produce $CO_2$. This obviously results in incorrectly measured values.

### 2. Obtain a blood sample from an arterial line (NBRC code: IB7e, IIIE2b) [Difficulty: R, Ap]

The steps that are commonly followed when an arterial blood sample is obtained include the following:

a. Tell a conscious patient that you are going to take a blood sample from the arterial catheter.
b. Put gloves on both hands.
c. Remove the dead-ender cap from the sample (side) port on the three-way stopcock between the catheter and the IV tubing.
d. Screw a sterile 5- to 10-mL syringe to the sample port for removal of the IV solution from the catheter (use a smaller syringe with a neonate).
e. Turn off the stopcock to the IV tubing (Fig. 3-1).
f. Pull a waste sample of IV solution and blood into the syringe; the amount to be withdrawn and discarded depends on the dead space volume from the tip of the catheter to the side port. (Studies indicate that between 2.5 and 6 times this volume should be removed—typically 5 mL in an adult and less in a neonate.)
g. Turn off the stopcock to all ports by turning it halfway between any two.
h. Attach a preheparinized sterile syringe to the sample port, turn the stopcock open to the syringe, and withdraw about 2 to 3 mL of arterial blood for analysis.
i. Turn off the stopcock to all ports by turning it halfway between any two.
j. Remove the blood sample syringe, and cap off the syringe to seal it.
k. Place the blood sample into an ice water bath.
l. Turn the stopcock toward the catheter; fast-flush the IV solution so that any blood left in the sample port is forced out onto a sterile gauze pad.
m. Turn the stopcock toward the sample port so the IV solution runs into the catheter.
n. Fast-flush any blood in the catheter back into the patient.
o. Screw the dead-ender cap onto the sample port.
p. Remove gloves, and properly dispose of them and any waste materials.

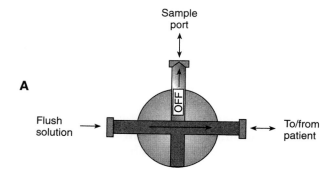

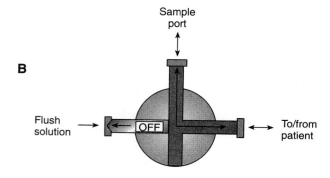

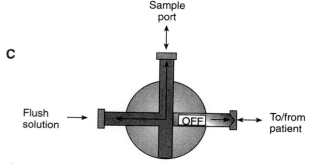

**Fig. 3-1** A three-way stopcock for use in an arterial line system. **A,** Normal operating position of the stopcock that allows fluid to flow to the patient (and the blood pressure to be monitored if assembled for continuous blood pressure monitoring). **B,** Stopcock position that allows blood to be withdrawn from the patient through the sample port. The flush solution port is closed. **C,** Stopcock position for flush solution to go to the sample port to clear out any blood. When the stopcock is turned to a 45-degree angle between any two ports, all of the ports are closed. *(From Scanlan CL: Analysis and monitoring of gas exchange. In Scanlan CL, Wilkins RL, Stoller JK, editors: Egan's fundamentals of respiratory care, ed 7, St Louis, 1999, Mosby.)*

## 3. Perform an arterial puncture to obtain a blood sample for analysis
### (NBRC code: IB7e, IIIE2a) [Difficulty: R, Ap]

A number of possible variations exist in an arterial puncture. A general but thorough list of the steps and important related information follow.

a. Check for a valid physician order.
b. Check the patient's chart for pertinent information on supplemental $O_2$ that is being used, bleeding disorders such as hemophilia, and the use of anticoagulant medications. The patient's clotting time must be checked because a hematoma results if extra time is not spent holding the puncture site. If a change in the patient's supplemental $O_2$ level has occurred, make sure that the change was made at least 15 min before the arterial blood sample was drawn.
c. Collect necessary equipment.
  1. Ice water in a cup
  2. A 3-mL glass or plastic syringe
  3. Appropriate short-bevel needle(s) [23- to 24-gauge for radial or dorsalis pedis puncture and 22-gauge for brachial or femoral puncture]
  4. Heparin, if needed
  5. Some 70% isopropyl alcohol or iodophor swabs to clean the puncture site and a sterile 4 × 4 gauze pad to be held over the puncture site to aid in clotting
  6. A seal for the needle or syringe to prevent room air contamination
  7. Clean gloves to protect both of the practitioner's hands from any contact with spilled blood
  8. Eye goggles
d. Introduce yourself and your department to the patient; identify the patient, explain what you will do, and gain the patient's confidence to ensure full cooperation.
e. Select the puncture site. The choices, presented in sequence from most to least favorable, are radial, brachial, dorsalis pedis, and femoral. (If the radial site is selected, try to puncture the left wrist if the patient is right-handed or vice versa.)
f. If a radial or pedal site is selected, the modified Allen test must be performed to ensure adequate collateral flow, in case the artery should become clotted because of the procedure.
  1. Radial artery site: Fig. 3-2 shows the basic procedure. Circulation to the hand is stopped by pressing closed both the radial and ulnar arteries. Release of pressure over the ulnar artery should result in hand flushing within 10 to 15 sec. This is a positive test result and proves that the ulnar artery has adequate circulation to the hand. If the hand does not flush within 15 sec of release of the ulnar artery, the circulation is inadequate and the radial artery of that wrist must *not* be punctured. Another site must be evaluated for puncture.
  2. Dorsalis pedis artery site: Press down on the dorsalis pedis artery to occlude it. Press on the nail of the great toe so that it blanches. Release the pressure on the nail, and watch for a rapid return

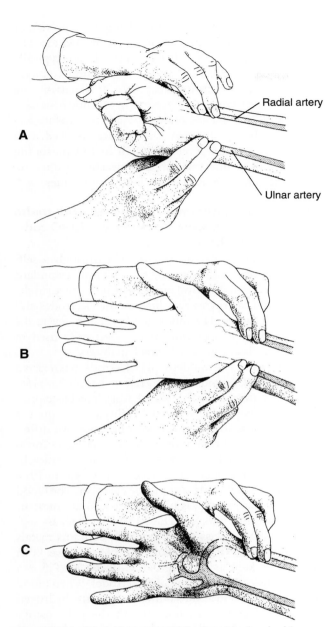

**Fig. 3-2** Modified Allen test. **A,** The hand is clenched into a tight fist, and pressure is applied to the radial and ulnar arteries. **B,** The hand is opened (but not fully extended); the palm and fingers are blanched. **C,** Removal of pressure on the ulnar artery should result in flushing of the entire hand. *(From Shapiro BA, Peruzzi WT, Kozelowski-Templin R: Clinical application of blood gases, ed 5, St Louis, 1994, Mosby.)*

of color. This positive test finding confirms good blood flow through the posterior tibial and lateral plantar arteries. Drawing a sample from the site is safe. A slow return of blood flow indicates poor circulation; another site must be chosen.

g. Prepare the equipment and the puncture site by using sterile technique.
   1. If necessary, draw up the heparin solution, flush the syringe with it, and discard the excess.
   2. If a radial or brachial site is selected, the joint should be hyperextended with a folded towel to help stabilize it.
   3. Clean the site by wiping the area with an alcohol or iodophor swab in a widening spiral motion that starts at the desired puncture site.
   4. Put on gloves and goggles.
   5. Some prefer to anesthetize the puncture site with a 0.8- to 1.0-mL injection of 2% lidocaine (Xylocaine) into the skin; others believe that this is unnecessary because the injection itself causes pain.

h. Draw the blood sample.
   1. Hold the syringe like a pencil. The radial and dorsalis pedis arteries should be entered at a 45-degree angle; the brachial and femoral arteries should be entered at a 90-degree angle (Fig. 3-3). Use the first two fingers of your free hand to palpate the pulse and hold the artery still. The bevel of the needle should be up as it enters the skin.
   2. Tell the patient that he or she will "feel a stick."
   3. The needle should enter the skin quickly to minimize pain. Carefully advance the needle into the artery. A pulsatile flow is seen with each heartbeat. If unsuccessful, withdraw the needle to the skin, change the angle as needed, and reinsert into the artery.
   4. Withdraw about 1 to 2 mL of blood before you remove the needle.
   5. Press the sterile gauze onto the puncture site for 2 to 5 min. Check the site to ensure that clotting has occurred, and hold longer if needed. An assistant may help with this.
   6. While you are holding the site, seal the syringe or carefully cover the needle.
   7. Roll the syringe to mix the heparin, and place the syringe into the ice water. (Failure to put the blood sample into ice water results in a decrease in the $PaO_2$ and pH values and an increase in the $PaCO_2$ value.)
   8. Label the syringe with the date, time, patient's name, $O_2$ percentage, and, if abnormal, the patient's temperature. Some departments may also add the patient's age and position when the sample was drawn because of the effects that these may have on oxygenation.
   9. Have the sample analyzed as soon as possible.
   10. Properly dispose of gloves and waste materials before you wash your hands.

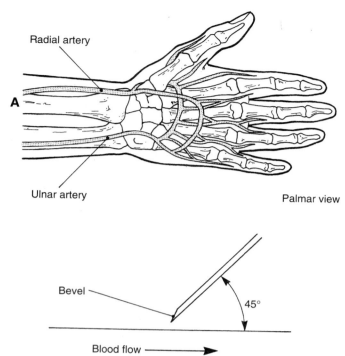

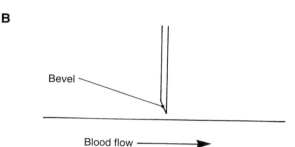

**Fig. 3-3 A,** Radial arterial position in the lower arm and wrist. **B,** Bevel and needle positioning for radial arterial puncture *(top)* and other arterial punctures *(bottom)*. *(From Lane EE, Walker JF: Clinical arterial blood gas analysis, St Louis, 1987, Mosby.)*

### Exam Hint

**C**ommonly tested areas involve the ABG technique and possible hazards to it. Patient hazards include blood vessel trauma, hematoma, arterial clot formation, arteriospasm, and infected puncture site. In addition, the therapist may receive a needle puncture injury.

## MODULE C
### Analyze blood gas values

## 1. Point-of-care blood gas analyzer
### a. Select the appropriate point-of-care blood gas analyzer (NBRC code: IIA10) [Difficulty: R, Ap]

A point-of-care (POC) blood gas analyzer can be used as an alternative to a centrally located analyzer. This is especially helpful when a patient is being transported, or when the data are very quickly needed at the bedside. The blood gas values of $PaO_2$, $PaCO_2$, and pH are typically obtained from either a POC analyzer or a standard blood gas analyzer. These units are acceptable for all patient care situations *except* when CO poisoning is known or suspected. Neither blood gas analyzer is able to measure carboxyhemoglobin (COHb). A CO-oximeter is needed to measure the patient's level of COHb in CO poisoning cases. Some POC analyzers can also measure serum electrolytes and other commonly needed patient values.

### b. Put the equipment together and make sure that it works properly (NBRC code: IIA10) [Difficulty: R, Ap]

Point-of-care analyzers can be powered through a self-contained battery or by plugging the unit into a standard alternating current electrical outlet. The units have single-use disposable cartridges that include the electrodes and calibration reagents. The following discussion covers the basic principles of operation of the electrodes used in POC and standard centrally located analyzers.

*pH Electrode.* The modern pH electrode has existed since the mid-1950s and is usually referred as the *Sanz electrode* (named after its principal inventor). The basic principle behind the pH analyzer is its ability to measure the voltage (potential for electrical flow) between two different solutions. The different hydrogen ion ($H^+$) concentrations between the solutions reflect their relative pH levels. The reference electrode is immersed in a solution with a pH of 6.840 that fills a glass or plastic chamber. The blood sample, of unknown pH, is placed in a separate measuring chamber called a *cuvette*. These two chambers are separated by a special glass membrane that contains metals and sodium ions ($Na^+$), thus making it pH sensitive. Both chambers are kept at a stable 37° C (98.6° F) (Fig. 3-4 shows a representation of the pH electrode). When blood or a QC material is introduced into the cuvette, hydrogen ions may replace the sodium ions in the pH-sensitive glass if the two pH levels are different. The replacement is proportionate to the difference between the two pH levels.

*$PCO_2$ Electrode.* The $CO_2$-pressure ($PCO_2$) electrode is a modified pH electrode that was first designed in the mid-1950s by Stowe, then further perfected by Severinghaus. Accordingly, these units are now referred to as *Severinghaus*, or sometimes *Stowe-Severinghaus*, *electrodes*. Fig. 3-5 depicts the electrode in cross section with a reference half-cell and a measuring half-cell enclosed within pH-sensitive glass and electrically connected by an electrolyte contact bridge. The blood sample is introduced into a cuvette that is heated to 37° C. The principle of operation is based on the amount of $CO_2$ found in the blood sample that diffuses through the silicon elastic membrane. The $CO_2$ chemically combines with the bicarbonate solution to change the pH of the solution by the release of $H^+$. This

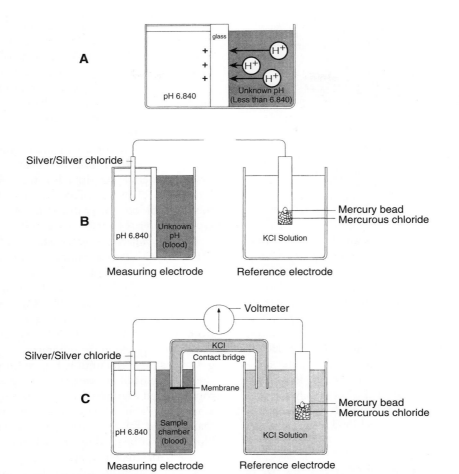

**Fig. 3-4** Key components of the pH electrode. **A,** A voltage develops across the pH-sensitive glass when a difference exists in the hydrogen ion concentration between the two solutions. **B,** Two separate half-cells are used for the measuring electrode and the reference electrode. **C,** The addition of a KCl contact bridge and voltmeter completes the electrical circuit and enables measurement of the pH of the patient's blood sample. *(From Shapiro BA, Harrison RA, Cane RD, Kozelowski-Templin R: Clinical application of blood gases, ed 4, Chicago, 1989, Mosby.)*

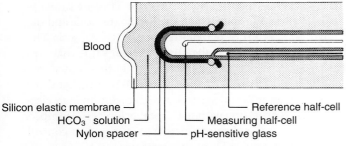

**Fig. 3-5** Schematic illustration of the modern $PCO_2$ electrode. Note that the space between the silicon membrane and the nylon spacer is greatly enlarged for clarity. *(From Shapiro BA, Harrison RA, Cane RD, Kozelowski-Templin R: Clinical application of blood gases, ed 4, Chicago, 1989, Mosby.)*

$H^+$ change creates a voltage difference between the measuring and reference half-cells that is proportionate to the amount of $CO_2$ found in the patient's blood sample.

***$PO_2$ Electrode.*** This unit is completely different from the others mentioned and was developed in the late 1950s by Clark; thus, it is usually called a *Clark electrode.* It is also sometimes known as a *polarographic electrode* because of the basis of its operation. Fig. 3-6 shows key features of the unit. A phosphate-KCl buffer solution surrounds the silver anode. A thin membrane separates the blood-filled cuvette from direct contact with the electrode but allows $O_2$ molecules to slowly diffuse through to contact the platinum wire cathode. The whole unit is heated to 37° C. The term *polarographic* comes from the addition of about −0.7 volts to the cathode to make it slightly "polarized" or negative compared with the anode. This addition ensures that $O_2$ is chemically reduced (gains electrons)

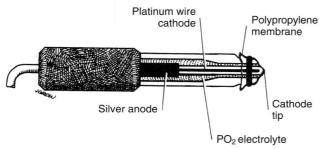

**Fig. 3-6** Schematic illustration of the Clark electrode for measuring $PO_2$. *(From Shapiro BA, Harrison RA, Cane RD, Kozelowski-Templin R: Clinical application of blood gases, ed 4, Chicago, 1989, Mosby.)*

rapidly at the cathode. This creates an electrical current that is directly proportionate to the number of reduced $O_2$ molecules.

The $O_2$ pressure ($PO_2$) that must be measured is derived from $O_2$ dissolved in the plasma and not from the hemoglobin found in the erythrocytes (red blood cells). The reported value for the saturation of $O_2$ in the hemoglobin ($SaO_2$) is calculated using a mathematical table. Under normal conditions, the calculated $SaO_2$ value is the same as or close to the true $SaO_2$ value. CO poisoning is the only commonly seen clinical situation during which a calculated saturation can be incorrectly high. If CO poisoning is suspected or known, the patient's blood sample should be analyzed on a CO-oximeter unit.

### c. Perform quality control procedures for a blood gas analyzer (NBRC code: IIC1) [Difficulty: R, Ap]

*Quality control.* Quality control refers to the creation and application of a measurement and documentation system to confirm the accuracy (precision) and reliability of all blood gas measurements. *Accuracy* or *precision* means that the measured physiologic values truly reflect the actual physiologic values. *Reliability* means that a high degree of confidence exists that the accuracy of the measured values represents the patient's actual physiologic values. Both are critically important if the blood gas results are to be used to make correct clinical decisions.

*Quality assurance.* Quality assurance refers to the broader concern that the results of the blood gas measurement are not only accurate and reliable but also clinically useful. To help ensure this, the Clinical Laboratory Improvement Amendments of 1988 (CLIA '88) require that the department must have written policies and procedures on items such as record keeping, equipment maintenance, staff training, and error correction. If a hospital has two blood gas analyzers, it is common practice for a patient's blood sample to be run through both. If the patient values match, additional assurance that they are correct is provided. If significant variance occurs, then both units must be checked for proper calibration accuracy.

*Calibration.* Calibration, the systematic standardization of the graduations of the blood gas analyzer against known values, is done to ensure consistency. Proper calibration of the electrodes is essential for accuracy of blood gas values. Some general calibration steps are discussed later. The manufacturer's guidelines must be followed for each specific step in calibration.

*Quality control materials.* A variety of QC reagent materials are available for use in calibrating the electrodes for $PO_2$, $PCO_2$, and pH. Their uses vary, and each of the following materials has its advantages, disadvantages, and limitations. The manufacturer of a particular brand or model of blood gas analyzer may require that a specific type of material be used in its units.

*Aqueous buffers* are water based and are used to check pH and $PCO_2$ measurements; they cannot be used to check $PO_2$ measurements. Commercially prepared *gases* are used to check $PO_2$ and $PCO_2$ measurements; they cannot be used to check pH. $CO_2$ mixes of 0%, 5%, 10%, and 12% may be used; $O_2$ mixes of 0%, 12%, 20%, 20.95% from room air, 21%, and 100% may be used. *Tonometered liquids* are exposed in the laboratory to known $O_2$ and $CO_2$ gas mixes until the liquids have been saturated and have the same partial pressures as the gases. Three types of tonometered liquids exist. First, *human* or *animal serum* or *whole blood* is the most accurate method available and is mainly used for $PO_2$ and $PCO_2$. Whereas whole human blood cannot be used for pH, a bovine blood product can be used for all three values. Second, *assayed liquids* are non–water-based liquids that have been pretonometered by the manufacturer and are available in sealed glass vials. They can be used for assessment of $PO_2$, $PCO_2$, and pH; they are very popular because of their speed and simplicity. Third, *oxygenated fluorocarbon–based emulsions* (prefluorinated compounds) can be used for $PO_2$, $PCO_2$, and pH measurement and are considered to be as accurate as whole blood without its associated risks.

*Levey-Jennings charts.* Levey-Jennings charts (also known as *Shewhart/Levey-Jennings* or *QC charts*) are used to record the results of each calibration procedure. They are similarly designed, with time plotted on the horizontal scale and the analyte ($PO_2$, $PCO_2$, or pH) plotted on the vertical scale. The vertical scale for each analyte has a central value that represents what is normally expected. On both sides of this normal value are standard deviation (SD) points that show movement away from what is expected. An analyte electrode that is operating within acceptable limits is described as *in control*. An analyte is generally considered in control when it lies within 2 SDs of the normal value.

An *out-of-control* situation exists when a single calibration value or series of calibration values are outside of established limits. A *random error* is an unpredictable aberration in precision that occurs when the QC material is sampled. A *systematic error* shows an accuracy problem and is much more serious. It must be investigated, corrected,

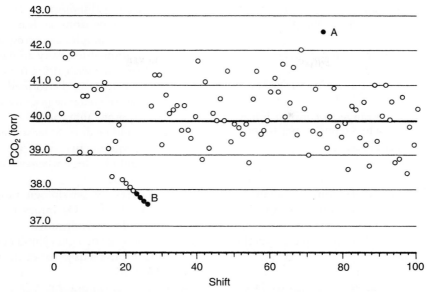

**Fig. 3-7** Levey-Jennings quality control chart for PaCO$_2$. The central horizontal line represents the mean value of 40 torr. The next lower and higher horizontal lines show 1 standard deviation (1 SD) value from the mean. The second most distant lower and higher horizontal lines show 2 SD values from the mean. The most distant horizontal lines show 3 SD values from the mean. The bottom number scale represents 8-hr work shifts. Open circles represent calibration values within 2 SDs of the mean, which are considered in control. Black circles represent out-of-control calibration values. *A* represents a random error; *B* represents a systematic error. *(From Shapiro BA, Peruzzi WT, Kozelowski-Templin R: Clinical application of blood gases, ed 5, St Louis, 1994, Mosby.)*

and documented. Fig. 3-7 shows an example of both a random error and a systematic error. Rules have been established for determining whether the error is random or systematic (Table 3-1).

***pH Electrode.*** Note: These and the following guidelines are based on CLIA standards or widely reported industry standards. The various brands and models of blood gas analyzers may have different frequencies of calibration requirements, depending on their US Food and Drug Administration–approved manufacturers' studies.

a. One-point calibration
  1. Should be done before every sample is analyzed if one-point calibration is not automatically performed every 30 min
  2. Performed with the near-normal QC material of 7.384 ± 0.005 pH used to set the balance potentiometer
  3. Recommended every 30 min
  4. Should be rechecked after a suspicious pH result; the blood sample should then be rerun
b. Two-point calibration
  1. Should be done at least once every 8 hr when patient samples are being analyzed
  2. Recommended every 25 patient samples
  3. Performed with the slope potentiometer set with a QC material of 6.840 ± 0.005 pH (same pH as the reference electrode solution)

| TABLE 3-1 | Westgard's Rules for Determining When an Analyzer Is Not Functioning Properly |
|---|---|
| **Rule name** | **Levey-Jennings chart** |
| **RANDOM ERROR** | |
| 1–2 SDs | Measurement is more than 2 SDs but not more than 3 SDs from the mean |
| 1–3 SDs | Measurement is more than 3 SDs from the mean |
| R*–4 SDs | Two consecutive measurements are 4 or more SDs apart |
| **SYSTEMATIC ERROR** | |
| 2–2 SDs | Two consecutive measurements are either 2 SDs above or 2 SDs below the mean |
| 4–1 SDs | Four consecutive measurements are either 1 SD above or 1 SD below the mean |
| 7-trend | Seven consecutive measurements are on only one side of the mean; each measurement is progressively farther out of control |
| 10-mean | Ten consecutive measurements are on only one side of the mean |

Modified from Lane EE, Walker JF: *Clinical arterial blood gas analysis,* St Louis, 1987, Mosby.
*= Repeat.
SDs, Standard deviations.

4. Performed with the balance potentiometer set with a QC material of $7.384 \pm 0.005$ pH
  c. Three-point calibration
    1. Should be done at least every 6 months on existing equipment
    2. Should be done whenever a new electrode is put into use
    3. Covers the physiologic range to confirm linearity: QC materials of $6.840 \pm 0.005$, $7.384 \pm 0.005$, and $7.874 \pm 0.005$ pH are used

***$PCO_2$ electrode***
a. One-point calibration
  1. Should be done before every sample is analyzed if one-point calibration is not automatically performed every 30 min
  2. Performed with $5\% \pm 0.03\%$ $CO_2$ used to set the balance potentiometer
  3. Recommended every 30 min
  4. Should be rechecked after a suspicious $PCO_2$ result; the blood sample should then be rerun

The $CO_2$ can be directly in contact with the electrode, tonometered with an aqueous material or blood, or premixed in aqueous buffers, assayed liquids, or fluorocarbon-based emulsion.

---

**Exam Hint**

**T**he solving of the following equation has been tested on past exams. Remember that more than one $CO_2$ percentage can be used. Note that the atmospheric pressure of a gas may be listed by the equivalent terms of *torr* or *mm Hg*. For example, a $PaO_2$ of 95 mm Hg is the same as a $PaO_2$ of 95 torr. However, it is important to note that on the NBRC exams, the term *torr* is used.

The predicted $PCO_2$ value at a given $CO_2$ percentage is calculated with this formula:

$$PCO_2 = (P_B - PH_2O) \times \% \, CO_2$$

$PCO_2$ = Predicted $PCO_2$ in torr
$P_B$ = Barometric pressure at the institution where the analysis is being performed
$PH_2O$ = Water vapor pressure based on the patient's temperature; 47 torr at 37° C (98.6° F)
$\% \, CO_2$ = Percentage of $CO_2$ (also listed as $FCO_2$)
Example for *one-point* (balance) potentiometer calibration at sea level where:
$P_B$ = 760 torr
$PH_2O$ = 47 torr
$\% \, CO_2$ = 5%
  1. $PCO_2 = (760 - 47) \times 0.05$
  2. $PCO_2 = 713 \times 0.05$
  3. $PCO_2 = 35.65$ or 36 torr
Therefore, set the $PCO_2$ control at 36 torr.

---

b. Two-point calibration
  1. Should be done at least once every 8 hr when patient samples are being analyzed
  2. Recommended every 25 patient samples
  3. Performed with $10\% \pm 0.03\%$ $CO_2$ to set the slope potentiometer. Performed with $5\% \pm 0.03\%$ $CO_2$ to set the balance potentiometer
c. Three-point calibration
  1. Should be done at least every 6 months on existing equipment
  2. Should be done whenever a new electrode is put into use
  3. Covers the physiologic range to confirm linearity; three $PCO_2$ values between 0 and 80 torr should be determined
  4. Room air or a gas cylinder containing $0\% + 0.03\%$ $CO_2$ can be used to set the 0 point

***$PO_2$ Electrode***
a. One-point calibration
  1. Should be done before every sample is analyzed if one-point calibration is not automatically performed every 30 min
  2. Performed with $12\% \pm 0.03\%$ $O_2$ used to set the balance potentiometer; some analyzers are designed to use $20\% \pm 0.03\%$ $O_2$ from a gas cylinder or to draw room air ($20.95\%$ $O_2$) into the unit
  3. Recommended every 30 min
  4. Should be rechecked after a suspicious $PO_2$ result; the blood sample should then be rerun

The $O_2$ can be directly in contact with the electrode, tonometered with an aqueous material or blood, or premixed in aqueous buffers, assayed liquids, or fluorocarbon-based emulsion.

---

**Exam Hint**

**T**he solving of the following equation has been tested on past exams. Remember that more than one $O_2$ percentage can be used.

The predicted $PO_2$ value at a given $O_2$ percentage is calculated with this formula:

$$PO_2 = (P_B - PH_2O) \times \% \, O_2$$

$PO_2$ = Predicted $PO_2$ in torr
$P_B$ = Barometric pressure at the institution where the analysis is being performed
$PH_2O$ = Water vapor pressure based on the patient's temperature; 47 torr at 37° C (98.6° F)
$\% \, O_2$ = Percentage of $O_2$ (also listed as $FO_2$)

Example for *one-point* (balance) potentiometer calibration at sea level where:

$PO_2$ = Predicted $PO_2$ in torr

$P_B$ = 760 torr

$PH_2O$ = 47 torr

% $O_2$ = 12%

1. $PO_2 = (760 - 47) \times 0.12$
2. $PO_2 = (713) \times 0.12$
3. $PO_2 = 85.56$ or 86 torr

Therefore, set the $PO_2$ control at 86 torr.

b. Two-point calibration
   1. Should be done at least once every 8 hr when patient samples are being analyzed
   2. Should be done whenever readjustment of one-point calibration is greater than 3 torr
   3. Recommended every 25 patient samples
   4. Performed with 0% + 0.03% $O_2$ to set the slope potentiometer
   5. Performed with 12% ± 0.03% $O_2$ to set the balance potentiometer; some analyzers are designed to use 20% ± 0.03% $O_2$ from a gas cylinder or to draw room air (20.95% $O_2$) into the unit
c. Three-point calibration
   1. Should be done at least every 6 months on existing equipment
   2. Should be done whenever a new electrode is put into use. Should be done to confirm linearity whenever the $PO_2$ value could be over 150 torr, assuming that the balance point is set on room $O_2$ content; the third point should be set on 100% + 0.03% $O_2$ from a gas cylinder

*Miscellaneous topics*

a. Calibration gas cylinders. For economic reasons, the low-percentage $O_2$ and $CO_2$ gases are placed together into one cylinder, and the high-percentage $O_2$ and $CO_2$ gases are placed together into a second cylinder. Box 3-1 summarizes the normal precision of the electrodes discussed and the gases used in their calibration. A cylinder that contains 100% $O_2$ and 0% $CO_2$ could be used for three-point calibration.
b. Temperature correction. Temperature correction refers to mathematical adjustment of a patient's $PaO_2$, $PaCO_2$, and pH values if his or her temperature is not 37° C. As has previously been discussed, blood gas analyzers are calibrated at 37° C (normal body temperature). If the patient has a fever, the $O_2$ and $CO_2$ partial pressures in the blood ($PO_2$ and $PCO_2$, respectively) will be greater than those found during the blood gas analysis. Conversely, the hypothermic patient will have lower $O_2$ and $CO_2$ partial pressures in the blood than those found during the blood gas analysis. The pH value will shift in the opposite direction of the $PCO_2$ value. This small shift in values is usually ignored.

---

**BOX 3-1   Electrode Precision and Calibration Gases**

**ELECTRODES**

pH ±0.01 unit

$PCO_2$ ±2% (approximately ±1 mm Hg at 40 torr)

$PO_2$ ±2% (approximately ±1.5 mm Hg at 80 torr)

If the $PO_2$ is higher than 150 torr, the precision is approximately ±5%–10%, unless three-point calibration is performed

**CALIBRATION GASES**

"Low" gas: 0% $O_2$ (+0.03%), 5% $CO_2$ (±0.03%), balance $N_2$

"High" gas: 12% or 21% $O_2$, 10% $CO_2$ (both ±0.03%), balance $N_2$

Suggested three-point gases: 100% $O_2$ (−0.03%), 0% $CO_2$ (+0.03%)

---

$N_2$, Nitrogen; $PCO_2$, pressure of carbon dioxide; $PO_2$, pressure of oxygen.

However, because some physicians may specify that their patients' blood gases should be temperature corrected, the patient's temperature should be listed on the blood gas slip. A simple mathematical process can temperature-correct the blood gas results. Most modern analyzers perform it automatically when they have been programmed to do so.

d. **Troubleshoot any problems with the point-of-care blood gas analyzer (NBRC code: IIA10) [Difficulty: R, Ap]**

Remember to flush the electrode membrane after each use, if possible, to prevent protein buildup. If such buildup occurs, the response time is longer than normal. Follow the manufacturer's guidelines to change an electrode membrane as needed. Make sure no air bubbles are under the membrane or within the tubing through which the blood travels. Rerun the calibration for any of the electrodes, and reanalyze the sample if the result is suspicious. The electrode should not be used if it does not calibrate close to the reference buffer solutions or gases.

With a *random error* situation, the practitioner likely made a simple error when introducing the material or running the analyzer. Common problems include an air bubble injected into the unit and incomplete flushing of the previous sample. Usually, the problem can be corrected by flushing out any residual blood, then carefully injecting more of the current patient blood sample. Run the analyzer again to get new patient values. The same patient sample can also be run through another analyzer to compare the two sets of results for closeness.

A *systematic error* usually indicates a problem with the analyzer or QC materials or processes. Examples of systematic errors include misanalyzed $CO_2$ or $O_2$ standards for calibration, contaminated QC materials, and deteriorated $O_2$, $CO_2$, or pH electrode function. Each of these must be investigated until the problem is found and corrected. The unit cannot be used again until it is proven to work properly and give accurate results.

### e. Perform blood gas analysis (NBRC code: IB7f, IIIE3b) [Difficulty: R, Ap]

Modern blood gas analyzers are simple to operate. Follow the manufacturer's guidelines on inserting the blood sample. Perform the specified steps in analysis, and print the results. Many units run self-diagnoses if any problems exist.

## 2. CO-oximeter

### a. Perform quality control procedures on the CO-oximeter (NBRC code: IIC1) [Difficulty: R, Ap]

A CO-oximeter would come preassembled by the manufacturer. Practical experience with a unit is recommended so the clinician can gain an understanding of how to add a patient blood sample and perform calibration duties (Fig. 3-8 shows a schematic drawing of a CO-oximeter). A thallium-neon hollow cathode lamp emits light in the infrared-visible range. A device called a *monochromator* contains four filters and rotates through the light beam. Each filter allows only one specific wavelength to pass through it. These four monochromatic wavelengths

correspond to 626.6 nm and to the three isosbestic points shown in Fig. 3-9. This last wavelength, which is poorly absorbed by all four hemoglobin moieties, is used to find the maximal difference in absorption so that the relative amounts of the hemoglobin species can be determined. When a blood sample is placed into the cuvette, the same four wavelengths are passed through it. The amount of absorbance at each wavelength is measured and compared with the absorbance at each wavelength by a reference sample solution (see the next section). The computer integrates the data and calculates the total hemoglobin (THb) and amounts of the four hemoglobin moieties.

THb should be calibrated when the unit is installed, at regular intervals suggested by the manufacturer, after the sample tubing is changed, after the cuvette is disassembled or changed, and when a suspicious reading occurs. This procedure involves filling the cuvette with a special dye produced by the manufacturer, then analyzing it by following the prescribed steps.

Routine calibration is done every 30 min. The unit obtains and stores absorbance readings at the four different wavelengths from a "blank" solution in the reference detector. When the same "blank" solution is added to the sample cuvette, the same four wavelengths are measured. The absorption levels are normally identical. The same procedure is done after every patient sample is analyzed.

The following examples describe common problems with a CO-oximeter and their solutions:

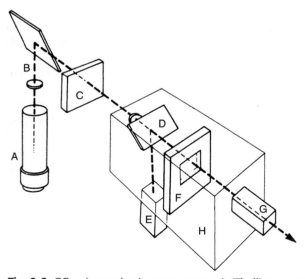

**Fig. 3-8** CO-oximeter basic components. **A,** Thallium-neon hollow cathode light source; **B,** lens and mirror; **C,** monochromator with four specific wavelength filters; **D,** light beam splitter that diverts half of the light to the reference wavelength detector and half to the cuvette; **E,** reference detector; **F,** patient sample cuvette; **G,** sample wavelength detector; and **H,** temperature-regulated block set at 37° C. *(From Shapiro BA, Peruzzi WT, Kozelowski-Templin R: Clinical application of blood gases, ed 5, St Louis, 1994, Mosby.)*

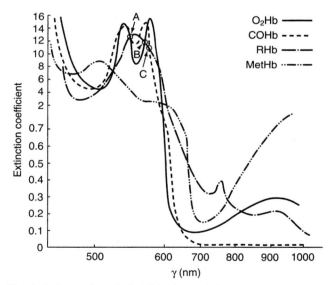

**Fig. 3-9** Spectral analysis of the hemoglobin moieties (species). **A,** The triple isosbestic point at 548 nm for $O_2Hb$, COHb, and RHb. **B,** The double isosbestic point at 568 nm for $O_2Hb$ and RHb. **C,** The double isosbestic point at 578 nm for RHb and COHb. A fourth wavelength at 626.6 nm is used for comparison purposes. $O_2Hb$, Oxyhemoglobin; COHb, carboxyhemoglobin; RHb, reduced hemoglobin; MetHb, methemoglobin. *(From Shapiro BA, Peruzzi WT, Kozelowski-Templin R: Clinical application of blood gases, ed 5, St Louis, 1994, Mosby.)*

1. Incomplete hemolysis of the blood sample causes the light to scatter off cell fragments and lipids. Sickle cells (as in sickle cell anemia) are difficult to disrupt and may cause false $O_2Hb$ and COHb readings if extra time is not taken for hemolysis. Follow the manufacturer's guidelines on the procedure for hemolyzing red blood cells.

2. Greater than 10% MetHb may cause errors in the measurement of all hemoglobin moieties. SHb also causes false readings. Additional information may need to be gathered from the chart or laboratory on the patient's levels of these abnormal hemoglobin moieties. CO-oximetry should probably not be performed on blood samples with abnormal levels of MetHb or SHb.

3. Intravenous dyes, such as methylene blue, Evans blue, and indocyanine green used in various cardiac studies, can absorb the same wavelengths of light used to identify the various forms of hemoglobin. Their presence results in measurement of a lower than actual level of $O_2Hb$. Check the patient's chart for a record of the dyes that are being used. CO-oximetry should probably not be used for blood gas analysis on patients who have these dyes in their systems.

4. Failure to reprogram the analyzer for FHb instead of adult hemoglobin may produce false results. Remember to check the chart for the patient's age. Reprogram the analyzer for FHb on any infant who is only a few weeks old.

5. The presence of lipid particles in the blood causes light scattering and results in a reading that is falsely high in the value of THb and the percentage of MetHb, and falsely low in the percentages of $O_2Hb$ and COHb. Follow the laboratory's guidelines regarding when a patient's blood lipid value is too high for accurate use of the CO-oximeter.

6. The presence of air bubbles or incomplete hemolysis of blood in the cuvette causes an absorbance error. Air bubbles need to be flushed out and the blood sample inserted again and reanalyzed. Make sure that all blood samples are hemolyzed according to the manufacturer's guidelines.

7. A blood clot(s) in the sample tubing prevents blood from flowing through to the cuvette. If a sample cannot be inserted into the unit, suspect and check for a blood clot. Obviously, any clotted tubing should be removed and replaced, and it must be confirmed that the CO-oximeter is working properly.

### b. Perform CO-oximetry (NBRC code: IB7f, IIIE3b) [Difficulty: R, Ap]

Most hospitals have a CO-oximeter in addition to a blood gas analyzer. A CO-oximeter should be used to analyze a blood gas sample whenever CO poisoning is known or suspected. A CO-oximeter also gives a complete analysis of relative amounts of different types of patient hemoglobin.

A CO-oximeter, also called a *spectrophotometric oximeter*, is the most accurate method available for measuring the four different hemoglobin moieties (species or variations in the hemoglobin molecule). These hemoglobin species include the following:

1. Oxyhemoglobin ($HbO_2$ or $O_2Hb$), which carries $O_2$ to the tissues, and reduced hemoglobin (HbR or RHb), which has given up its $O_2$ and picked up $CO_2$

2. Carboxyhemoglobin (HbCO or COHb), which is nonfunctional because of the tightness with which CO binds to the hemoglobin

3. Methemoglobin (HbMet or MetHb), which is nonfunctional because the Hb molecule is unable to combine reversibly with $O_2$

4. Sulfhemoglobin (HbS or SHb), which is nonfunctional and similar to HbMet

5. In addition, a CO-oximeter can measure the fetal hemoglobin (HbF or FHb) found in a newborn infant instead of adult $O_2Hb$

Each of these hemoglobin moieties has a spectroscopic "fingerprint" of unique, absorbed lightwave frequencies. Fig. 3-9 shows the spectral analysis of the various forms of hemoglobin.

Follow the manufacturer's guidelines on rewarming the blood sample to body temperature, hemolyzing the sample, and inserting it into the measurement cuvette. Failure to do so could result in incorrect patient values.

The principle of operation of a CO-oximeter is comparison of the relative absorbances of four wavelengths of light by $O_2Hb$, RHb, and COHb. This procedure compares the absorptions at the three isosbestic points (where the moieties being compared have equal absorption) and a wavelength point with the greatest difference in absorption between the two moieties. Through computer integration of the data, the relative proportions of $O_2Hb$, RHb, and COHb are determined. If the total is less than 100% of the hemoglobin present, the difference has to be MetHb (or, rarely, SHb). The unit then provides the following: data on THb; percentages for $O_2Hb$, RHb, COHb, and MetHb; and total amounts for them provided as grams per deciliter of blood. Some units also calculate $O_2$ content.

### Exam Hint

If a patient is known or suspected of having carbon monoxide poisoning, a CO-oximeter should be used for blood gas analysis. A standard or point-of-care blood gas analyzer or pulse oximeter should not be used. These instruments cannot detect or measure carbon monoxide.

## MODULE D

**Interpret blood gas analysis results to determine how the patient is responding to respiratory care**

### 1. Review the chart for any blood gas results (NBRC code: IA4) [Difficulty: R]

Look in the chart for any blood gas results, including arterial, capillary, or mixed venous values. Any patient may have had an arterial sample analyzed, and a neonate may have had an arterialized capillary sample analyzed. A patient with a pulmonary artery catheter may have had a mixed venous sample analyzed.

### 2. Interpret the results of arterial blood gas analysis (NBRC code: IB8d, IIIE4) [Difficulty: R, Ap]

A number of authors have written extensively on how ABGs should be interpreted. The system proposed by Shapiro and associates (1994) has been found to be practical and relatively easy to understand. Most of the following discussion and tables are based on this system. Anyone who is studying for the NBRC examination who has learned another system, however, is not at any disadvantage.

The NBRC examination includes specific questions about blood gas interpretation. The examination also includes blood gas results in other questions that relate to any respiratory care technique or procedure, such as $O_2$ therapy and mechanical ventilation. The examinee must be proficient in blood gas interpretation to do well on NBRC examinations.

*Assessment of oxygenation.* Hypoxemia or hypoxia can be rapidly life threatening. Table 3-2 shows normal $PaO_2$ values for the newborn, child to adult, and older adult when room air (almost 21% $O_2$) is inhaled at sea level. These values decrease progressively as altitude increases. However, under most clinical conditions, this is not a factor unless one is working at high altitudes.

Generally, any patient is seriously hypoxemic if the $PaO_2$ is less than 60 torr on room air. Table 3-3 shows guidelines on judging the seriousness of hypoxemia. The most obvious way to correct hypoxemia, once it is recognized, is to give supplemental $O_2$. The clinician must realize that $O_2$ alone will not correct the hypoxemia if the patient is hypoventilating (increased $PaCO_2$), has heart failure, or is unable to carry or make use of the $O_2$. In general, try to keep the patient's $PaO_2$ at between 60 and 100 torr.

Shapiro and associates (1994) suggested the following formula, where $F_IO_2$ is the fraction of inspired oxygen, for determining whether the patient will be hypoxemic on room air: "If $PaO_2$ is less than $F_IO_2 \times 5$, the patient can be assumed to be hypoxemic on room air."

Fig. 3-10 shows a normal $O_2Hb$ dissociation curve. The saturation value is important because it shows how much hemoglobin is saturated with $O_2$. Several important points of correlation exist between the $SaO_2$ and the $PaO_2$. (Calculated saturation values can be misleadingly high if the patient has inhaled CO. In this situation, saturation should be directly measured on a CO-oximeter–type blood gas analyzer.)

| TABLE 3-2 | Age-Based Acceptable Levels of Partial Pressure of Oxygen in Arterial Blood ($PaO_2$) When Room Air (21% Oxygen) Is Breathed at Sea Level |
|---|---|
| **Age** | **$PaO_2$** |
| **NEWBORN** | |
| Acceptable range | 40 to 70 torr |
| **CHILD TO ADULT** | |
| Normal | 97 torr |
| Acceptable range | >80 torr |
| Hypoxemia | <80 torr |
| **OLDER ADULT** | |
| 60-year-old | >80 torr |
| 70-year-old | >70 torr |
| 80-year-old | >60 torr |
| 90-year-old | >50 torr |

Modified from Shapiro BA, Peruzzi WT, Kozelowski-Templin R: Clinical application of blood gases, ed 5, Chicago, 1994, Mosby–Year Book.

| TABLE 3-3 | Evaluation of Hypoxemia | |
|---|---|---|
| **CONDITIONS: ROOM AIR IS INSPIRED; THE PATIENT IS YOUNGER THAN 60 YEARS OLD*** | | |
| **Hypoxemia** | **$PaO_2$** | **$SaO_2$** |
| Mild | 60–79 torr | 90%–94% |
| Moderate | 40–59 torr | 75%–89% |
| Severe | <40 torr | <75% |
| **CONDITIONS: SUPPLEMENTAL $O_2$ IS INSPIRED; THE PATIENT IS YOUNGER THAN 60 YEARS OLD** | | |
| **Hypoxemia** | **$PaO_2$** | |
| Uncorrected | Less than room air acceptable limit | |
| Corrected | Within room air acceptable limit (<100 torr) | |
| Excessively corrected | >100 torr | |

Modified from Shapiro BA, Peruzzi WT, Kozelowski-Templin R: Clinical application of blood gases, ed 5, Chicago, 1994, Mosby–Year Book.
*Subtract 1 torr of $O_2$ from limits of mild and moderate hypoxemia for each year over 60. A $PaO_2$ of less than 40 torr indicates severe hypoxemia in any patient at any age.

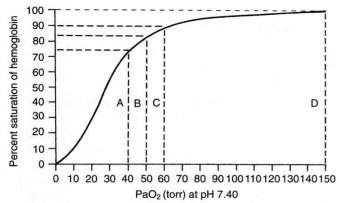

**Fig. 3-10** The oxygen (oxyhemoglobin) dissociation curve plots the relationship between hemoglobin saturation (*y* axis) and plasma $PaO_2$ (*x* axis). **A,** 75% saturation and a $PaO_2$ of 40 torr are normally seen in venous blood. **B,** 85% saturation and a $PaO_2$ of 50 torr are the minimal levels allowed in a *chronically* hypoxemic patient. **C,** 90% saturation and a $PaO_2$ of 60 torr are the minimal levels allowed in an *acutely* hypoxemic patient. **D,** Hemoglobin in the pulmonary capillaries adjacent to normal alveoli will become 100% saturated when the $PaO_2$ reaches 150 torr. *(Modified from Lane EE, Walker JF: Clinical arterial blood gas analysis, St Louis, 1987, Mosby.)*

Fig. 3-11 shows a number of factors that can influence the $O_2Hb$ dissociation curve and illustrates how $O_2$ loads onto and unloads from hemoglobin. In a patient with normal oxygenation, these factors are not clinically significant. However, when the $PaO_2$ is less than 60 torr and the $SaO_2$ is less than 90%, these factors can become an important consideration. As Fig. 3-11 shows, a left-shifted $O_2Hb$ dissociation curve results in a lower $PaO_2$ at any given saturation, which results in delivery of even less $O_2$ to the tissues.

***Assessment of carbon dioxide and pH.*** The pH is the next important value to be interpreted because extreme acidemia/acidosis and alkalemia/alkalosis can be life threatening. Interpretation of the $CO_2$ value is important because the value has a direct effect on the pH and indirectly affects the $O_2$ level. A high or low $PaCO_2$ level, by itself, is not life threatening.

Table 3-4 shows normal values for $PaCO_2$ and pH with acceptable ranges around the mean or average. Table 3-5 shows the most widely acceptable therapeutic ranges for $PaCO_2$ and pH. Values outside of these ranges present a progressively greater risk to the patient. Table 3-6 shows the definitions of Shapiro and associates (1994) for alkalemia and acidemia from a respiratory cause. An *acute* change in the patient's ventilation causes the following when one is starting from a $PaCO_2$ of 40 torr:

   a. If the $PaCO_2$ increases by 20 torr, the pH will decrease by 0.10 unit.

   b. If the $PaCO_2$ decreases by 10 torr, the pH will increase by 0.10 unit.

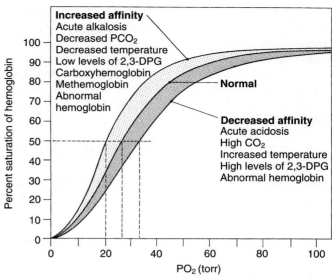

**Fig. 3-11** Conditions associated with altered affinity of hemoglobin for $O_2$. $P_{50}$ is the $PaO_2$ at which hemoglobin is 50% saturated (normally, 26.6 torr). A low $P_{50}$ represents increased affinity of hemoglobin for $O_2$; a high $P_{50}$ is seen with decreased affinity. Note that variation from normal is associated with decreased (low $P_{50}$) or increased (high $P_{50}$) availability of $O_2$ to tissues *(dashed lines)*. The shaded area shows the entire oxyhemoglobin dissociation curve under the same circumstances. 2,3-DPG, 2,3-Diphosphoglycerate; $PCO_2$, pressure of carbon dioxide; $PO_2$, pressure of oxygen. *(From Lane EE, Walker JF: Clinical arterial blood gas analysis, St Louis, 1987, Mosby.)*

| TABLE 3-4 | Normal Laboratory Ranges for Partial Pressure of Carbon Dioxide in Arterial Blood ($PaCO_2$) and pH | | |
|---|---|---|---|
| | **Mean** | **1 SD** | **2 SDs** |
| $PaCO_2$ | 40 | 38–42 torr | 35–45 torr |
| pH | 7.40 | 7.38–7.42 | 7.35–7.45 |

Modified from Shapiro BA, Peruzzi WT, Kozelowski-Templin R: Clinical application of blood gases, ed 5, Chicago, 1994, Mosby–Year Book. *SD*, Standard deviation.

| TABLE 3-5 | Acceptable Clinical Ranges for Partial Pressure of Carbon Dioxide in Arterial Blood ($PaCO_2$) and pH |
|---|---|
| $PaCO_2$ | 30–50 torr* |
| pH | 7.30–7.50 |

Modified from Shapiro BA, Peruzzi WT, Kozelowski-Templin R: Clinical application of blood gases, ed 5, Chicago, 1994, Mosby–Year Book. *This is the range for patients with an acute change. It does not apply to patients with long-standing disease, such as chronic obstructive pulmonary disease. These patients may have $PaCO_2$ values greater than 50 torr.

Thus, the body can be seen as better able to compensate with metabolic buffers for a respiratory acidosis than a respiratory alkalosis.

Metabolic effects are evaluated through interpretation of either the bicarbonate ($HCO_3^-$) value or the base excess/base deficit (BE/BD) value. Both reveal whether any metabolic effect exists on the pH. Normal values are as follows:

   a. $HCO_3^-$: 24 mEq/L
   b. BE/BD: 0 mEq/L; ±1 mEq/L is often listed as the normal range

Values that indicate metabolic alkalosis of a primary or secondary nature are as follows:

   a. $HCO_3^-$ greater than 24 mEq/L
   b. BE greater than 0 or greater than +1 mEq/L

Values that indicate metabolic acidosis of a primary or secondary nature are as follows:

   a. $HCO_3^-$ less than 24 mEq/L
   b. BE less than 0 or less than −1 mEq/L (some laboratories report this as a BD or a negative BE)

Tables 3-7 to 3-9 show definitions of terms and classifications of the various acid-base states. As has been stated earlier, other systems can be used for interpreting blood gases. All are probably satisfactory for interpretation purposes and for preparation for NBRC examinations.

### Exam Hint

**E**xpect to see several arterial blood gas questions that require the interpretation of acid-base balance and oxygenation. For example, identify that a COPD patient has an elevated carbon dioxide level and a normal pH with a compensated respiratory acidosis. Also, expect to see ABG values included in questions about adjustment of both oxygen therapy and the mechanical ventilator. Note that the NBRC uses BE as a negative value in its examination questions.

### 3. Interpret the results of CO-oximetry blood gas analysis (NBRC code: IB8d, IIIE4) [Difficulty: R, Ap]

The CO-oximeter–type blood gas analyzer gives values for $O_2Hb$, RHb, COHb, and MetHb/SHb. Each of these hemoglobin moieties can be displayed in terms of grams per deciliter and percentage of the whole, and they can be added together for a THb. Table 3-10 shows normal adult hemoglobin values. The amounts of COHb and MetHb should be subtracted from the THb to find the amount of functional hemoglobin. Any increase in the COHb and/or MetHb level to above those listed is abnormal and results in even less normal hemoglobin available to carry $O_2$. The patient who suffers from CO poisoning is at greatest risk. A COHb level of 30% or greater saturation can be fatal. By subtraction, the $O_2Hb$ ($SaO_2$) level can be no greater than 70% with a resulting $PaO_2$ of less than 40 torr.

The following example shows how one should calculate the amount of functional hemoglobin and saturation for a patient with normal COHb and MetHb levels:

| TABLE 3-6 | Naming Unacceptable Values for Partial Pressure of $CO_2$ in Arterial Blood ($PaCO_2$) and pH |
|---|---|
| $PaCO_2$ >45 torr | Respiratory acidosis/alveolar hypoventilation/ventilatory failure |
| pH <7.35 | Acidemia |
| $PaCO_2$ <35 torr | Respiratory alkalosis/alveolar hyperventilation |
| pH >7.45 | Alkalemia |

Modified from Shapiro BA, Peruzzi WT, Kozelowski-Templin R: Clinical application of blood gases, ed 5, Chicago, 1994, Mosby–Year Book.

| TABLE 3-7 | Clinical Terminology for Arterial Blood Gas Measurements |
|---|---|
| **Clinical terminology** | **Clinical findings** |
| Respiratory acidosis/alveolar hypoventilation/ventilatory failure | $PaCO_2$ >45 torr |
|    Acute ventilatory failure | $PaCO_2$ >45 torr; pH <7.35 |
|    Chronic ventilatory failure | $PaCO_2$ >45 torr; pH 7.36–7.40 |
| Respiratory alkalosis/alveolar hyperventilation | $PaCO_2$ <35 torr |
|    Acute alveolar hyperventilation | $PaCO_2$ <35 torr; pH >7.45 |
|    Chronic alveolar hyperventilation | $PaCO_2$ <35 torr; pH 7.41–7.45 |
| Acidemia | pH <7.35 |
| Acidosis | Pathophysiologic condition in which the patient has a significant base deficit (plasma bicarbonate below normal) |
| Alkalemia | pH >7.45 |
| Alkalosis | Pathophysiologic condition in which the patient has a significant base excess (plasma bicarbonate above normal) |

Modified from Shapiro BA, Peruzzi WT, Kozelowski-Templin R: Clinical application of blood gases, ed 5, Chicago, 1994, Mosby–Year Book.

| TABLE 3-8 | Evaluation of Ventilatory and Metabolic Effects on Acid-Base Status |
|---|---|

**EVALUATION OF $PaCO_2$**

| PaCO₂ >45 torr | Respiratory acidosis/alveolar hypoventilation/ventilatory failure |
|---|---|
| PaCO₂ 35-45 torr | Acceptable alveolar ventilation |
| PaCO₂ <35 torr | Respiratory alkalosis/alveolar hyperventilation |

**EVALUATION OF $PaCO_2$ IN CONJUNCTION WITH pH**

*Acceptable alveolar ventilation (PaCO₂ from 35 to 45 torr)*

| pH >7.50 | Metabolic alkalosis |
|---|---|
| pH 7.30-7.50 | Acceptable ventilatory and metabolic pH |
| pH <7.30 | Metabolic acidosis |

*Alveolar hypoventilation (PaCO₂ >45 torr)*

| pH 7.40-7.50 | *Partially compensated* metabolic alkalosis |
|---|---|
| pH 7.30-7.50 | *Chronic* ventilatory failure |
| pH <7.30 | *Acute* ventilatory failure |

*Alveolar hyperventilation (PaCO₂ <35 torr)*

| pH >7.50 | *Acute* alveolar hyperventilation |
|---|---|
| pH 7.40-7.50 | *Chronic* alveolar hyperventilation |
| pH 7.30-7.40 | *Compensated* metabolic acidosis |
| pH <7.30 | *Partially compensated* metabolic acidosis |

Modified from Shapiro BA, Peruzzi WT, Kozelowski-Templin R: Clinical application of blood gases, ed 5, Chicago, 1994, Mosby–Year Book.
*PaCO₂,* Partial pressure of CO₂ in arterial blood.
Some authors use a narrower pH range for these classifications.

15.00 g THb
− 0.225 g COHb
14.775 g
− 0.150 g MetHb
14.625 g functional hemoglobin

100.0% potential saturation of O₂Hb in arterial blood
− 1.5% saturation of COHb
98.5%
− 1.5% saturation of MetHb
97.0% saturation of arterial blood (SaO₂ of 97%)

The following example represents a patient with an elevated COHb and a normal MetHb level:

15.0 g THb
− 3.0 g COHb
12.0 g
− 0.15 g MetHb
11.85 g functional hemoglobin

100.0% potential saturation of O₂Hb in arterial blood
− 20.0% saturation of COHb
80.0%
− 1.5% saturation of MetHb
78.5% saturation of arterial blood (SaO₂ of 78.5%)

| TABLE 3-9 | Primary Blood Gas Classifications |
|---|---|

| | PaCO₂ | pH | Bicarbonate | BE |
|---|---|---|---|---|
| **VENTILATORY IMBALANCE** | | | | |
| Acute alveolar hypoventilation | I | D | N | N |
| Chronic alveolar hypoventilation | I | N | I | I |
| Acute alveolar hyperventilation | D | I | N | N |
| Chronic alveolar hyperventilation | D | N | D | D |
| **METABOLIC IMBALANCE** | | | | |
| Uncompensated acidosis | N | D | D | D |
| Partially compensated acidosis | D | D | D | D |
| Uncompensated alkalosis | N | I | I | I |
| Partially compensated alkalosis | I | I | I | I |
| Compensated acidosis or alkalosis | I or D | N | I or D | I or D |

Modified from Shapiro BA, Peruzzi WT, Kozelowski-Templin R: Clinical application of blood gases, ed 5, Chicago, 1994, Mosby–Year Book. *BE,* Base excess; *D,* decreased; *I,* increased; *N,* normal range; *PaCO₂,* partial pressure of CO₂ in arterial blood.

| TABLE 3-10 | Normal Hemoglobin Values for Adults |
|---|---|

| Total hemoglobin (THb) | Men: 13.5–18.0 g/dL<br>Women: 12.0–16.0 g/dL<br>15.0 g/dL is often listed as an average for both |
|---|---|
| Oxyhemoglobin | 94%–100% of THb (reported as SaO₂ of 94% to 100%) |
| Carboxyhemoglobin | Nonsmokers: <1.5% (0.225 g/dL) of THb<br>Smokers: 1.5%–10% of THb |
| Methemoglobin | 0.5%–3% (0.075–0.45 g/dL) of THb |
| Oxygen content (arterial sample) | 15–23 g/dL |

*g/dL,* Grams per deciliter (sometimes listed as g/100 mL ); *SaO₂,* O₂ saturation in arterial blood.

**Exam Hint**

**U**se a CO-oximeter to evaluate a patient's oxygenation when carbon monoxide poisoning is known or suspected. CO poisoning would be confirmed by a significantly lower saturation value on a CO-oximeter than that found on a standard or point-of-care oxygen analyzer or a pulse oximeter. Remember that standard or point-of-care oxygen analyzers and pulse oximeters cannot identify or measure carboxyhemoglobin.

**TABLE 3-11** Normal and Abnormal Mixed Venous Blood Gas Values

**NORMAL VALUES**

Average: $S\bar{v}O_2$ 75%; $P\bar{v}O_2$ 40 torr; $P\bar{v}CO_2$ 46 torr; pH 7.35
Range: $S\bar{v}O_2$ 76%-70%; $P\bar{v}O_2$ 43-37 torr; $P\bar{v}CO_2$ 46-44 torr; pH 7.36-7.34

**CRITICALLY ILL PATIENT**

| | $P\bar{v}O_2$ (torr) | | $S\bar{v}O_2$ (%) | |
| --- | --- | --- | --- | --- |
| | Average | Range | Average | Range |
| Excellent cardiovascular reserves | >37 | 40-35 | >70 | 75-68 |
| Limited cardiovascular reserves | >32 | 35-30 | 60 | 68-56 |
| Failure of cardiovascular reserves | <30 | <30 | <56 | <56 |

Modified from Shapiro BA, Peruzzi WT, Kozelowski-Templin R: Clinical application of blood gases, ed 5, St Louis, 1994, Mosby.

### 4. Mixed venous blood gases

#### a. Review the patient's chart for mixed venous blood gas results (NBRC code: IA4) [Difficulty: R]

A mixed venous blood sample can be taken from the pulmonary artery of any patient who has a pulmonary artery (Swan-Ganz) catheter (see Chapter 5). This true mixed venous sample should not be confused with a blood sample taken from an arm vein or other venous site. The symbol $P\bar{v}$ is the prefix for venous blood gas values of $O_2$, $CO_2$, and so forth. A patient typically has the following mixed venous blood gas values: $S\bar{v}O_2$, 75%; $P\bar{v}O_2$, 40 torr; $P\bar{v}CO_2$, 46 torr; and pH, 7.35. (Table 3-11 gives details on normal venous blood gas values and their interpretation in patients with cardiovascular disease.)

#### b. Interpret the results of mixed venous blood gas analysis to evaluate the patient's response to respiratory care (NBRC code: IB8d, IIIE4) [Difficulty: R, Ap]

In the critically ill patient, measuring the mixed venous blood gases is as important as measuring the ABGs. Venous blood gas values reveal what has happened as the arterial blood has passed through the body. $O_2$ has been extracted and $CO_2$ has been added to the blood. The difference between the arterial and venous $O_2$ levels reflects $O_2$ consumption by the body and cardiac output.

Because of this, the most critical venous blood gas values to be measured are the $S\bar{v}O_2$ and the $P\bar{v}O_2$. Generally, a $P\bar{v}O_2$ value of less than 30 torr or an $S\bar{v}O_2$ of less than 56% indicates that the patient has tissue hypoxia. Both values can be obtained by analyzing a mixed venous blood sample taken through a pulmonary artery catheter. If the patient has a fiberoptic catheter, the $S\bar{v}O_2$ value can be monitored continuously. This is extremely helpful if the patient is unstable or is having frequent changes in inspired $O_2$ or ventilator settings.

## MODULE E
### Pulse oximetry

#### 1. Check the patient's chart for previous pulse oximetry results (NBRC code: IA6d) [Difficulty: R, Ap]

Pulse oximetry ($SpO_2$) is generally indicated when a patient's oxygenation must be monitored. An $SpO_2$ of 92% or greater indicates that the patient is adequately oxygenated. Past values should be compared with current readings to assess the patient's progress or response to treatment.

#### 2. Make a recommendation to perform pulse oximetry (NBRC code: IB9) [Difficulty: R, Ap]

Pulse oximetry is indicated in the following situations: during anesthesia and intraoperative monitoring of oxygenation; postoperatively when the patient is still sedated; when the patient is receiving sedatives or analgesics that can blunt the airway protective reflexes; during bronchoscopy; during a sleep study; and for evaluation of the effectiveness of $O_2$ therapy. An exception to the use of $SpO_2$ should be made when CO poisoning is known or suspected.

#### 3. Get an appropriate pulse oximeter and related equipment (NBRC code: IIA21) [Difficulty: R]

Each pulse oximeter reports a percentage on a light-emitting diode (LED) display. Many newer units also display the patient's pulse rate. More expensive units print out a copy of the $SpO_2$ percentage and pulse rate for placement in the patient's chart, if required. A variety of sensors fit the feet or hands of infants, an adult's fingers, the bridge of the nose, the forehead, and the ear lobe. A sensor that is designed to fit the selected site should be selected.

#### 4. Put the equipment together and make sure that it works properly (NBRC code: IIA21) [Difficulty: R]

Follow the manufacturer's suggestions for setup. Newer pulse oximetry systems visually display the strength of the pulse for ease in finding the best place for the probe (Fig. 3-12). Keep bright light out of the patient site and transducer. Fig. 3-13 shows how to properly apply the finger probe.

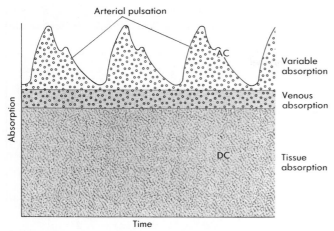

Fig. 3-12 Pulse oximetry signal strength. The strong surge of blood through the artery with each heartbeat results in variable absorption of the light emitted by the pulse oximeter. Venous and tissue absorption of light is stable when the heart is at rest. This absorption difference is used to find the patient's artery and measure the heart rate. *AC* refers to variable absorption; *DC* refers to stable absorption. *(From Ruppel G: Manual of pulmonary function testing, ed 6, St Louis, 1994, Mosby.)*

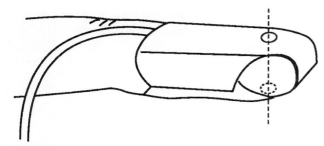

Fig. 3-13 Pulse oximetry transducer properly placed on a finger. Fold the OXISENSOR over the end of the digit. Align the other end of the OXISENSOR so that the two alignment marks are directly opposite each other. Press the OXISENSOR into the skin. Wrap the adhesive flaps around the digit. *(Courtesy of Nellcor Puritan Bennett Corp, Pleasanton, Calif.)*

### 5. Troubleshoot any problems with the equipment (NBRC code: IIA21) [Difficulty: R]

The pulse signal is not strong if the patient has poor circulation at the site of the oximeter probe. This can occur if the patient is hypothermic or hypotensive or is receiving a vasoconstricting medication. If the pulse signal is weak, the $SpO_2$ values may not be accurate. See Table 3-12 for common sources of error and their solutions.

### 6. Perform pulse oximetry on your patient (NBRC code: IB7b, IIIE3a) [Difficulty: R, Ap]

$SpO_2$ has gained wide acceptance because it offers a way to continuously and noninvasively monitor a patient's oxygenation by following the percentage of hemoglobin saturated with $O_2$. The reported $SpO_2$ percentage is the percentage of $O_2Hb$.

Pulse oximetry makes practical use of two physical principles. The first is spectrophotometry, which is used to analyze the transmission of two wavelengths of light through the blood and body tissues. One wavelength is 660 nm, and the other is between 920 and 940 nm, depending on the manufacturer. The 660-nm wavelength can be seen as red and is preferentially absorbed by $O_2Hb$. The 920- to 940-nm wavelength is not visible because it is in the infrared range and is preferentially absorbed by RHb.

The second principle is plethysmography, which is used to find and then evaluate the amplitude of the arterial pulse waveform. See Fig. 3-12 for the plethysmographic arterial waveform. When the pulse oximetry sensor is placed on a patient site, such as the fingertip, the two wavelengths of light shine through the blood, tissues, and bone within the finger. The sending LED and the receiving (photodiode) sensors must be placed opposite each other. Most units have a signal strength display that indicates when the photodiode is receiving a strong signal and the patient's pulse has been detected. The microprocessor is designed to detect a baseline level of light absorption by the tissues and venous blood (containing more RHb) and the light absorption of arterial blood (containing more $O_2Hb$). It can then compare the absorptions of the two wavelengths to determine the level of saturated $O_2Hb$, which is displayed as saturation by $SpO_2$.

Because pulse oximetry samples only two wavelengths of light, the technology is unable to recognize the presence or quantity of the nonfunctional hemoglobin species of COHb and MetHb. Instead, an ABG should be drawn and sent to the laboratory to be passed through a CO-oximeter for complete fractional hemoglobin analysis. Even healthy persons have small amounts of COHb and MetHB. For this and other technical reasons, manufacturers report the following $SpO_2$ values for general accuracy at 1 SD for a general population: ±2% from 100% to 70% saturation, and ±3% from 70% to 50% saturation. Because of these limitations, the following clinical guidelines have been documented by a number of authors:

a. Do not use pulse oximetry on patients with significant levels of COHb or MetHB.

b. If in doubt about abnormal types of hemoglobin, analyze an ABG through a CO-oximeter, and compare the true $SaO_2$ with the $SpO_2$ from pulse oximetry. Pulse oximetry can be used if the correlation of values is within 4%.

c. Question the $SpO_2$ value when the displayed heart rate is different from the actual heart rate.

d. Do not use pulse oximetry when the $SpO_2$ reading is less than 70%.

e. Pulse oximetry can be used on a term neonate or a 1500-g or larger neonate. Smaller neonates should have oxygenation measured by a transcutaneous $O_2$ monitor because hyperoxygenating a small neonate

**TABLE 3-12** Sources of Error in Pulse Oximetry

| Sources of error | Remedy |
| --- | --- |
| Light interference: Xenon lamp, fluorescent light, infrared (bilirubin) light, probe fell off of patient | Cover the probe with an opaque wrap; put the probe back in place on the patient |
| Low perfusion: Low blood pressure, hypothermia, vasoconstricting drugs | Use ear lobe, bridge of nose, or forehead instead of finger or toe; discontinue use if still unreliable |
| Motion artifact | Secure the probe site; ensure that the $SpO_2$ reading is synchronized with the heart rate |
| Darkly pigmented patient | Use lightly pigmented site such as tip of finger or toe; $SpO_2$ value may overestimate $PaO_2$; discontinue use if still unreliable |
| Artificial or painted fingernails | Remove acrylic nails; remove black, blue, green, metallic, or frosted nail polish; use a different site |
| Venous pulsation being read as an arterial pulsation | Loosen a tight sensor; change the finger sensor site every 2-4 hr; loosen the cause of a tourniquet-like effect |
| The following vascular dyes will cause low $SpO_2$ readings: Methylene blue, indigo carmine, indocyanine green | Do not use $SpO_2$ |

$PaO_2$, Partial pressure of $O_2$ in arterial blood; $SpO_2$, pulse oximeter.

**TABLE 3-13** Recommended Clinical Ranges for True Values in Saturation of $O_2$ in the Hemoglobin ($SaO_2$), Values in Pulse Oximetry ($SpO_2$),* and Their Correlation With Values in Partial Pressure of $O_2$ in Arterial Blood ($PaO_2$)

| | $SaO_2$ | $SpO_2$ | Approximate PaO (torr) |
| --- | --- | --- | --- |
| **ADULT** | | | |
| Acute hypoxemia | 90%-95% | 92%-95%[†] | 60-95 |
| Chronic hypoxemia | 85%-90% | 87%-92% | 50-60 |
| **NEONATE** | | | |
| <1500 g or in the first week of life | About 97% | 92%-96% | 60-70 |
| >1500 g or after the first week of life | 90%-96% | 90%-96% | 50-70 |
| >1 month of age with chronic lung disease | 85%-90% | 87%-92% | 50-60 |

Note: The clinical goal with most neonates is to prevent both hypoxemia, defined as a $PaO_2$ <45 torr, and hyperoxia, defined as a $PaO_2$ >90 torr.
*Based on the patient having normal carboxyhemoglobin and methemoglobin levels. Elevated level(s) result in an erroneously high $SpO_2$ reading and unsuspected hypoxemia.
[†]Black patients should have an $SpO_2$ of 95% maintained to ensure adequate oxygenation.

is too easy when small changes in saturation can result in wide swings in $PO_2$. The risk of retinopathy of prematurity (formerly called *retrolental fibroplasia*) from hyperoxia is too great in the small neonate.

Table 3-13 lists common clinical ranges for $SpO_2$ values. For the aforementioned reasons, the minimum safe values are 2% higher than the corresponding $SaO_2$ value by CO-oximetry. It is important that the patient have good pulsatile blood flow to the measurement site so that an accurate reading can be obtained.

### 7. Interpret your patient's pulse oximetry value (NBRC code: IB8a) [Difficulty: R, Ap]

The previously healthy patient with cardiopulmonary failure should have the $SpO_2$ value kept at 92% or greater to ensure adequate oxygenation. The patient with chronic obstructive pulmonary disease can probably tolerate an $SpO_2$ value of as low as 87%. The $SpO_2$ for the neonate should be kept between 92% and 96%. Saturations below these values indicate hypoxemia in most patients.

Note the site where the saturation was measured, which is especially important in neonates who may have congenital heart defects. A higher saturation in the right fingers or right ear lobe compared with the rest of the body is seen with patent ductus arteriosus. A higher saturation in the fingers and ear lobes compared with the toes is seen with coarctation of the aorta.

---

### Exam Hint

The patient with CO poisoning should *not* be evaluated with a pulse oximeter because the units are unable to distinguish $O_2Hb$ from $COHb$. The pulse oximeter will only measure the $O_2Hb$, and a higher-than-true $O_2Hb$ saturation will be reported. These patients should be evaluated for oxygenation only by means of an arterial blood gas sample analyzed on a CO-oximeter blood gas analyzer.

---

### 8. Chart your patient's pulse oximetry value (NBRC code: IIIA1b4) [Difficulty: R, Ap]

Charting should be performed as required by the hospital's policies.

### MODULE F
**Transcutaneous oxygen monitoring**

Note: Transcutaneous monitoring (TCM) involves the continuous monitoring of $O_2$, $CO_2$, or both gases as they diffuse through the skin. Each gas has its own electrode, and a combined electrode is used for both gases.

### 1. Review the patient's chart for a transcutaneous oxygen value (NBRC code: IA6d) [Difficulty: R, Ap]

Transcutaneous monitoring ($PtcO_2$, $tcPO_2$, or $TcO_2$) enables a patient's oxygenation to be followed on a continuous basis. In practice, neonates are monitored much more often than adults. Check the chart for a record of the patient's $PtcO_2$ values. Comparison of the $PaO_2$ with the $PtcO_2$ is particularly important. Note also what the $PtcO_2$ values are when the inspired $O_2$ is changed, the patient is suctioned, or changes are made in continuous positive airway pressure (CPAP) or mechanical ventilation. Avoid earlier clinical situations that resulted in hypoxemia.

Heating the electrode speeds up the diffusion of $O_2$ through the skin and provides a closer correlation with the patient's $PaO_2$ value. Always follow the manufacturer's recommendations for the proper electrode temperature. The temperature generally ranges from 42.5° C for a 1000-g infant to 44° C for a 3500-g infant. A pediatric patient can tolerate a temperature of 44° C, whereas an adult can have an electrode temperature of 45° C. Remember, however, that the $PtcO_2$ value is *not* the same

as the $PaO_2$ value. Current recommendations are that any unit should give $PtcO_2$ values within ±15% of the $PaO_2$ over the operating range of the instrument. The values should then correlate within ±15% as the patient's condition changes. This should always be confirmed.

An ABG should be drawn for $PaO_2$ every time that $PtcO_2$ monitoring is started. The $PaO_2$-$PtcO_2$ gradient can then be calculated as the difference between the two. For example, if the patient's $PaO_2$ is 100 torr, the $PtcO_2$ should be no less than 85 torr. If the $PtcO_2$ decreases to 70 torr, the $PaO_2$ should have decreased to no lower than 85 torr. Because of this close correlation, the patient can be trend monitored with some assurance of accuracy. In addition, ABGs do not need to be drawn as frequently for the $PaO_2$. This trending relationship holds true for changes in the patient's pulmonary condition. It does not, however, hold true when the patient has cardiovascular problems, such as hypotension, hypothermia, peripheral vascular disease, or cardiogenic shock with decreased tissue perfusion.

### 2. Recommend transcutaneous oxygen monitoring for additional data (NBRC code: IB9) [Difficulty: R, Ap]

$PtcO_2$ monitoring has been used for the following purposes:
   a. Monitoring of oxygenation of an unstable neonate during transportation within the hospital or between two hospitals
   b. Intraoperative and postoperative monitoring of oxygenation
   c. Monitoring of oxygenation during changes in the inspired $O_2$ and in mechanical ventilation, as well as for detection of hypoxemia during an equipment failure
   d. Detection of a right-to-left shunt (when a neonate has a PDA, the $PtcO_2$ is higher in the right upper chest than in the left upper chest, abdomen, or thighs)
   e. Detection of coarctation of the aorta (when this defect is present, the $PtcO_2$ is higher in the right and left upper chest than in the abdomen or thighs)
   f. Determination of the congenital heart disease patient's response to an $O_2$-challenge test

### 3. Get the necessary equipment to perform transcutaneous oxygen monitoring (NBRC code: IIA21) [Difficulty: R]

The electrode used for monitoring the patient's $PtcO_2$ level is a miniaturized and modified Clark-type polarographic electrode similar to that used in the blood gas analyzer (Fig. 3-14). Some authors describe it as a *Huch* or *Hellige electrode*, named after the two researchers who modified the original Clark electrode for their work with pediatric patients.

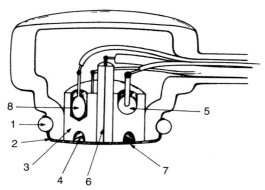

**Fig. 3-14** Schematic drawing of the modified Clark electrode used to monitor transcutaneous $O_2$ tension. **1**, O-ring to hold the membrane to the electrode; **2**, polypropylene membrane permeable to $O_2$; **3**, silver anode that surrounds the platinum cathode; **4**, electrolyte chamber with solution held in place by the polypropylene membrane; **5**, heating element; **6**, platinum cathode; **7**, electrolyte solution of sodium bicarbonate and sodium chloride held between the membrane and the electrode; and **8**, negative temperature coefficient resistor that serves to regulate the temperature of the sensor. *(From Shapiro BA, Peruzzi WT, Kozelowski-Templin R: Clinical application of blood gases, ed 5, St Louis, 1994, Mosby.)*

### 4. Put the transcutaneous oxygen monitor together and make sure it works properly (NBRC code: IIA21) [Difficulty: R]

Always follow the manufacturer's recommendations for assembly and care of the equipment. Select the proper electrode for the monitor based on the physician's order for evaluating $PtcO_2$, $PtcCO_2$, or both at the same time.

Two-point calibration must be performed before the $PtcO_2$ electrode is placed on the patient. Usually, the first calibration point is a "zero" point because the electrode is exposed to 0% $O_2$ in a nitrogen-filled chamber. This point is usually quite stable. The second calibration point is found when the electrode is exposed to room air (20.95% or 0.2095 $O_2$). Always follow the manufacturer's written procedures during the calibration process.

Expose the electrode to room air to determine whether it matches the calculated calibration value. Adjust the instrument to match the calibration $PtcO_2$ if necessary. It is recommended that the room air calibration point be rechecked every 24 hr when in continuous use, after the membrane is changed, and after the electrolyte solution is changed. A variation of up to ±5 torr is acceptable and can be corrected by adjusting the reading on the instrument. If the variation is greater than ±5 torr, the zero-point and room air calibration procedures should be repeated.

### 5. Troubleshoot any problems with the equipment (NBRC code: IIA21) [Difficulty: R]

Problems usually associated with too much electrode drift include the following: electrode or membrane surfaces contaminated by debris (e.g., blood or sweat), an improperly applied membrane, a worn-out membrane, an air bubble beneath the membrane, improper gas exposed to the membrane during the calibration, exhausted electrolyte solution in the electrode, and inaccurate calibration values. After the problem is corrected, the calibration procedure should be repeated.

An airtight seal is necessary between the skin and electrode for accurate readings. An air leak results in an increase in the $PtcO_2$ reading (and a fall in the transcutaneous $CO_2$ reading). The following steps should be taken to ensure that the skin site and electrode are prepared and an airtight seal is achieved:

a. Cleanse the skin; usually cleansing with an alcohol swab is enough to remove perspiration, but oily skin should be cleansed with soap and water.
b. Adults may need to have hair shaved at the site.
c. Adults may have some of the dead skin cells removed by placing sticky adhesive tape against the site and pulling it off.
d. Prepare the electrode according to the manufacturer's guidelines; this normally includes placing a drop of the electrolyte solution on the electrode surface and placing a gas-permeable membrane with a double-adhesive ring over the electrode.
e. Press the other side of the adhesive ring against the monitoring site for an airtight seal.
f. As the electrode warms the skin, patient values will fluctuate; stabilization usually requires several min, after which patient values should be clinically useful.

## MODULE G
### Transcutaneous carbon dioxide monitoring

### 1. Review the patient's chart for a transcutaneous carbon dioxide value (NBRC code: IA6d) [Difficulty: R, Ap]

Transcutaneous $CO_2$ ($PtcCO_2$, $tcPCO_2$, or $TcCO_2$) monitoring enables any patient's ventilation status to be followed on a continuous basis. In practice, neonates are monitored much more often than adults. Check the chart for a record of the patient's $PtcCO_2$ values. Correlating these values with any ABG values is particularly important because it allows comparison of the $PaCO_2$ and $PtcCO_2$ values. In addition, note what the $PtcCO_2$ values are when changes are made in CPAP or mechanical ventilation. Avoid clinical situations that resulted in earlier hypoventilation.

The information on skin site selection and preparation and patient precautions that was presented earlier in the discussion of $PtcO_2$ monitors applies here as well. As with the $PtcO_2$ electrode, it has been found that heating the $PtcCO_2$ electrode speeds up the diffusion of $CO_2$ through the skin. Always follow the manufacturer's recommendations for proper electrode temperature. The temperature is generally 44° C in both neonates and adults.

Remember that the $PtcCO_2$ value is *not* the same as the $PaCO_2$ value. An ABG should be drawn for $PaCO_2$ every time transcutaneous $CO_2$ monitoring is started. Unlike in $PtcO_2$ monitoring, the correlation between $PaCO_2$ and $PtcCO_2$ is as good in adult as in neonatal patients and is not as influenced by changes in the patient's skin blood flow.

The net effect of heating the $CO_2$ electrode and skin is $PtcCO_2$ readings that are 1.2 to 2 times (120% to 200%) greater than $PaCO_2$ values. Commonly, an average multiplier of 1.6 is found. The actual value varies among patients and can be found by dividing the $PtcCO_2$ by the $PaCO_2$.

For example, a patient has a $PaCO_2$ of 40 torr and a $PtcCO_2$ of 64 torr. Calculate the gradient between the arterial and transcutaneous values.

$$Gradient = PtcCO_2/PaCO_2 = 64/40 = 1.6$$

As long as the patient's cardiovascular status is fairly stable, the $PaCO_2$ can be calculated by dividing the $PtcCO_2$ by 1.6. For example, if the patient's $PtcCO_2$ increases to 80 torr, calculate the $PaCO_2$.

$$PaCO_2 = 80(PtcCO_2)/1.6 = 50 \, torr$$

Rather than perform these calculations every time the patient's status changes, some practitioners divide the $CO_2$ values found during the calibration procedure by 1.6. This results in "real" $PaCO_2$ values that are given continuously on the monitor. This change must be clearly communicated to all staff members to avoid confusion between the original $PtcCO_2$ values and values that have been reduced for the purpose of "arterializing" them.

### 2. Recommend transcutaneous carbon dioxide monitoring for additional data (NBRC code: IB9) [Difficulty: R, Ap]

$PtcCO_2$ monitoring has been used for the following purposes:

   a. Monitoring of ventilation of an unstable infant during transportation within the hospital or between two hospitals

   b. Intraoperative and postoperative monitoring of ventilation

   c. Monitoring of ventilation during changes in mechanical ventilation, such as tidal volume, rate, minute ventilation, or mechanical dead space

   d. Detection of hypoventilation during accidental disconnection from the ventilator

### 3. Get the necessary equipment to perform transcutaneous carbon dioxide monitoring (NBRC code: IIA21) [Difficulty: R]

The electrode used for monitoring the patient's $PtcCO_2$ level is a miniaturized and modified Stow-Severing-

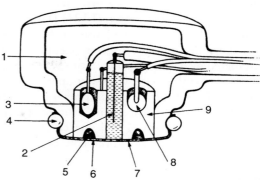

**Fig. 3-15** Schematic drawing of the modified Stow-Severinghaus electrode used to monitor transcutaneous $CO_2$ tension. **1,** Epoxy resin; **2,** glass electrode with a chlorinated silver wire, a buffer solution (the inner liquid), and a pH-sensitive glass membrane; **3,** negative temperature coefficient resistor that serves to regulate the temperature of the sensor; **4,** O-ring to hold the membrane to the electrode; **5,** electrolyte chamber with solution held in place by the polypropylene membrane; **6,** electrolyte solution of sodium bicarbonate and sodium chloride held between the membrane and the electrode; **7,** polypropylene membrane permeable to $CO_2$; **8,** heating element; and **9,** silver/silver chloride reference electrode. *(From Shapiro BA, Peruzzi WT, Kozelowski-Templin R: Clinical application of blood gases, ed 5, St Louis, 1994, Mosby.)*

haus–type electrode similar to the ABG electrode (Fig. 3-15).

### 4. Put the transcutaneous carbon dioxide monitor together and make sure it works properly (NBRC code: IIA21) [Difficulty: R]

Always follow the manufacturer's recommendations for assembly and care of the equipment. Select the proper electrode for the monitor based on the physician's order for evaluating $PtcCO_2$, $PtcO_2$, or both at the same time.

Two-point calibration must be performed before the $PtcCO_2$ electrode is placed on the patient. Usually, the electrode is exposed to 5% and 10% $CO_2$ from prepared cylinders. Always follow the manufacturer's written procedures during the calibration process. Expose the electrode to 10% $CO_2$ in a sealed chamber to determine whether it matches the calculated calibration value. Adjust the instrument to match the calibration $PtcCO_2$ if necessary. Next, expose the electrode to 5% $CO_2$ in the sealed chamber. Again, adjust the instrument to match the calibration $PtcCO_2$ if necessary. Rechecking the two-point calibration points every 24 hr is recommended during continuous use, after the membrane is changed, and after the electrolyte solution is changed. A variation of up to ±4 torr is acceptable and can be corrected by adjusting the instrument reading. If the variation is greater than ±4 torr, two-point calibration procedures should be repeated.

**5. Troubleshoot any problems with the equipment (NBRC code: IIA21) [Difficulty: R]**

Problems usually associated with too much electrode drift include the following: electrode or membrane surfaces contaminated by debris (e.g., blood or sweat); an improperly applied membrane; a worn-out membrane; an air bubble beneath the membrane; improper gas exposed to the membrane during calibration; exhausted electrolyte solution in the electrode; and inaccurate calibration values. After the problem has been corrected, the calibration procedure should be repeated.

## MODULE H
### Respiratory care plan

**1. Analyze the available information to determine the patient's pathophysiologic state (NBRC code: IIIH1) [Difficulty: R, Ap, An]**

ABG analysis remains the "gold standard" by which all other values are judged. Typically, the arterial sample is analyzed through a standard blood gas analyzer. A CO-oximeter is needed if the patient has CO poisoning. Mixed venous and capillary blood sample analysis is limited in clinical application but very helpful in the right patient situation. However, these offer only momentary insight into the patient's condition.

Pulse oximetry and $PtcO_2$ monitoring offer continuous information on the patient's oxygenation. $PtcCO_2$ monitoring allows continuous monitoring of the patient's ventilation. As with all technology, these units have advantages, disadvantages, and limitations. The respiratory therapist is responsible for making the correct choices. Some unstable patients can best be monitored through the combination of periodic evaluation of ABGs and these noninvasive continuous monitoring systems.

Many patients with pneumonia or other pulmonary conditions will have significant hypoxemia despite receiving supplemental oxygen. This gap between the alveolar oxygen level and the arterial oxygen level is called the alveolar-arterial oxygen pressure difference $[P(A - a)O_2]$. Measurement of this gap or difference gives an important indication of the seriousness of the patient's condition. Perform the following to determine the alveolar-arterial $O_2$ pressure difference $[P(A - a)O_2]$:

a. Note the patient's inspired $O_2$ percentage.
b. Draw and analyze an ABG sample. Note the patient's $PaO_2$ and $PaCO_2$.
c. Note the patient's temperature. This is needed to determine the patient's $PH_2O$. The value of 47 torr is used if the patient's temperature is normal. Check published tables for the $PH_2O$ if the patient's temperature is higher or lower than normal.
d. Measure the local $P_B$ in torr.
e. If possible, calculate the patient's respiratory exchange ratio. If this cannot be done, use the standard value of 0.8.

f. Calculate the patient's $PAO_2$. The formula presented here is the most commonly used of several versions:

$$PAO_2 = [(P_B - PH_2O)F_IO_2] - \frac{PaCO_2}{0.8}$$

Where:

$PAO_2$ = Pressure of alveolar $O_2$

$P_B$ = Barometric pressure of air; 760 torr at sea level (decreases as the altitude increases)

$PH_2O$ = Pressure of water vapor in the lungs; 47 torr at 37° C (98.6° F) (remember that $PH_2O$ increases if the patient has a fever and decreases if the patient is hypothermic)

$F_IO_2$ = Fractional concentration (percentage) of inspired $O_2$; use the percentage of $O_2$ that the patient is breathing

$\frac{PaCO_2}{0.8}$ = Effect of $CO_2$ and the patient's metabolism.

The factor of 0.8 is based on how much $O_2$ a normal person uses and how much $CO_2$ is produced per minute. The symbols for this metabolic value are *R* for respiratory exchange ratio and *RQ* for respiratory quotient. The following calculation is based on a normal person's metabolism:

$$R \text{ or } RQ = \frac{VCO_2}{VO_2} = \frac{200 \, mL/min}{250 \, mL/min} = 0.8$$

Because many sick patients react unexpectedly, the factor has a range of 0.6 to 1.1, depending on $O_2$ consumption and $CO_2$ production. Assume that the factor is 0.8 unless you are told otherwise or the measurement is different.

g. Subtract the patient's $PaO_2$ from the $PAO_2$ to determine the $P(A - a)O_2$.

When you are interpreting the patient's value, remember that the $P(A - a)O_2$ in a normal young person should be no greater than 15 torr. The difference slowly increases as a normal person ages. Lung disease causes the value to increase significantly. Following are some examples of conditions in which measurement of the $P(A - a)O_2$ aids in diagnosis or treatment:

a. Patients who are hypoxemic because they are hypoventilating (increased $CO_2$) have a normal $P(A - a)O_2$ when they are breathing room air. Hypoxemia can be corrected by increased ventilation. Supplemental $O_2$ results in an expected increase in $PaO_2$.

b. Any condition with a low ventilation-to-perfusion ratio reveals an elevated $P(A - a)O_2$ when the patient is breathing room air. Supplemental $O_2$ results in an increase in $PaO_2$, but it is not as dramatic as that seen in the hypoventilating patient. Examples include asthma, bronchitis, emphysema, or any other condition with unequal distribution of air into and out of the lungs with relatively normal perfusion.

c. Any shunt-producing disease or condition. Examples include ARDS and right-to-left anatomic shunt, such as ventricular septal defect. The $P(A - a)O_2$ becomes greater as the $O_2$ percentage is increased. It is commonly accepted that a $P(A - a)O_2$ of greater than 350 torr, when 80% to 100% $O_2$ is administered, indicates refractory hypoxemia. The patient probably needs to be supported by a mechanical ventilator.

d. Any disease that produces a diffusion defect. Pulmonary fibrosis from any cause results in a wider than normal $P(A - a)O_2$. Supplemental $O_2$ results in an increase in the $PaO_2$, but it is not as great an increase as would be expected.

The following examples are offered to aid in calculation of $P(A - a)O_2$ and interpretation of the results.

## EXAMPLE 1

You are working in a major teaching hospital in Miami. The patient's physician asks you to calculate the $P(A - a)O_2$ on a 30-year-old patient. The following conditions exist:

$P_B = 760$ torr

$PH_2O = 47$ torr (because the patient's temperature is 37° C [98.6° F])

$F_IO_2 = 0.21$ (because the patient is breathing room air)

$PaCO_2 = 40$ torr from ABGs

$PaO_2 = 90$ torr from ABGs

$R = 0.8$

1. $PAO_2 = [(P_B - PH_2O) F_IO_2] - PaCO_2/0.8$
2. $PAO_2 = [(760 - 47) 0.21] - 40/0.8$
3. $PAO_2 = [(713) 0.21] - 50$
4. $PAO_2 = [150] - 50$
5. $PAO_2 = 100$ torr
6. $P(A - a)O_2 = 100 - 90 = 10$ torr

Interpretation: A $P(A - a)O_2$ of 10 torr is normal for a patient of this age. It is normal to see a difference between the alveolar and arterial $O_2$ levels that starts out in the range of 4 to 12 mm Hg and slowly increases with age.

## EXAMPLE 2

You are working in a major teaching hospital in Denver. You are asked to calculate the $P(A - a)O_2$ on a 40-year-old patient. The following conditions exist:

$P_B = 710$ torr

$PH_2O = 50$ torr (because the patient's temperature is 38° C [100° F])

$F_IO_2 = 0.35$ (because the patient is breathing 35% $O_2$ by mask)

$PaCO_2 = 55$ torr from ABGs

$PaO_2 = 65$ torr from ABGs

$R = 0.85$

1. $PAO_2 = [(P_B - PH_2O) F_IO_2] - PaCO_2/0.85$
2. $PAO_2 = [(710 - 50) 0.35] - 55/0.85$
3. $PAO_2 = [(660) 0.35] - 65$
4. $PAO_2 = [231] - 65$
5. $PAO_2 = 166$ torr
6. $P(A - a)O_2 = 166 - 65 = 101$ torr

Interpretation: The difference of 101 torr is elevated even though this patient is older than the patient in Example 1.

## 2. Determine the appropriateness of the prescribed therapy and goals for the patient's pathophysiologic state (NBRC code: IIIH3) [Difficulty: R, Ap, An]

As part of the patient care team, the respiratory therapist may need to evaluate the patient's blood gas values and other parameters to make a recommendation. For example, if the patient has CO poisoning, the best treatment is 100% $O_2$ by nonrebreather mask. Pure $O_2$ reduces the half-life of COHb to 60 to 90 min. A pulse oximeter should *not* be used to measure this patient's $O_2$Hb saturation. These units are unable to identify COHb and give misleadingly high $O_2$Hb saturation values.

Be prepared to make a recommendation on adjusting the patient's inspired $O_2$ based on the $PaO_2$ (or related) value. Also be prepared to make a recommendation on adjusting the patient's mechanical ventilation settings for tidal volume, rate, minute volume, or mechanical dead space based on the $PaCO_2$ (or related) value.

## BIBLIOGRAPHY

Aloan CA, Hill TV, editors: *Respiratory care of the newborn and child*, ed 2, Philadelphia, 1997, Lippincott-Raven.

American Academy of Pediatrics: Task force on transcutaneous oxygen monitors, *Pediatrics* 83(1):122, 1989.

American Association for Respiratory Care: Clinical practice guideline: Transcutaneous blood gas monitoring for neonatal and pediatric patients, *Respir Care* 39(12):1176, 1994.

American Association for Respiratory Care: Clinical practice guideline: Capillary blood gas sampling for neonatal and pediatric patients, *Respir Care* 39(12):1180, 1994.

American Association for Respiratory Care: Clinical practice guideline: Oxygen therapy in the acute care hospital, *Respir Care* 36(12):1410, 1991.

American Association for Respiratory Care: Clinical practice guideline: Pulse oximetry, *Respir Care* 36(12):1406, 1991.

American Association for Respiratory Care: Clinical practice guideline: Sampling for arterial blood gas analysis, *Respir Care* 37(8):913, 1991.

American Association for Respiratory Care: Clinical practice guideline: In-vitro pH and blood gas analysis and hemoximetry, *Respir Care* 38(5):505, 1993.

Barnes TA, editor: *Textbook of respiratory care practice*, ed 2, St Louis, 1994, Mosby.

Barnhart SL, Czervinske MP: *Perinatal and pediatric respiratory care*, Philadelphia, 1995, WB Saunders.

Blanchette T, Dziodzio J, Harris K: Pulse oximetry and normoximetry in neonatal intensive care, *Respir Care* 36(1):25, 1991.

Bohn DJ: Ask the Expert, *Respiratory tract*, 9 Feb 1988.

Branson RD, Hess DR, Chatburn RL, editors: *Respiratory care equipment*, ed 2, Philadelphia, 1999, Lippincott Williams & Wilkins.

Burton GC, Hodgkin JE, Ward JJ, editors: *Respiratory care: a guide to clinical practice*, ed 4, Philadelphia, 1997, Lippincott-Raven.

Cairo JM, Pilbeam SP: *Mosby's respiratory care equipment*, ed 7, St Louis, 2004, Mosby.

Czervinske MP: Arterial blood gas analysis and other cardiopulmonary monitoring. In Koff PB, Daily KE, Schroeder JS: *Techniques in bedside hemodynamic monitoring*, ed 4, St Louis, 1989, Mosby.

Eitzman D, Neu J: *Neonatal and pediatric respiratory care*, ed 2, St Louis, 1993, Mosby.

Elser RC: Quality control of blood gas analysis: A review, *Respir Care* 31(9):807, 1986.

Federal government releases CLIA '88 final regulations, *AARC Times* 16(4):76, 1992.

Fell WL: Sampling and measurement of blood gases. In Lane EE, Walker JF, editors: *Clinical arterial blood gas analysis*, St Louis, 1987, Mosby.

Fink JB, Hunt GE, editors: *Clinical practice in respiratory care*, Philadelphia, 1999, Lippincott-Raven.

Garza D, Becan-McBride K: *Phlebotomy handbook*, ed 4, Stamford, Conn, 1996, Appleton & Lange.

Instrumentation Laboratories: *Operator's manual for the IL282 CO-oximeter*, Lexington, Mass.

Jubran A, Tobin MJ: Reliability of pulse oximetry in titrating supplemental oxygen therapy in ventilator-dependent patients, *Chest* 97:1420, 1990.

Lane EE, Walker JF: *Clinical arterial blood gas analysis*, St Louis, 1987, Mosby.

Levitzky MG, Cairo JM, Hall SM: *Introduction to respiratory care*, Philadelphia, 1990, WB Saunders.

Madama VC: *Pulmonary function testing and cardiopulmonary stress testing*, ed 2, Albany, 1998, Delmar.

Mahoney JJ, Hodgkin JE, Van Kessel AL: Arterial blood gas analysis. In Burton GG, Hodgkin JE, Ward JJ, editors: *Respiratory care: a guide to clinical practice*, ed 4, Philadelphia, 1997, Lippincott-Raven.

Martin RJ: Transcutaneous monitoring: Instrumentation and clinical applications, *Respir Care* 35(6):577, 1990.

Mathews P, Conway L: Arterial blood gases and noninvasive monitoring of oxygen and carbon dioxide. In Wyka KA, Mathews PJ, Clark WF, editors: *Foundations of respiratory care*, Albany, 2002, Delmar.

Mohler JG, Collier CR, Brandt W: Blood gases. In Clausen JL, editor: *Pulmonary function testing guidelines and controversies*, Orlando, 1984, Grune & Stratton.

Moran RF: Assessment of quality control of blood gas/pH analyzer performance, *Respir Care* 26(6):538, 1981.

Moran RF: CLIA regulations. I. The cure might be worse than the disease, *AARC Times* 14(11):41, 1990.

Moran RF: CLIA regulations. II. An analysis of some technical requirements, *AARC Times* 14(12):25, 1990.

Nelson CM, Murphy EM, Bradley JK, et al: Clinical use of pulse oximetry to determine oxygen prescriptions for patients with hypoxemia, *Respir Care* 31(8):673, 1986.

Novametrics Medical Systems, *Product literature on transcutaneous monitoring*, Wallingford, Conn.

Peters JA, Hodgkin JE, Collier CA: Blood gas analysis and acid-base physiology. In Burton GG, Hodgkin JE, Ward JJ, editors: *Respiratory care: a guide to clinical practice*, ed 3, Philadelphia, 1991, JB Lippincott.

Ruppel G: *Manual of pulmonary function testing*, ed 8, St Louis, 2003, Mosby.

Salyer JW: Pulse oximetry in the neonatal intensive care unit, *Respir Care* 36(1):17, 1991.

Scanlan CL, Wilkins RL: Analysis and monitoring of gas exchange. In Wilkins RL, Stoller JK, Scanlan CL, editors: *Egan's fundamentals of respiratory care*, ed 8, St Louis, 2003, Mosby.

Shapiro BA, Kacmarek RM, Cane RD, et al, editors: *Clinical application of respiratory care*, ed 4, St Louis, 1991, Mosby.

Shapiro BA, Peruzzi WT, Templin R: *Clinical application of blood gases*, ed 5, St Louis, 1994, Mosby.

Sonnesso G: Are you ready to use pulse oximetry? *Nursing* 21(8):60, 1991.

Walton JR, Shapiro BA: Value and application of temperature-compensated blood gas data, *Respir Care* 25(2), 1980.

Welch JP, DeCesare R, Hess D: Pulse oximetry: Instrumentation and clinical applications, *Respir Care* 35(6):584, 1990.

Whitaker K: *Comprehensive perinatal & pediatric respiratory care*, ed 2, Albany, 1997, Delmar.

White GC: *Equipment theory for respiratory care*, ed 3, Albany, 1999, Delmar.

## SELF-STUDY QUESTIONS

1. Before drawing a blood gas sample from the radial artery, you should perform which test of adequate perfusion?
   A. Allen test
   B. Modified Allen test
   C. Blood pressure measurement
   D. $P(A - a)O_2$

2. A patient is brought into the emergency room after being rescued from a house fire. She is unconscious and has facial burns. The physician believes that she is suffering from smoke inhalation. What would you recommend as the best way to evaluate her?
   A. ABGs analyzed through a CO-oximeter
   B. Pulse oximetry
   C. ABGs analyzed through a standard blood gas analyzer
   D. $PtcO_2$ monitor

3. You are ordered to draw a blood sample from your patient's radial artery. You test for adequate circulation by having the patient make a fist while you put pressure over his ulnar and radial arteries. The patient's hand is then opened, and pressure is released from the ulnar artery. His hand color returns within 15 sec. This would indicate that
   A. The patient's radial circulation is adequate
   B. The patient's radial circulation is inadequate
   C. The patient's ulnar circulation is adequate
   D. The patient's ulnar circulation is inadequate

4. You are working in the intensive care unit when you notice that an arterial blood sample has been sitting out for 20 min. It was not put in ice water. You could expect the blood gas analysis to be affected in which ways?
   I. Increased $PaO_2$
   II. Increased $PaCO_2$
   III. Decreased $PaO_2$
   IV. Decreased $PaCO_2$
   V. Increased pH
   VI. Decreased pH
   A. I, II, and VI
   B. III, IV, and V
   C. II, III, and VI
   D. III, IV, and VI

5. You would recommend an arterial puncture to obtain a sample for blood gas analysis under which of the following conditions?
   I. To measure the patient's $PaO_2$ after a change in his inspired $O_2$
   II. Suspected CO poisoning
   III. To measure the patient's $PaCO_2$ after a change in his minute volume
   IV. After the patient has been admitted into the emergency room with a tension pneumothorax
   V. During a cardiopulmonary resuscitation attempt
   A. I
   B. I and III
   C. II and IV
   D. All of the above

6. Safety guidelines for the protection of the therapist who is drawing an ABG sample include which of the following?
   I. Wash your hands before drawing the sample.
   II. Put a glove on the hand used to draw the sample.
   III. Put a glove on the hand with which you feel the pulse.
   IV. Put gloves on both hands.
   V. Wear eyeglasses or goggles.
   A. IV and V
   B. I and V
   C. II
   D. III

7. A 50-year-old patient has a $PaO_2$ of 72 torr when breathing room air. You would interpret this as
   A. Normal for a person of his age
   B. Mild hypoxemia
   C. Moderate hypoxemia
   D. Severe hypoxemia

8. An acute rise in $PaCO_2$ from 40 to 50 torr would result in the following change in pH:
   A. Rise of 0.10 unit
   B. Fall of 0.05 unit
   C. Fall of 0.10 unit
   D. Rise of 0.05 unit

9. Interpret the following blood gas drawn from a patient who is breathing 40% $O_2$: $PaO_2$, 54 torr; $SaO_2$, 87%; pH, 7.37; $PaCO_2$, 62 torr; bicarbonate, 38 mEq/L; and base excess, +11 mEq/L.
   I. Corrected hypoxemia
   II. Uncorrected hypoxemia
   III. Metabolic alkalosis
   IV. Uncompensated metabolic acidosis
   V. Compensated respiratory acidosis
   A. I and IV
   B. I and III
   C. II and IV
   D. II and V

10. Interpret the following blood gas drawn when the patient was breathing in 35% $O_2$: $PaO_2$, 86 torr; $SaO_2$, 90%; pH, 7.29; $PaCO_2$, 37 torr; bicarbonate, 17 mEq/L; and base excess, −8 mEq/L.
    I. Corrected hypoxemia
    II. Uncorrected hypoxemia
    III. Compensated metabolic acidosis
    IV. Uncompensated metabolic acidosis
    V. Compensated respiratory acidosis
    A. II and IV
    B. I and IV
    C. II and V
    D. I and III

11. Interpret the following blood gas drawn from a patient who is breathing 21% $O_2$: $PaO_2$, 117 torr; $SaO_2$, 98%; pH, 7.57; $PaCO_2$, 20 torr; bicarbonate, 24 mEq/L; and base excess, +1 mEq/L.
    I. Normal oxygenation
    II. Excessively corrected hypoxemia
    III. Uncompensated respiratory alkalosis
    IV. Uncompensated metabolic acidosis
    V. Compensated respiratory and metabolic alkalosis
    A. II and III
    B. II and IV
    C. I and III
    D. I and IV

12. Interpret the following blood gas drawn from a patient who is breathing 60% $O_2$: $PaO_2$, 72 torr; $SaO_2$, 94%; pH, 7.18; $PaCO_2$, 50 torr; bicarbonate, 18 mEq/L; and base excess, −10 mEq/L.
    I. Uncorrected hypoxemia
    II. Corrected hypoxemia
    III. Uncorrected respiratory acidosis
    IV. Uncorrected metabolic acidosis
    V. Combined metabolic and respiratory acidosis
    A. I and V
    B. II and V
    C. II and III
    D. II and IV

13. Interpret the following blood gas drawn from a patient who is breathing 24% $O_2$: $PaO_2$, 57 torr; $SaO_2$, 91%; pH, 7.45; $PaCO_2$, 22 torr; bicarbonate, 16 mEq/L; and base excess, −6 mEq/L.
    I. Corrected hypoxemia
    II. Uncorrected hypoxemia
    III. Compensated respiratory alkalosis
    IV. Uncompensated respiratory alkalosis
    V. Combined metabolic and respiratory acidosis
    A. I and III
    B. I and IV
    C. II and III
    D. II and V

14. Which of the following would indicate that a patient's tissues are adequately oxygenated?
    A. $PaO_2$, 85 torr
    B. $P\bar{v}O_2$, 30 torr
    C. $S\bar{v}O_2$, 75%
    D. $SaO_2$, 90%

15. Blood gas analyzer calibration values are considered to be *in control* if they are
    A. Within 1 SD of the norm
    B. Within 2 SDs of the norm
    C. Within 3 SDs of the norm
    D. Within 4 SDs of the norm

16. A 50-year-old patient with emphysema seems to be tiring after 30 min into a weaning attempt on a Briggs adapter (T piece). The best way to evaluate her ventilatory status is by
    A. Checking her $PaO_2$ value
    B. Measuring a $PtcCO_2$ value
    C. Checking her $PaCO_2$ value
    D. Performing a bedside vital capacity

17. Your patient has Guillain-Barré syndrome and pneumonia. The patient has just been placed on 35% $O_2$ by mask. The physician asks for your suggestion on the best way to evaluate the patient's overall ability to breathe. You would recommend
    A. Doing a full set of pulmonary function tests
    B. Drawing an arterial blood sample for analysis
    C. Performing pulse oximetry
    D. Performing pulse oximetry and a force vital capacity measurement

18. You are called to evaluate a patient who is using a pulse oximeter. Upon entering the room, you notice a black woman with an oximeter probe on her right ear lobe. The monitor shows a weak pulse signal and a fluctuating $SpO_2$ value. Which of the following would you do in an attempt to correct the problem?
    I. Try monitoring from a fingertip.
    II. Switch to a probe over the bridge of the nose.
    III. Cover the probe with an opaque wrap.
    IV. Switch the probe to the left ear lobe.
    A. II
    B. I and III
    C. II and IV
    D. III

19. You are working with a postanesthesia patient who is on a $PtcCO_2$ monitor. The correlation factor between the $PaCO_2$ and $PtcCO_2$ is 1.4. The patient's previous $PtcCO_2$ was 63 torr. The nurse has called you because it is now 75 torr. The patient's approximate $PaCO_2$ would be calculated as
    A. 63 torr
    B. 75 torr
    C. 54 torr
    D. 105 torr

20. A 50-year-old male patient is being treated for a pulmonary embolism. He is receiving 50% $O_2$ by mask. The results of a $P(A − a)O_2$ study indicate that his alveolar-arterial difference is 205 torr. What is the best interpretation of this study?
    A. It should be repeated because these results are not physiologically possible.
    B. It is within the normal range.
    C. The alveolar-arterial difference is increased.
    D. The patient's condition is improving.

## ANSWER KEY AND RATIONALE

1. **B.** A modified Allen test is used to determine whether adequate perfusion exists through the ulnar artery in case the radial artery should become occluded. This would ensure that the hand is still well perfused. Allen test is used to determine adequate perfusion through the radial artery. Adequate arm blood pressure does not ensure adequate perfusion of the hand, should the radial artery become blocked. The $P(A - a)O_2$ test does not measure local perfusion.

2. **A.** Blood gas analysis through a CO-oximeter gives the most accurate results in that the unit can detect COHb. The other three choices cannot measure COHb. Additionally, pulse oximetry and $PtcO_2$ monitoring do not give $CO_2$ or pH values.

3. **C.** The described test and its results are of a positive modified Allen test. This positive result means that the patient has adequate ulnar circulation.

4. **C.** When a blood sample is not quickly cooled in ice water, the living tissue will continue to consume $O_2$ and produce $CO_2$. The increased $CO_2$ level will decrease the pH value.

5. **D.** All of the listed conditions would warrant a blood gas analysis because they all deal with significant oxygenation and/or $CO_2$ removal issues.

6. **A.** Standard precautions necessitate that gloves be worn on both hands when blood may be contacted by either hand. Additionally, the eyes should be protected from possible blood splashes.

7. **B.** Review Table 3-3 for the categories of hypoxemia.

8. **B.** Shapiro and associates (1994) have stated that an acute rise in $CO_2$ of 10 mm Hg results in a drop in pH of 0.05 unit.

9. **D.** A $PaO_2$ of less than 80 torr is uncorrected hypoxemia. A compensated respiratory acidosis is indicated by the increased $PaCO_2$ coupled with an increased bicarbonate and increased base excess found with a normal pH. Review Tables 3-2 and 3-8.

10. **B.** A $PaO_2$ of greater than 80 torr with supplemental $O_2$ is corrected hypoxemia. An uncompensated metabolic acidosis is indicated by the normal $PaCO_2$ coupled with decreased bicarbonate and decreased base excess found with an acidotic pH. Review Tables 3-2 and 3-8.

11. **C.** Normal oxygenation is indicated because the patient's $PaO_2$ is elevated as a result of hyperventilation ($PaCO_2$ of 20 torr). An uncompensated respiratory alkalosis is indicated by the low $PaCO_2$ coupled with normal bicarbonate and normal base excess found with an alkalotic pH. Review Tables 3-2 and 3-8.

12. **A.** A $PaO_2$ of less than 80 torr is uncorrected hypoxemia. A combined metabolic and respiratory acidosis is indicated by the increased $PaCO_2$ coupled with decreased bicarbonate and decreased base excess found with an acidotic pH. Review Tables 3-2 and 3-8.

13. **C.** A $PaO_2$ of less than 80 torr is uncorrected hypoxemia. A compensated respiratory alkalosis is indicated by the decreased $PaCO_2$ coupled with decreased bicarbonate and decreased base excess found with a normal pH. Review Tables 3-2 and 3-8.

14. **C.** As shown in Table 3-11, an $S\bar{v}O_2$ value of 75% is normal and correlates with normal tissue oxygenation. A $PvO_2$ of 30 torr indicates tissue hypoxia. Normal ABG values do not necessarily correspond to normal tissue oxygenation values.

15. **B.** Two SDs are considered "in control" with a blood gas analyzer. See Fig. 3-7.

16. **C.** The patient's $PaCO_2$ value best correlates with her ventilatory status and level of fatigue. The other tests are of value but give less direct evidence of her ability to breathe effectively.

17. **B.** The results of an ABG inform you of the patient's oxygenation and $PaCO_2$. Pulse oximetry gives information only on oxygenation. Pulmonary function tests do not give any information on the patient's $PaO_2$ and $PaCO_2$. Additionally, a full set of pulmonary function tests can be very tiring for the patient.

18. **B.** Some pulse oximeters get inaccurate readings through the skin of darkly pigmented patients. Blocking outside light with an opaque wrap or moving the probe to a lightly pigmented area such as a fingertip (without nail polish) often results in accurate readings.

19. **C.** The patient's approximate $PaCO_2$ value is found by dividing the $PtcCO_2$ by the correlation factor of 1.4. Review the example calculations in this chapter.

20. **C.** A $P(A - a)O_2$ value should be 15 torr or less in a normal person. Therefore, this patient's alveolar-arterial difference is increased. Review the example calculations in this chapter.

# 4 | Pulmonary Function Testing

A review of the most recent Entry Level Examinations has shown an average of 7 questions (5% of the exam) that cover pulmonary function testing.

## MODULE A
### Review the patient's record

### 1. Pulmonary function results (NBRC code: IA3) [Difficulty: R]

Be prepared to review the results of all types of pulmonary function tests.

### 2. Respiratory monitoring (e.g., rate, tidal volume, minute volume, I:E ratio, inspiratory and expiratory pressures, vital capacity) (NBRC code: IA6a, IA6b) [Difficulty: R, Ap]

Patients at risk of respiratory failure, such as those with a neurologic disease, should have their breathing monitored regularly. Information on spirometry tests is presented in the following section.

### 3. Lung compliance (NBRC code: IA6c) [Difficulty: R, Ap]

Lung compliance ($C_L$) is usually measured in patients with stiff lungs (as found with pulmonary fibrosis) or overly compliant lungs (as found with emphysema).

### 4. Airway resistance (NBRC code: IA6c) [Difficulty: R, Ap]

Patients with asthma or chronic bronchitis may have airway resistance (Raw) measured as part of bronchodilator therapy management. The patient's Raw decreases if medication in the proper type and amount is taken.

### 5. Work of breathing (NBRC code: IA6c) [Difficulty: R, Ap]

Work of breathing (WOB) is the patient's subjective feeling about his or her difficulty in breathing. A normal person with no cardiopulmonary disease does not feel any difficulty in breathing at rest. However, a patient with cardiopulmonary disease, such as COPD or congestive heart failure, feels an increased work of breathing, even at rest.

## MODULE B
### Spirometry tests

### 1. Perform spirometry tests (NBRC code: IIIE7) [Difficulty: R, Ap]

The following spirometry tests can be performed at the bedside for basic patient monitoring and in the pulmonary function testing laboratory as part of a detailed diagnostic study of the patient.

### 2. Tidal volume
#### a. Perform the procedure (NBRC code: IB7c) [Difficulty: R, Ap]

The tidal volume ($V_T$) is the volume of gas breathed out with each respiratory cycle. Realize that individual $V_T$s are rarely identical. Fig. 4-1 shows several $V_T$s before and after a nonforced (slow) vital capacity (VC). For that reason, it is recommended that the $V_T$s be accumulated for a minute (thus providing a minute volume [$\dot{V}_E$]) and the respiratory rate ($f$) counted. An average $V_T$ is found by dividing the $\dot{V}_E$ by $f$. If this cannot be done, find the average volume of at least six breaths. The average, predicted $V_T$ for a resting, afebrile, alert adult should be about

$$3 \text{ to } 4 \text{ mL/lb of ideal body weight} \quad or$$
$$7 \text{ to } 9 \text{ mL/kg of ideal body weight}$$

For example, the predicted $V_T$ range of a 154-lb (70-kg) patient would be calculated as follows:

$$3 \text{ to } 4 \text{ mL/lb} \times 154 \text{ lb} = 462 \text{ to } 616 \text{ mL}$$
$$7 \text{ to } 9 \text{ mL/kg} \times 70 \text{ kg} = 490 \text{ to } 630 \text{ mL}$$

The patient should be allowed to relax before the test is performed so that the measured volume is accurate and is not increased because of any undue stress or excitement. Keeping the instructions and demonstration simple and easy to follow helps reduce the patient's anxiety. Some patients cannot tolerate a full minute's $V_T$ measurement. In that case, obtain the average by measuring the accumulated $V_T$s for as long as possible and dividing by the number of respirations.

#### b. Interpret the results (NBRC code: IB8b) [Difficulty: R, Ap]

A $V_T$ that is larger or smaller than expected for the patient's size necessitates further evaluation. A small $V_T$ may be seen in patients who have a low metabolic rate, are asleep or in a coma, have neuromuscular diseases that

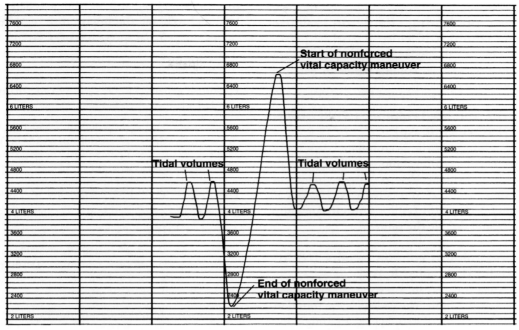

**Fig. 4-1** Tracing of tidal volumes and nonforced vital capacity.

prevent deep breathing, or are alkalotic. A large $V_T$ is seen in patients with a high metabolic rate, fever, dead space–producing diseases, increased intracranial pressure, or acidotic conditions.

### c. Monitor tidal volume (NBRC code: IA6b) [Difficulty: R, Ap]

Tidal volume should be monitored on a regular basis in patients with the previous conditions and in those who are being weaned from mechanical ventilation.

### 3. Inspiratory:expiratory ratio

### a. Review monitoring data on inspiratory:expiratory (I:E) ratio (IA6b) [Difficulty: R, Ap]

The inspiratory:expiratory (I:E) ratio is the ratio of the patient's inspiratory time ($T_I$) to the expiratory time ($T_E$). It can be simply measured at the bedside with a stopwatch. Or, it can be more accurately measured in the pulmonary function testing laboratory during spirometry testing.

### b. Monitor I:E ratio (NBRC code: IIIE8) [Difficulty: R, Ap]

Make sure that the patient is relaxed and is breathing in the normal pattern so accurate results will be obtained. Measure several of the patient's $T_I$ and $T_E$ readings to figure an average for each. For a more complete analysis of the patient's breathing pattern, a spirometer that gives a printout will be needed.

**Exam Hint**

**T**he National Board of Respiratory Care (NBRC) is known to test the examinee's ability to calculate (1) the $T_I$ and $T_E$ from a given I:E ratio and $f$, and (2) the I:E ratio from a given $T_I$ and $T_E$. These examples should help.

1. Calculate the patient's $T_I$ and $T_E$ when the I:E ratio is 1:2 and $f$ is 12/min.
   
   a. $\dfrac{60\,\text{sec/min}}{12\,\text{breaths/min}} = 5\,\text{sec/respiratory cycle}$
   
   b. $\dfrac{5\,\text{sec/respiratory cycle}}{3\,\text{parts of I and E}} = 1.66\,\text{sec for one part}$
   
   c. $T_I = 1\,\text{part} = 1.66\,\text{sec}$
   
   d. $T_E = 2\,\text{parts} = 3.32\,\text{sec}$

2. Calculate the neonatal patient's I:E ratio when the $T_I$ is 0.3 sec and the $T_E$ is 0.9 sec.
   
   a. $\text{I:E} = \text{I/E} = 0.3\,\text{sec}/0.9\,\text{sec}$
   
   b. $\text{I/E} = 1/3$ (The I:E ratio is 1:3.)

### c. Interpret the I:E ratio results (NBRC code: IIIE8) [Difficulty: R, Ap]

A normal, spontaneously breathing patient has an I:E ratio of 1:2 to 1:4. A prolonged $T_I$ is often seen in patients with an upper airway obstruction. A prolonged $T_E$ is often seen in patients with asthma or chronic obstructive pulmonary disease (COPD). Any abnormal I:E ratio should be investigated.

## 4. Minute volume

### a. Review monitoring data on minute volume (IA6b) [Difficulty: R, Ap]

The $\dot{V}_E$ is the volume of gas exhaled in 1 min. Often, it will vary in the same way as tidal volume varies in patients with cardiopulmonary problems.

### b. Perform minute volume (NBRC code: IB7c) [Difficulty: R, Ap]

$\dot{V}_E$ is found by adding up the accumulated $V_T$s for a minute, thereby usually yielding a more stable value than is attained with individual $V_T$s. A simple handheld spirometer is often used to accumulate the $V_T$ breaths. If the patient cannot perform the test for a minute, measure breaths for 30 sec and double the value.

### c. Interpret minute volume results (NBRC code: IB8b) [Difficulty: R, Ap]

The predicted range for a $\dot{V}_E$ in a resting, afebrile, alert adult should be 5 to 10 L/min. The wide range is found in part because it is a product of two factors: $V_T$ and $f$. One or both of these factors may be normal, abnormally high, or abnormally low. For these reasons, the $\dot{V}_E$ must be evaluated, along with the $V_T$ and $f$, before any conclusion can be reached about the patient's condition.

## 5. Alveolar ventilation

### a. Review monitoring data on alveolar ventilation (IA6b) [Difficulty: R, Ap]

Alveolar ventilation ($V_A$) is the amount of $V_T$ that reaches the alveoli. It can be calculated on a breath-to-breath basis. However, the patient's breathing is usually monitored for a minute to calculate the minute alveolar ventilation ($\dot{V}_A$). This results in a more stable value in that each individual tidal volume breath can vary considerably.

### b. Perform the alveolar ventilation procedure (NBRC code: IB7c) [Difficulty: R, Ap]

Alveolar ventilation is calculated by subtracting the physiologic dead space (anatomic plus alveolar dead space) from the measured exhaled $V_T$. For a bedside test, only the estimated anatomic dead space, which is estimated at 1 mL/lb or 2.2 mL/kg of lean body weight, can be subtracted. The alveolar dead space measurement requires sophisticated equipment, which is usually available only in a laboratory that tests pulmonary function. Clinically normal people have very little alveolar dead space.

*Example.* A 154-lb/70-kg person has a measured $V_T$ of 500 mL and an estimated anatomic dead space of about 154 mL. The calculated $\dot{V}_A$ = 500 mL − 154 mL = 346 mL.

### c. Interpret the alveolar ventilation results (NBRC code: IB8b) [Difficulty: R, Ap]

The following examples show how the patient's $\dot{V}_A$ can vary considerably because of changes in the $f$ and $V_T$, even though the $\dot{V}_E$ remains unchanged. These examples are included to show the importance of $\dot{V}_A$ in the patient's values for partial pressure of $CO_2$ in arterial blood ($PaCO_2$).

*Examples*

1. Normal patient: $f$ = 12; $V_T$ = 500 mL; anatomic dead space = 154 mL

$$\dot{V}_E = 12 \times 500\,mL = 6000\,mL$$
$$\dot{V}_A = 12 \times (500\,mL - 154\,mL)$$
$$= 12 \times 346\,mL$$
$$= 4152\,mL$$

This patient should have a normal $CO_2$ level.

2. Tachypneic patient: $f$ = 24; $V_T$ = 250 mL; anatomic dead space = 154 mL

$$\dot{V}_E = 24 \times 250\,mL = 6000\,mL$$
$$\dot{V}_A = 24 \times (250\,mL - 154\,mL)$$
$$= 24 \times 96\,mL$$
$$= 2304\,mL$$

This patient should have a high $CO_2$ level.

3. Bradypneic patient: $f$ = 6; $V_T$ = 1000 mL; anatomic dead space = 154 mL

$$\dot{V}_E = 6 \times 1000\,mL = 6000\,mL$$
$$\dot{V}_A = 6 \times (1000\,mL - 154\,mL)$$
$$= 6 \times 846\,mL$$
$$= 5076\,mL$$

This patient should have a low $CO_2$ level.

## 6. Measure and interpret the patient's maximal inspiratory pressure at the bedside

### a. Review monitoring data on maximal inspiratory pressure (IA6a, IA6b) [Difficulty: R, Ap]

The maximal inspiratory pressure (MIP), also known as negative inspiratory force (NIF), is the greatest amount of negative pressure the patient can create when inspiring against an occluded airway. Factors that affect the test results include strength of the diaphragm and accessory muscles of inspiration, lung volume when the airway is occluded, ventilatory drive, and the length of time the airway is occluded. MIP is most commonly used to determine whether mechanically ventilated patients should be weaned and to help monitor the strength of patients with a neuromuscular disease.

### b. Perform the maximal inspiratory pressure procedure (NBRC code: IB7g) [Difficulty: R, Ap]

A study of the literature reveals that a number of measurement devices have been assembled and that different bedside techniques have been used to determine the effort of patients who are breathing naturally or while intubated and on a mechanical ventilator. Branson and

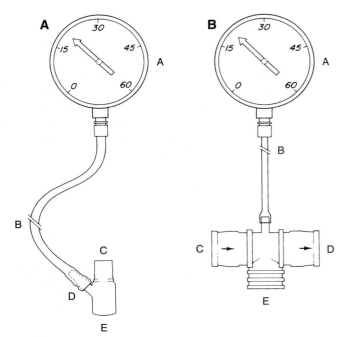

**Fig. 4-2** Two systems for measuring maximal inspiratory pressure (MIP) on a patient with an artificial airway. *A,* Simple occlusion. *A,* Pressure manometer; *B,* Connecting tubing; *C,* Port to be occluded during the MIP; *D,* Connection of the adapter to the manometer; *E,* Port to connect to the patient's airway. *B,* One-way valve. *A,* Pressure manometer; *B,* Connecting tubing; *C,* Inspiratory port to be occluded during the MIP effort; *D,* Expiratory port; *E,* Port to be connected to the patient's artificial airway. *(From Kacmarek RM, Cycyk-Chapman MD, Young-Palazzo PJ, et al: Determination of maximal inspiratory pressure: A clinical study and literature review, Respir Care 34:868, 1989.)*

associates (1989) and Kacmarek and associates (1989) make a strong case for using a double one-way valve to connect the intubated patient to the manometer (Fig 4-2). Use of the one-way valve lets the patient exhale but prevents inhalation when the practitioner occludes the opening. This forces the patient to inhale from closer to RV with each breathing effort. In addition, the use of a double one-way valve allows the test to be performed on an unconscious and uncooperative patient. Investigators in the two studies also recommend that the patient should make inspiratory efforts for 15 to 20 sec. Steps in the MIP procedure for a normally breathing patient include the following:

a. Obtain a pressure gauge capable of measuring pressure of at least −60 cm $H_2O$.
b. Have the patient sit upright. Place a note in the chart if the patient is lying down.
c. Describe the procedure to the patient.
d. Simulate a demonstration of the procedure.
e. Place nose clips over the patient's nose. Have the patient seal his or her lips and teeth around the mouthpiece and breathe through the open port.
f. Tell the patient to exhale completely. Seal the port when residual volume (RV) has been reached.
g. Tell the patient to breathe in as hard as possible and hold for 1 to 3 sec.
h. Reteach if necessary.
i. Repeat until at least three good efforts have been made. Record the greatest stable value seen after the first second of effort. This eliminates any artifact created by the cheeks or by chest wall movement.

### c. Interpret the maximal inspiratory pressure results (NBRC code: IB8e) [Difficulty: R, Ap]

Patients of either sex and any age should be able to generate at least −60 cm $H_2O$. This is enough to ensure that the patient has enough strength and coordination to protect the airway, take a deep breath, and cough effectively. Patients with neuromuscular disease, disease of the respiratory muscles, a thoracic injury or abnormality, or chronic obstructive lung disease tend to have decreased strength. The patient who cannot generate at least −20 cm $H_2O$ is at risk and probably does not have the strength to cough effectively. Depending on the blood gas values and other physical parameters, the patient may need to be intubated and maintained on a mechanical ventilator.

Black and Hyatt (1969) published the following MIP prediction formulas for spontaneously breathing, nonintubated adult subjects between 20 and 86 years of age who are breathing from RV. The values are expressed in centimeters of water pressure. The older the patient, the lower is the predicted MIP.

|  | Lower limits of normal |
|---|---|
| Men: 143 − (0.55 × age) | −75 cm $H_2O$ |
| Women: 104 − (0.51 × age) | −50 cm $H_2O$ |

### d. Monitor the patient's maximal inspiratory pressure (NBRC code: IIIE8) [Difficulty: R, Ap]

A patient who is being weaned from mechanical ventilation or who has a deteriorating neuromuscular condition should have MIP measured on a frequent basis. If the patient cannot generate at least −20 cm $H_2O$, the physician should be notified. Mechanical ventilation is probably needed.

Monitoring of any patient for signs of undue stress and hypoxemia, such as tachycardia, bradycardia, ventricular dysrhythmia, hypertension, hypotension, or decreasing saturation on pulse oximetry, is important. If any of these is seen, the procedure should be stopped and the patient reoxygenated and ventilated. Some patients make their best effort on the first or second inspiration with decreasing effort as they continue trying, probably because of fatigue. Stop the procedure and record the best effort.

## Exam Hint

**E**xpect to see at least one question in which the MIP value is used to help determine if a patient is getting stronger or weaker. If the patient's MIP is at least $-20\,cm\,H_2O$ (for example, $-35\,cm\,H_2O$), and other conditions are acceptable, the patient can be weaned from the mechanical ventilator. Conversely, if the patient's MIP is not at least $-20\,cm\,H_2O$ (for example, $-15\,cm\,H_2O$), and other conditions are unacceptable, the patient should not be weaned from the mechanical ventilator.

### 7. Maximal expiratory pressure
#### a. Review monitoring data on maximal expiratory pressure (IA6b) [Difficulty: R, Ap]

The maximal expiratory pressure (MEP), also known as maximal expiratory force (MEF), is the greatest amount of positive pressure the patient can create when expiring from total lung capacity (TLC) against an occluded airway. Factors that affect the test results include patient cooperation and effort, strength of the expiratory muscles, lung volume when the airway is occluded, ventilatory drive, and the length of time the airway is occluded. It is used to determine whether mechanically ventilated patients should be weaned and to monitor the strength of patients with neuromuscular disease.

#### b. Perform the maximal expiratory pressure procedure (NBRC code: IB7g) [Difficulty: R, Ap]

As with the MIP test, a study of the literature reveals that a number of measurement devices have been assembled, and that different bedside techniques have been used to determine the effort of a patient who is breathing naturally and one who is intubated and breathing by way of a mechanical ventilator. A strong case can be made for the use of a double one-way valve to connect the intubated patient to the manometer (see Fig. 4-2). Use of the one-way valves lets the patient inhale but prevents exhalation when the practitioner occludes the expiratory opening. This forces the patient to exhale from closer to TLC with each breathing effort. However, the expiratory efforts should not be held for longer than 3 sec. In addition, the use of a double one-way valve allows the test to be performed on an unconscious and uncooperative patient. This test is similar to Valsalva's maneuver, and the high intrathoracic pressure can cause reduced cardiac output.

Steps in the MEP procedure for a normally breathing patient include the following:
a. Obtain a pressure gauge that is capable of measuring at least $+60\,cm\,H_2O$.

b. Have the patient sit upright. Place a note in the chart if the patient is lying down.
c. Describe the procedure to the patient.
d. Simulate a demonstration of the procedure.
e. Place nose clips over the patient's nose. Have the patient seal his or her lips and teeth around the mouthpiece and breathe through the open port.
f. Tell the patient to inhale completely. Seal the port when total lung capacity (TLC) has been reached.
g. Tell the patient to breathe out as hard as possible and hold for 1 to 3 sec.
h. Reteach if necessary.
i. Repeat until at least three good efforts have been made. Record the greatest stable value seen after the first second of effort. This eliminates any artifact created by the cheeks or by chest wall movement.

Monitoring of any patient for signs of undue stress and hypoxemia, such as tachycardia, bradycardia, ventricular dysrhythmia, hypotension, or decreasing saturation on pulse oximetry, is important. If any of these is seen, the procedure should be stopped and the patient reoxygenated and ventilated.

#### c. Interpret the maximal expiratory pressure results (NBRC code: IB8e) [Difficulty: R, Ap]

Clinically normal people of either sex and any age should be able to generate at least $+80\,cm\,H_2O$. Patients with neuromuscular disease, thoracic injury or abnormality, or COPD tend to have decreased strength. A MEP value of $+40\,cm\,H_2O$ is probably enough to ensure that the patient has enough strength and coordination to cough effectively to clear secretions. However, depending on the blood gas values and other physical parameters, the patient may need to be intubated and maintained on a mechanical ventilator.

Black and Hyatt (1969) published the following MEP prediction formulas for spontaneously breathing, nonintubated adult subjects between 20 and 86 years old who are breathing from TLC. These values are expressed in centimeters of water pressure. The older the patient, the lower is the predicted MEF.

|  | Lower limit of normal |
|---|---|
| Men: $268 - (1.03 \times age)$ | $+ 140\,cm\,H_2O$ |
| Women: $170 - (0.53 \times age)$ | $+ 95\,cm\,H_2O$ |

### 8. Vital capacity
#### a. Review monitoring data on vital capacity (IA6a) [Difficulty: R, Ap]

The vital capacity (VC) is the greatest volume of gas the patient can exhale after the lungs have been completely filled. Because there is no need to blow out quickly, this is sometimes called a *slow* or *nonforced vital capacity* (see Fig. 4-1). The forced vital capacity (FVC) is the greatest volume

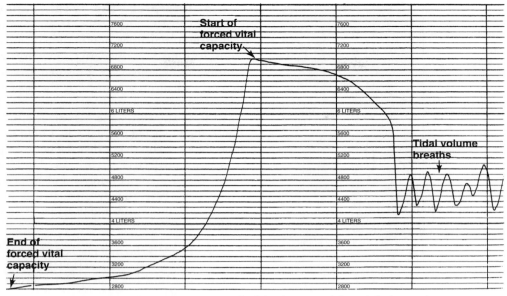

**Fig. 4-3** A volume-time tracing of tidal volumes and forced vital capacity.

of gas the patient can exhale *as rapidly as possible* after the lungs have been completely filled. Normally, the same volume is found in a slow VC and a forced VC.

The VC is commonly measured at the bedside in patients with neuromuscular disease and those who are being weaned from mechanical ventilation. A VC that is increasing toward the normal, predicted patient value is a good sign because it indicates that the patient is recovering. If the VC is decreasing, it is likely that the patient is becoming weaker and will not be able to cough out secretions effectively. Mechanical ventilation may be needed.

### b. Perform the vital capacity test (NBRC code: IB7c, IB7m, IIIE7) [Difficulty: R, Ap]

Careful instructions, demonstrations, and coaching are needed to ensure that the patient's efforts are the best possible. If the measurement instrument does not give a printout, simply record the patient's volume efforts in the chart. This is usually the case with a bedside slow VC. In the pulmonary function testing (PFT) laboratory, a printout of the data and the flow tracing will be obtained.

### c. Monitor vital capacity graphic tracings (NBRC code: IA6a) [Difficulty: R, Ap]

When a FVC is obtained in the PFT laboratory, at least *three* proper efforts must be obtained and printed out. (Fig. 4-3 shows the tracing of a properly performed FVC). The tracings enable the efforts to be compared for the best patient effort. The best effort is then recorded and is used for other types of tests to be discussed later. For example, see Fig. 4-4 in which the FVC has been subdivided into a series of volumes exhaled in 1-sec intervals. Because of

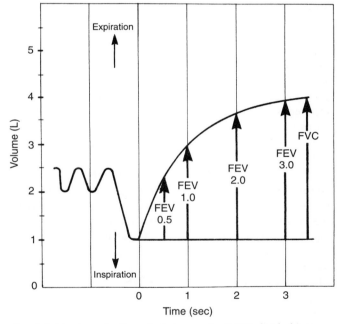

**Fig. 4-4** Tracing of a forced vital capacity (FVC) divided into $FEV_{0.5}$, $FEV_1$, $FEV_2$, and $FEV_3$. FEV, Forced expiratory volume. *(From Ruppel G: Manual of pulmonary function testing, ed 6, St Louis, 1994, Mosby.)*

this, the tracing is often referred to as a *volume-time curve*. Notice that the start of the effort is smooth and without interruption. The initial fast flow of gas from the upper airway is seen as the nearly vertical part of the tracing. The rest of the tracing is smooth with no coughing or other interruptions in the patient's effort. The tracing becomes

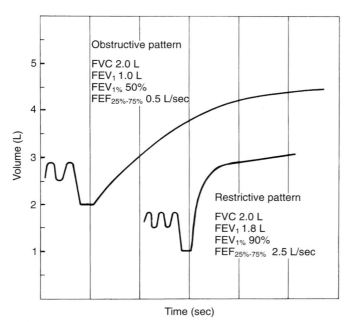

**Fig. 4-5** Forced vital capacity (FVC) tracings showing an obstructed flow pattern and a restrictive flow pattern. FEV, Forced expiratory volume; FVC, forced vital capacity. *(From Ruppel G: Manual of pulmonary function testing, ed 4, St Louis, 1986, Mosby.)*

progressively more horizontal as the end of the effort is reached. Encourage the patient to try to push out as much air as possible as the end approaches. Guidelines require that the patient keep pushing so that the total effort lasts at least 6 sec.

Fig. 4-3 was made on a chain-compensated, water-seal spirometry system. Notice how the tracing progresses from the right to the left. The Stead-Wells system shows the same tracing "upside down" compared with the chain-compensated system. The tracing starts on the left and moves to the right (see Fig. 4-4; Fig. 4-5). Other tracings could show either the chain-compensated or the Stead-Wells tracings in a mirror image or opposite shape.

---

### Exam Hint

**T**he NBRC can show an FVC tracing from any system and expect it to be interpreted. The start of the FVC effort can be determined by the near-vertical portion of the tracing and the relatively small expiratory reserve volume (ERV) compared with the inspiratory reserve volume (IRV). The examinee must be able to determine the various volumes and capacities from a spirometry tracing.

---

### b. Interpret the vital capacity results (NBRC code: IB8c, IB8i) [Difficulty: R, Ap]

Normally, racial differences in the FVC must be taken into consideration. Most modern pulmonary function systems automatically adjust the measured values for racial differences when programmed by the operator. If not, the predicted values should be mathematically adjusted by the therapist. Morris and associates (1971) reported the following predicted normal values in liters for the FVC in the white patient. (Note that the body temperature, pressure, saturated [BTPS] correction has been calculated into these equations. Morris and associates, and other researchers, have already calculated a standard patient and room temperature and barometric pressure into their formulas.)

Men: $[(0.148 \times \text{height in inches}) - (0.025 \times \text{age})] - 4.24$
  (1 standard deviation [1 SD] 0.58)
Women: $[(0.115 \times \text{height in inches}) - (0.024 \times \text{age})] - 2.85$
  (1 SD 0.52)

***Example.*** Calculate the predicted FVC of a 50-year-old white man who is 6 ft (72 in) tall.

$$
\begin{aligned}
\text{FVC} &= [(0.148 \times \text{height in inches}) - (0.025 \times \text{age})] - 4.24 \\
&= [(0.148 \times 72) - (0.025 \times 50)] - 4.24 \\
&= [10.656 - 1.25] - 4.24 \\
&= 9.406 - 4.24 \\
&= 5.166\,\text{L}
\end{aligned}
$$

Blacks have a smaller lung capacity than whites of the same height. Because of this, a 10% to 15% adjustment should be made for the predicted FVC and TLC of a black patient. In other words, the predicted values for a black patient would be 85% to 90% those of a comparable white patient. Adjustments for Hispanic and Asian populations are not as well documented. It has been reported that the predicted FVC values should be adjusted down by 20% to 25% for Asians.

A measured FVC that is at least 80% of the predicted FVC is considered to be within normal limits for adults of all races. The $FEV_1$ and TLC measurements have also been included in this "80% of predicted" rule. Knudson and associates (1987) and Paoletti and associates (1985) suggest that normal values for most tests should be determined by finding the "percent of predicted" above which 95% of the population would be seen (the so-called "normal 95th percentile"). Even though this method would find 5% (1 in 20) of healthy nonsmokers to be abnormal, for instance, it offers more realistic predicted values. A decline in the FVC with age is normal.

Restrictive problems such as advanced pregnancy, obesity, ascites, neuromuscular disease, sarcoidosis, and chest wall or spinal deformity commonly result in a small FVC. Patients with chronic obstructive lung disease such as emphysema, bronchitis, asthma, cystic fibrosis, and bronchiectasis can have a small FVC. Fig. 4-6 shows a com-

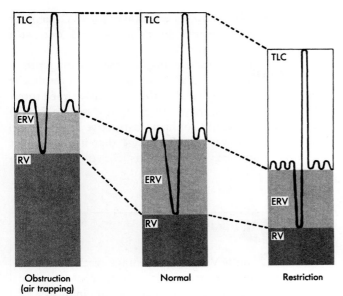

**Fig. 4-6** Tracings for obstructed, normal, and restricted patients. ERV, expiratory reserve volume; RV, residual volume; TLC, total lung capacity. *(Modified from Ruppel G: Manual of pulmonary function testing, ed 6, St Louis, 1994, Mosby.)*

parison of the spirometry tracings of normal, obstructed, and restricted patients.

One must understand the four normal lung volumes and four normal lung capacities before an understanding of how they shift with restrictive and obstructive diseases can be attained. See Fig. 4-7 for normal volumes and capacities and their relationships to each other. In general, with restrictive lung diseases, all volumes and capacities are decreased from predicted. The key findings are that the total lung capacity, functional residual capacity, and residual volume are less than 80% of predicted. In general, with obstructive lung diseases, all volumes and capacities are increased from predicted. The key findings are that the total lung capacity, functional residual capacity, and residual volume are more than 120% of predicted.

(The limitations of this text prevent discussion of back extrapolation to find the start of a less-than-perfect effort, or calculations for converting volumes and flows from atmospheric temperature, pressure, saturated [ATPS] to BTPS. However, most pulmonary function textbooks include discussion of these topics.)

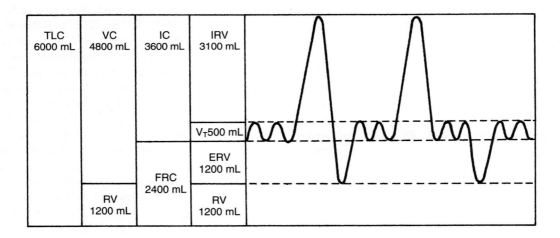

Volumes: Four primary

A. Tidal volume ($V_T$). The volume of gas inspired *or* expired during normal respiration.
B. Inspiratory reserve volume (IRV): The maximum volume of gas that can be inspired beyond a normal inspiration.
C. Expiratory reserve volume (ERV): The maximum volume of gas that can be exhaled after a normal expiration.
D. Residual volume (RV): The volume of gas remaining in the lungs after a maximum expiration.

Capacities: Four, which include two or more primary volumes

A. Total lung capacity (TLC): The total amount of gas contained in the lungs after maximum inspiration. Includes all four primary volumes (TLC = $V_T$ + IRV + ERV + RV).
B. Vital capacity (VC): The maximum amount of gas that can be exhaled after a maximum inspiration. Includes three primary volumes (VC = $V_T$ + IRV + ERV).
C. Inspiratory capacity (IC): The maximum amount of gas that can be inspired after a normal expiration. Includes two primary volumes (IC = $V_T$ + IRV).
D. Functional residual capacity (FRC): The total amount of gas remaining in the lungs after normal expiration. Includes two primary volumes (FRC = ERV + RV).

**Fig. 4-7** Lung volumes and capacities for a clinically normal young man.

## 9. Timed, forced expiratory volumes

### a. Perform the timed, forced expiratory volume (timed FEV) procedure (NBRC code: IB7d, IB7m) [Difficulty: R, Ap]

Timed FEVs effectively "cut" the FVC into sections according to how much volume the patient forcibly exhales in 0.5, 1, 2, and 3 sec ($FEV_{0.5}$, $FEV_1$, $FEV_2$, and $FEV_3$, respectively). Some patients with severe obstructive lung disease require several additional seconds to completely exhale. In these cases, simply keep measuring the volume exhaled in each additional second.

Some bedside units give a numerical value for some or all of the timed intervals. However, it is best for the therapist to have a spirometer that produces a printout of the patient's FVC effort. See Fig. 4-4 (from a Stead-Wells system) for an FVC tracing that is subdivided into 0.5-, 1-, 2-, and 3-sec intervals.

### b. Interpret the timed, forced expiratory volume results (NBRC code: IB8c) [Difficulty: R, Ap]

Obviously, every person exhales different volumes for these time intervals because FVCs vary among patients. The method that should be used to standardize this test is to divide the $V_TS$ by the FVC volume, then convert the fraction into a percentage. This value is called the *FEV_{timed %}*. These values can then be standardized for all individuals, even though FVCs vary from one person to the next. The following are predicted values for normal patients:

$FEV_{0.5}$ = 50% to 60% of the FVC
$FEV_1$ = 75% to 85% of the FVC
$FEV_2$ = 94% of the FVC
$FEV_3$ = 97% of the FVC

These values normally decrease slightly in the elderly patient. Most patients with normal lungs and airways are still able to completely exhale their FVC within 4 sec. Patients with restrictive lung diseases typically exhale their FVC more quickly than expected. This abnormal finding occurs because these patients tend to have a smaller-than-normal FVC, along with stiff lungs that recoil to their resting volume more quickly than would be expected. See Fig. 4-5 for comparison of the FVC curves of a patient with restrictive lung disease and one with obstructive lung disease.

Patients with obstructive lung disease take longer than expected to exhale their FVC (see Fig. 4-5). As a result, the percentages of FVC exhaled in the previously timed intervals are lower than normal. An $FEV_1$ of less than 65% to 70% of the FVC would confirm obstructive lung disease. Obviously, the lower the percentage that is exhaled for any timed interval, the worse is the obstruction to exhalation.

## 10. Peak flow

### a. Perform the peak flow procedure (NBRC code: IB7c, IB7m, IIIE7) [Difficulty: R, Ap]

The peak flow (PF), referred to by some authors as the *peak expiratory flow rate* (PEFR), is the greatest flow rate seen in a patient's forced expiratory effort. It is usually seen at the beginning of the FVC effort. Instructions for the test should emphasize that the patient must "blast" the air out as hard and quickly as possible. Encouraging the patient to completely empty the lungs to RV is unnecessary.

The patient's effort is easily directly measured from a handheld peak flowmeter. Usually, at least three efforts are necessary before two are found that are acceptably close. Recording of the patient's effort in liters per second (L/sec) is reasonable because the effort takes place in about that time. However, do not be confused by some measurement instruments and prediction equations that give the value in liters per *minute*. Simply multiply or divide by 60 to convert your patient's effort from one time to the other. For example, a young man's PF could be recorded as 10 L/sec or 600 L/min.

### b. Interpret the peak flow results (NBRC code: IB8b) [Difficulty: R, Ap]

Cherniack and Raber (1972) have published formulas for predicting PF in liters per second. The PF is directly related to height and indirectly related to age. Therefore, it would be expected that the taller the patient, the greater would be the flow. PF would be expected to decrease with age and is a rather nonspecific measurement of airway obstruction. It measures flow through the upper airways and is reduced in patients with an upper airway problem such as tumor, vocal cord paralysis, or laryngeal edema.

The PF test is most often given to patients who are having an asthma attack as a quick and easy measurement of small-airways obstruction. Asthma management guidelines state that if an asthma patient's PF is 80% to 100% of predicted, or personal best, he or she is in the "green zone." This means that the patient's medications are adequately controlling the asthma. If the PF is 50% to 79% of predicted or personal best, he or she is in the "yellow zone." This means that the patient's medications are not adequately controlling the asthma. Increased doses are indicated if ordered by the physician. If the PF is less than 50% of predicted or personal best, he or she is in the "red zone." The patient is in trouble and should get medical help as soon as possible.

## MODULE E
### Special purpose pulmonary function tests

1. **Spirometry before and after an aerosolized bronchodilator has been inhaled**
   a. **Perform the before and after aerosolized bronchodilator procedure (NBRC code: IB7m) [Difficulty: R, Ap]**

Following are common indications for the procedure:
1. Patient is known to have asthma or another type of chronic obstructive lung disease.
2. Patient has an $FEV_{1\%}$ of less than 70% (unless elderly).
3. Effectiveness of a new bronchodilator is being evaluated.

The most commonly administered tests are the PF and $FEV_{1\%}$ from an FVC. Either one or both should be measured before the bronchodilator is given to determine the patient's initial airway condition. Then, a fast-onset sympathomimetic-type drug is given. This medication can be given by intermittent positive-pressure breathing (IPPB), handheld nebulizer, or metered-dose inhaler, as long as the method is done properly. Wait about 10 to 15 min for the medication to take effect and for the patient's blood gas values to return to normal. Repeat the PF and/or the $FEV_{1\%}$ test. The percentage of improvement is calculated by using this formula:

$$\% \text{ of change} = \frac{\text{after-drug airflow} - \text{before-drug airflow}}{\text{before-drug airflow}} \times 100$$

   b. **Interpret the before and after aerosolized bronchodilator results (NBRC code: IB8i) [Difficulty: R, Ap]**

The medication is shown to be effective if the patient has both a 12% improvement in PF and/or $FEV_{1\%}$ and a 200-mL increase in exhaled volume. (Note: The old standard of at least a 15%–20% increase may still be used by some practitioners.) Patients with asthma who improve much more than this are not uncommon. Other patients may not have this much improvement but do show increases

in airflow and FVC and say that they feel better. In these cases, the physician may decide to continue the medication.

### Exam Hint

**A** post-bronchodilator increase in PF or a $FEV_{1\%}$ of at least 15% show reversible small-airways obstruction. This would indicate that a patient with asthma or COPD is responding to the inhaled bronchodilator.

2. **Flow-volume loops**
   a. **Review monitoring data on flow-volume loops (IA6b) [Difficulty: R, Ap]**

The flow-volume loop is a graphic display of the flow and volume generated during a forced expiratory vital capacity (FEVC) immediately followed by a forced inspiratory vital capacity (FIVC). It identifies inspiratory or expiratory flow at any lung volume.

   b. **Perform the flow-volume loop procedure (NBRC code: IB7m) [Difficulty: R, Ap]**

As with the FVC test, the patient should be coached to inhale completely and blast the air out until he or she is completely empty. When the patient has exhaled to residual volume (RV), coach him or her to inhale as quickly as possible until the lungs are completely full. There should be no hesitation at the start; nor should there be any leaks, closing of the glottis, or coughing throughout the entire procedure.

The expiratory half of the curve is called the *maximal expiratory flow volume (MEFV) curve.* It begins at TLC and ends at RV. The inspiratory half of the curve is called the *maximal inspiratory flow volume (MIFV) curve.* It begins at RV and ends at TLC. Ideally, the two halves of the loop meet at the TLC. Flow is recorded in liters per second and is graphed on the vertical (ordinate, or *y*) axis. Volume is recorded in liters and is graphed on the horizontal (abscissa, or *x*) axis. Both flow and volume should be BTPS adjusted.

   c. **Interpret the flow-volume loop results (NBRC code: IB8i, IIIE7) [Difficulty: R, Ap]**

Flow-volume loops have gained great popularity because the shape of the curve is diagnostic of the patient's condition. In addition, peak inspiratory and peak expiratory flows can be determined. If the effort can be timed, all the parameters found on the previously discussed volume-time curves can be found on the flow-volume loop. The following examples show a normal flow-volume loop and representative abnormal loops.

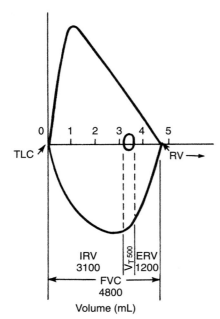

**Fig. 4-8** Flow-volume loop tracing of a normal adult showing the positions and values of lung volumes. ERV, expiratory reserve volume; FVC, forced vital capacity; IRV, inspiratory reserve volume; RV, residual volume; TLC, total lung capacity.

***Normal.*** A normal flow-volume loop is shown in Figs. 4-8 and 4-9. In Fig. 4-8, the various volumes are measured on the horizontal scale. The $V_T$ of 500 mL is the small loop within the larger VC loop. The ERV and IRV are shown on both sides of the $V_T$. The FVC is shown as the total of all three volumes. Finally, TLC and RV are marked.

Fig. 4-9 shows the same normal flow-volume loop where the various flows are measured on the vertical scale. Starting from TLC with the FEVC, the PEFR is seen as the greatest flow generated, at about 9 L/sec. Starting from RV with the FIVC, the peak inspiratory flow rate (PIFR) is seen as the greatest flow generated, at about 7 L/sec. The PEFR is normally greater than the PIFR.

In determining the instantaneous flow at any FVC lung volume, the FVC must be divided by 4 to yield the 25th, 50th, and 75th percentile points. In Fig. 4-9, the FVC is 4800 mL. Dividing by 4 gives 1200 mL per quarter of the FVC. These points are marked on the horizontal volume scale. If a vertical (dashed) line is drawn through these three points to the flow-volume tracing, the instantaneous flows at these volumes can be found. The following *expiratory flows* are reported:

a. Flow at 75% of the FEVC = $\dot{V}_{max75\%}$ (maximal flow with 75% of the FVC remaining) or $FEF_{25\%}$ (forced expiratory flow with 25% of the FVC exhaled)
b. Flow at 50% of the FEVC = $\dot{V}_{max50\%}$ (maximal flow with 50% of the FVC remaining) or $FEF_{50\%}$ (forced expiratory flow with 50% of the FVC exhaled)

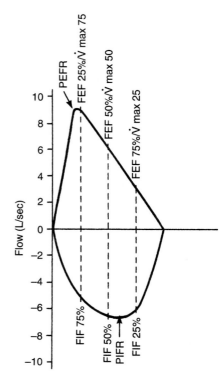

**Fig. 4-9** Flow-volume loop tracing of a normal adult showing the positions and values of the various inspiratory and expiratory flows. Flow values are determined by means of a horizontal line drawn from the intersection of the loop tracing and the FIF or FEF point in question. For example, the PEFR is 9 L/sec. FEF, forced expiratory flow; FIF, forced inspiratory flow; PEFR, peak expiratory flow rate; PIFR, peak inspiratory flow rate.

c. Flow at 25% of the FEVC = $\dot{V}_{max25\%}$ (maximal flow with 25% of the FVC remaining) or $FEF_{75\%}$ (forced expiratory flow with 75% of the FVC exhaled)

The following *inspiratory flows* are reported:

a. Flow at 25% of the FIVC = $FIF_{25\%}$ (forced inspiratory flow with 25% of the FVC inhaled)
b. Flow at 50% of the FIVC = $FIF_{50\%}$ (forced inspiratory flow with 50% of the FVC inhaled)
c. Flow at 75% of the FIVC = $FIF_{75\%}$ (forced inspiratory flow with 75% of the FVC inhaled)

The PEFR and $FEF_{25\%}$ or $\dot{V}_{max75\%}$ values should be about the same because they all measure flow through the large upper airways. Either test is a good gauge of the patient's effort because the value obtained will be low if the patient is not trying hard. The $FIF_{50\%}$ is normally greater than the $FEF_{50\%}$.

***Small-airways disease.*** Examples of conditions that result in small-airways disease (less than 2 mm in diameter) include asthma, chronic bronchitis, bronchiectasis, cystic fibrosis, and emphysema. The obstruction can result from bronchospasm, mucus plugging, or damage to the alveoli and small airways, leading to their collapse on expiration.

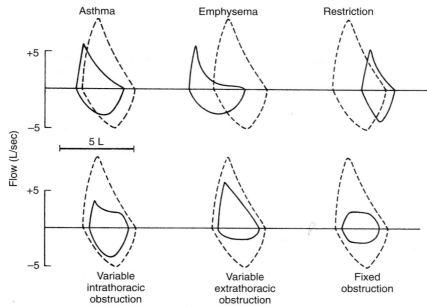

**Fig. 4-10** A series of abnormal flow-volume loop tracings superimposed over a dashed line tracing of a normal loop. *(From Ruppel G: Manual of pulmonary function testing, ed 6, St Louis, 1994, Mosby.)*

Fig. 4-10 shows representative flow-volume loops of asthma and emphysema superimposed over a normal flow-volume loop. Notice that both loops are shifted to the left toward the TLC because the RVs are increased. Also, notice that the flows are decreased to a greater extent than normal as the patient exhales closer to the RV. This "scooped out" appearance is characteristic of small-airways disease. Having the patient inhale a bronchodilator, then repeating the flow-volume loop shows the degree of reversibility. Some computer-based systems allow the before-and-after bronchodilator loops to be superimposed to show in greater detail the amount of improvement.

**Restriction.** A restriction can be caused by the following: a pulmonary condition such as fibrosis; a thoracic condition such as pleural effusion, pneumothorax, hemothorax, or kyphoscoliosis; obesity; advanced pregnancy; or ascites that pushes up on the diaphragm. Only fibrosis and kyphoscoliosis are permanent. Fig. 4-10 shows a representative flow-volume loop for a patient with restrictive lung disease. Notice that the volume is small and is shifted to the right toward the small RV.

**Variable intrathoracic obstruction.** A variable intrathoracic obstruction can be caused by a tumor or a foreign body that is partially blocking a bronchus. Fig. 4-10 shows a representative flow-volume curve. Note that the FVC volume is almost normal and that a greatly decreased PEFR exists.

**Variable extrathoracic obstruction.** A variable extrathoracic obstruction can be caused by vocal cord paralysis, laryngeal tumor, or a foreign body that is partially

obstructing the upper airway. Fig. 4-10 shows a representative flow-volume curve. Note that the FVC volume is almost normal with a greatly reduced inspiratory flow. This same pattern is commonly seen in patients with obstructive sleep apnea. The $FEF_{50\%}$ will be greater than the $FIF_{50\%}$.

**Fixed large-airway obstruction.** A fixed large-airway obstruction is usually caused by a tumor in the trachea or a mainstem bronchus. Fig. 4-10 shows a representative flow-volume loop. Again, the FVC volume is close to normal. Note the abnormally reduced inspiratory and expiratory flow rates. The tracing looks almost "squared off" with $FEF_{50\%}$ and $FIF_{50\%}$ values that are about the same.

### 3. Maximal voluntary ventilation
#### a. Perform the maximal voluntary ventilation procedure (NBRC code: IB7m) [Difficulty: R, Ap]

Maximal voluntary ventilation (MVV) is the volume of air that is exhaled in a specified period during a repetitive maximal respiratory effort. MVV is most commonly done to evaluate a patient's ability to perform a stress test. It may also be used as a preoperative screening test to help determine the patient's chance of pulmonary complications.

The patient should breathe at a volume greater than the $V_T$ but less than the VC with a rate between 70 and 120/min. The minimal time for the test is 5 sec with a recommended time of 12 sec. Fig. 4-11 shows two different tracings of the MVV effort. The total volume exhaled in the given time period is mathematically adjusted for 1 min so that the derived value is expressed in liters per minute.

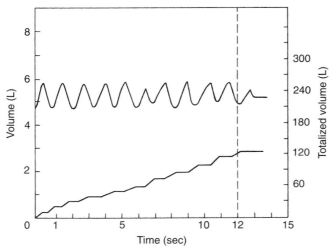

**Fig. 4-11** Two tracings of the same maximal voluntary ventilation effort. The saw-toothed tracing shows each individual volume effort and the respiratory rate. The stair-stepped tracing shows the cumulative volume during the effort. *(From Ruppel G: Manual of pulmonary function testing, ed 6, St Louis, 1994, Mosby.)*

This adjustment is made by multiplying a 5-sec effort by 12 or a 12-sec effort by 5. The derived value is then BTPS corrected to give the final value.

### b. Interpret the results (NBRC code: IB8i) [Difficulty: R, Ap]

Results of the MVV test are among the more difficult data to evaluate because any one or more of several problems can result in a low test value. These include poor patient effort, weakened condition of the respiratory muscles, decreased lung-thoracic compliance ($C_{LT}$), decreased neurologic control over the drive to breathe, and increased airway and tissue resistance. Also, because more than one problem can exist, a decreased MVV value does not pinpoint the exact difficulty.

A healthy young man can have an MVV of 150 to 200 L/min. Women tend to have smaller values, and the values for both sexes decline with age. Because of the many factors involved in the MVV, normal predicted values may vary by as much as ±30%. Therefore, unless a patient has an MVV value that is less than 70% of predicted, results cannot really be considered abnormally low. Cherniack and Raber (1972) have published equations that can be used for predicting the MVV in liters per minute.

### 4. Lung compliance

#### a. Perform the lung compliance procedure (NBRC code: IB7g, IIIE7) [Difficulty: R, Ap]

Lung compliance ($C_L$) is the volume change per unit of pressure change in the lungs. It is recorded in liters or milliliters per centimeter of water pressure (L[mL]/cm $H_2O$). A $C_L$ test is indicated in a patient with a known or

suspected condition that causes the lungs to be either overly compliant (as with emphysema) or noncompliant (as with pulmonary fibrosis).

The patient must swallow a 10-cm-long balloon to the midthoracic level. A catheter connects the proximal end of the balloon to a pressure transducer outside of the patient. Air is injected into the balloon, and the transducer is calibrated to accurately measure changes in intrathoracic pressure as the patient breathes. The patient is placed into a body plethysmograph that is then sealed. The body plethysmograph unit (sometimes called the *body bubble*) is a sealable chamber that is large enough for an adult to sit inside. Auxiliary equipment includes a differential pressure pneumotachometer, monitor/storage oscilloscope, computer, and recording device. The plethysmograph can be used to measure the following: the FRC (also called the thoracic gas volume) and, from that, the RV and TLC, the $C_L$, and Raw.

The patient is then told to breathe through the differential pressure pneumotachometer so that lung volumes can be measured. The patient is instructed to slowly inhale from the resting level (FRC) to TLC. As this is being done, the pneumotachometer shutter is periodically closed to measure the intrathoracic pressure drop at increasing volumes (Fig. 4-12). As the patient slowly exhales from TLC, the shutter is again periodically closed for measurement of increasing intrathoracic pressure as the patient returns to FRC volume. $C_L$ is usually calculated from the pressure and volume points of FRC and FRC +500 mL (for a $V_T$).

### b. Interpret the lung compliance results (NBRC code: IB8e) [Difficulty: R, Ap]

Normal $C_L$ in an adult is 0.2 L/cm $H_2O$. Through other methods, the normal adult's thoracic compliance ($C_T$) has been determined to also be 0.2 L/cm $H_2O$. However, because the lungs tend to collapse to a smaller size and the thorax cage tends to expand out, the two opposing forces offset each other somewhat. Because of this, the $C_{LT}$ is calculated as 0.1 L (100 mL)/cm $H_2O$. A number of diseases and conditions can affect the $C_L$, $C_T$, and $C_{LT}$. Patients with emphysema are known to have a higher-than-normal $C_L$. Their lungs are overly distended. Decreased $C_L$ is seen in pulmonary fibrosis (from sarcoidosis, silicosis, or asbestosis), lung tumor, pulmonary edema, atelectasis, pneumonia, and decreased surfactant. Decreased $C_T$ is seen in patients with kyphoscoliosis, pectus excavatum, obesity, enlarged liver, or advanced pregnancy. All of these conditions result in small, stiff lungs.

### 4. Airway resistance

#### a. Perform the airway resistance procedure (NBRC code: IB7g, IIIE7) [Difficulty: R, Ap]

Airway resistance (Raw) is the difference in pressure between the alveoli and the mouth that develops as air flows into and out of the lungs. It is recorded in centime-

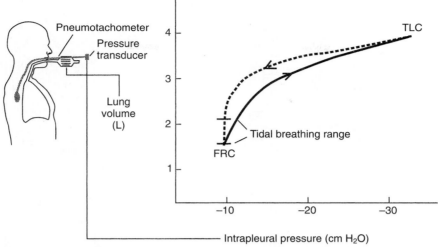

**Fig. 4-12** Measurement of lung compliance with the esophageal balloon technique. A balloon is swallowed to the midthoracic level, filled with air, and connected to a pressure transducer to measure intrapleural pressure. The patient sits within a body plethysmograph to measure inspiratory and expiratory volumes. FRC, Functional residual capacity; TLC, total lung capacity. *(From Ruppel G: Manual of pulmonary function testing, ed 6, St Louis, 1994, Mosby.)*

ters of water pressure per liter of gas moved per second (cm $H_2O$/L/sec). The test is performed on patients with a known or suspected condition of increased Raw, including asthma, emphysema, and chronic bronchitis (COPD). The test confirms the patient's condition; after this, the proper dose of bronchodilator medications to help manage the problem is determined.

The patient is placed in a plethysmograph that is then sealed. He or she is instructed to breathe through a differential pressure pneumotachometer. With the pneumotachometer shutter open, the patient is told to pant several $V_Ts$ of about 500 mL at a rate of 1 breath/sec. Data on flow rate, $V_T$, mouth pressure changes, and chamber pressure changes are recorded and graphed (Fig. 4-13). Then, at the patient's resting FRC volume, the shutter is closed. The patient is told to continue panting at the same volume and rate, and the data are recorded and graphed again. The computer integrates the data to calculate the patient's Raw during $V_T$ breathing.

### b. Interpret the airway resistance results (NBRC code: IB8e) [Difficulty: R, Ap]

Raw is the pressure difference developed per unit of flow. This pressure is necessary to overcome the friction of moving the $V_T$ through the airways to the lungs. It can be thought of as the ratio of alveolar pressure to airflow. It is calculated by this formula:

$$Raw = \frac{atmospheric\ pressure - alveolar\ pressure}{airflow\ (in\ L/second)}$$

Ruppel (2003) reports the normal adult's Raw as ranging from 0.6 to 2.4 cm $H_2O$/L/sec. The standard inspiratory

and expiratory flow rate during the test is 0.5 L/sec (500 mL/sec), which standardizes air turbulence during the test. The usual components of Raw found in an adult are as follows:

a. Upper airway including the nose and mouth = 50%
b. Trachea and bronchi larger than 2 mm in diameter = 30%
c. Airways smaller than 2 mm in diameter = 20%

An increased Raw is abnormal and is most readily noticed if the problem is in the upper airway, trachea, or major bronchi because most resistance is normally found at these sites. Patients with asthma, bronchitis, and emphysema have most of their resistance in airways that are 2 mm or smaller in diameter. Because of this, significant disease must be present before a Raw is large enough to alert the therapist or physician to the problem. Fig. 4-14 parts **B, C,** and **D** show normal and increased expiratory resistance curves. Madama (1998) lists the following Raw values and their severity:

| Raw (cm $H_2O$/L/sec) | Severity |
|---|---|
| 2.8–4.5 | Mild |
| 4.5–8 | Moderate |
| >8 | Severe |

### 6. Diffusing capacity
#### a. Perform the diffusing capacity procedure (NBRC code: IB7m) [Difficulty: R, Ap]

The diffusing capacity ($D_L$ or $D_{L\ CO}$) tests look at the capacity for carbon monoxide (CO) to diffuse through the lungs into the blood. CO is used because its high affinity for hemoglobin virtually eliminates blood as a barrier to

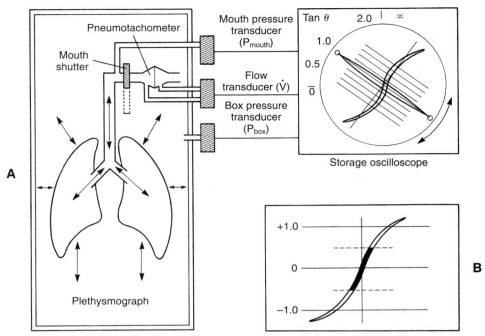

**Fig. 4-13** Measurement of airway resistance. **A,** Body plethysmograph in which the patient sits during the test. $V_T$ panting against an open and then closed pneumotachometer shutter is displayed on the storage oscilloscope. **B,** Printout of the pressure changes as the patient pants a $V_T$ of 500 mL/sec. *(From Ruppel G: Manual of pulmonary function testing, ed 6, St Louis, 1994, Mosby.)*

diffusion. The measured value can then be correlated with the ability of $O_2$ to diffuse through the lungs. This test is indicated when the extent of lung disability that is causing hypoxemia must be known. This is most common in patients with emphysema but is also important in patients with fibrotic lung disease.

The single-breath CO diffusing capacity test ($D_{L\,CO}^{SB}$) is the only version of the test with a widely adopted standard technique for administration. It is recorded in milliliters of CO per minute per millimeter of mercury at 0° C, 760 mm Hg, and dry (STPD).

Following are key steps in the procedure. A reservoir or spirometer is filled with a mix of 0.3% CO, 10% He, 21% $O_2$, and the balance of $N_2$ (Fig. 4-15). The patient is connected to the apparatus and breathes room air while being instructed about the test. After the patient is told to exhale completely (to RV), the practitioner switches the patient to the gas mix. The patient is instructed to rapidly inhale an inspiratory vital capacity (IVC). A shutter automatically closes so that the patient cannot exhale for 10 sec. This allows time for some of the CO to diffuse into the patient's bloodstream. After the patient holds his or her breath, the shutter opens and the patient is told to exhale to resting volume. The equipment is designed to automatically let 750 to 1000 mL of exhaled gas pass through to the spirometer. The next 500 mL of gas is

diverted into the end-tidal gas sampler. This sample is then analyzed for percentages of He and CO. The remainder of the patient's exhaled volume is passed through into the spirometer. The various measured parameters are integrated into the equations in the computer to obtain the patient's $D_{L\,CO}^{SB}$ value.

This test is done only after the patient has been measured for both RV and TLC because the patient's lung volume directly affects the diffusibility of CO.

### b. Interpret the results (NBRC code: IB8I) [Difficulty: R, Ap]

Interpretation is limited to the results of the $D_{L\,CO}^{SB}$ test. Ruppel (2003) reports the average resting normal adult $D_{L\,CO}^{SB}$ as 25 mL CO/min/mm Hg STPD. (All $D_L$ values are reported in standard temperature pressure dry conditions.) Gaensler and Wright (1966) reported $D_{L\,CO}^{SB}$ prediction equations with mL CO/min/mm Hg STPD values. Other authors have developed their own prediction equations.

In general, patients who show $D_{L\,CO}^{SB}$ results within ±20% of predicted values (80% to 120% of predicted) are considered to be within normal limits. A patient who has actual results significantly below the predicted values has a problem with lung diffusion. Fig. 4-16 shows a number

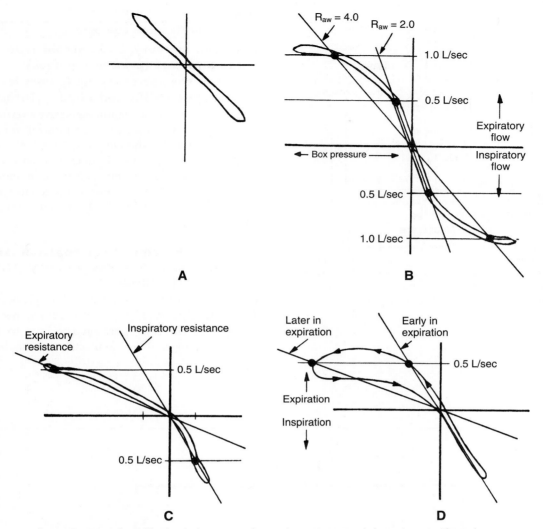

**Fig. 4-14** Examples of body plethysmography tracings. **A,** Normal thoracic gas volume loop. **B,** Normal inspiratory and expiratory loop for airway resistance (Raw). Note that it is symmetrical. This patient has a Raw of 2 cm $H_2O$/L/sec at the standard flow of 0.5 L/sec. As the flow increases, the Raw increases as a result of the increased turbulence. So, the Raw of 4 cm $H_2O$/L/sec seen at the flow of 1 L/sec should not be recorded as the patient's value. **C,** Patient who has an expiratory resistance greater than inspiratory resistance. In this case, both resistances should be recorded in the chart, or just the expiratory resistance should be recorded if only one can be recorded. **D,** Significant difference between early and late expiratory resistance. This is commonly seen in patients with obstructive airways disease such as emphysema. Record the late resistance because it better represents the patient's disease condition. *(From Zarins LP, Clausen JL: Body plethysmography. In Clausen JL, editor: Pulmonary function testing guidelines and controversies, Orlando, 1984, Grune & Stratton.)*

of common conditions that can lead to poor lung diffusion. Additionally, use of the patient's actual hemoglobin level in the diffusion equation is important, and the patient should not be allowed to smoke for several hours before taking the test. The patient should breathe room air for at least 4 min before the test is repeated.

The fact that diffusibility is directly related to lung volume is well known and is the reason that blacks have lower diffusion rates than whites. To eliminate this as a factor in interpretation of the $D_L$ value, the diffusion value must be divided by the TLC. Blacks have the same normal values as whites when this calculation is performed.

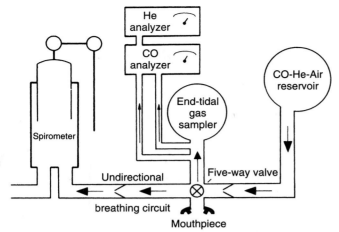

**Fig. 4-15** Schematic drawing of the components and breathing circuit used when a single-breath lung diffusion test is performed. Analysis of the patient's exhaled helium (He) and carbon monoxide (CO) percentages is critical to the test. *(From Ruppel G: Manual of pulmonary function testing, ed 6, St Louis, 1994, Mosby.)*

## MODULE F

### Pulmonary function equipment

### 1. Water, mercury, and aneroid-type manometers (pressure gauges)

#### a. Get the necessary equipment for the procedure (NBRC code: IIA17) [Difficulty: R]

Mercury or water-type manometers have a vertical column of the liquid, as in a sphygmomanometer, for measuring blood pressure. An aneroid (spring-loaded) unit is most commonly used because it does not have to be kept upright to measure accurately. Aneroid manometers can be calibrated in either millimeters of mercury (mm Hg) or centimeters of water (cm $H_2O$) pressure and look like a Bourdon gauge.

#### b. Put the equipment together and make sure that it works properly (NBRC code: IIA17) [Difficulty: R]

The gauges just mentioned come preassembled by the manufacturer. The pressure source need only be attached to the inlet port on the unit to measure a pressure change. This connection must be airtight,

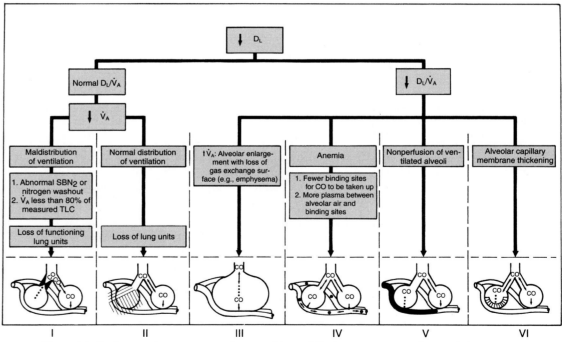

**Fig. 4-16** Six factors that can cause decreased lung diffusion. Factors I and II result in a decrease in diffusing capacity ($D_L$) that is in proportion to the decrease in alveolar volume. Factors III, IV, V, and VI result in a decrease in $D_L$ that is greater than the decrease in alveolar volume. Therefore, these latter conditions are more harmful to the patient's pulmonary function and well-being. SBN$_2$, Single breath N$_2$ washout; TLC, total lung capacity; $\dot{V}_A$, minute alveolar ventilation. *(Modified from Ayers LN, Whipp BJ, Ziment I: A guide to the interpretation of pulmonary function tests, ed 2, New York, 1978, Roerig.)*

or a leak will occur and the measured pressure will be less than actual. Accuracy of the unit can be checked by opening the inlet port to room air and reading the pressure. A reading of zero should be seen (indicating no pressure change from atmospheric). A known pressure is then applied to the gauge, often by attaching it to a sphygmomanometer and pumping up the pressure to a known level such as 50 mm Hg. The pressure gauge should show the same.

### c. Troubleshoot any problems with the equipment (NBRC code: IIA17) [Difficulty: R]

If, during the calibration procedure, the set pressure does not match the pressure in the gauge, a leak may exist in the system, or the pressure gauge may be miscalibrated. Tighten all connections and attempt to calibrate again. Do not use a pressure gauge that cannot be calibrated.

## 2. Inspiratory and/or expiratory force meters (pressure gauges)
### a. Get the necessary equipment for the procedure (NBRC code: IIA17) [Difficulty: R]

The MIP and MEP tests are usually recorded in centimeters of water pressure. However, millimeters of mercury could be used. If a centimeters of water pressure gauge is used, it should be able to record a negative and/or positive pressure of at least 100 cm $H_2O$. However, a unit that can record ±60 cm $H_2O$ would probably be adequate.

### b. Put the equipment together and make sure that it works properly (NBRC code: IIA17) [Difficulty: R]

No standard setup exists for pressure gauges. See Fig. 4-2 for possible assembly. The system can be sealed and pressure checked with a known force to make sure that the pressure manometer is accurate and all the connections are airtight.

### c. Troubleshoot any problems with the equipment (NBRC code: IIA17) [Difficulty: R]

If, during the calibration procedure, the set pressure does not match the pressure in the gauge, a leak may exist in the system, or the pressure gauge may be miscalibrated. Tighten all connections and attempt to calibrate again. Do not use a pressure gauge that cannot be calibrated. The one-way valves must function so that the patient can exhale or inhale only as needed for the test.

## 3. Bedside spirometry screening equipment
### a. Get the necessary equipment for the procedure (NBRC code: IIA24) [Difficulty: R, Ap]

### b. Put the equipment together and make sure that it works properly (NBRC code: IIA17) [Difficulty: R]
### c. Troubleshoot any problems with the equipment (NBRC code: IIA17) [Difficulty: R]

A bedside spirometry screening unit must be small enough to be transported easily and durable enough to not be damaged or lose its calibration as it is moved. These units are usually able to provide only forced vital capacity information and data that are taken from the FVC. A variety of pneumotachometer-type units are available. See the following discussion for the differences.

## 4. Pneumotachometer respirometers
### a. Get the necessary equipment for the procedure (NBRC code: IIA18) [Difficulty: R, Ap]
### b. Put the equipment together and make sure that it works properly (NBRC code: IIA18) [Difficulty: R, Ap]
### c. Troubleshoot any problems with the equipment (NBRC code: IIA18) [Difficulty: R, Ap]

All pneumotachometers convert one type of physical information or signal to another. Two common types–differential pressure (flow sensing) and heat transfer—are discussed next. Either type should be acceptable for performing bedside spirometry. Make sure that the unit you select is capable of performing the ordered test and of printing out a hard copy of the patient's test results and spirometry tracings, if these are required for the chart.

***Differential-pressure (flow sensing) pneumotachometer.*** Some articles refer to a differential-pressure pneumotachometer as a *Fleisch-type* device. These units have a resistive element (tubes or mesh screen) in the flow tube. The faster the flow of gas through the flow tube, the greater is the pressure difference before and after resistance. Hoses connect the flow tubes before and after the resistive element to the differential pressure transducer. The transducer converts this pressure difference into an electrical signal. A microprocessor calculates various patient values from this information (Fig. 4-17).

Assembly necessitates the addition of the patient's mouthpiece to the inspiratory port so that no air leak exists. The expiratory port should be kept completely open so that the only obstruction to the patient's airflow comes from the resistive element. A volume calibration check is performed by forcing a known amount of air from a supersyringe (certified-volume standard syringe) through the pneumotachometer. Minimally, several repetitions of a known 3-L volume should reveal identical measured volumes. As long as the measured volumes are within ±3% or 50 mL (whichever is less), the unit is acceptably accurate.

| TABLE 4-1 | Lung Volumes and Capacities Seen in Various Disorders | | | | | | |
|---|---|---|---|---|---|---|---|
| **Disorder** | **VC** | **IC** | **ERV** | **FRC** | **RV** | **TLC** | **RV:TLC** |
| Asthma or airway disease | D | N | D | N,I | I | N,I* | I |
| Emphysema | N | N | N | I | I | I | N,I |
| Diffuse parenchymal disease | | | | | | | |
| Early | N | N | N | D | N | N | N |
| Advanced (all volumes and capacities are equally reduced) | | | | | | | |
| Space-occupying lesions | N | N | N | N | D | N | D |
| Obesity | N | N | D | N,I† | N | N | I |
| Thoracic/skeletal disease | D | D | D | D | N | D | I |

Modified from Snow MG: Determination of functional residual capacity, Respir Care 34(7):586, 1989.

D, Decreased; ERV, expiratory reserve volume; FRC, functional residual capacity; I, increased; IC, inspiratory capacity; N, normal; RV, residual volume; TLC, total lung capacity; VC, vital capacity.

*When airway resistance is greater than about 3.5 cm $H_2O$/L/sec.

†When the weight:height (pounds:inches) ratio is greater than 5:1.

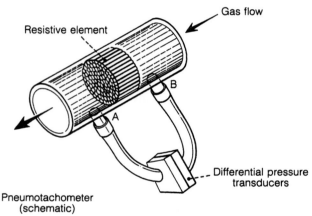

Fig. 4-17 Cutaway view of a differential-pressure pneumotachometer. Flow is measured as the pressure drops between **A** and **B,** which are ports leading to a differential-pressure transducer. The resistive element may consist of a mesh screen, a network of parallel capillary tubes, or other devices. *(From Beauchamp RK: Pulmonary function testing procedures. In Barnes TA, editor: Respiratory care practice, Chicago, 1988, Mosby.)*

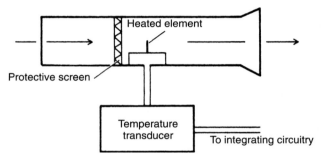

Fig. 4-18 Cutaway view of a heat-transfer pneumotachometer. *(From Ruppel G: Manual of pulmonary function testing, ed 6, St Louis, 1994, Mosby.)*

Common problems with accuracy include the following: an air leak around the mouthpiece; cracked, disconnected, or obstructed pressure-relaying hoses; water condensation or mucus on the resistive element; and obstructed upstream or downstream port. The resistive element is usually heated to minimize any condensation.

***Heat-transfer pneumotachometer.*** Some articles refer to a heat-transfer pneumotachometer as a *thermistor-type device* or a *hot wire anemometer.* These units have a heated thermistor that is cooled as the gas flows past it. The temperature transducer automatically increases and measures the flow of electricity to the thermistor to keep it at the required temperature. A microprocessor calculates

various patient values from this information. The earlier discussion on assembly, calibration, and troubleshooting applies to the heat-transfer–type pneumotachometer, except that no pressure-relaying hoses exist (Fig. 4-18).

## MODULE D
### Respiratory care plan

### 1. Analyze the available information to determine the patient's pathophysiologic state (NBRC code: IIIH1) [Difficulty: R, Ap, An]

Even though a physician must legally determine the patient's diagnosis, a therapist must be able to understand the cause, pathophysiology, diagnosis, treatment, and prognosis for patients with cardiopulmonary disorders. Interpretation of patient data as tested by the NBRC was discussed earlier. A summary of key findings is shown in Table 4-1. Following is a brief categorization of conditions that may be diagnosed by pulmonary function testing.

### a. Obstructive airways disease

The patient with severe obstructive lung disease shows low gas flow at all time intervals. Especially note that a less than predicted $FEV_3$ and $FEF_{25\%-75\%}$ are early markers of small-airways disease. The RV is commonly increased because of air trapping. This increases the FRC and often the TLC. Despite increased lung volume, the patient's diffusing ability is decreased. Examples of conditions that cause obstructive lung disease include asthma, emphysema, bronchitis, and bronchiolitis. Excessive mucus, foreign body, and airway tumor also cause bronchospasm and air trapping. Many patients with asthma and some patients with chronic bronchitis will show improved expiratory flows after inhaling a bronchodilator medication.

### b. Restrictive lung disease

In restrictive lung disease, all lung volumes and capacities are reduced and lung diffusion is reduced. Expiratory flows such as $FEV_1$ are increased. Examples of conditions that cause restrictive lung disease include pulmonary fibrosis, pulmonary edema, hemothorax or pneumothorax, acute or infant respiratory distress syndrome, chest wall deformities, obesity, and various neuromuscular disorders.

### 2. Determine the appropriateness of the prescribed therapy and goals for the patient's pathophysiologic state (NBRC code: IIIH3) [Difficulty: R, Ap, An]

Obviously, the patient's care plan depends on the diagnosis and degree of limitation of the patient. If the patient has reversible small-airways disease, he or she should be counseled to stop smoking and avoid all airborne irritants. Inhaled and/or parenteral bronchodilators should be prescribed to relax the airways as much as possible.

If the patient has restrictive lung disease, he or she should also be counseled to avoid any airborne irritants. Whether any medications or other procedures can be performed to offer some relief depends on the specific cause of the patient's disorder.

## BIBLIOGRAPHY

American Association for Respiratory Care: Clinical practice guideline: Spirometry, *Respir Care* 36(12):1414, 1991.

American Association for Respiratory Care: Clinical practice guideline: Single-breath carbon monoxide diffusing capacity, *Respir Care* 38(5):511, 1993.

American Association for Respiratory Care: Clinical practice guideline: Single-breath carbon monoxide diffusing capacity, 1999 update, *Respir Care* 44(1):91, 1999.

American Association for Respiratory Care: Clinical practice guideline: Static lung volumes, *Respir Care* 39(8):830, 1994.

American Association for Respiratory Care: Clinical practice guideline: Infant/toddler pulmonary function tests, *Respir Care* 40(7):761, 1995.

American Association for Respiratory Care: Clinical practice guideline: Bronchial provocation, *Respir Care* 37(8):902, 1992.

American Association for Respiratory Care: Clinical practice guideline: Body plethysmography: 2001 revision & update, *Respir Care* 46(5):506-513, 2001.

American Association for Respiratory Care: Clinical practice guideline: Assessing response to bronchodilator therapy at point of care, *Respir Care* 40(12):1300, 1995.

American Thoracic Society: Standardization of spirometry: 1987 update, *Am Rev Respir Dis* 136:1285, 1987.

Ayers LN, Whipp BJ, Ziment I: *A guide to the interpretation of pulmonary function tests,* ed 2, New York, 1978, Roerig.

Bates DV, Macklem PT, Christie RV: *Respiratory function in disease,* ed 2, Philadelphia, 1971, WB Saunders.

Beauchamp RK: Pulmonary function testing procedures. In Barnes TA, editor: *Respiratory care practice,* Chicago, 1988, Mosby.

Black LF, Hyatt RE: Maximal respiratory pressures: normal values and relationship to age and sex, *Am Rev Respir Dis* 99:696, 1969.

Branson RD, Hurst JM, Davis K Jr, et al: Measurement of maximal inspiratory pressure: A comparison of three methods, *Respir Care* 34(9):789, 1989.

Buist SA, Ross BB: Predicted values for closing volumes using a modified single-breath nitrogen test, *Am Rev Respir Dis* 111:405, 1975.

Cairo JM: Assessment of pulmonary function. In Cairo JM, Pilbeam SP, editors: *Mosby's respiratory care equipment,* ed 7, St Louis, 2004, Mosby.

Cherniack RM: *Pulmonary function testing,* ed 2, Philadelphia, 1992, WB Saunders.

Cherniack RM, Raber MD: Normal standards for ventilatory function using an automated wedge spirometer, *Am Rev Respir Dis* 106:38, 1972.

Clausen JL, editor: *Pulmonary function testing guidelines and controversies,* Orlando, 1984, Grune & Stratton.

Clausen JL: Clinical interpretation of pulmonary function test, *Respir Care* 34(7):638, 1989.

Crapo RO: Reference values for lung function tests, *Respir Care* 34(7):626, 1989.

Douce FH: Pulmonary function testing. In Wilkins RL, Stoller JK, Scanlan CL, editors: *Egan's fundamentals of respiratory care,* ed 8, St Louis, 2003, Mosby.

Enright PL, Hodgkin JE: Pulmonary function tests. In Burton GG, Hodgkin JE, Ward JJ, editors: *Respiratory care: A guide to clinical practice,* ed 4, Philadelphia, 1997, Lippincott-Raven.

Gaensler EA, Wright GW: Evaluation of respiratory impairment, *Arch Environ Health* 12:146, 1966.

Gardner RM: Pulmonary function laboratory standards, *Respir Care* 34(7):651, 1989.

Goldman HI, Becklake MR: Respiratory function tests: Normal values at median altitudes and the prediction of normal results, *Am Rev Tuberculosis* 79:457, 1959.

Gursel G, Adams AB: Pulmonary function testing. In Hess DR, MacIntyre NR, Mishoe SC, et al, editors: *Respiratory care principles & practice,* Philadelphia, 2002, WB Saunders.

Hess D: Measurement of maximal inspiratory pressure: A call for standardization, *Respir Care* 34:857, 1989.

Holland SA: Pulmonary function testing. In Wyka KA, Mathews PJ, Clark WF, editors: *Foundations of respiratory care*, Albany, 2002, Delmar.

Hunt GE: Diagnostic procedures at the bedside. In Fink JB, Hunt GE, editors: *Clinical practice in respiratory care*, Philadelphia, 1999, Lippincott Williams & Wilkins.

Kacmarek RM, Cycyk-Chapman MC, Young-Palazzo PJ, et al: Determination of maximal inspiratory pressure: A clinical study and literature review, *Respir Care* 34:868, 1989.

Knudson RJ, Kaltenborn WT, Knudson DE, et al: The single-breath carbon monoxide diffusing capacity, *Am Rev Respir Dis* 135:805, 1987.

Knudson RJ, Lebowitz MD, Holberg CJ, et al: Changes in the normal maximal expiratory flow-volume curve with growth and aging, *Am Rev Respir Dis* 127:725, 1983.

Kory RC, Callahan R, Syner JC: The Veterans Administration-Army cooperative study of pulmonary function. I. Clinical spirometry in normal men, *Am J Med* 30:243, 1961.

MacIntyre NR: Diffusing capacity of the lung for carbon monoxide, *Respir Care* 34(6):489, 1989.

Madama VC: *Pulmonary function testing and cardiopulmonary stress testing*, ed 2, Albany, 1998, Delmar.

Morris JF, Koski A, Johnson LC: Spirometric standards for healthy nonsmoking adults, *Am Rev Respir Dis* 103:57, 1971.

National Institutes of Health, *Practical guide for the diagnosis and management of asthma*, Pub No 97- 4053, October 1997, US Department of Health and Human Services.

Paoletti P, Viegi G, Pistelli G, et al: Reference equations for the single-breath diffusing capacity, *Am Rev Respir Dis* 132:806, 1985.

Ruppel G: *Manual of pulmonary function testing*, ed 8, St Louis, 2003, Mosby.

Single breath carbon monoxide diffusing capacity (transfer factor): Recommendations for a standard technique, *Am Rev Respir Dis* 136:1299, 1987.

Snow MG: Determination of functional residual capacity, *Respir Care* 34(7):586, 1989.

Sue D: Exercise testing and the patient with cardiopulmonary disease. In Goldman AL, editor: *Problems in pulmonary disease* 2(1):1, Spring 1986.

Wanger J: *Pulmonary function testing*, ed 2, Baltimore, 1996, Williams & Wilkins.

Zamel N, Altose MD, Speir WA Jr: Statement on spirometry, *Chest* 3:547, 1983.

## SELF-STUDY QUESTIONS

1. Which of the following statements is true of the MEP test?
   - I. −20 to −25 cm $H_2O$ is usually adequate.
   - II. +20 to +25 cm $H_2O$ is usually adequate.
   - III. +40 cm $H_2O$ is usually adequate.
   - IV. It is a good indicator of the patient's ability to cough.
   - V. The patient should hold the effort for 1 to 3 sec.
   - A. I and II
   - B. III and IV
   - C. III
   - D. III, IV, and V

2. The predicted FVC value for blacks is
   - A. 10% to 15% larger than that for whites
   - B. The same as that for whites
   - C. 10% to 15% less than that for whites
   - D. 20% to 25% less than that for whites

3. Which of the following test results is needed to calculate TLC?
   - I. FRC
   - II. RV
   - III. $V_T$
   - IV. ERV
   - V. IC
   - VI. VC
   - A. I and III
   - B. II and VI
   - C. II and V
   - D. I and V, or II and VI

4. A normal MEFV loop test would show
   - A. $FEF_{50\%}$ less than $FIF_{50\%}$
   - B. Predicted lung diffusion ability
   - C. $FEF_{50\%}$ greater than $FIF_{50\%}$
   - D. A normal FRC

5. A patient with a neuromuscular disease has been having serial bedside spirometry performed. Over the past 4 hr, her VC and MIP values have been decreasing. How should this be interpreted?
   - A. Her strength is improving.
   - B. She is not performing to the best of her ability.
   - C. She has undiagnosed asthma.
   - D. Her condition is worsening.

6. A patient has been scheduled for a battery of pulmonary function tests. He tells you that he is so nervous about the testing that he has smoked four cigarettes in the last 2 hr. Which of the following tests is most likely to be adversely affected by this?
   - A. FRC
   - B. Lung diffusion
   - C. Raw
   - D. FVC

7. Before a patient does an FVC test, the pneumotachometer should have the following done:
   - A. The gas analyzer should be calibrated.
   - B. A $CO_2$-absorbing material should be placed in line with the circuit.
   - C. A 3-L volume should be pumped into and out of the circuit to check for leaks.
   - D. The kymograph speeds should be checked.

8. To help in the diagnosis of asthma, you would recommend all of the following tests EXCEPT
   A. Diffusion study
   B. Flow-volume loop
   C. Before-and-after bronchodilator study
   D. Raw

9. A patient has just been tested for $C_L$ in a body plethysmograph. Her compliance was determined to be 0.2 L (200 mL)/cm $H_2O$. Based on this, she most likely has
   A. Asthma
   B. Pulmonary fibrosis
   C. Emphysema
   D. Normal lungs

10. Calculate a patient's inspiratory time and expiratory time when he has an I:E ratio of 2:1 and a respiratory rate of 15/min.
    A. 2.7 sec for inspiration and 1.3 sec for expiration
    B. 3.3 sec for inspiration and 1.7 sec for expiration
    C. 1.3 sec for inspiration and 2.7 sec for expiration
    D. 1.7 sec for inspiration and 3.3 sec for expiration

11. When a patient performs an MEP test, it is important that he or she
    A. Blow out all air before starting the effort
    B. Breathe in a $V_T$ and blow out hard
    C. Inhale to TLC and blow out hard
    D. Exhale a $V_T$ breath and inhale as hard as possible

12. A patient weighs 45 kg (100 lb). Her predicted $V_T$ would be
    A. 550 mL
    B. 450 mL
    C. 350 mL
    D. 250 mL

13. You receive an order to calculate your patient's alveolar ventilation. His respiratory rate is 16, and his average $V_T$ is 580 mL. He weighs 170 lb. His alveolar ventilation is
    A. 2720 mL
    B. 410 mL
    C. 750 mL
    D. 510 mL

14. Your patient has an $FEV_{1\%}$ that calculates out to be 80% of his FVC. On the basis of this finding, the patient probably
    A. Is having an asthma attack
    B. Has a laryngeal tumor
    C. Has a fibrotic lung disease
    D. Is clinically normal

Note: Refer to the following figure for Questions 15 and 16.

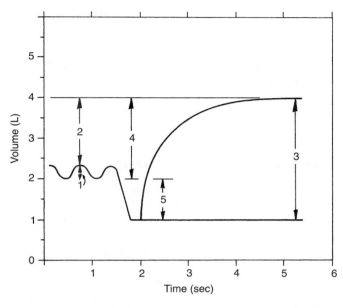

15. Which section of the spirometry tracing represents the FVC?
    A. 2
    B. 3
    C. 4
    D. 5

16. Which section of the spirometry tracing represents the $V_T$?
    A. 1
    B. 2
    C. 3
    D. 4

17. The VC is made up of
    I. RV
    II. FRC
    III. ERV
    IV. $V_T$
    V. IRV
    A. II and IV
    B. III and IV
    C. I, II, and III
    D. III, IV, and V

18. Which of the following is true of the PF measurement?
    I. It is usually seen at the end of the patient's FVC effort.
    II. It increases with height.
    III. It increases with age.
    IV. It decreases with age.
    V. It is usually seen at the beginning of the patient's FVC effort.
    A. I, II, and III
    B. II, IV, and V
    C. I, II, and IV
    D. IV and V

19. You are having your patient perform the MIP test. His three attempts produce these results: $-15\,cm$ $H_2O$, $-45\,cm$ $H_2O$, and $-20\,cm$ $H_2O$. The best explanation for these values is that
    A. The patient is starting from FRC
    B. The equipment has a large leak
    C. The patient is starting from RV
    D. The patient is not trying his best every time

20. The physician wants to know whether a new bronchodilator would be helpful to his asthmatic patient. He orders a before-and-after bronchodilator study. The patient has the following peak flow values: $7.5\,L/min$ before the medication and $9.4\,L/min$ after the medication. Calculate her percentage change.
    A. 25%
    B. 1.25%
    C. −25%
    D. 80%

## ANSWER KEY AND RATIONALE

1. **D.** The MEP test is a measure of expiratory muscle strength. A value of $+40\,cm$ $H_2O$ usually indicates enough strength for spontaneous breathing and the ability to cough effectively. The pressure should be sustained for a short time to ensure that the measurement is accurate.

2. **C.** Blacks have been shown to have an FVC that is between 10% and 15% less than age- and height-matched whites. Review the FVC discussion.

3. **D.** Review Fig. 4-7 for volumes and capacities.

4. **A.** Flow at the midpoint of expiration is normally less than flow at the midpoint of inspiration because the small airways are beginning to close at the halfway point of an expiratory effort. A flow-volume loop test cannot measure lung diffusion or RV to calculate FRC.

5. **D.** A progressively declining VC and MIP indicate that the patient is getting weaker and her condition is getting worse. If her condition were improving, these tests would show increasing values. It is up to the respiratory therapist to ensure that the patient is performing the tests properly. If done properly, the test results will be valid. The MIP test is not used to help in the diagnosis of asthma because it measures strength, not flow.

6. **B.** The unit should be calibrated before use. The lung diffusion test would be most affected in that the CO in the cigarette smoke would bind to the hemoglobin of the patient's blood. This results in a lower-than-true test result. The other tests are not affected by CO.

7. **C.** $CO_2$ buildup is not a problem with the FVC test because the patient does not rebreathe his or her own gas for very long. A gas analyzer and kymograph are not used with an FVC test.

8. **A.** A patient with asthma will probably have a normal diffusion study between attacks. The other three tests are all sensitive to an airway resistance problem.

9. **C.** Emphysema is the only condition listed wherein the $C_L$ would be increased. Normal compliance is $0.1\,L$ ($100\,mL$)/cm $H_2O$.

10. **A.** Review the calculation at the beginning of the chapter.

11. **C.** It has been determined that blowing out from TLC results in the greatest expiratory force. This is the recommended procedure.

12. **C.** $V_T$ is estimated as 3 to $4\,mL/lb$ or 7 to $9\,mL/kg$ of ideal body weight, which results in a range of about 300 to $400\,mL$.

13. **B.** Alveolar ventilation is estimated by subtracting the patient's ideal body weight in pounds (170) from the $V_T$ ($580\,mL$).

14. **D.** The patient exhaled a normal percentage of his or her VC in 1 sec. The other conditions would all result in a low value. Review the normal values discussed earlier in the chapter.

15. **B.** The FVC is the largest capacity that can be measured by spirometry. Review Fig. 4-7.

16. **A.** The $V_T$ would be seen as the repeated smallest volumes. Review Fig. 4-7.

17. **D.** The VC is made up of these three volumes. Review Fig. 4-7.

18. **B.** PF is directly related to height and indirectly related to age. When done properly, the PF will be seen at the start of an FVC effort because that is when air is emptied from the upper airway.

19. **D.** Inconsistent high and low pressures are most likely the result of inconsistent effort. A leak would result in a consistently low value. A patient should have a consistent value starting from either RV or FRC.

20. **A.** Review the calculation earlier in the chapter.

# 5

# Advanced Cardiopulmonary Monitoring

A review of the most recent Entry Level Examinations has shown an average of 2 questions (1% of the exam) that cover advanced cardiopulmonary monitoring.

## MODULE A

### Cardiopulmonary monitoring procedures

1. **Capnography (exhaled carbon dioxide monitoring)**
   a. **Review capnography data in the patient's chart (NBRC code: IA6d) [Difficulty: R, Ap]**

Capnography is the analysis of graphic and numeric data that shows the pattern and amount of the patient's exhaled carbon dioxide ($CO_2$). Usually, the patient's pressure of end-tidal carbon dioxide ($PetCO_2$) is monitored. Following are indications for capnography:

- General anesthesia to monitor the patient's recovery and return of spontaneous breathing
- Mechanical ventilation to monitor the effect of changing tidal volume, rate, or mechanical dead space
- Checking for the presence of exhaled carbon dioxide to confirm tracheal rather than esophageal intubation
- Screening for changes in exhaled carbon dioxide because of changes in the patient's condition such as pulmonary embolism and chronic obstructive pulmonary disease (COPD)
- Monitoring the success or failure of CPR attempts based on the production of carbon dioxide

It is wise to look for previous capnography data before measuring the patient's exhaled $CO_2$ level again. Look for numerical values and a printout of the tracing of exhaled $CO_2$. Be prepared to compare the previous information with the new data to help you in evaluating the patient's condition. Comparing the patient's partial pressure of $CO_2$ in arterial blood ($PaCO_2$) values with the capnography information is useful in monitoring the patient's status. However, do not expect them to be the same.

   b. **Perform the bedside procedure (NBRC code: IB7b, IIIB3c) [Difficulty: R, Ap]**

The capnometer is a device that measures the concentration of $CO_2$ in a gas sample from a patient. The principle of operation of most bedside units is based on the absorption of infrared light by $CO_2$ in a narrow wavelength band ($4.3\,\mu$). Infrared light at this wavelength is passed through the gas sample to a receiving unit. The difference between what is sent out and what is received is directly related to how much $CO_2$ is in the gas sample. In other words, the greater the difference between the sent and received infrared light, the greater the concentration of $CO_2$ in the gas sample.

The capnometer is calibrated by comparison of a gas sample without $CO_2$ (possibly room air) with a second gas sample that contains a known amount of $CO_2$. The first gas sample without $CO_2$ should give a "zero" reading (adjust the calibration control to zero if needed). The second sample usually contains 5% to 10% $CO_2$. The capnometer should read out a $CO_2$ level that matches the amount in the known gas sample (adjust the calibration control as necessary). The exhaled alveolar $CO_2$ level can be read as a percentage or fraction ($F_ACO_2$) or as partial pressure ($P_ACO_2$) in either torr or millimeters of mercury (mm Hg).

The capnograph is a strip chart recorder that provides a copy of the patient's exhaled $CO_2$ curve. At least two paper speeds are useful for different purposes. The fast speed is most useful for evaluating sudden changes in the patient's condition; each breath is easily seen (Fig. 5-1). The slow speed is most useful for trend monitoring (Fig. 5-2).

Two different gas sampling methods exist: mainstream and sidestream. The mainstream method involves placing the infrared sensing unit at the airway; usually, it is attached directly to the endotracheal/tracheostomy tube. If the patient is on a ventilator, the sampling adapter must be placed between the endotracheal tube and the ventilator circuit (with or without mechanical dead space). All inspired and expired gas passes through the sensor (Fig. 5-3).

The sidestream method uses a capillary tube placed so that a small sampling of the patient's exhaled gas can be drawn into the capnometer for analysis. The patient's entire breath does not need to pass through the sampling adapter; therefore, the device can be used in an unintubated patient by taping the sampling catheter a short distance into a nostril. If the patient is on a ventilator, the sampling adapter must be placed between the

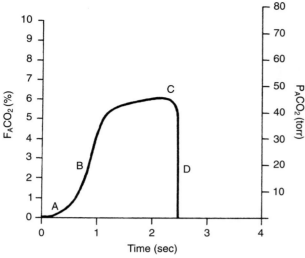

**Fig. 5-1** Normal capnograph tracing taken at a fast speed. The percentage of exhaled alveolar $CO_2$ is shown on the left vertical scale as $F_ACO_2$. The partial pressure of exhaled alveolar $CO_2$ is shown on the right vertical scale as $P_ACO_2$. The tracing of exhaled gas can be divided into these four components: **A,** Beginning of exhalation, which shows no $CO_2$ in the upper airway anatomic dead space; **B,** addition of alveolar gas, rich in $CO_2$, to the anatomic dead space gas causes a rapid rise in measured $CO_2$; **C,** pure alveolar gas with a stable amount of $CO_2$ causes a plateau—the end-tidal $CO_2$ point is shown at **C** just before inspiration; **D,** inspiration with a rapid drop in $CO_2$ to zero. A fast-speed tracing is more useful for determining the cause of a patient's changing condition than a slow-speed tracing.

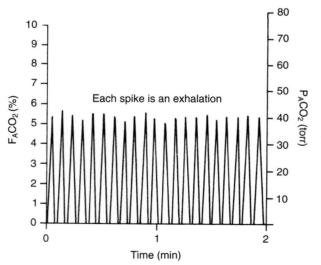

**Fig. 5-2** Normal capnograph tracing taken at a slow speed. The percentage of exhaled alveolar $CO_2$ is shown on the left vertical scale as $F_ACO_2$. The partial pressure of exhaled alveolar $CO_2$ is shown on the right vertical scale as $P_ACO_2$. The slow speed results in a blending of parts **A, B,** and **C** of the fast-speed tracing (see Fig. 5-1). Each spike is part **C** of the curve and marks an exhalation. A slow-speed tracing is more useful in trend monitoring of a patient than is a fast-speed tracing.

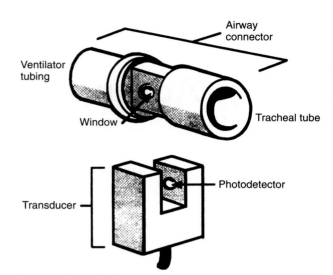

**Fig. 5-3** Schematic drawing of a mainstream exhaled-$CO_2$ analyzer sensor. The infrared sensor is attached to the patient's airway so that all of the exhaled and inhaled gases pass through it. *(From Szaflarski NL, Cohen NH: Use of capnography in critically ill patients, Heart Lung 20:363, 1991.)*

endotracheal tube and the ventilator circuit (with or without mechanical dead space). Remember that the patient's exhaled tidal volume ($V_T$) and minute volume ($\dot{V}_E$) will be reduced by the amount drawn into the capnometer (Fig. 5-4).

### c. Interpret the results from the procedure (NBRC code: IB8a, IIIA1b4) [Difficulty: R, Ap]

It is known that carbon dioxide diffuses from a higher concentration in the tissues to the venous blood and to the lungs to be exhaled. Fig. 5-5 shows the normal physiology behind capnography. This diffusion or "flow" of $CO_2$ results in a measurable gradient or difference. In a normal, upright-sitting person, a close relationship is seen between carbon dioxide levels in the venous blood, exhaled carbon dioxide gas, and arterial blood. The carbon dioxide level at the end of exhalation is most commonly monitored for patient care. This is called the *end-tidal carbon dioxide pressure (PetCO$_2$)*. When ventilation and perfusion match well, as in a normal upright person, the gradient between the arterial carbon dioxide level ($PaCO_2$) and the $PetCO_2$ is between 1 and 5 torr. The gradient will show the $PetCO_2$ to be less than the $PaCO_2$. This is because the $PetCO_2$ is an average of exhaled carbon dioxide from all lung areas.

Box 5-1 lists normal values of capnography. Three factors influence the use of capnography and the interpretation of results. First is the patient's metabolism. The average resting adult produces about 200 mL of $CO_2$/min. Fever and exercise increase this value. Hypothermia, sleep, and sedation decrease $CO_2$ production.

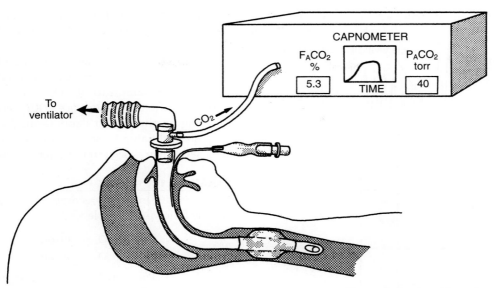

**Fig. 5-4** Representation of a sidestream capnometry system. A capillary tube is placed into the ventilator circuit to sample the exhaled and inhaled gases.

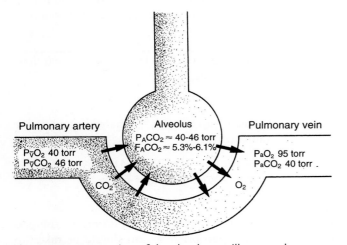

**Fig. 5-5** Representation of the alveolar-capillary membrane showing the diffusion of $O_2$ and $CO_2$ and the arterialization of venous blood. Also shown are alveolar $CO_2$ values measured by capnography.

---

**BOX 5-1   Normal Blood Gas and Capnography Values (based on a sea level barometric pressure of 760 torr)***

$PaCO_2$ is approximately 40 torr.

$P\bar{v}CO_2$ is approximately 46 torr.

Pressure of exhaled alveolar $CO_2$ ($P_ACO_2$) ranges from approximately 35 to 43 torr with the breathing cycle.

The pressure of exhaled end-tidal $CO_2$ (PetCO$_2$) ranges from 35 to 43 torr. This shows that the $CO_2$ level varies between the arterial and mixed venous blood levels. This value is often correlated with the $PaCO_2$.

The percent of exhaled $CO_2$ ($F_ACO_2$) ranges from 5% to approximately 6% with the breathing cycle.

The percent of end-tidal $CO_2$ ($F_ACO_2$) is approximately 5% to 6% and correlates with the $PaCO_2$.

---

*Both $P_ACO_2$ and $F_ACO_2$ may be seen listed as end-tidal $CO_2$. End-tidal $CO_2$ may be abbreviated as ETCO$_2$, et $CO_2$, or PET$_{CO2}$.

$F_ACO_2$, Percentage of $CO_2$ level; $PaCO_2$, partial pressure of $CO_2$ in arterial blood; $P_ACO_2$, partial pressure of alveolar $CO_2$ level; $P\bar{v}CO_2$, partial pressure of carbon dioxide in mixed venous blood.

---

Second, although it is not a major factor, is the patient's cardiac output. Sepsis, which might double a patient's cardiac output, reduces the $PCO_2$ by only a few millimeters of mercury (mm Hg). Cardiogenic shock, which reduces cardiac output, raises the partial pressure of $CO_2$ ($PCO_2$) by only a few millimeters of mercury.

Third, and most important, is alveolar ventilation. Doubling of alveolar ventilation under steady-state conditions for $CO_2$ production results in halving of the $PCO_2$ in arterial blood and alveolar gas. However, a reduction in alveolar ventilation to half of its previous level results in doubling of the $PaCO_2$ and the $P_ACO_2$ (Fig. 5-6).

Tidal volume ($V_T$) and respiratory rate are directly related to alveolar ventilation. Of the two, $V_T$ is more important because it relates to the patient's dead space ($V_D$)/$V_T$ ratio ($V_D/V_T$). A decrease in the patient's $V_T$ results in less alveolar ventilation and a rise in $PCO_2$. Conversely, an increase in the $V_T$ results in greater alveolar ventilation and a drop in the $PCO_2$.

Capnography is most accurate and correlates best with the $PaCO_2$ if the patient's ventilation and perfusion match. The greater the ventilation and perfusion mismatching, or the more unstable the pulmonary perfusion,

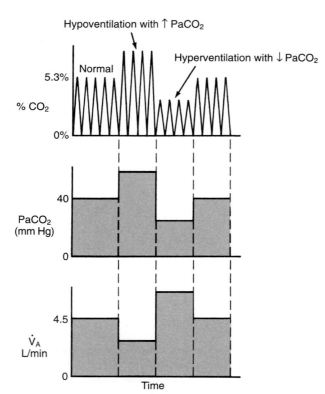

**Fig. 5-6** Relationship between alveolar ventilation ($\dot{V}_A$), partial pressure of carbon dioxide ($CO_2$) in arterial blood ($PaCO_2$), and exhaled $CO_2$ percentage. *(From Pilbeam SP: Mechanical ventilation: Physiological and clinical applications, ed 3, St Louis, 1998, Mosby.)*

the wider or less reliable is the gradient between the patient's arterial $CO_2$ and alveolar $CO_2$ levels. The following procedures should be done to enhance understanding of the patient's condition and interpretation of the capnography results.

***Pressure of arterial–end-tidal alveolar carbon dioxide gradient.*** The pressure of arterial–end-tidal alveolar $CO_2$ gradient [P(a – et)$CO_2$] is useful because, once it has been reliably determined, the patient with a stable cardiopulmonary condition can have his/her ventilatory condition monitored by capnography alone. This occurs most widely in a sedated patient or one with a head injury who has normal cardiopulmonary function. The unstable patient's $PaCO_2$ level will still need to be checked regularly.

Most patients who use capnography are lying flat in bed and do not have normal ventilation and perfusion matching. It has been reported that the possible P(a – et)$CO_2$ gradient ranges from –6 to +20 torr in unstable patients with cardiopulmonary abnormalities. For example, the patient who is breathing shallowly may have an end-tidal $CO_2$ that is significantly less than the arterial $CO_2$. This shallow-breathing patient is blowing out upper airway dead space (low in carbon dioxide) rather than alveolar gas (high in carbon dioxide).

For confirmation of the patient's breathing efforts, the P(a – et)$CO_2$ gradient should be calculated. Follow these steps:

a. Simultaneously draw an arterial blood gas (ABG) sample for $PaCO_2$ measurement and take an end-tidal gas sample for $P_ACO_2$ measurement.

b. The difference is the P(a – et)$CO_2$ gradient. Depending on the patient's condition, the gradient could show the alveolar sample with a higher or lower $CO_2$ level than is seen in the arterial sample.

## EXAMPLE 1

A patient is seen in the recovery room after surgery and has the following $PCO_2$ levels:

$$\begin{aligned} PaCO_2 &= 40\,\text{torr} \\ PetCO_2 &= \underline{-36\,\text{torr}} \\ P(a-et)CO_2 &= \phantom{-}4\,\text{torr gradient} \end{aligned}$$

The usefulness of this gradient is seen when one is monitoring the patient's spontaneous breathing during weaning or making ventilator changes in the $V_T$ and/or $\dot{V}_E$. It may be possible to avoid drawing so many ABG samples.

## EXAMPLE 2

The patient in Example 1 is seen later and has the following capnography reading:

$$PetCO_2 = 54\,\text{torr}$$

The patient's $PaCO_2$ can be easily estimated by adding the following gradient:

$$\begin{aligned} PetCO_2 &= 54\,\text{torr} \\ P(a-et)CO_2\ \text{gradient} &= \underline{+4\,\text{torr}} \\ \text{Estimated}\ PaCO_2 &= 58\,\text{torr} \end{aligned}$$

It could be concluded that the patient is not breathing as deeply as before. Appropriate action should be taken to awaken the patient, further reverse the anesthesia, or begin artificial ventilation. (NOTE: If the gradient were reversed from alveolar to arterial, the patient's $PaCO_2$ could still be mathematically estimated.)

Review the components of a fast-speed capnography tracing in Fig. 5-1 to understand a normal person's expiratory pattern. Fig. 5-7 shows eight different abnormal fast-speed capnography tracings. As the patient returns to normal, the tracing should approach that shown in Fig. 5-1.

***Residual volume alveolar-arterial carbon dioxide gradient.*** If the patient is cooperative and exhales maximally to residual volume (RV), this measurement will provide more clinically useful information. The usual P(a – RV)$CO_2$ gradient in a normal person is less than 7 torr. The wider the gradient, the greater the amount of ventilation-to-perfusion ($\dot{V}/\dot{Q}$) mismatching there is. A gradient of more than 13 torr is considered to be markedly abnormal.

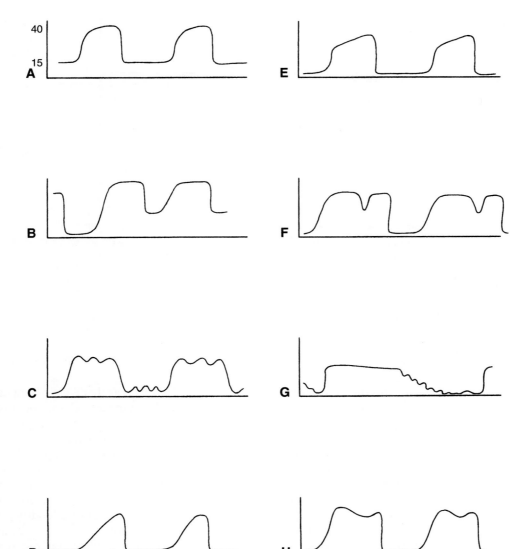

**Fig. 5-7** A series of abnormal fast-speed capnography tracings. **A,** A mechanically ventilated patient with a malfunctioning exhalation valve. Note how the baseline $CO_2$ level is elevated because the patient's exhaled breath is being measured during an inspiration. Correction of the exhalation valve should result in normal inhalation and exhalation. **B,** This rapidly rising baseline gas pressure and failure to return to baseline are usually seen when moisture or secretions block the capillary tube. Clearing the obstruction enables the patient's gas to again reach the analyzer. **C,** Distortions in the tracing from incomplete exhalation. These could be caused by hiccups, chest compressions during CPR, or inconsistent tidal volume efforts during an asthma attack. **D,** An obstructive lung disease patient with ventilation and perfusion mismatching. There is no alveolar plateau with a stable $CO_2$ level. Inhaling a bronchodilator should result in return of the tracing to closer to normal. **E,** A patient with restrictive lung disease showing no plateau of alveolar gas emptying, because the alveoli do not empty evenly. **F,** A sudden drop in $CO_2$ level in the middle of an exhalation indicating the patient attempted inspiration. This "cleft" is usually seen when a patient who has been pharmacologically paralyzed begins to regain movement. **G,** Uneven $CO_2$ levels seen at the end of exhalation can be caused by (1) the patient's heartbeat pumping fresh blood and $CO_2$ to the emptying lungs (the cardiogenic oscillations should match the heart rate), or (2) the ventilator's exhalation valve fluttering open and closed. **H,** The alveolar plateau is biphasic. This has been seen in patients with lungs that are different in compliance and ventilation:perfusion matching (e.g., single lung transplantation).

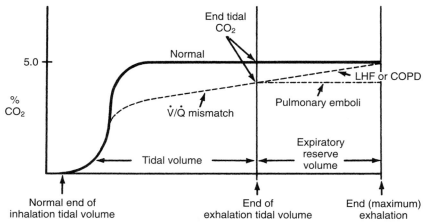

**Fig. 5-8** Comparison of several fast-speed capnograph tracings showing how the exhaled $CO_2$ level changes as the patient exhales to residual volume (RV). A normal tracing *(solid line)* is matched against abnormal tracings of pulmonary emboli, left heart failure (LHF), and chronic obstructive pulmonary disease (COPD) *(dotted line)*. The normal patient has the same end-tidal $CO_2$ as RV $CO_2$, showing good matching of ventilation and perfusion. LHF and COPD patients have a narrowing of the gradient as RV is approached. The patient with a pulmonary embolism keeps the same gradient at the RV as that found at the end of the tidal volume. $\dot{V}/\dot{Q}$, Ventilation-to-perfusion ratio. *(From Pilbeam SP: Mechanical ventilation: Physiological and clinical applications, ed 3, St Louis, 1998, Mosby.)*

This may be the case in patients with chronic obstructive pulmonary disease (COPD), pulmonary emboli, left heart failure (LHF), or hypotension.

When the normal (solid line) tracing in Fig. 5-8 is compared with the $\dot{V}/\dot{Q}$ mismatching (dashed line) tracing, note the increased gradient at end-tidal $CO_2$. With continued exhalation to RV, patients with LHF and COPD have a narrowing of the gradient. This could be used clinically to follow the progress and response to treatment of these patients. The patient with large pulmonary emboli does *not* have such a narrowing of the gradient as he or she exhales to RV. This patient's gradient narrows to normal as the embolism is resolved and the physiologic dead space returns to normal.

## 2. Review the patient's chart for information on any previously measured dead space:tidal volume ratio tests (NBRC code: IA6d) [Difficulty: R, Ap]

Review previous data before repeating the test to understand if the patient was abnormal. Be prepared to compare the previous information with the new data to help you as you evaluate the patient's current condition. This test is most commonly done to document the $V_D$ (wasted ventilation) in a patient with a pulmonary embolism. The following discussion should help in interpretation of the patient's results.

The normal adult's $V_D/V_T$ ratio ranges from 0.2 (20%) to 0.4 (40%). Anatomic dead space is normally greater in men than in women. The normal 3-kg neonate's $V_D:V_T$ ratio is 0.3 (30%). Physiologic dead space (also known as *respiratory dead space*) is gas that is ventilated into the lungs but does not take part in gas exchange because the alveoli are not perfused, or they are underperfused for the amount of gas that they receive.

Physiologic dead space is made up of the following:
a. Anatomic dead space, or the gas in the connecting airways from the nose and mouth to the terminal bronchioles. Generally, it is assumed to be about 1 mL/lb or 2.2 mL/kg of ideal body weight.
b. Alveolar dead space, or the gas in nonfunctioning alveoli that are ventilated but not perfused. It is minimal in a normal person. The previous "normal" adult example has the expected amount of dead space for his or her weight.

The following conditions or pulmonary disorders can cause the ratio to vary from the normal range:
1. Decreased $V_D/V_T$ ratio
   a. Lung resection or pneumonectomy because the airways are removed; the patient maintains his or her $V_T$ in other lung segments
   b. Asthma attack because the airways are narrowed
   c. Insertion of an endotracheal or tracheostomy tube because the upper airway is bypassed
   d. Exercise in the normal person because the increased blood pressure increases perfusion of the apices (zone 1)
2. Increased $V_D/V_T$ ratio
   a. Vascular tumor because of decreased perfusion to ventilated alveoli
   b. Pulmonary embolism because of lack of blood flow to ventilated alveoli. Consider this if the

patient is a candidate for a pulmonary embolism and suddenly deteriorates
3. Increased dead space effect with ventilation greater than perfusion (V > Q)
   a. Rapid, shallow ventilations because the upper airway dead space is overventilated compared with the alveoli
   b. Mechanical dead space added to the ventilator circuit. This is an intentional effort to have the patient retain some of his or her exhaled $CO_2$ to correct for a respiratory alkalosis
   c. COPD (e.g., bronchitis, bronchiectasis, cystic fibrosis, emphysema) because varying degrees of bronchospasm, mucus plugging, and tissue destruction lead to increased ventilation and perfusion mismatching

Many clinicians believe that a $V_D/V_T$ ratio of 0.6 (60%) or greater is an indication for mechanical ventilation of the patient. A person wasting 60% or more of his or her ventilation will soon tire out from the work of breathing (WOB) and will go into ventilatory failure.

### Exam Hint

**R**emember that a pulmonary embolism is the most likely cause of a sudden increase in dead space. A patient with COPD will have a chronically increased dead space value.

### Math Review

Previous versions of the Entry Level Examination have required the calculation of a patient's $V_D/V_T$ ratio. The following sample calculations are included to aid in the understanding of how the results are found. The procedure is the mathematical comparison of a person's $V_D$ with $V_T$. Steps in the procedure follow (Fig. 5-9):
1. Determine the *average* exhaled $CO_2$ ($P_{\bar{E}}CO_2$) value by either of these methods:
   a. Collect the patient's entire exhaled gas sample over several minutes in a large, airtight bag. Count the number of breaths that occurred. Calculate the average $V_T$ breath by dividing the total exhaled volume by the total rate. Put all or part of this gas sample through the blood gas analyzer for the $PCO_2$ value.
   b. Pass the patient's exhaled gas through a capnometer that provides an average value (not end-tidal $CO_2$). A number of breaths should be averaged for greater $PCO_2$ accuracy. Measure or calculate the patient's average $V_T$ over the time of the test.
2. Draw an arterial sample at the same time as either step 1a or 1b. Have the blood sample analyzed for $PaCO_2$.
3. Calculate the results using either of two methods.

**Determine the decimal fraction or percentage of dead space.**

Place both $CO_2$ values into this formula, which is derived from the original Bohr formula:

$$V_D/V_T \,(\text{or } V_D) = \frac{PaCO_2 - P_{\bar{E}}CO_2}{PaCO_2}$$

In which:

$V_D/V_T$ or $V_D$ = The patient's physiologic dead space
$PaCO_2$ = The patient's arterial $CO_2$ pressure
$P_{\bar{E}}CO_2$ = The patient's average exhaled $CO_2$ pressure

The following example is based on a normal adult:

$$PaCO_2 = 45 \text{ torr}$$
$$P_{\bar{E}}CO_2 = 18 \text{ torr}$$
$$V_D = \frac{(45-18)}{45}$$
$$= \frac{27}{45} = .6$$

The patient's $V_D$ fraction can be recorded as .6 or 60%. (Note that this equation must be used when the patient's tidal volume is not known.)

**Determine the dead space volume.**

Place both $CO_2$ values into this formula, which is derived from the original Bohr formula:

$$V_D/V_T \,(\text{or } V_D) = \frac{PaCO_2 - P_{\bar{E}}CO_2}{PaCO_2} \times V_E$$

In which:

$V_D/V_T$ or $V_D$ = The patient's physiologic dead space
$V_{\bar{E}}$ = Average exhaled $V_T$
$PaCO_2$ = The patient's arterial $CO_2$ pressure
$P_{\bar{E}}CO_2$ = The patient's average exhaled $CO_2$ pressure

The following example is based on a normal adult:

$$V_{\bar{E}} = 500 \text{ mL}$$
$$PaCO_2 = 40 \text{ torr}$$
$$P_{\bar{E}}CO_2 = 28 \text{ torr}$$
$$V_D = \frac{(40-28)}{40}$$
$$= \frac{12}{40} \times 500 \text{ mL} = 0.3 \times 500 \text{ mL}$$
$$= 150 \text{ mL (Note that this equation must be used when the patient's tidal volume is known.)}$$

The patient's $V_D/V_T$ ratio is 150/500, 0.3, or 30%, depending on how it is written.

### 3. Perform the procedure for mixed venous blood sampling (NBRC code: IIIE2b) [Difficulty: R, Ap]

A patient with a functioning pulmonary artery catheter (PAC) can have a sample of blood withdrawn through it and analyzed for the mixed venous $O_2$ ($P\bar{v}O_2$) value (and the other blood gas values as well). See Fig. 5-10 for an example of a catheter. As always, the $P\bar{v}O_2$ value(s) should be reviewed before measuring is done again. (See Chapter

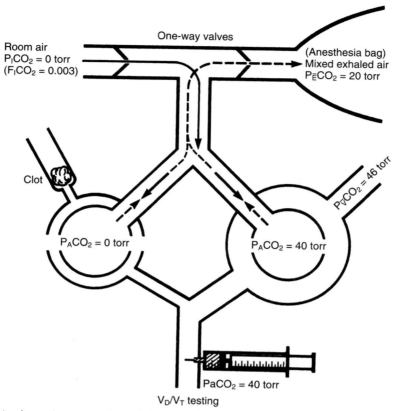

One-way valves

Room air
$P_ICO_2 = 0$ torr
$(F_ICO_2 = 0.003)$

(Anesthesia bag)
Mixed exhaled air
$P_\overline{E}CO_2 = 20$ torr

Clot

$P\overline{v}CO_2 = 46$ torr

$P_ACO_2 = 0$ torr

$P_ACO_2 = 40$ torr

$PaCO_2 = 40$ torr

$V_D/V_T$ testing

**Fig. 5-9** A schematic presentation of the procedure for gathering patient samples for calculating the dead space-to-tidal volume ratio ($V_D/V_T$). An anesthesia or other airtight bag is used to gather all exhaled gas to determine the average exhaled $CO_2$ pressure ($P_\overline{E}CO_2$). An arterial sample is collected for partial pressure of $CO_2$ in arterial blood ($PaCO_2$). $F_ICO_2$, percentage of average inhaled $CO_2$ pressure; $P_ACO_2$, partial pressure of $CO_2$ in alveolar gas; $P_ICO_2$, average inhaled $CO_2$ pressure; $P\overline{v}CO_2$, partial pressure of carbon dioxide in mixed venous blood. *(From Pilbeam SP: Mechanical ventilation: physiological and clinical applications, ed 2, St Louis, 1992, Mosby.)*

3 for additional information on mixed venous blood gas values.) There are currently three ways to perform the bedside procedure.

1. Perform the procedure through the distal port of a PAC as the catheter is being inserted.

This method is used when one is trying to determine if a ventricular septal defect exists. The procedure is commonly done on neonates with suspected congenital heart defect but may be used in adults as well. Blood samples are withdrawn serially from the distal port of the catheter as blood passes through the right atrium, the right ventricle, and sometimes the pulmonary artery of the patient. The venous blood sampling procedure is the same as described in Chapter 3 for obtaining an arterial blood sample through an arterial line.

Normally, the $P\overline{v}O_2$ and venous $O_2$ saturation ($S\overline{v}O_2$) values are the same in all blood samples. The patient with a ventricular septal defect shows an *increase* in $P\overline{v}O_2$ and $S\overline{v}O_2$ values in the right ventricle or pulmonary artery sample compared with the right atrium sample. This

occurs because the oxygenated blood from the left ventricle is forced though the ventricular septal defect to raise the $O_2$ value of the right ventricular blood.

2. Use a PAC with reflectance oximetry capability. These catheters have fiberoptic bundles built into them and use technology similar to that used in pulse oximeters (Fig. 5-11). The monitoring unit sends several wavelengths of light down the transmitting fiberoptic bundle to be shined on the passing blood in the pulmonary artery. Oxyhemoglobin ($HbO_2$) in the red blood cells absorbs some of the light, and the rest is reflected off. The receiving fiberoptic bundle picks up some of this light and transmits it back to the monitoring unit.

$S\overline{v}O_2$ is determined by the monitoring unit on the basis of the light waves transmitted and what was received. Care must be taken when this catheter is used in patients with elevated carboxyhemoglobin (COHb) or methemoglobin (MetHb) levels. As with pulse oximetry, COHb and MetHb cannot be measured. Thus, inaccurately high readings for $S\overline{v}O_2$ are seen.

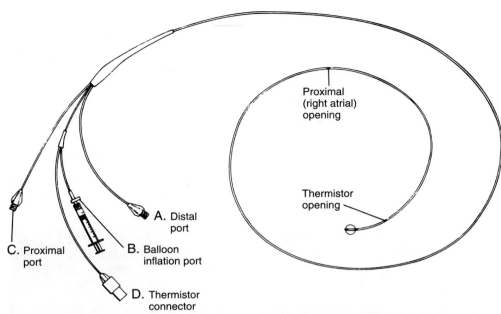

**Fig. 5-10** A 7-French quadruple lumen thermodilution pulmonary artery catheter. **A,** Distal port goes to the tip of the catheter. It is used for measuring pulmonary artery pressure, pulmonary capillary wedge pressure (PCWP), and partial pressure of $O_2$ in mixed venous blood. **B,** Balloon inflation port is used to inflate the balloon for inserting the catheter and obtaining a PCWP reading. **C,** Proximal port is used for measuring central venous pressure and for injecting iced saline for a thermodilution cardiac output study. The iced saline exits from the right atrial opening. **D,** Thermistor connector attaches to the cardiac output computer. A bimetallic wire runs through the catheter to the thermistor opening, where it is exposed to temperature changes of the blood and cold injectate. (Note: Not all catheters are capable of measuring cardiac output. Some catheters have other special features such as continuously measuring venous $O_2$ saturation or cardiac pacemaker leads.) *(From Oblouk Darovic G: Hemodynamic monitoring, Philadelphia, 1987, WB Saunders.)*

An actual mixed venous blood sample can be taken with this catheter through the distal port, as described above. The advantage of the reflectance oximetry system is that it provides continuous monitoring of your patient's $S\bar{v}O_2$ level. In addition, high and low saturation alarms can be set. If the tip should become lodged in the wall of the artery, or if a clot should form at the tip, the $S\bar{v}O_2$ will drop or fluctuate dramatically. The alarms should warn the clinician of a problem with the equipment.

3. Use the distal port of a "standard" PAC.

A true mixed venous blood sample is obtained by withdrawal of blood from the distal port of the catheter. This is the same lumen that is used for PAP and PCWP readings. The blood sampling procedure is similar to that described in Chapter 3, with the following revisions. A 5- to 10-mL syringe is used with sterile technique to pull out the heparinized solution in the lumen until about 1 to 2 mL of blood is removed. A second preheparinized syringe is then used to withdraw about 2 mL of mixed venous blood. It is important that the IV solution and blood be withdrawn at a rate no faster than 0.5 mL/sec. Drawing any faster could pull preoxygenated blood back through the capillary bed and give falsely elevated $O_2$ values. After

the blood is sampled, the lumen must be fast-flushed with the heparinized solution to prevent the blood from clotting. Flush for several seconds until the solution flows freely. This blood sample may be reliably analyzed for $S\bar{v}O_2$, $P\bar{v}O_2$, and $P\bar{v}CO_2$.

## 4. Interpret the results of the mixed venous blood sample (NBRC code: IB8d, IIIE4) [Difficulty: R, Ap]

This topic is discussed in some detail in Chapter 3. The normal values follow:

$P\bar{v}O_2$ of 40 torr (range of 37 to 43 torr)
$S\bar{v}O_2$ of 75% (range of 70% to 76%)

Mixed venous blood $O_2$ values are useful for following the patient's $O_2$ consumption. A $P\bar{v}O_2$ value of less than 30 torr or an $S\bar{v}O_2$ value of less than 56% is considered to show tissue hypoxia. Quick steps must be taken to reverse this. Increase the inspired $O_2$ percentage as needed. Low stroke volume and cardiac output can be increased by administering the drug digitalis (Lanoxin) or other inotropic agents. Low blood pressure can be increased by giving vasopressors such as dopamine HCl (Intropin).

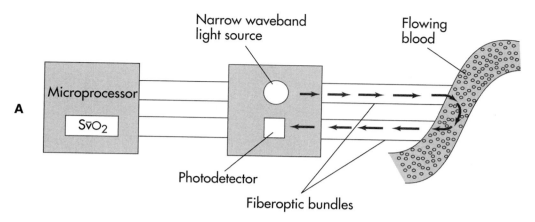

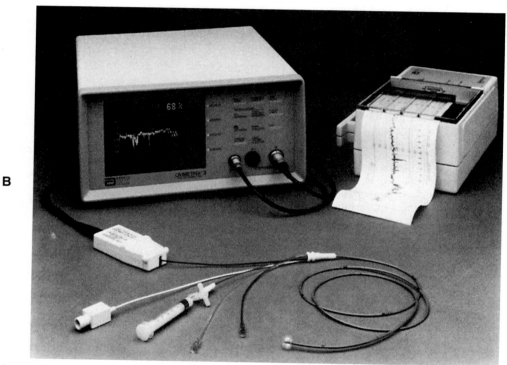

**Fig. 5-11** Mixed venous oxygen saturation ($S\bar{v}O_2\%$) can be monitored continuously by reflection spectroscopy in the appropriate pulmonary artery catheter. **A,** Detail of the fiber optic bundles in the catheter. Specific wavelengths of light are directed at passing blood. Some of the light is absorbed by the passing red blood cells and some is reflected back to the photodetector. The microprocessor calculates the $S\bar{v}O_2\%$. **B,** Components of the system include (1) microprocessor that connects to the catheter, displays $S\bar{v}O_2\%$ values, and has high and low saturation alarms; (2) strip chart recorder to copy the saturation values over time; and (3) reflective spectroscopy-type pulmonary artery catheter. The catheter can also be used for measuring pulmonary artery pressure, pulmonary capillary wedge pressure, and cardiac output; and taking a mixed venous blood gas sample. (*A from Ruppel GL: Manual of pulmonary function testing, ed 8, St. Louis, 2003, Mosby. B courtesy Hospira, Inc., Lake Forest, IL.*)

## MODULE B
### Respiratory care plan

### 1. Analyze the available information to determine the patient's pathophysiologic state (NBRC code: IIIH1) [Difficulty: R, Ap, An]

Review the previous discussion for information related to cardiac and pulmonary problems. A variety of problems can cause the patient's exhaled carbon dioxide level to vary from normal. Heart failure can result in a drop in the patient's mixed venous oxygen level.

### 2. Determine the appropriateness of the prescribed respiratory care plan and recommend modifications when indicated.

### a. Determine the appropriateness of the prescribed therapy and goals for the patient's pathophysiologic state (NBRC code: IIIH3) [Difficulty: R, Ap, An]

### b. Recommend changes in the therapeutic plan if supportive data exist (NBRC code: IIIH4) [Difficulty: Ap, An]

Be prepared to recommend changes in the patient's ventilatory support when capnography shows an abnormality. If the patient has an increased level of dead space, be prepared to increase ventilatory support. If a pulmonary embolism is the cause of the increased dead space, a clot-dissolving medication may be indicated. Proper management of a patient with heart failure will usually result in an increase in the mixed venous oxygen level.

## BIBLIOGRAPHY

American Association for Respiratory Care: Clinical practice guideline: Capnography/capnometry during mechanical ventilation–2003 revision & update, *Respir Care* 48(5):534, 2003.

Anton WR, Raghu G: Measuring end-tidal carbon dioxide tension at maximal exhalation to improve its utility during T-piece weaning trials, *Respir Care* 35(11):1082, 1990.

Bakow ED: A limitation of capnography, *Respir Care* 27(2):167, 1982.

Branson RD, Campbell RS: Cardiovascular monitoring. In Branson RD, Hess DR, Chatburn RL, editors: *Respiratory care equipment*, ed 2, Philadelphia, 1999, Lippincott, Williams & Wilkins.

Cairo JM: Assessment of physiologic function. In Cairo JM, Pilbeam SP: *Mosby's respiratory care equipment*, ed 7, St Louis, 2004, Mosby.

Carlon GC, Ray C Jr, Miodownik S, et al: Capnography in mechanically ventilated patients, *Crit Care Med* 16(5):550, 1988.

Clark DB, Marshall SG: Mixed venous oxygen saturation measurement. II. General and specific clinical applications, *Respir Ther* 81, Nov/Dec 1986.

Daily EK, Schroeder JS: *Techniques in bedside hemodynamic monitoring*, ed 4, St Louis, 1989, Mosby.

Deshpande VM, Pilbeam SP, Dixon RJ: *A comprehensive review in respiratory care*, East Norwalk, Conn, 1988, Appleton & Lange.

Divertie MB, McMichan JC: Continuous monitoring of mixed venous oxygen saturation, *Chest* 85(3):423, 1984.

Fahey PJ, Harris K, Vanderwarf C: Clinical experience with continuous monitoring of mixed venous oxygen saturation in respiratory failure, *Chest* 86(5):748, 1984.

Fink JB, Hunt GE, editors: *Clinical practice in respiratory care*, Philadelphia, 1999, Lippincott-Raven.

Harris K: Noninvasive monitoring of gas exchange, *Respir Care* 32(7):544, 1987.

Hess D: Capnometry and capnography: technical aspects, physiologic aspects, and clinical applications, *Respir Care* 35(6):557, 1990.

Hess D: Respiratory care monitoring. In Burton GG, Hodgkin JE, Ward JJ, editors: *Respiratory care: a guide to clinical practice*, ed 4, Philadelphia, 1997, Lippincott.

Hess DR, Branson RD: Noninvasive respiratory monitoring equipment. In Branson RD, Hess DR, Chatburn RL, editors: *Respiratory care equipment*, ed 2, Philadelphia, 1999, Lippincott, Williams & Wilkins.

Hunt GE: Diagnostic procedures at the bedside. In Fink JB, Hunt GE, editors: *Clinical practice in respiratory care*, Philadelphia, 1999, Lippincott-Raven.

Jaquith SM: The oximetrix opticath: What is it and how can it facilitate nursing management of the critically ill patient? *Crit Care Nurse* 4(3):55, 1984.

Kandel G, Aberman A: Mixed venous oxygen saturation: Its role in the assessment of the critically ill patient, *Arch Intern Med* 143:1400, 1983.

Kinasewitz GT: Use of end-tidal capnography during mechanical ventilation, *Respir Care* 25(2):169, 1982.

Krider SJ: Cardiac output assessment. In Wilkins RL, Sheldon RL, Krider SJ, editors: *Clinical assessment in respiratory care*, ed 3, St Louis, 1995, Mosby.

Krider SJ: Invasively monitored hemodynamic pressures. In Wilkins RL, Sheldon RL, Krider SJ, editors: *Clinical assessment in respiratory care*, ed 3, St Louis, 1995, Mosby.

Malinowski T: Respiratory monitoring in the intensive care unit. In Wilkins RL, Krider SJ, Sheldon RL, editors: *Clinical assessment in respiratory care*, ed 3, St Louis, 1990, Mosby.

Marini JJ: Obtaining meaningful data from the Swan-Ganz catheter, *Respir Care* 30(7):572, 1985.

Mathews PJ, Gregg BL: Monitoring and management of the patient in the ICU. In Scanlan CL, Wilkins RL, Stoller JK, editors: *Egan's fundamentals of respiratory care*, ed 7, St Louis, 1999, Mosby.

McMichan JC: Continuous monitoring of mixed venous oxygen saturation in clinical practice, *Mt Sinai J Med* 51(5):569, 1984.

Nuzzo PF, Anton WR: Practical applications of capnography, *Respir Ther* 12, Nov/Dec 1986.

Oblouk Darovic G: *Hemodynamic monitoring*, ed 2, Philadelphia, 2000, WB Saunders.

Paulus DA: Invasive monitoring of respiratory gas exchange: Continuous measurement of mixed venous oxygen saturation, *Respir Care* 32(7):535, 1987.

Pilbeam SP: *Mechanical ventilation, physiological and clinical applications*, ed 3, St Louis, 1998, Mosby.

Ramage JE Jr: Hemodynamic and gas exchange monitoring. In Hess DR, MacIntyre NR, et al, editors, *Respiratory Care Principles & Practice*, Philadelphia, 2002, WB Saunders.

Ruppel G: *Manual of pulmonary function testing*, ed 6, St Louis, 1994, Mosby.

Scanlan CL, Wilkins RL: Analysis and monitoring of gas exchange. In Wilkins RL, Stoller JK, Scanlan CL, editors: *Egan's fundamentals of respiratory care*, ed 8, St Louis, 2003, Mosby.

Shapiro BA, Kacmarek RM, Cane RD, et al, editors: *Clinical application of respiratory care*, ed 4, St Louis, 1991, Mosby.

Shapiro BA, Peruzzi WT, Templin R, et al: *Clinical application of blood gases*, ed 5, Chicago, 1994, Mosby.

Whitaker K: *Comprehensive perinatal & pediatric respiratory care*, ed 2, Albany, 1997, Delmar.

White GC: *Equipment theory for respiratory care*, ed 3, Albany, 1999, Delmar.

Wiedemann HP: Invasive monitoring techniques in the ventilated patient. In Kacmarek RM, Stoller JK, editors: *Current respiratory care*, Toronto, 1988, BC Decker.

## SELF-STUDY QUESTIONS

1. Your patient has a $V_D/V_T$ ratio of 0.68. Based on these results, which of the following would you recommend?
   A. Give the patient supplemental $O_2$.
   B. Coach the patient in hyperinflation therapy.
   C. Put the patient on a mechanical ventilator.
   D. Give the patient an IPPB treatment.

2. A patient with thrombophlebitis in his leg suddenly complains of shortness of breath. What test would be best to help determine the problem?
   A. Peak flow
   B. Pulse oximetry
   C. $V_D/V_T$ ratio
   D. Flow-volume loop

3. A patient has an end-tidal $CO_2$ of 30 torr and a $P(a - et)CO_2$ gradient of 4 torr. The alveolar to end-tidal gradient is in the usual direction. Based on this, his $PaCO_2$ would be estimated as
   A. 26 torr
   B. 30 torr
   C. 4 torr
   D. 34 torr

4. Your patient is known to have advanced COPD. When checking his $V_D/V_T$ ratio, you would expect it to be
   A. Unaffected by his condition
   B. Increased
   C. Normal
   D. Decreased

5. A patient with heart failure and pulmonary edema has an initial $P\bar{v}O_2$ value of 35 torr. After being mechanically ventilated and given digitalis, the $P\bar{v}O_2$ value is found to be 41 torr. How should this be interpreted?
   A. Improved tissue oxygenation
   B. No clinical change
   C. Decreased tissue oxygenation
   D. Worsening heart failure

6. The following capnograph on a patient in the recovery room could be interpreted as
   A. Normal
   B. V/Q mismatching
   C. Pulmonary fibrosis
   D. Cardiopulmonary arrest

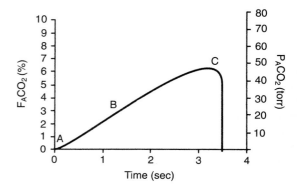

7. While you are working in the critical care unit, a nurse asks you to assess a patient. The patient has a $PvO_2$ value of 29 torr. This indicates that the patient
   A. Is normal
   B. Is suffering some tissue hypoxia
   C. Is not consuming the normal amount of $O_2$
   D. Is hypercarbic

8. A patient is being mechanically ventilated and has a reflectance oximetry pulmonary artery catheter in place. What should the patient's $S\bar{v}O_2$ target be set at?
   A. 40%
   B. 50%
   C. 75%
   D. 90%

9. The normal $P(a - et)CO_2$ gradient is
   A. 0–1 torr
   B. 1–5 torr
   C. More than 15 torr
   D. About 40 torr

10. A neonatal patient is suspected of having a ventricular septal defect. What could be done to confirm or rule out this condition?
    A. Perform capnography to monitor the $PetCO_2$.
    B. Perform a $V_D/V_T$ calculation.
    C. Check the $P\bar{v}O_2$ from the pulmonary artery.
    D. Check the $P\bar{v}O_2$ from the right atrium and right ventricle.

11. A patient has a $PaCO_2$ of 52 torr and $PetCO_2$ of 66 torr. Calculate her $P(a - et)CO_2$.
    A. 118 torr
    B. 66 torr
    C. 52 torr
    D. −14 torr

## ANSWER KEY AND RATIONALE

1. **C.** A $V_D/V_T$ ratio of 0.68 (68%) indicates that most of the patient's breathing efforts are wasted. Many practitioners would believe that a value this high justifies putting the patient on a ventilator. An IPPB treatment would temporarily give the patient some relief but is not a long-term solution. Hyperinflation therapy or supplemental $O_2$ will not help the patient's condition.

2. **C.** A pulmonary embolism (PE) should be suspected in a patient with thrombophlebitis who experiences sudden shortness of breath. If this is the case, the $V_D/V_T$ ratio would be increased. The peak flow test is not helpful in determining if the patient had a PE. Although the patient's pulse oximetry value will probably drop with a PE, this is not specific for a PE. The flow-volume loop will not show any change related to a pulmonary embolism.

3. **A.** The difference between the $PetCO_2$ of 30 torr and $P(a - et)CO_2$ gradient of 4 torr is 26 torr. Review the math examples in the chapter.

4. **B.** Patients with COPD have significant ventilation-to-perfusion mismatches. This results in increased dead space ventilation and shunt-like effects. The COPD patient would not be expected to have normal or decreased dead space.

5. **A.** After treatment, the patient's $P\bar{v}O_2$ value has increased to 41 torr. This is in the normal range and would indicate that the patient has normal tissue oxygenation. If the patient had worsening heart failure or decreased tissue perfusion, the $P\bar{v}O_2$ value would have decreased to less than the original value of 35 torr.

6. **B.** The figure best fits that of mismatching of ventilation and perfusion. Review the example tracings in Fig. 5-7.

7. **B.** This low value indicates that tissue hypoxia is present. Review the earlier discussion and normal values for $P\bar{v}O_2$.

8. **C.** An $S\bar{v}O_2$ of 75% would be normal and indicate normal tissue oxygenation. Values of less than 75% saturation would indicate tissue hypoxia. A saturation of 90% is far higher than that needed in venous blood.

9. **B.** When ventilation and perfusion match well, as in a normal person, the gradient between the arterial carbon dioxide level and the average exhaled carbon dioxide level is between 1 and 5 torr. A carbon dioxide level of less than this would indicate that no ventilation or no $CO_2$ is being produced. Gradients of greater than 1 to 5 torr have been found in patients with significant ventilation/perfusion mismatching.

10. **D.** If the patient has a ventricular septal defect, the oxygen level from the right atrium to the right ventricle will be increased. This is because high-oxygen blood from the left ventricle will leak through the defect into the right ventricle. Capnography and dead space values will not point specifically to a hole in the ventricular septum. It is insufficient to check the $P\bar{v}O_2$ only from the pulmonary artery. This value will not provide a comparison with the oxygen value before the right ventricle.

11. **D.** Subtracting the $PetCO_2$ of 66 torr from the $PaCO_2$ of 52 torr results in a gradient difference of −14 torr. Review the examples from earlier in the chapter if necessary.

# 6 | Oxygen Therapy

A review of the most recent Entry Level Examinations has shown an average of 12 questions (9% of the exam) that cover oxygen therapy.

## MODULE A

### Ensure that the patient is adequately oxygenated

1. **Oxygen administration**

   a. **Minimize hypoxemia by positioning the patient properly** (NBRC code: IIID6) [Difficulty: R]

Usually, a patient who is short of breath when lying supine should be repositioned to sit more upright in a Fowler's or semi-Fowler's position. This seems to work best in patients with bilateral pulmonary problems such as congestive heart failure or pneumonia. If the patient cannot sit up and the lung problem is one-sided, roll the patient so that the more functional lung is down. The good lung should be positioned up in the following exceptions:

1. Undrained pulmonary abscess that should not be drained into the good lung
2. Neonatal congenital diaphragmatic hernia in which the good lung should not be compressed by the bowel in the chest cavity
3. Pulmonary interstitial emphysema in which, when the patient lies on the bad lung, the air leak and functional residual capacity can be reduced

In either case, always ask the patient whether the new position helps to make breathing easier. If not, reposition the patient until breathing is more comfortable with less shortness of breath.

   b. **Administer oxygen as needed and make a recommendation to change the fractional inspired oxygen concentration or oxygen flow to spontaneously breathing patients** (NBRC code: IIID4b, IIIG2c) [Difficulty: R, Ap]

Oxygen ($O_2$) must be administered in doses (up to 100%) that are adequate to treat hypoxemia or decrease the patient's work of breathing or work of the heart. Because the US Food and Drug Administration has declared supplemental $O_2$ to be a drug, a physician's order must be issued before it can be given to a patient, or before a change can be made in the patient's oxygen percentage. The only exceptions occur when recognized protocols within an institution permit $O_2$ to be given under certain limited conditions. For example, all patients with a diagnosed heart attack may be given a nasal cannula at 2 L/min, or all patients undergoing CPR may receive 100% $O_2$.

See Chapter 3 (Module A) for a listing of indications for drawing blood for an arterial blood gas (ABG) measurement. This list shows most of the conditions that justify the need for supplemental $O_2$. The general goal of giving supplemental $O_2$ is to keep the patient's $PaO_2$ level at between 60 and 100 torr. Exceptions include CO poisoning, severe anemia, and CPR, wherein the hope is to fully saturate the hemoglobin and increase the plasma $O_2$ content as much as possible. $O_2$ should not be given without proof of hypoxemia or another clinical justification. When those conditions have been corrected, the $O_2$ percentage should be adjusted accordingly.

Supplemental $O_2$ is not given without risk. Following is a list of $O_2$-related problems that may be clinically seen:

***$O_2$-induced hypoventilation.*** Although this is a controversial issue, it is wise to watch for this when supplemental oxygen is given to a COPD patient with a low oxygen level and an elevated $CO_2$ level. A common clinical goal is to keep the $PaO_2$ level at between 50 and 60 torr. Check the patient's arterial blood gas values frequently for the $O_2$ and $CO_2$ levels.

***Retinopathy of prematurity (ROP) (formerly called retrolental fibroplasia, or RLF).*** This type of blindness is found in some premature neonates who were given high levels of supplemental $O_2$. The exact cause is not completely understood but is related primarily to the degree of prematurity. Keeping the $PaO_2$ in the range of 50 to 60 torr the first week and 50 to 70 torr after that should help to prevent the problem.

***Denitrogenation absorption atelectasis.*** Giving greater than 80% $O_2$ can result in atelectasis of underventilated alveoli after the $O_2$ has been taken up by the blood.

***Central nervous system abnormalities.*** A patient who is breathing 100% $O_2$ in a hyperbaric chamber can have muscle tremors and seizures.

***Pulmonary $O_2$ toxicity.*** In general, it appears that patients can breathe up to 50% $O_2$ for prolonged periods without significant damage. If clinically possible, many practitioners try to limit patients to no more than 48 to 72 hr of breathing greater than 50% $O_2$.

### c. Measure the patient's oxygen percentage or oxygen liter flow (NBRC code: IIIE9) [Difficulty: R]

Always measure the patient's $O_2$ percentage ($F_1O_2$), if possible. The gas sample should be taken as close as possible to the patient to minimize the chance of dilution from room air. Record the $O_2$ percentage on the ABG order slip, in the department records, and in the patient's chart if needed. As discussed in Chapter 3, the $O_2$ percentage must be known before the patient's $PaO_2$ level can be interpreted.

The $O_2$ liter flow is all that can be recorded with these devices: nasal cannula, nasal catheter, simple mask, partial-rebreather mask, nonrebreather mask, and transtracheal $O_2$ catheter. A direct relationship exists between the liter flow and the $O_2$ percentage, but it is not predictably accurate.

### d. Prevent the patient from becoming hypoxemic by using proper technique (NBRC code: IIID7) [Difficulty: R, Ap]

Use caution and plan ahead to minimize any time that the $O_2$ supply to the patient is cut off or reduced. When equipment of any kind is changed, have the replacement set up and tested for proper function before the current setup is replaced.

Suctioning the airway is known to reduce the patient's $O_2$ level, which can result in dangerous arrhythmia. Remember to increase the patient's inspired $O_2$ percentage for about 1 min before, during, and for at least 1 min after suctioning. Giving 100% $O_2$ for short periods like this is acceptable and safe. Remember to reduce the $O_2$ percentage or liter flow to the previous level once the patient is stable after the procedure. Reanalyze the percentage if possible.

### 2. Perform quality control procedures for oxygen analyzers (NBRC code: IIC2) [Difficulty: R]

Because so many different models are available, consult an equipment book or the manufacturer's literature for details of the various analyzers. All portable, handheld analyzers fall into one of the following categories: electric, physical/paramagnetic, or electrochemical.

Calibration is done on all analyzers by sampling room air, adjusting a calibration control if necessary to have the unit show 21% $O_2$, sampling 100% $O_2$, and adjusting a calibration control if necessary to have the unit show 100% $O_2$. Always follow the manufacturer's guidelines for setup and calibration.

*Electric analyzers.* These analyzers basically operate by comparing the cooling effects of an $O_2$-enriched gas sample on a heated wire with the cooling effects of a room air gas sample on a heated wire. The $O_2$-enriched gas cools faster than the room air gas, which is known as the principle of thermal conductivity. Each sample must be drawn into the analyzer through a capillary line. These analyzers are designed to work only in $O_2$ and $N_2$ gas mixes. Do not use them around flammable gases such as those found in anesthesia. Failure to calibrate could be caused by a weak battery, a plugged capillary line, or a defect in an electrical component.

*Physical/paramagnetic analyzers.* These analyzers work on the principle that $O_2$ is attracted toward a magnetic field (paramagnetic property). The more $O_2$ is present in a sample gas, the more altered the magnetic field will be. These units can be used with all types of gases and are safe in the operating room with flammable and explosive anesthetics. A silica gel–filled container is in line with the capillary tube to dry out the sample gas before it gets to the analyzing chamber. Failure to calibrate could be caused by water or a defect in the analyzing chamber, a weak battery, or a plugged capillary line.

*Electrochemical analyzers: Polarographic and galvanic fuel cells.* Electrochemical analyzers make use of the fact that each $O_2$ molecule accepts up to two electrons and becomes chemically reduced. The more $O_2$ is present in the gas sample, the greater is the number of electrons that are released from an oxidizing electrolyte solution. This is measured as an electrical current that is proportionate to the $O_2$ percentage. These analyzers can continuously monitor and display the $O_2$ percentages. Both types are safe by themselves in the presence of flammable gases, but the added alarm systems are electrically powered and may make the units unsafe. Polarographic analyzers use a battery to polarize the gas-sampling probe. Because of this, they have a faster response time than do the galvanic fuel–cell types. Galvanic fuel–cell analyzers do not need a battery for power. However, they usually include battery-powered alarms.

Failure to calibrate either type could be caused by a weak battery, an exhausted supply of chemical reactant in the gas-sampling probe, or an electronic failure. The galvanic units must have their probes kept dry for accurate reading. Both types are pressure sensitive. High altitude causes them to display a lower-than-true $O_2$ percentage, and high pressure as seen in a ventilator circuit with positive end-expiratory pressure causes the units to display a higher-than-true $O_2$ percentage.

## MODULE B

### Storage, hardware, and distribution of medical gases

1. **Oxygen and other gas cylinders**
   a. **Get the necessary equipment for the procedure (NBRC code: IIA9) [Difficulty: R]**
   b. **Put the equipment together and make sure that it works properly (NBRC code: IIA9) [Difficulty: R]**
   c. **Troubleshoot any problems with the equipment (NBRC code: IIA9) [Difficulty: R]**

*Oxygen and other gas cylinders.* The different types of gases in cylinders are identified by the color code of the cylinder and the cylinder's label. Note that only E-cylinders have mandatory color coding. Color codings on the other cylinders are voluntary but are usually followed by the manufacturers. However, you should always read the label to be sure of the contents of the cylinder. The most important cylinder colors to remember are those for $O_2$ and air, but Table 6-1 includes all of the colors for the sake of completeness.

### Exam Hint

The NBRC is known to ask the examinee to calculate how long a certain cylinder lasts at a given gas flow. On past exams, only the durations of E-, H-, and K-sized $O_2$ cylinders have had to be calculated.

To review how to calculate the duration of flow of a type of cylinder, see Table 6-2 and the following equation and examples.

$$\text{Minutes of flow (divide by 60 to calculate hours)} = \frac{\text{gauge pressure in psig} \times \text{cylinder factor}}{\text{liter flow}}$$

1. Calculate the duration of flow of an E-cylinder with a 1500 pounds per square inch gauge (psig) that is running at 6 L/min.

   Minutes of flow
   $$= \frac{1500 \text{ psig} \times .28}{6} = \frac{420}{6}$$
   Minutes of flow = 70 (1.16 hours, or 1 hour and 10 minutes)

2. Calculate the duration of flow of an H-cylinder with 1950 psig that is running at 9 L/min.

   Minutes of flow
   $$= \frac{1950 \text{ psig} \times 3.14}{9} = \frac{6123}{9}$$
   Minutes of flow = 680.33 (11.34 hours, or 11 hours and 20 minutes)

| TABLE 6-1 | Color Codes for Gas Cylinders |
|---|---|
| **Gas** | **Color** |
| Oxygen | Green (white for international) |
| Air | Yellow |
| Helium | Brown |
| Helium and oxygen | Brown and green (check the label for the percentage of each gas) |
| Carbon dioxide | Gray |
| Carbon dioxide and oxygen | Gray and green (check the label for the percentage of each gas) |
| Nitrous oxide | Light blue |
| Cyclopropane | Orange |
| Ethylene | Red |

| TABLE 6-2 | Oxygen Cylinder Duration of Flow Factors |
|---|---|
| **Cylinder size** | **Factor (L/psig)** |
| E | 0.28 |
| H | 3.14 |
| K | 3.14 |
| D | 0.16 |
| M | 1.36 |
| G | 2.41 |

*psig,* Pounds per square inch gauge.

Following are related gas delivery systems:

*Bulk storage systems.* The bulk liquid $O_2$ (LOX)-storage system is the main source of a hospital's $O_2$. A reducing valve is used to decrease the gas pressure to 50 psig before it is piped throughout the hospital for easy access. Alarms sound if the pressure falls too low or goes too high. Pressure relief valves open if the pressure is greater than 75 psig. Zone valves are located throughout the hospital to turn off the gas if a leak develops or a fire occurs.

*Manifolds.* A manifold is a piping system that connects the bulk storage system and the hospital gas-piping system with a bank of H- or K-cylinders. These freestanding cylinders are a backup source of $O_2$ in case the bulk system fails. A 24-hour supply of gas must be available. The manifold system includes a reducing valve to decrease the gas pressure to 50 psig. Check valves are built into the manifold so that a leak in one cylinder connection does not result in leaking out from all of the gas cylinders.

2. **Adjunct hardware: Reducing valves, flowmeters, regulators, and high-pressure hose connectors**
   a. **Get the necessary equipment for the procedure** (NBRC code: IIA9) [Difficulty: R]
   b. **Put the equipment together and make sure that it works properly** (NBRC code: IIA9) [Difficulty: R]
   c. **Troubleshoot any problems with the equipment** (NBRC code: IIA9) [Difficulty: R]

*Reducing valves.* Reducing valves are used to reduce the high pressure seen in a bulk $O_2$ storage system, manifold, or gas cylinder. One or more stages (pressure-reducing steps) can be used to reach the working pressure of 50 psig. Single-stage reducing valves reach the pressure in a single step. Multiple-stage reducing valves give finer control over pressure and flow by dropping pressure in the first stage to about 200 psig and to 50 psig in the second stage. Occasionally, three stages are seen. All reducing valves (and regulators) have the following safety features built into them:

   a. A frangible disk that breaks to release gas pressure in case of mechanical failure or breakage
   b. A fusible plug that melts to release gas pressure in the event of a fire
   c. American Standard Compressed Gas Cylinder Valve Outlet and Index Connections (usually called the American Standard system), which prevent the accidental connection of the wrong reducing valve (or regulator) onto a large gas cylinder
   d. The pin-index safety system, which is a special section of the American Standard System that applies to E-sized and smaller gas cylinders. It is designed to prevent an accidental connection of the wrong gas with a reducing valve or regulator. These reducing valves and regulators are designed with a specifically pinned yoke to wrap around the valve stem of a gas cylinder. A soft plastic O-ring washer is included to help ensure a tight seal. Fig. 6-1 shows the location of the pinholes in the cylinder valve face. Table 6-3 shows the gases and pinhole positions. It is important to know the positions for $O_2$ and air; the others are included in Table 6-3 for the sake of completeness.

It is necessary to "crack" or blow some gas out of a cylinder before any reducing valve or regulator is put onto it to prevent any dust or debris from being forced into the reducing valve or regulator, which might cause a fire.

*Flowmeters.* Flowmeters are designed to regulate and indicate flow. They come with the following safety features so that they cannot be attached to the wrong reducing valve, regulator, high-pressure hose, or appliance:

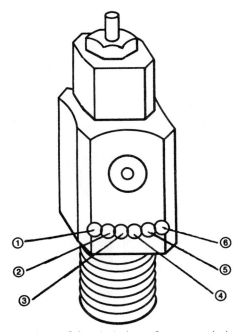

**Fig. 6-1** Locations of the pin-index safety system holes in the cylinder valve face. *(From Branson RD, Hess DR, Chatburn RL: Respiratory care equipment, ed 2, Philadelphia, 1999, Lippincott Williams & Wilkins.)*

| TABLE 6-3 | Pin-Index Safety System Gases and Pinhole Locations |
|---|---|
| **Gas** | **Pinhole locations** |
| Oxygen | 2–5 |
| Air | 1–5 |
| Oxygen/carbon dioxide (≤7%) | 2–6 |
| Oxygen/carbon dioxide (>7%) | 1–6 |
| Oxygen/helium (not >80% helium) | 2–4 |
| Oxygen/helium (helium >80%) | 4–6 |
| Nitrous oxide | 3–5 |
| Ethylene | 1–3 |
| Cyclopropane | 3–6 |

   a. Diameter-index safety system (DISS) inlets and outlets that are specific to the various gases so that a mixup cannot be made with the wrong appliance or connector. The DISS system applies to flowmeters that attach to all American Standard and DISS reduction valves.
   b. Flowmeters with quick-connect inlet adapters instead of DISS inlets. These quick-connects are designed specifically for the hospital's piped-in $O_2$ and air outlets. They are not interchangeable between gases or between manufacturers. Occasionally, a piped-in $O_2$ outlet jams open and lets gas rapidly escape. Insert the proper flowmeter into the

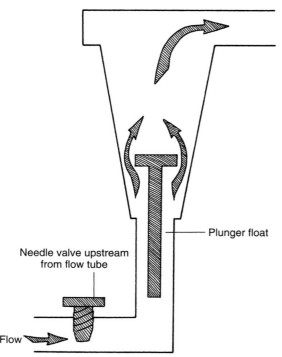

**Fig. 6-2** Kinetic-type non–backpressure-compensated (pressure-uncompensated) flowmeter. *(Modified from McPherson SP, Spearman SB: Respiratory care equipment, ed 4, St Louis, 1990, Mosby.)*

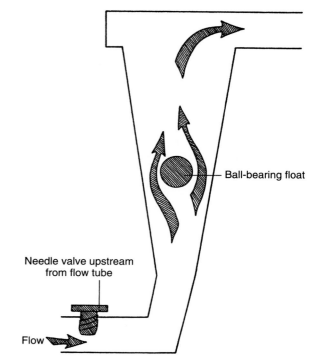

**Fig. 6-3** Thorpe-type non–backpressure-compensated (pressure-uncompensated) flowmeter. *(Modified from McPherson SP, Spearman SB: Respiratory care equipment, ed 4, St Louis, 1990, Mosby.)*

outlet and turn the flowmeter off. This stops the leak until the defective wall outlet can be repaired. Flowmeters are usually categorized by how they react to backpressure. The fact that three different manufactured types of flowmeters exist that may or may not be backpressure compensated further complicates matters. The three types follow:

a. Non–backpressure-compensated (pressure-uncompensated) flowmeters *inaccurately* indicate the flow through them in the face of backpressure. Figs. 6-2 and 6-3 show non–backpressure-compensated kinetic and Thorpe types of flowmeters, respectively. Note that the Thorpe and kinetic flowmeters have the flow-control valve upstream from the meter. They read accurately if they are kept upright and do not have to "push" against any backpressure. If laid on their sides, the plunger and ball bearing will not indicate the set flow. They will both read a *lower* flow than what is actually delivered when they are faced with a backpressure.

b. The Bourdon flowmeter is designed like the Bourdon gauge in the reducing valve (Fig. 6-4). The facepiece is marked in liters of flow rather than pressure. It is the flowmeter of choice in a transport situation because it can be laid flat with no effect on its flow if no backpressure exists. These flowmeters

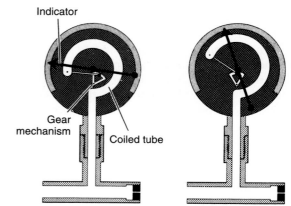

**Fig. 6-4** Bourdon-type non–backpressure-compensated (pressure-uncompensated) flowmeter. *(From McPherson SP, Spearman SB: Respiratory care equipment, ed 4, St Louis, 1990, Mosby.)*

display a *higher* flow than what is actually delivered when they are faced with a backpressure.

c. Backpressure-compensated (pressure-compensated) flowmeters accurately indicate the flow through them in the face of backpressure. For this reason, they should be used whenever possible. Figs. 6-5 and 6-6 show backpressure-compensated kinetic and Thorpe types of flowmeters, respectively. Note that

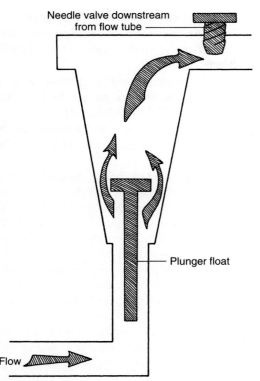

**Fig. 6-5** Kinetic-type backpressure-compensated (pressure-compensated) flowmeter. *(Modified from McPherson SP, Spearman SB: Respiratory care equipment, ed 4, St Louis, 1990, Mosby.)*

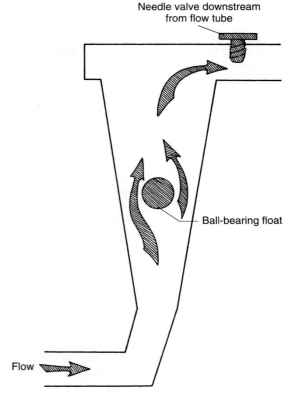

**Fig. 6-6** Thorpe-type backpressure-compensated (pressure-compensated) flowmeter. *(Modified from McPherson SP, Spearman SB: Respiratory care equipment, ed 4, St Louis, 1990, Mosby.)*

both of these flowmeters have the flow-control valve downstream from the meter. Therefore, they read accurately in the face of backpressure as long as they are kept upright. Besides facilitating reading of the label, this simple test will enable the practitioner to tell whether a flowmeter is backpressure compensated:

1. Make sure the flowmeter is turned off.
2. Plug the flowmeter into a gas outlet.
3. If the float or ball bearing bounces, the flowmeter is backpressure compensated.

**Exam Hint**

Choose a backpressure-compensated flowmeter in all situations except during patient transport when the $O_2$ tank and flowmeter might be laid flat.

***Regulators.*** Regulators combine a reducing valve and a flowmeter. Everything that has been discussed so far relates to regulators. Bourdon gauge reducing valves are usually seen and can have either a second Bourdon gauge added as a flowmeter or a Thorpe or kinetic flowmeter. As has been mentioned earlier, a backpressure-compensated flowmeter should be used in all situations except for patient transport.

***Pulse-dose systems.*** A pulse-dose $O_2$ delivery system is used in the home care setting to reduce the patient's use of $O_2$ and to save money. The unit takes the place of a regulator and flowmeter on the $O_2$ source. Some units are designed for a low-pressure LOX system, whereas others are designed for a high-pressure E-cylinder of $O_2$. Be careful to avoid placing a low-pressure unit onto a high-pressure gas source because this may damage the unit. In all units, the distal end of a regular nasal cannula is attached to a pressure sensor on the pulse-dose system. The pressure sensor senses a drop in pressure as the patient inspires. The sensor then triggers a solenoid valve that delivers a burst of $O_2$ to the cannula. A pulse-dose unit can be adjusted to change several factors, such as how long the $O_2$ is delivered, how much is delivered, and if the patient receives $O_2$ on every breath or every second or third breath.

Make sure the patient can feel a flow of gas from the cannula after he or she starts to inhale. The gas should stop during exhalation. Check the patient's pulse-oximetry value at rest and during exercise to ensure that desaturation does not occur. Adjust the pressure sensor or solenoid if needed to meet the patient's $O_2$ needs.

If the patient cannot feel any $O_2$ flowing, consider the following: (1) The source of $O_2$ might be empty, (2) tubing might be disconnected or kinked, or (3) the sensor is not detecting the patient's effort. The patient or therapist can switch to a second $O_2$ source and look for disconnections or kinks in the tubing. The therapist will have to adjust the nasal cannula or pulse-dose unit to correct for a sensitivity problem. Do not use a system that is malfunctioning and cannot be adjusted.

***High-pressure hose connectors.*** These connectors and other adapters connect high-pressure hoses, flowmeters, and $O_2$ appliances. They have DISS inlets and outlets so that the connectors cannot be cross-fitted onto the wrong equipment and cannot let gases be mixed.

### 3. Perform quality control procedures for gas-metering devices: Flowmeters and regulators (NBRC code: IIC4) [Difficulty: R]

It is critical that an accurately known flow be sent through a flowmeter when a quality control procedure is being performed so that the flowmeter can be checked for accuracy. This should be done with no backpressure. When backpressure is placed against a flowmeter, the following is seen:

a. Non–backpressure-compensated (pressure-uncompensated) Thorpe and kinetic flowmeters will show an inaccurately *low* flow in the face of backpressure. In other words, they will show less flow than is actually being delivered. With complete occlusion, the flowmeter will show zero flow.

b. Bourdon regulators (Bourdon reducing valve and flowmeter) will show an inaccurately *high* flow in the face of backpressure. In other words, they will show more flow than is actually being delivered.

c. Backpressure-compensated (pressure-compensated) Thorpe and kinetic flowmeters show an accurate flow in the face of backpressure. If the gas flow is restricted, the ball bearing or plunger float will drop to mark the reduced flow. If the flow is completely blocked off, the float will drop to zero and will show no flow.

Reducing valves and regulators must have a known pressure directed against them that enables checking for accuracy. The known pressure should be seen on the regulator gauge. Any flowmeter or regulator that is not reading accurately should not be used until after it has been repaired.

### 4. Air/oxygen proportioners (blenders)

**a. Get the necessary equipment for the procedure** (NBRC code: IIA9) [Difficulty: R]

**b. Put the equipment together and make sure that it works properly** (NBRC code: IIA9, IIIF2d2) [Difficulty: R]

**c. Troubleshoot any problems with the equipment** (NBRC code: IIA9) [Difficulty: R]

These units are designed to change the ratio of $O_2$ and air to blend the specific percentage of $O_2$ from 21% to 100% (Fig. 6-7). To most accurately deliver the desired $O_2$ percentage, both source gases must be pressurized to 50 psig. The $O_2$ percentage will remain close to that desired level, even if a small drop occurs in one or both line pressures. Always analyze the $O_2$ percentage to confirm its accuracy. The blended gas can be sent directly to a ventilator or other device that uses 50 psig or through an added flowmeter.

Keep the gas inlets and outlets clear of any debris. All current units give an audible whistle if one or both line pressures drop to an unsafe level (often about 30 psig). If

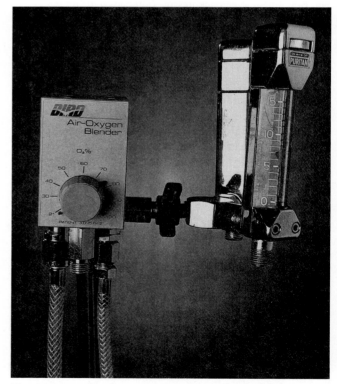

**Fig. 6-7** Example of an oxygen blender. Note the high-pressure air and oxygen hoses entering the bottom of the unit, the dial to set the oxygen percentage (75%), and the blended oxygen outlet to the right. In this case, a wye connector has been attached with two oxygen flowmeters. *(From Cairo JM, Pilbeam SP: Mosby's respiratory care equipment, ed 7, St Louis, 2004, Mosby.)*

the unit has a water trap at the compressed air inlet, keep it emptied of any condensate.

## MODULE C
### Administration of oxygen therapy

**1. Oxygen tents**

   **a. Get the necessary equipment for the procedure** (NBRC code: IIA12) [Difficulty: R]

   **b. Put the equipment together and make sure that it works properly** (NBRC code: IIA12) [Difficulty: R]

   **c. Troubleshoot any problems with the equipment** (NBRC code: IIA12) [Difficulty: R]

Oxygen tents were formerly used for adults but are now used only for children who are too large and active for an oxygen hood. The tent is used to control the environment by providing cooled aerosol, humidity, and controlled $O_2$ percentage (Fig. 6-8). In addition, the following procedures should be observed:

   a. Set an $O_2$ flowmeter to deliver 8 to 10 L/min to small tents and 12 to 15 L/min to large tents. Flows of 30 L/min or greater are needed to keep the $O_2$ percentage close to the 50% maximum that can be reliably maintained. (Commonly, 35% to 50% $O_2$ can be kept in a tent.)

   b. The $O_2$ should flow through a nebulizer or ultrasonic unit to provide the needed humidity. Try to keep the relative humidity at 60% or greater to minimize any risk of a fire caused by a spark inside the tent.

   c. The tent must be cooled to prevent the patient from overheating the enclosed space. Also, if the infant who is put into a tent has croup, the cooled air is therapeutic. Be careful not to chill the infant.

   d. An $O_2$ analyzer should be continuously monitoring how much $O_2$ is inside the tent. The analyzer probe should be placed at the same level as the infant's nose. Keep the tent sealed and the bottom edges tucked under the mattress to try to keep the $O_2$ percentage as high and stable as possible. The child should not be allowed to have any electrically powered toys inside the tent to minimize the risk of a spark and fire.

**2. Air-entrainment devices and masks**

   **a. Get the necessary equipment for the procedure** (NBRC code: IIA1b) [Difficulty: R, Ap]

   **b. Put the equipment together and make sure that it works properly** (NBRC code: IIB1b) [Difficulty: R, Ap]

   **c. Troubleshoot any problems with the equipment** (NBRC code: IIB2b) [Difficulty: R, Ap]

Air-entrainment masks are designed to provide the patient with a controlled $O_2$ percentage at a flow rate high enough to meet all of the patient's needs (Fig. 6-9). To ensure this, the total flow through the mask must be equal to or greater than the patient's peak inspiratory flow rate (PIFR). These masks are sometimes called Venturi masks, Venti masks, jet-mixing, and high airflow with $O_2$ enrichment systems. See Table 6-4 for specific information on available air-entrainment masks.

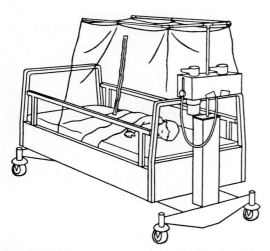

**Fig. 6-8** Child in an oxygen tent. *(From Gaebler G, Blodgett D: Gas administration. In Blodgett D, editor: Manual of pediatric respiratory care procedures, Philadelphia, 1982, Lippincott.)*

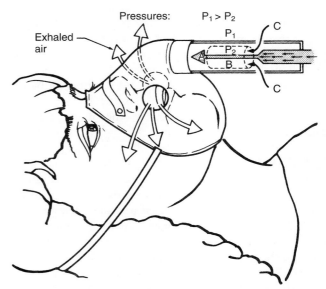

**Fig. 6-9** Adult wearing an air-entrainment mask. **A,** High-velocity jet; **B,** area of reduced lateral pressure (Bernoulli's principle); and **C,** room air entrainment. *(From White GC: Basic clinical lab competencies for respiratory care, an integrated approach, Albany, NY, 1988, Delmar.)*

| | Approximate | | Oxygen Flow Rate | |
| Oxygen (%) | Air/Oxygen Ratio | Total Ratio Parts | (L/min)* | Total Flow (L/min) |
|---|---|---|---|---|
| 24 | 25:1 | 26 | 4 | 104 |
| 28 | 10:1 | 11 | 4 | 44 |
| 30 | 8:1 | 9 | 6 | 54 |
| 35 | 5:1 | 6 | 8 | 48 |
| 40 | 3:1 | 4 | 10 | 40 |
| 45 | 2:1 | 3 | 15 | 45 |
| 50 | 1.7:1 | 2.7 | 15 | 40.5 |

**TABLE 6-4** Specifications for Air-Entrainment Devices and Masks

*These flow rates were selected to ensure that the minimum total flow through the system would be at least 40 L/min. Manufacturers may recommend other minimal $O_2$ flow rates.

These masks are recommended in any clinical situation in which a known, certain $O_2$ percentage must be given to the patient who has a variable respiratory rate, inspiratory:expiratory (I:E) ratio, tidal volume ($V_T$), or minute volume ($\dot{V}_E$). Common situations include a patient with chronic obstructive pulmonary disease (COPD) and a patient in respiratory failure with the need for increasing $O_2$ percentages. Because it is difficult to ensure that the patient's PIFR is matched by gas flow through the mask, the following guidelines are recommended:

a. Make sure that the total flow through the mask is at least 40 L/min in a resting patient. More flow may be needed if the patient is breathing rapidly.

b. Provide the patient with a total flow that is four to six times his or her measured $\dot{V}_E$.

c. Total flow through the mask can be raised by increasing the $O_2$ flow. This should not significantly change the $O_2$ percentage because more room air is entrained to keep the same ratio. However, to be certain, analyze the $O_2$ percentage inside the mask to ensure that it is prescribed properly. The total flow through the mask can be calculated by adding the total of the ratio parts and multiplying by the $O_2$ flow rate.

The following examples review the math for air-entrainment mask calculations:

## EXAMPLE 1

A patient is on a 28% air-entrainment mask with an $O_2$ flow of 4 L/min. His condition worsens, and he increases his $\dot{V}_E$ to 15 L/min. To ensure that he still receives his prescribed $O_2$ percentage, someone makes a recommendation to increase the $O_2$ liter flow to 6 L/min. The new total flow through the mask can be calculated as follows:

1. A 28% air-entrainment mask has an air:$O_2$ ratio of 10:1.
2. The sum of the ratio parts is 10 + 1 = 11.
3. Total flow = 11 × 6 L/min $O_2$ flow = 66 L/min.
4. This flow is more than four times the patient's current $\dot{V}_E$. He should have all of his flow needs met.

5. The delivered $O_2$ percentage should be reanalyzed to make certain that it is as prescribed.

## EXAMPLE 2

A patient is wearing a 40% air-entrainment mask with the manufacturer's suggested 8 L/min of $O_2$ running into it. Her PIFR is about 48 L/min (0.75 L/sec). To what should her $O_2$ flow be changed to ensure that the total gas flow is greater than her PIFR? The new $O_2$ flow to the mask can be calculated as follows:

1. A 40% air-entrainment mask has an air:$O_2$ ratio of 3:1.
2. The sum of the ratio parts is 3 + 1 = 4.
3. Divide the sum of the ratio parts into the PIFR: 48/4 = 12.
4. Increase the $O_2$ flow from 8 to 12 L/min.

### Exam Hint

**O**n past examinations, examinees had to calculate a change in the $O_2$ flow needed to increase the total flow to a level that met or exceeded a patient's peak inspiratory flow rate (PIFR), which ensures that the proper $O_2$ percentage is delivered.

Some patients may complain that the gas coming through the mask is dry. To resolve this problem, some manufacturers have designed an aerosol adapter to add to the jet. A separate bland aerosol that enters the jet stream is then added to the room air. Make sure that the adapter fits properly and does not interfere with or block the jet or room air entrainment ports.

Two different types of air-entrainment devices are based on the physical principles seen in the Bernoulli effect. The two different types should be examined for an understanding of what can go wrong with them and how they can be fixed.

*Variable jet diameter.* Notice that the jets have different diameters, but the room air entrainment ports are the same size. The smaller the jet diameter, the lower the O₂ percentage. This occurs because as the jet becomes smaller, more room air is brought into the entrainment ports to dilute the O₂ and raise the total flow.

Make sure that the jets are not obstructed by mucus or anything else, or the O₂ percentage will be decreased. An obstruction downstream from the jet prevents as much room air as is normal from being brought into the mask, which results in an increase in the O₂ percentage and a decrease in total flow.

*Variable air-entrainment ports.* Notice that the jet size is fixed, but the room air entrainment ports have different sizes. The smaller the entrainment ports, the higher is the O₂ percentage. This occurs because less room air can be entrained to dilute the O₂.

Make sure that the entrainment ports are not obstructed by the patient's sheet or by anything else, or the O₂ percentage will increase. An obstruction downstream from the jet also prevents as much room air as is normal from being brought into the mask, which results in an increase in the O₂ percentage and a decrease in the total flow.

### 3. Nasal cannula
   **a. Get the necessary equipment for the procedure** (NBRC code: IIA1a) [Difficulty: R]
   **b. Put the equipment together and make sure that it works properly** (NBRC code: IIA1a) [Difficulty: R]
   **c. Troubleshoot any problems with the equipment** (NBRC code: IIA1a) [Difficulty: R]

The nasal cannula is an O₂ delivery tube modified with two short prongs to deliver O₂ to the nostrils (Fig. 6-10). They come in neonatal, pediatric, and adult sizes based on the diameter of the prongs. Care must be taken to make sure that the nares are patent and are not plugged by a common cold, deviated septum, or other unseen problem. This low-flow O₂ delivery device is very widely used because it is more comfortable for many patients than an air entrainment or other type of facemask.

If a humidifier is to be used, make sure it is properly filled with sterile water and that the O₂ bubbles through it. Check the high-pressure pop-off valve for pressure release and a whistling sound. Before placing the cannula on the patient, check to see that the O₂ is flowing through the tubing. If available, use a cannula with curved prongs. These direct the gas flow toward the back of the nasal passages for better natural humidification and patient comfort. Take care not to pull the elastic restraining band too tightly around the head. Some brands loop the O₂ tubing over the ears to be drawn up snugly under the chin,

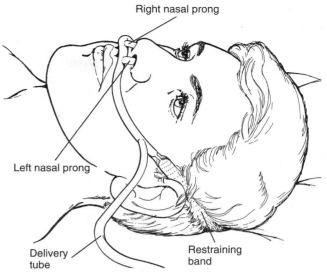

**Fig. 6-10** Adult wearing a nasal cannula. *(From Scanlan CL, Heuer A: Medical gas therapy. In Scanlan CL, Wilkins RL, Stoller JK, editors: Egan's fundamentals of respiratory care, ed 7, St Louis, 1999, Mosby.)*

| TABLE 6-5 | Estimated Delivered Oxygen Percentage in Adults Based on the Oxygen Liter Flow Through a Nasal Cannula | |
| --- | --- |
| **Oxygen (L/min)** | **Estimated delivered oxygen (%)** |
| 1 | 24 |
| 2 | 28 |
| 3 | 32 |
| 4 | 36 |
| 5 | 40 |
| 6 | 44 |

which is often more comfortable than the types with the elastic band.

The problem with a nasal cannula is the unreliability of the delivered O₂ percentage. Variations in the patient's respiratory rate, I:E ratio, $V_T$, and $\dot{V}_E$ result in different inhaled O₂ percentages. This is clearly unacceptable in an unstable patient in whom PaO₂ values are being used to help the clinician to judge the changing cardiopulmonary status. Because of this clinical limitation, this device and the other low-flow O₂ delivery systems in the discussions that follow should be used only with stable patients. In the adult, the delivered O₂ percentage can be *estimated* at 4% for each liter of O₂ per minute (Table 6-5). Flows are usually limited to 6 L/min to avoid excessive irritation to the nasal passages.

Flows are usually limited to no more than 1 to 2 L/min in infants and 4 L/min in older children. The pulse oximetry value or PaO₂ level should be checked in patients of any age whenever a flow change is made, or the patient's condition changes significantly.

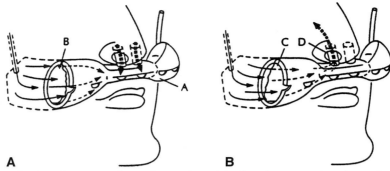

**A** **B**

**Fig. 6-11** The Oxymizer reservoir nasal cannula and its functions. **A,** When the patient exhales, oxygen is accumulating in the reservoir *(A)* formed by the inflated diaphragm *(B)* and the back wall of the Oxymizer. **B,** When the patient inhales, the diaphragm *(C)* collapses, and the oxygen-enriched air from the reservoir is released to the patient *(D)*. *(Courtesy of Chad Therapeutics, Chatsworth, Calif.)*

The traditional cannulas previously described are commonly used in hospitals for short-term patient use. However, in the home setting for long-term use, using one of the newer cannulas with a built-in $O_2$ reservoir is more economical because less $O_2$ is used.

*Oxygen-conserving nasal cannula.* $O_2$-conserving nasal cannulas are used with patients who need long-term $O_2$ therapy and wish to reduce their costs. When this cannula is combined with a pulse-dose $O_2$ delivery system, the patient's $O_2$ delivery costs can be significantly cut. At least two different types of $O_2$-conserving cannulas exist. Fig. 6-11 shows a reservoir nasal cannula and how it operates. It has an 18-mL reservoir that fills when the patient exhales and gives up its $O_2$ bolus during the next inspiration. Fig. 6-12 shows a pendant nasal cannula with its reservoir hanging on the chest. Both types can have the same problems with tubing disconnections or kinks that can be found with any type of cannula. The only problem unique to both of these units is failure of the diaphragm that moves back and forth as the reservoir fills and empties. This membrane may wear out after about a week, which may prevent the reservoir from filling or emptying properly. Watch as the patient breathes to make sure that the diaphragm is moving properly. If not, replace the cannula.

4. **Oxygen masks: Simple oxygen mask, partial-rebreathing mask, nonrebreathing mask, and face tent**
   a. **Get the necessary equipment for the procedure (NBRC code: IIA1a) [Difficulty: R]**
   b. **Put the equipment together and make sure that it works properly (NBRC code: IIA1a) [Difficulty: R]**
   c. **Troubleshoot any problems with the equipment (NBRC code: IIA1a) [Difficulty: R]**

*Simple oxygen mask.* This mask, like all others, is designed to fit over the patient's nose and mouth and act

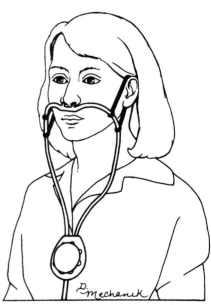

**Fig. 6-12** A patient wearing a pendant reservoir nasal cannula made by Chad Therapeutics. *(From Scanlan CL, Heuer A: Medical gas therapy. In Scanlan CL, Wilkins RL, Stoller JK: Egan's fundamentals of respiratory care, ed 7, St Louis, 1999, Mosby.)*

as an $O_2$ reservoir for the next breath (Figs. 6-13 and 6-14). Various adult and pediatric sizes are available, and the patient should wear one that best fits the facial contours and size of the face. This enhances comfort and may increase the inspired $O_2$ percentage by decreasing the amount of inspired room air. Exhaled breath escapes through the exhalation ports. The patient's breathing pattern affects the amount of room air that is breathed in through the same exhalation ports. These ports are also important in case the $O_2$ flow to the mask is cut off. Because the $O_2$ reservoir in the mask is not large enough to meet the patient's $V_T$, the inspired $O_2$ percentage is unpredictable. $O_2$ flows of between 5 and 10 L/min should provide *approximately* 35% to 60% inspired $O_2$. The pulse

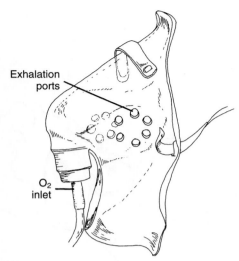

**Fig. 6-13** Close-up view of a simple oxygen ($O_2$) mask. *(From McPherson SP, Spearman SB: Respiratory care equipment, ed 4, St Louis, 1990, Mosby.)*

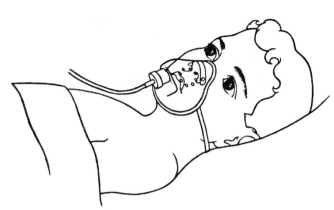

**Fig. 6-14** Child wearing a simple oxygen mask. *(From Gaebler G, Blodgett D: Gas administration. In Blodgett D, editor: Manual of pediatric respiratory care procedures, Philadelphia, 1982, Lippincott.)*

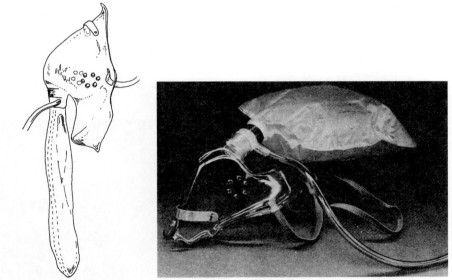

**Fig. 6-15** Outside view of a partial-rebreathing mask. *(From McPherson SP, Spearman SB: Respiratory care equipment, ed 4, St Louis, 1990, Mosby.)*

oximetry value or $PaO_2$ level should be checked whenever a flow change is made, or the patient's condition changes significantly.

A bubble humidifier is often added so that the gas is not dry. Make sure that it works properly and that $O_2$ is flowing through the tubing before you put it on the patient. This and all other masks use an adjustable elastic strap that goes behind the head to hold it in place. Make sure that the mask fits snugly but not so tight as to cut off circulation.

***Partial-rebreathing mask.*** The partial-rebreathing mask has a 500- to 1000-mL plastic bag added to the mask that acts as an $O_2$ reservoir for the next breath (Figs. 6-15 to 6-17). Child- and adult-sized masks are commonly available. The first third of the patient's exhaled gas from the anatomic dead space is exhaled back into this bag when properly applied. This gas is close to pure $O_2$ and contains no $CO_2$. Additional exhaled breath escapes through the exhalation ports. The patient's breathing pattern affects the amount of room air that is breathed in through the same exhalation ports. These ports are also important in case the $O_2$ flow to the mask is cut off. The added reservoir of $O_2$ results in the patient's receiving a higher percentage of $O_2$ than is obtained with a simple $O_2$ mask. An $O_2$ flow of between 6 and 10 L/min should provide *approximately* 35% to 80% inspired $O_2$.

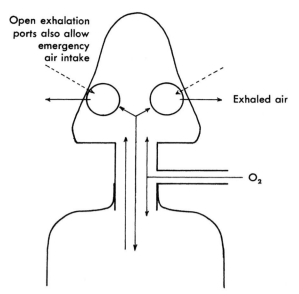

Open exhalation ports also allow emergency air intake

Exhaled air

$O_2$

**Fig. 6-16** Cutaway view of a partial-rebreathing mask showing gas flow. $O_2$, Oxygen. *(From Thalken FR: Medical gas therapy. In Scanlan CL, Spearman CB, Sheldon RL, editors: Egan's fundamentals of respiratory care, ed 5, St Louis, 1990, Mosby.)*

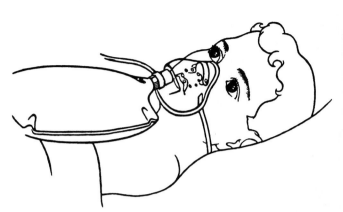

**Fig. 6-17** Child wearing a partial-rebreathing mask. *(From Gaebler G, Blodgett D: Gas administration. In Blodgett D, editor: Manual of pediatric respiratory care procedures, Philadelphia, 1982, Lippincott.)*

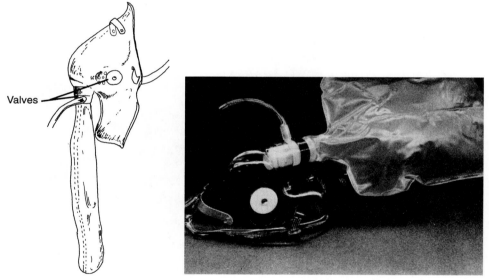

Valves

**Fig. 6-18** Outside view of a nonrebreathing mask. *(From McPherson SP, Spearman SB: Respiratory care equipment, ed 4, St Louis, 1990, Mosby.)*

A bubble humidifier is often added so that the gas is not dry. Make sure that it works properly, that the $O_2$ is flowing through the tubing, and that the reservoir bag has been filled before you put it on the patient. Adjust the flow as needed to ensure that the reservoir does not collapse by more than one third on inspiration. This also ensures that the mask and reservoir are filled with as much $O_2$ as possible. A pulse oximetry value or $PaO_2$ level should be checked whenever a flow change is made, or the patient's condition changes significantly.

***Nonrebreathing mask.*** The nonrebreathing mask initially looks like the partial-rebreathing mask with its plastic bag added as an $O_2$ reservoir for the next breath (Figs. 6-18 and 6-19). However, notice that a one-way valve has been added between the mask and the reservoir bag. This allows the bag to be filled with pure $O_2$ for the next breath. No exhaled gas can enter the reservoir. Two (sometimes one) one-way valves are added to the exhalation ports on the mask. These ensure that the patient breathes in only $O_2$ and not room air. Exhaled breath

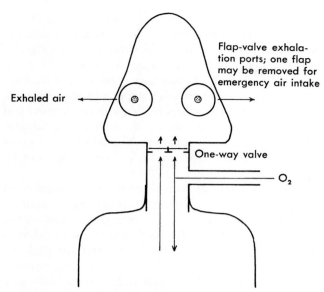

**Fig. 6-19** Cutaway view of a nonrebreathing mask showing gas flow. *(From Thalken FR: Medical gas therapy. In Scanlan CL, Spearman CB, Sheldon RL, editors: Egan's fundamentals of respiratory care, ed 5, St Louis, 1990, Mosby.)*

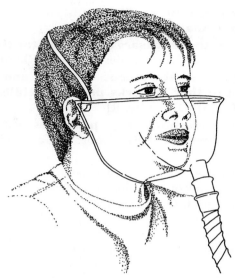

**Fig. 6-20** Young adult wearing a face tent.

> **Exam Hint**
>
> **E**xpect to see a question that deals with collapsing of the reservoir bag on inspiration. Solve the problem by increasing the $O_2$ flow to the mask and bag.

escapes through the exhalation ports, as with the partial-rebreathing mask. Although not shown, an emergency pop-in valve can be used that allows room air to be drawn into the mask if the $O_2$ supply should be cut off.

Adult and pediatric sizes are available. The mask should conform to fit as well as possible the patient's facial contours and size. As has been mentioned earlier, this enhances comfort and may increase the inspired $O_2$ percentage by decreasing the amount of inspired room air. It is theoretically possible for 100% $O_2$ to be delivered with this mask if the $O_2$ flow is high enough and the mask is airtight over the face. However, experience has shown that the disposable masks that are usually available in the hospital do not prevent room air from being drawn in. $O_2$ flows of between 8 and 10 L/min should provide *approximately* 60% to 80% (or more) inspired $O_2$.

A bubble humidifier is often added so that the gas is not dry. Make sure that it works properly, the $O_2$ is flowing through the tubing, and the reservoir bag has been filled before you put it on the patient. Adjust the flow as needed to ensure that the reservoir does not collapse by more than one third on inspiration. This ensures that the mask and reservoir are filled with $O_2$, and that the patient's $V_T$ comes completely from the reservoir bag. The patient's pulse oximetry value or $PaO_2$ level should be checked whenever a flow change is made, and when the patient's condition changes significantly.

*Face tent.* These masks are designed to fit around the patient's neck, under the jaw, and around the cheeks in front of the ears. The front edge should be higher than the level of the patient's nostrils (Fig. 6-20). Face tents are sometimes used to provide $O_2$ to a patient who cannot wear a mask or cannula because of oral and nasal trauma, burns, or surgery. The patient who uses a face tent should be sitting as upright as possible because $O_2$ is heavier than air and tends to settle in the mask around the patient's nose and mouth, if the fit is tight. If the patient is lying flat or if the mask fits loosely, the $O_2$ will simply "pour" down out of it. This makes it difficult for the clinician to know with any certainty what inspired $O_2$ percentage is available to the patient. Flows of 5 to 10 L/min $O_2$ are commonly used with adults.

A face tent is usually ordered with the $O_2$ run through a humidifier or nebulizer so that the gas is not dry. Make sure that the humidifier or nebulizer is filled with sterile water, the high pressure pop-off works, and gas is flowing through the tubing before it is put on the patient. Try to analyze the $O_2$ percentage close to the patient's nose and mouth with as much accuracy as possible. A pulse oximetry value or $PaO_2$ level should be checked whenever a change in the $O_2$ percentage is made, or when the patient's condition changes significantly.

## 5. Tracheostomy appliances: Mask/collar and Briggs adapter/T-piece

   **a. Get the necessary equipment for the procedure (NBRC code: IIA1a) [Difficulty: R]**

   **b. Put the equipment together and make sure that it works properly (NBRC code: IIA1a) [Difficulty: R]**

   **c. Troubleshoot any problems with the equipment (NBRC code: IIA1a) [Difficulty: R]**

*Tracheostomy mask/collar.* The adult or pediatric tracheostomy mask or collar fits over a tracheostomy tube or stoma to provide $O_2$ and aerosol (Fig. 6-21). Because the patient's upper airway is bypassed, a nebulizer is used for humidity. It is usually an air-entrainment type, so the $O_2$ percentage can be adjusted. Make sure that the nebulizer is filled with sterile water and that adequate mist is flowing through to the mask before you place it on the patient.

Because the tracheostomy mask is an open system without reservoir, guaranteeing the patient's inspired $O_2$ percentage is difficult. Set the gas flow high enough to make a "cloud" of aerosol around the tracheostomy. If an excess of aerosol can be seen around the tracheostomy during inspiration, the desired $O_2$ percentage is probably being delivered. Analyze the $O_2$ percentage from inside the mask for as much accuracy as possible. A pulse oximetry value or $PaO_2$ level should be checked whenever a flow change or an $O_2$ percentage change is made, or when the patient's condition changes significantly.

*Briggs adapter/T-piece.* The Briggs adapter or T-piece is designed to provide air or supplemental $O_2$ and aerosol to an endotracheal or tracheostomy tube. It has one 15-mm inner diameter opening that fits over any endotracheal or tracheostomy tube adapter. The other two openings are 22-mm outer diameter openings, so aerosol tubing can be added (Fig. 6-22). A nebulizer is commonly used for humidity because the patient's upper airway is bypassed. Make sure that the nebulizer is filled with sterile water and that adequate mist is flowing through to the adapter before you place it on the patient. The nebulizer is usually an air-entrainment type, so the $O_2$ percentage can be adjusted.

An added length of aerosol tubing downstream from the adapter acts as a reservoir to ensure the inspired $O_2$ percentage. A reservoir of 50 to 100 mL of aerosol tubing is commonly needed for the adult. Care must be taken to adjust the gas flow high enough to meet the patient's PIFR. The proper gas flow can be determined by watching the aerosol flow past the adapter and reservoir. Make sure during inspiration that the aerosol is still flowing past the tracheostomy/endotracheal tube and into the reservoir. Inadequate flow could cause the patient to rebreathe gas from the reservoir. This recently exhaled gas is high in $CO_2$ and low in $O_2$.

> **Exam Hint**
>
> **I**f the aerosol cannot be seen during a patient's inspiration, increase the aerosol flow to either a tracheostomy mask or a Briggs adapter/T-piece.

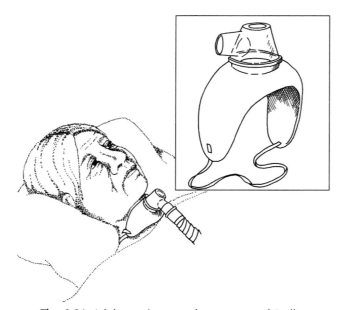

**Fig. 6-21** Adult wearing a tracheostomy mask/collar.

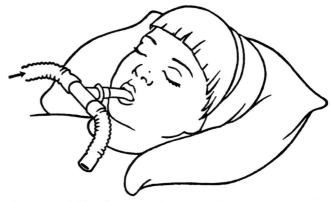

**Fig. 6-22** Child with intubated airway with a Briggs adapter/T-piece and aerosol tubing added to the endotracheal tube. *(From Gaebler G, Blodgett D: Gas administration. In Blodgett D, editor: Manual of pediatric respiratory care procedures, Philadelphia, 1982, Lippincott.)*

## MODULE D
### Respiratory care plan

**1. Analyze the available information to determine the patient's pathophysiologic state (NBRC code: IIIH1) [Difficulty: R, Ap, An]**

Look for signs of hypoxemia, and be prepared to recommend a change in the patient's $O_2$ delivery system or $O_2$ percentage to correct the problem. Tachycardia and tachypnea are common in hypoxemic patients. Proper $O_2$ therapy should relieve the problem so that the patient's vital signs return toward normal. An abnormal heart rhythm as a result of hypoxemia should return to normal with relief of the problem. Check the patient's pulse oximetry or $PaO_2$ value whenever a change in the inspired $O_2$ percentage or a significant change in the patient's clinical condition occurs.

**2. Determine the appropriateness of the prescribed respiratory care plan and recommend modifications when indicated.**

 **a. Review the interdisciplinary patient and family care plan (NBRC code: IIIH2b) [Difficulty: R, Ap]**

 **b. Review the planned therapy to establish the therapeutic plan (NBRC code: IIIH2a) [Difficulty: R, Ap]**

 **c. Determine the appropriateness of the prescribed therapy and goals for the patient's pathophysiologic state (NBRC code: IIIH3) [Difficulty: R, Ap, An]**

 **d. Recommend changes in the therapeutic plan if supportive data exist (NBRC code: IIIH4) [Difficulty: Ap, An]**

 **e. Change the oxygen percentage (NBRC code: IIIF2d1) [Difficulty: R, Ap]**

 **f. Change the flow of oxygen (NBRC code: IIIF2d1) [Difficulty: R, Ap]**

 **g. Change the method of administering the oxygen (NBRC code: IIIF2d1) [Difficulty: R, Ap]**

Every patient's $O_2$ percentage or flow must be tailored to meet the patient's clinical goals. Usually, this means keeping the acutely hypoxemic patient at a $PaO_2$ level of between 60 and 100 torr and an $SpO_2$ value of between 90% and 97%. Exceptions, when the blood $O_2$ level is kept as high as possible, include cardiopulmonary resuscitation and the treatment of carbon monoxide (CO) poisoning.

Another exception is the COPD patient who is hypoxemic and hypercarbic. Usually, these patients' conditions are maintained with moderate hypoxemia. The $PaO_2$ level should be between 50 and 60 torr, and the $SpO_2$ value between 85% and 90%. It is imperative that the $O_2$ be kept in this relatively narrow range. Further hypoxemia will result in pulmonary hypertension and cor pulmonale. Cardiac arrhythmia or arrest and death can occur if the hypoxemia is severe (<40 mm Hg). $O_2$ levels in the normal range (>60 mm Hg) may result in blunting of the hypoxic drive, which could result in bradypnea and even greater $CO_2$ retention with corresponding acidemia. When the $CO_2$ pressure level exceeds 80 to 90 torr, many patients become drowsy or somnolent. Treatment involves decreasing the $F_IO_2$ to lower the $PaO_2$ level to 50 to 60 torr. This in turn stimulates the hypoxic drive so that the patient increases his or her ventilation.

**3. Discontinue treatment based on the patient's response (NBRC code: IIIG1f) [Difficulty: R, Ap]**

If the patient's cardiopulmonary condition has improved to the point that hypoxemia is no longer present, the supplemental oxygen can be stopped. See the previous discussion for typical clinical considerations.

---

### Exam Hint

**K**now the advantages, disadvantages, and possible $O_2$ ranges for the various $O_2$ appliances. Be prepared to make recommendations to change from one appliance to another or to change the $O_2$ percentage or flow.

---

### BIBLIOGRAPHY

American Association for Respiratory Care: Clinical practice guideline: Oxygen therapy in the acute care hospital, *Respir Care* 36:1410, 1991.

American Association for Respiratory Care: Clinical practice guideline: Oxygen therapy for adults in the acute care facility—2002 revision & update, *Respir Care* 47:717, 2002.

American Association for Respiratory Care: Clinical practice guideline: Selection of an oxygen delivery device for neonatal and pediatric patients—2002 revision & update, *Respir Care* 47:707, 2002.

American Association for Respiratory Care: Clinical practice guideline: Oxygen therapy in the home or extended care facility, *Respir Care* 37(8):918, 1992.

Bageant RA: Oxygen analyzers, *Respir Care* 21:410, 1976.

Cairo JM, Pilbeam SP: *Mosby's respiratory care equipment,* ed 7, St Louis, 2004, Mosby.

Eubanks DH, Bone RC: *Comprehensive respiratory care,* ed 2, St Louis, 1990, Mosby.

Gaebler G, Blodgett D: Gas administration. In Blodgett D, editor: *Manual of pediatric respiratory care procedures,* Philadelphia, 1982, Lippincott.

Heuer AJ, Scanlan CL: Medical gas therapy. In Wilkins RL, Stoller JK, Scanlan CL, editors: *Egan's fundamentals of respiratory care,* ed 8, St Louis, 2003, Mosby.

Hill KV: Oxygen therapy. In Aloan CA, Hill TV, editors: *Respiratory care of the newborn and child,* ed 2, Philadelphia, 1997, Lippincott-Raven.

Hunt GE: Gas therapy. In Fink JB, Hunt GE, editors: *Clinical practice in respiratory care,* Philadelphia, 1999, Lippincott-Raven.

Shapiro BA, Harrison RA, Cane RD, et al: *Clinical application of blood gases,* ed 4, Chicago, 1989, Mosby.

Shapiro BA, Kacmarek RM, Cane RD, et al, editors: *Clinical application of respiratory care,* ed 4, St Louis, 1991, Mosby.

Vines DL, Scanlan CL: Storage and delivery of medical gases. In Wilkins RL, Stoller JK, Scanlan CL, editors: *Egan's fundamentals of respiratory care,* ed 8, St Louis, 2003, Mosby.

Ward JJ: Equipment for mixed gas and oxygen therapy. In Branson RD, Hess DR, Chatburn RL, editors: *Respiratory care equipment,* ed 2, Philadelphia, 1999, Lippincott, Williams & Wilkins.

Ward JJ: Medical gas therapy. In Burton GC, Hodgkin JE, Ward JJ, editors: *Respiratory care: A guide to clinical practice,* ed 4, Philadelphia, 1997, Lippincott-Raven.

Whitaker K: *Comprehensive perinatal & pediatric respiratory care,* ed 2, Albany, 1997, Delmar.

White GC: *Equipment theory for respiratory care,* ed 3, Albany, NY, 1999, Delmar.

Youtsey JW: Oxygen and mixed gas therapy. In Barnes TA, editor: *Core textbook of respiratory care practice,* ed 2, St Louis, 1994, Mosby.

## SELF-STUDY QUESTIONS

1. Your home care patient has a problem with his $O_2$ concentrator and needs to change to his H-tank of $O_2$. If his nasal cannula is receiving a flow of 3 L/min and the tank pressure is 1300 psig, how long can the patient receive $O_2$?
   A. Longer than 22 hr
   B. Longer than 1300 hr
   C. 2 hr
   D. Longer than 120 hr

2. What is the most likely problem to watch for in a severe COPD patient who is receiving supplemental $O_2$?
   A. Pulmonary edema from $O_2$ toxicity
   B. Hypoventilation
   C. Retinopathy of prematurity (ROP)
   D. Hyperventilation

3. A patient has just been admitted through the emergency department with suspected CO poisoning. The physician wants her to receive the highest possible $O_2$ percentage. What would you recommend?
   A. Continuous positive-airway pressure mask at 5 cm $H_2O$ and 40% $O_2$
   B. Simple mask at 6 L/min flow
   C. Face tent at 8 L/min flow
   D. Nonrebreather mask with enough flow to keep the reservoir bag at least two-thirds full

4. You are making general rounds in the hospital when you find a patient whose reservoir tubing has fallen off his 40% T-piece. This would result in which of the following?
   A. Increased inspired $O_2$
   B. Increased inspired $CO_2$
   C. Decreased inspired $CO_2$
   D. Decreased inspired $O_2$

5. The risks of $O_2$ therapy include all of the following EXCEPT
   A. Pulmonary $O_2$ toxicity
   B. Denitrogen absorption atelectasis
   C. $O_2$-induced hyperventilation
   D. Retinopathy of prematurity (ROP)

6. Your patient is wearing a face tent because of recent facial surgery. It is set at 35% $O_2$. The nurse moves the patient from an upright to a supine position in bed. What effect will this have on her respiratory status?
   A. Increased $V_T$
   B. Increased inspired $O_2$
   C. Increased inspired $CO_2$
   D. Decreased inspired $O_2$

7. To minimize the risk of hypoxemia during a treatment or procedure, you would do which of the following?
   I. Increase the $O_2$ percentage by 20% above the normal setting before suctioning or changing equipment.
   II. Keep the $O_2$ percentage the same as if the patient is not hypoxemic at this time.
   III. Minimize the time that the patient would be breathing room air.
   IV. Increase the $O_2$ percentage to 100% before suctioning.
   V. Make sure the replacement equipment is working properly before you place it on the patient.
   A. I and III
   B. III, IV, and V
   C. II and V
   D. III and IV

8. Initially, the $O_2$ percentage found in an $O_2$ tent of a 2-year-old child was found to be stable at the ordered 35%. Now, less than that is found. All of the following should be tried EXCEPT
   A. Add an additional flowmeter and run them both at flush.
   B. Keep the tent canopy tightly tucked under the mattress.
   C. Keep the canopy flaps closed when the child is not receiving nursing care.
   D. Check the analyzer for proper function.

9. Your patient is wearing a partial-rebreathing mask. The reservoir bag almost totally collapses during inspiration. You would do which of the following?
   A. Tell the patient to breathe more slowly.
   B. Put a nasal cannula on the patient.
   C. Tell the patient to breathe more rapidly.
   D. Increase the $O_2$ flow.

10. When checking your home care patient's reservoir-type nasal cannula, you notice that the reservoir does not fill and empty in synchrony with the patient's breathing pattern. Based on this, you would
    A. Increase the $O_2$ flow to deliver the intended amount
    B. Replace the cannula
    C. Decrease the $O_2$ flow to unstick the reservoir membrane
    D. Switch the patient to an air-entrainment mask at approximately the same $O_2$ percentage as that given to the patient who received it by cannula

11. What $O_2$ delivery device would you recommend for a patient who has a variable respiratory rate, I : E ratio, and $V_T$?
    A. Nasal cannula
    B. Air-entrainment mask
    C. Simple $O_2$ mask
    D. Face tent

12. The physician asks you which $O_2$ delivery device would be best for a patient who needs about 75% $O_2$. You would recommend which of the following?
    A. Nonrebreathing mask
    B. Face tent
    C. Air-entrainment mask
    D. Simple $O_2$ mask

13. A patient has a nasal cannula and needs to be transported on a stretcher. The E-sized $O_2$ cylinder will need to be laid flat under the stretcher. What flowmeter would you recommend?
    A. Backpressure-compensated Thorpe
    B. Non–backpressure-compensated Thorpe
    C. Bourdon
    D. Backpressure-compensated kinetic

14. An E-cylinder of $O_2$ needs to be prepared for transport of a patient. You would look for a regulator with which pinhole locations?
    A. 1–5
    B. 2–6
    C. 3–5
    D. 2–5

15. What is the duration of flow of an E-cylinder with 1700 psig that is running at 5 L/min?
    A. 0.9 hr
    B. 1.6 hr
    C. 7.7 hr
    D. 13.7 hr

16. You are called to draw an arterial blood sample from a patient who is wearing a 35% air-entrainment mask. When you enter the room, you notice that his covers are drawn up over the air-entrainment ports of the mask. How would this affect the function of the mask?
    A. The total flow will be increased.
    B. There will be no effect.
    C. The $O_2$ percentage will be increased.
    D. The $O_2$ percentage will be decreased.

17. You are doing quality assurance on the department's flowmeters. After plugging in a backpressure-compensated Thorpe flowmeter, you set the flow at 10 L/min. The flowmeter outlet is partially and then completely obstructed. You would expect to see the following:
    A. The float will stay at the 10-L/min mark.
    B. The float will move upward in the flowmeter.
    C. The float will move upward and then downward in the flowmeter.
    D. The float will move downward and then drop to the bottom of the flowmeter, showing zero flow.

## ANSWER KEY AND RATIONALE

1. **A.** See the sample H-tank duration calculation given earlier in the chapter. Common errors include using the E-tank factor and failing to convert from minutes to hours by dividing by 60.

2. **B.** A patient with COPD who is hypercarbic and breathing on hypoxic drive should be given supplemental $O_2$ with great care. Too much $O_2$ will result in too high an arterial $O_2$ level and will blunt the hypoxic drive. Hypoventilation will result in a rising $CO_2$ level. Pulmonary edema from $O_2$ toxicity would necessitate a high percentage of $O_2$ for an extended period. ROP is seen only in premature infants. Hyperventilation is not caused by breathing of supplemental $O_2$.

3. **D.** A properly applied and used nonrebreathing mask should deliver at least 60% $O_2$. Continuous positive-airway pressure is not indicated in a patient with CO poisoning; more than 40% $O_2$ should be delivered. A simple mask or face tent does not deliver as much $O_2$ as is provided by a nonrebreathing mask.

4. **D.** The reservoir tubing holds $O_2$ from which the patient can inspire. Losing the reservoir results in inhalation of room air and a decrease in the overall $O_2$ percentage. When set up properly, any exhaled $CO_2$ is blown clear from the reservoir tubing before the next inspiration.

5. **C.** No known condition of $O_2$-induced hyperventilation exists. Do not confuse this with $O_2$-induced hypoventilation, which needs to be monitored in some COPD patients. See the rationale for Question 2.

6. **D.** Because the face tent is open on top and $O_2$ is heavier than room air, the $O_2$ in the face tent tends to "pour" out if the patient lies supine. When all is set up properly, $CO_2$ should not build up in a face tent, no matter the patient's position. A face tent should not influence a patient's $V_T$. Lying supine may result in decreased $V_T$.

7. **B.** The three listed items are all important for minimizing hypoxemia during a treatment or procedure. Increasing the $O_2$ by 20% will help to minimize hypoxemia, but it is appropriate to raise the percentage much higher.

8. **A.** Running two flowmeters at flush would put too much $O_2$ into the tent and would probably raise the percentage to a far greater extent than ordered. In addition, the noise level would be high, which could be harmful to the child's hearing. Closing any source of leaks would help keep the $O_2$ level stable. The analyzer may be malfunctioning and may be reporting a low value.

9. **D.** When properly operating, a partial-rebreathing–mask reservoir bag should not collapse during inspiration. Raise the $O_2$ flow so that the bag stays at least two-thirds full during inspiration. Hypoxic patients usually breathe in at whatever pattern and rate is most efficient for them. It may be counterproductive to try to have the patient breathe differently. A nasal cannula cannot deliver as high an $O_2$ percentage as can be delivered by the partial-rebreathing mask.

10. **B.** The reservoir membrane is defective, so the cannula should be replaced. The $O_2$ flow should not be increased because this would give the patient more $O_2$ than is intended. Decreasing (or increasing) the $O_2$ flow will not unstick a defective reservoir membrane. Changing to an air-entrainment mask would be a possible remedy if a replacement cannula did not exist.

11. **B.** An air-entrainment mask should provide enough flow of the prescribed $O_2$ percentage at any patient rate, $V_T$, and so forth. The other three devices do not provide enough flow to deliver a consistent, known $O_2$ percentage.

12. **A.** A properly fitting nonrebreathing mask with enough flow to keep the reservoir bag inflated will deliver the highest $O_2$ percentage of all available devices.

13. **C.** A Bourdon flowmeter is the only unit that will accurately indicate the flow when it is laid horizontally. The others read accurately only in a vertical position.

14. **D.** Review the information on pinholes in Table 6-3.

15. **B.** Review the sample E-tank duration calculation in this chapter. Common errors include using the H-tank factor and failure to convert from minutes to hours by dividing by 60.

16. **C.** Covering the air-entrainment ports on an air-entrainment mask will result in the patient's receiving a higher $O_2$ percentage than is desired. In addition, the total flow will be decreased.

17. **D.** A Thorpe-type flowmeter will read accurately if backpressure is placed upon the exit of gas. Thus, the flowmeter will read less, then zero, as the outlet is partially and then completely blocked.

# 7 Hyperinflation Therapy

A review of the most recent Entry Level Examinations has shown an average of 2 questions (1% of the exam) that cover hyperinflation therapy.

## MODULE A

**Perform coughing and deep-breathing procedures with the patient to help make breathing more effective**

### 1. Teach the patient the best techniques for breathing efficiently (NBRC code: IIID1a) [Difficulty: R]

Teach the following steps to patients with obstructive airways diseases:

a. Have the patient lie in a comfortable supine position; knees can be flexed.

b. Instruct the patient to relax physically as much as possible, especially the shoulders.

c. Use soothing music, meditation, or other techniques for mental relaxation.

d. Instruct the patient to concentrate on breathing more slowly.

e. Emphasize pursed-lip breathing wherein the patient with relaxed abdominal muscles breathes in slowly through the nose and out slowly through pursed (slightly opened) lips. Breathing with pursed lips keeps some backpressure on the airways so that they stay open longer. The technique helps to improve gas exchange so that the patient experiences less dyspnea.

### 2. Teach the patient techniques for strengthening the inspiratory muscles (NBRC code: IIID1b) [Difficulty: R]

In addition to the first three steps described previously, teach the following steps to patients with obstructive airways diseases:

a. The practitioner places his or her hands and the patient's hands gently over the area(s) where the patient is to concentrate the breathing effort. Usually, this is the abdominal area just below the sternum. This encourages the patient to use the diaphragm more effectively and to strengthen it. With diaphragmatic breathing, the hands move out during an inspiration.

b. The same hands-on technique can be used to aid in segmental breathing over an area that is underventilated or that has atelectasis.

c. Breathing *in* against an obstruction can also increase strength and endurance of inspiratory muscles. A variety of devices exist. One type of device is a mouthpiece with selectable, variably sized openings at the other end (Fig. 7-1). The patient breathes in through the largest opening and progresses to smaller openings as tolerated.

Increasing the strength and endurance of inspiratory muscles usually requires a training program similar to the following:

a. Plug the nose with nose clips.

b. Inspire a normal tidal volume ($V_T$) at a rate of 12 to 15 breaths/min through the largest opening.

c. Continue for 10 to 15 min per day for a total of 3 to 5 times/week in the first week. If the patient notices shortness of breath, a noticeably increased pulse rate, or increased fatigue, the exercise should be stopped until the symptoms are gone. Resume the exercise when the patient is comfortable again.

d. Gradually increase the duration to about 30 min/session or two 15-min sessions/day.

e. When this schedule can be easily tolerated 3 times/week, switch to the next smallest hole.

f. Repeat steps **a** to **e** as tolerated. The most beneficial exercise is tiring but not exhausting. The device may be adjusted to the next larger hole setting if the patient becomes too tired. The whole process usually takes 4 to 6 weeks before positive results are seen.

g. A maintenance program necessitates that exercise be done every other day.

### 3. Reinforce to the patient the need to breathe deeply (NBRC code: IIID1a) [Difficulty: R]

Explain to the patient that taking in deep breaths keeps the lungs inflated and healthy and decreases the chance that pneumonia will develop. Deep breathing and coughing are indicated in patients with atelectasis, pulmonary infiltrates, or pneumonia. These exercises should help to raise secretions. It is especially important to use deep breathing and coughing to prevent or limit atelectasis and pneumonia in patients who have just had abdominal surgery such as cholecystectomy or splenectomy. Ideally, the patient is taught these techniques before surgery is performed. If not, teach them postoperatively:

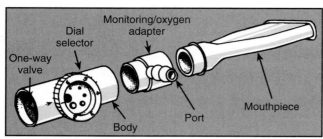

**Fig. 7-1** PFLEX inspiratory muscle trainer. The body of the device features a dial selector with inspiratory holes. The holes range from the 1 setting (largest opening) to the 6 setting (smallest opening). A one-way valve allows the patient to expire. The mouthpiece can be directly attached to the body, or a monitoring/oxygen adapter can be added between them. This adapter allows oxygen to be added to meet the patient's needs. An inspiratory force meter also can be added to determine the amount of negative pressure the patient is generating at each of the inspiratory hole settings. *(Courtesy of Respironics, HealthScan Asthma & Allergy Products, Inc., Cedar Grove, NJ.)*

a. To decrease the pain, minimize traction or tension on the incision by placing your or the patient's hands on both sides of the incision. Alternatively, the practitioner or the patient can hold a pillow against the incision.

b. Instruct the patient to breathe two or three times in through the nose and out through the mouth.

c. Instruct the patient to take in as deep a breath as possible and to perform a normal cough.

d. If the patient cannot cough normally because of pain, a serial or huff cough can be performed.

Teach the following cough techniques to the patient with obstructive airways disease:

a. Avoid an ineffective, shallow, hacking cough.

b. Position the patient in a sitting position, bent slightly forward, with feet on the floor or supported. The patient who must lie in bed can be positioned on the preferred side with the legs flexed at the knees and hips.

c. Instruct the patient to perform a midinspiratory cough.
   1. Breathe two or three times in through the nose and out through the mouth.
   2. Breathe in to a comfortable volume larger than the $V_T$, but not as deeply as possible.
   3. Briefly hold the breath.
   4. Cough hard, or perform a serial cough at relatively low flows. This should help to raise secretions without causing airway collapse.
   5. Squeezing the knees and thighs together at the instant of coughing helps to increase the airflow and volume.

Coaching is important because patients in pain or who are suffering from chronic lung disease tend to be uncooper-

ative and to not try hard. Give positive reinforcement when the patient does well. Correct any problems that the patient is having in trying to follow the instructions. Demonstrations are often helpful so that the patient can copy a good example.

## MODULE B
### Incentive spirometry

### 1. Teach the patient the proper techniques for incentive spirometry and evaluate the patient's ability to perform it (NBRC code: IIID1a) [Difficulty: R]

Incentive spirometry (IS) is a technique whereby a patient is encouraged to breathe deeply by seeing his or her inhaled volume on the spirometry device. The patient receives positive feedback by seeing that the volume gradually increases as his or her condition improves. IS is indicated in any patient who has developed or is likely to develop atelectasis and can perform the procedure. Those in which atelectasis is likely to be seen include postoperative thoracic or upper abdominal surgery patients, the aged, the obese, and patients with airway obstruction, inadequate sigh, and cardiopulmonary disease.

> **Exam Hint**
>
> **R**emember that incentive spirometry is the preferred treatment choice for atelectasis in patients who can perform it properly.

Because the goal of IS is to prevent or treat atelectasis, the patient should inhale a near-normal inspiratory capacity (IC). The patient can benefit more by holding the IC for several seconds, which is referred to as *sustained maximal inspiration (SMI)*. Before the operation, the co-operative surgical patient should have the IC measured at the bedside or calculated from a pulmonary function test in which vital capacity (VC) is measured (review Chapter 4 for IC information). The IC is measured again postoperatively.

Before you start the instruction, make sure that the patient is alert and cooperative enough to follow instructions. The patient's respiratory rate should be less than 25 breaths/min if the procedure is to be performed properly. Use the following steps in teaching IS:

a. Have the patient sit in semi-Fowler's position, on the edge of the bed, or up in a chair.

b. Set an initial goal of twice the patient's $V_T$.

c. Tell the patient the purpose of the treatment and how to perform it properly.

d. Simulate the procedure for the patient.

e. Put the unit within easy reach, and keep it upright.

f. Have the patient exhale normally (to functional residual capacity), seal the lips around the mouthpiece, and inspire maximally through the unit. The patient must inspire in a slow, controlled effort.

  g. Have the patient hold the IC for *at least* 3 sec before exhaling (the SMI) but no longer than 15 sec.

  h. Proceed to extend the patient's goal as tolerated and indicated earlier.

  i. The patient should perform the deep breath at least 10 times/hr while awake. A rest period with normal breathing should take place after each large breath.

Monitor your patient's progress in the following ways:

  a. If the patient cannot meet the initial goal, reconsider whether this is the best form of treatment. Intermittent positive-pressure breathing (IPPB) might be a better choice for providing a deep breath.

  b. Stop the treatment temporarily if the patient has signs of hyperventilation, such as dizziness or tingling of the fingertips. A few minutes of normal breathing should result in a normal feeling again. Have the patient take longer rest periods between maximal breaths.

  c. Stop the treatment if the patient complains of acute chest pain. It is possible to cause pulmonary barotrauma by breathing in as deeply as possible. Evaluate the patient's pulmonary condition, and call the physician if indicated.

## 2. Increase or decrease the patient's incentive spirometry goal (NBRC code: IIIF2b) [Difficulty: R, Ap]

See Table 7-1 for IS guidelines. The following guidelines are also suggested:

  a. Set the initial IC goal at twice the $V_T$.

  b. Increase the goal in 200-mL increments as the patient tolerates.

  c. Set a final IC goal of greater than 12 mL/kg of ideal body weight, or set a forced vital capacity (FVC) goal of greater than 15 mL/kg of ideal body weight.

  d. A normal person should have an IC of about 75% of his or her FVC. For example, a predicted FVC of

5.166 L was calculated for a male patient in Chapter 4. His predicted IC would be calculated as 5.166 L × 0.75 = 3.875 L. However, because of natural variations in people, he might inhale only 80% of this (3.1 L) and still be considered within normal limits. Use this as a guideline for anticipating a patient's maximum IC, and do not expect your patient to inhale a greater IC than is physically possible.

Consider increasing the IS goal if the patient is easily able to reach the set goal, or if the patient's breath sounds are diminished in the bases. Consider decreasing the IS goal if the patient cannot reach the set goal because it is too large, the patient is frustrated and discouraged at his or her inability to reach the set goal, or excessive surgical site pain prevents the patient from reaching the set goal.

## 3. Discontinue the patient's incentive spirometry treatment based on the patient's response (NBRC code: IIIG1f) [Difficulty: R, Ap]

Be prepared to discontinue the treatment if the patient is having an adverse reaction to it. Usually, incentive spirometry is a safe procedure. However, some patients will hyperventilate during the procedure and will feel dizzy or lightheaded. If this should happen, the patient should be told to stop the treatment for a few minutes. The dizziness should go away, and the patient should be able to resume the IS procedure. Direct the patient to continue to inhale deeply but at a slower rate.

## MODULE C
### Incentive spirometry equipment

## 1. Get the necessary equipment for the procedure (NBRC code: IIA13) [Difficulty: R]

## 2. Put the equipment together, make sure that it works properly, and identify and fix any problems with it (NBRC code: IIA13) [Difficulty: R]

Two basic types of IS equipment exist: flow displacement and volume displacement units.

  a. Flow displacement

With flow displacement units, patients breathe in a flow great enough to raise one or more plastic balls in calibrated cylinders (Fig. 7-2). The patient is encouraged to try to keep the ball (or balls) suspended by breathing in more deeply. Encourage the patient to breathe in *slowly* to suspend the balls for as long as possible. Have the patient watch as the balls are held up by the inspired breath to provide positive reinforcement for doing a good job. The patient is not helped by breathing in a fast, short breath and having the balls pop up and down. Volume is calculated by multiplying the flow per second needed to suspend the balls by the number of seconds that the balls are suspended. For example, 600 cc/sec × 2 sec = 1200 cc

| TABLE 7-1 Guidelines for the Use of Incentive Spirometry | |
|---|---|
| **Postoperative Bedside Spirometry** | **Treatment Modality** |
| IC > 80% of the preoperative value | No treatment needed unless radiographic or clinical evidence of atelectasis exists |
| IC at least 33% of the preoperative value or FVC of at least 10 mL/kg | IS is indicated |
| IC < 33% of the preoperative value or FVC < 10 mL/kg | IPPB is indicated |

FVC, Forced vital capacity; IC, inspiratory capacity; IPPB, intermittent positive-pressure breathing; IS, incentive spirometry.

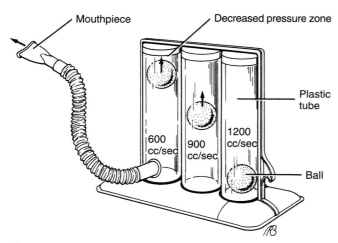

**Fig. 7-2** Triflo II incentive deep-breathing exerciser. *(From Eubanks DH, Bone RC: Comprehensive respiratory care, ed 2, St Louis, 1990, Mosby.)*

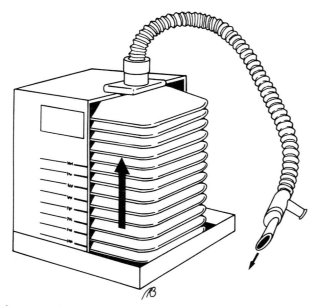

**Fig. 7-3** Volume incentive breathing exerciser. *(From Eubanks DH, Bone RC: Comprehensive respiratory care, ed 2, St Louis, 1990, Mosby.)*

IC. Assemble the device by attaching the flow tube to the unit and the mouthpiece to the flow tube.

   b. Volume displacement

With volume displacement units, patients breathe in a preset volume goal from the reservoir bellows (Fig. 7-3). Many of these units have a whistle built into them to warn if the breath is too fast. Patients who cannot generate enough inspiratory flow to use a flow displacement unit should use a volume displacement unit instead.

Some units also have a small built-in leak so that the patient must continue inspiring to keep the bellows suspended. Have the patient watch as the bellows is suspended for positive reinforcement for doing a good job. Volume is marked on the bellows container. If the unit has a built-in leak, multiply the volume inspired by the time the bellows is suspended. For example, 800 mL × 3 sec = 2400 mL IC. Assemble the device by attaching the flow tube to the unit and the mouthpiece to the flow tube.

### 3. Troubleshoot any problems with the equipment (NBRC code: IIA13) [Difficulty: R]

In either type of incentive spirometer, an obstruction to the flow tube or mouthpiece or a built-in leak in the calibrated cylinders stops airflow. With a flow displacement unit, no balls will rise despite the patient's inspiratory effort. With a volume displacement unit, the bellows will not rise despite the patient's inspiratory effort. Clearing the obstruction or sealing the leak allows either unit to work properly.

### MODULE D
#### Respiratory care plan

### 1. Analyze the available information to determine the patient's pathophysiologic state (NBRC code: IIH1) [Difficulty: R, Ap, An]

Review the information in Chapter 1 that deals with the interpretation of breath sounds and chest x-ray findings. As was discussed earlier, atelectasis is the primary problem that can be treated with IS.

### 2. Determine the appropriateness of the prescribed respiratory care plan and recommend modifications when indicated
#### a. Determine the appropriateness of the prescribed therapy and goals for the patient's pathophysiologic state (NBRC code: IIIH3) [Difficulty: R, Ap, An]

IS is the easiest and least expensive way to treat atelectasis if the patient can properly perform the procedure. See Table 7-1 for guidelines on the indications for IS or IPPB.

#### b. Recommend changes in the therapeutic plan if supportive data exist (NBRC code: IIIH4) [Difficulty: R, Ap]

The following should be considered in evaluation of the patient's response:

   1. The opening of atelectatic areas would be signaled by the return of normal rather than diminished or absent breath sounds.
   2. Acute chest pain could be the result of a pneumothorax from barotrauma. A chest x-ray film would be needed to confirm or deny the presence of a pneumothorax. Stop the treatment if a pneumothorax is suspected.

3. Be prepared to measure $V_T$, VC, and IC to determine the patient's goals and evaluate his or her progress.
4. The patient may have an increase in sputum production if the deep-breathing exercises and IS open up atelectatic areas. The patient may have a more productive cough because of a greater VC.

### c. Terminate the treatment based on the patient's response to therapy (NBRC code: IIIF1) [Difficulty: R, Ap, An]

A treatment can be stopped for one of three reasons. First, an adverse reaction or complication to the treatment can lead to cessation of treatment. For example, stop the treatment if the patient has a serious problem, such as chest pain, that may be the result of a pneumothorax. Inform the physician if clinical evidence of this is noted. The treatment may also need to be stopped if the patient repeatedly hyperventilates during the IS procedure. Other reasons to terminate the treatment include inadequate pain control, exacerbation of bronchospasm, hypoxemia from removal of the patient's oxygen mask, and fatigue. If these problems are corrected, it may be possible to begin IS treatment again.

Second, the treatment is no longer effective. If the patient cannot perform a proper IS treatment, another way to treat atelectasis should be found. This could include intermittent positive-pressure breathing (IPPB). See Chapter 14 for the discussion.

Third, the patient has recovered and no longer needs the treatment. As the postsurgical patient recovers, walks about, and performs proper coughing and deep-breathing exercises, any atelectasis will be corrected. In many cases, IS can be stopped within a week after surgery.

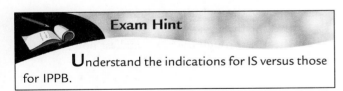

**Exam Hint**

**U**nderstand the indications for IS versus those for IPPB.

### BIBLIOGRAPHY

American Association for Respiratory Care: Clinical practice guideline: Incentive spirometry, *Respir Care* 36(12):1402, 1991.

Cairo JM: Lung expansion devices. In Cairo JM, Pilbeam SP: *Mosby's respiratory care equipment,* ed 2, St Louis, 2004, Mosby.

Douce FH: Incentive spirometry and other aids to lung inflation. In Barnes TA, editor: *Core textbook of respiratory care practice,* ed 2, St Louis, 1994, Mosby.

Eubanks DH, Bone RC: *Comprehensive respiratory care, a learning system,* ed 2, St Louis, 1990, Mosby.

Fink JB: Volume expansion therapy. In Burton GG, Hodgkin JE, Ward JJ, editors: *Respiratory care: A guide to clinical practice,* Philadelphia, 1997, Lippincott-Raven.

Fink JB: Bronchial hygiene and lung expansion. In Fink JB, Hunt GE, editors: *Clinical practice in respiratory care,* Philadelphia, 1999, Lippincott Williams & Wilkins.

Fink JB, Hess DR: Secretion clearance techniques. In Hess DR, MacIntyre NR, Mishoe SC: *Respiratory care principles & practice,* Philadelphia, 2002, WB Saunders.

Johnson NT, Pierson DJ: The spectrum of pulmonary atelectasis: Pathophysiology, diagnosis, and therapy, *Respir Care* 31:1107, 1986.

Mang H, Obermayer A: Imposed work of breathing during sustained maximal inspiration: Comparison of six incentive spirometers, *Respir Care* 34:1122, 1989.

Rutkowski JA: Hyperinflation therapy. In Wyka KA, Mathews PJ, Clark WF, editors: *Foundations of respiratory care,* Albany, 2002, Delmar.

Scuderi J, Olsen GN: Respiratory therapy in the management of postoperative complications, *Respir Care* 34:281, 1989.

Shapiro BA, Kacmarek RM, Cane RD, et al: *Clinical application of respiratory care,* ed 4, St Louis, 1991, Mosby.

Wilkins RL: Lung expansion therapy. In Wilkins RL, Stoller JK, Scanlan CL, editors: *Egan's fundamentals of respiratory care,* ed 8, St Louis, 2003, Mosby.

Wojciechowski WV: Incentive spirometers, secretion evacuation devices, and inspiratory muscle training devices. In Barnes TA, editor: *Core textbook of respiratory care practice,* ed 2, St Louis, 1994, Mosby.

### SELF-STUDY QUESTIONS

1. Your patient is quite weak and, despite repeated attempts to raise the ball marker on a flow displacement–type incentive spirometer, is unable to raise the ball near the goal. What would you recommend?
   A. Have her continue trying.
   B. Recommend that she be switched to IPPB.
   C. Change her to a volume displacement–type spirometer.
   D. Discontinue the treatment because it is not effective.

2. A patient with obstructive airways disease should be taught all of the following cough techniques EXCEPT
   A. Take two to three breaths in and out before coughing
   B. Breathe in a volume larger than the $V_T$ but less than the VC
   C. Perform a normal cough
   D. Perform a midinspiratory cough

3. IS is indicated when a patient's postoperative IC is what percentage of the preoperative IC?
   A. Between 30% and 50%
   B. Between 50% and 80%
   C. Between 80% and 90%
   D. Greater than 90%

4. A 16-year-old postoperative appendectomy patient has clear breath sounds and normal vital signs. What would you recommend to prevent atelectasis?
   A. CPAP at 5 cm $H_2O$
   B. PEP therapy
   C. IPPB
   D. IS

5. If pulmonary function results are not available, at what should the initial IS goal be set?
   A. The IC measured at the bedside
   B. The VC measured at the bedside
   C. Three times the $V_T$ measured at the bedside
   D. Twice the $V_T$ measured at the bedside

6. Your patient has an ideal body weight of 90 kg (200 lb). What would be his initial IC goal?
   A. His VC
   B. At least half of his VC
   C. At least 1080 mL
   D. At least 540 mL

7. It is recommended that IS be performed how often while the patient is awake?
   A. At least 5 times/hr
   B. At least 10 times/hr
   C. At least 20 times/hr
   D. At least 10 times/day

8. Your patient has just performed several excellent IS efforts. She complains of tingling fingers and dizziness. Your response would be to
   A. Have her continue with additional IS maneuvers
   B. Check her fingers and forehead for cyanosis
   C. Call her physician to cancel the treatment order
   D. Tell her to relax and breathe quietly until she feels normal again

9. Your patient has a flow displacement type of IS device. She is attempting to, but is unable to, inhale forcibly through it. What is the most likely problem?
   A. The airflow is obstructed.
   B. She is not really trying.
   C. The flow resistance is set too high.
   D. The bellows is in the locked-down position.

10. If IS has been successful, which breath sounds can be heard in the areas where atelectasis was noted before the treatment?
    A. Bronchial
    B. Absent
    C. Normal vesicular
    D. Tracheal

11. A patient's IS device is a flow displacement type. With good coaching, he can raise a ball with 900 cc/sec of flow. He can keep it elevated for 1.5 sec. What is his IC?
    A. 450 cc
    B. 900 cc
    C. 1350 cc
    D. 1800 cc

12. When you are helping a COPD patient learn to breathe more effectively, it is important to teach all of the following EXCEPT
    A. Exhale through pursed lips
    B. Exhale through blow bottles to increase expiratory muscle strength
    C. The patient should place his hands over the upper abdominal area to feel the movement of the diaphragm
    D. Inhale through an inspiratory muscle-training device.

13. Your patient has been using an inspiratory muscle-training device. He is currently on the third largest of six settings and has been comfortably breathing through it 4 days/week over the past 2 weeks. What would you now recommend that he do?
    A. Keep breathing through the same inspiratory hole.
    B. Breathe through the smallest hole.
    C. Breathe through the largest hole.
    D. Breathe through the next smallest hole.

## ANSWER KEY AND RATIONALE

1. **C.** Switching the patient from a flow displacement to a volume displacement incentive spirometer lets her see the results of her breathing efforts. This should help to motivate her to keep trying.

2. **C.** A patient with COPD should not attempt a normal cough because the high lung pressure generated may cause the airways to collapse. This could lead to air trapping.

3. **B.** Review Table 7-1 for the indications for IS.

4. **D.** IS is the most reasonable treatment for atelectasis at this time. The other three options are more equipment and labor intensive and therefore are more expensive.

5. **D.** An initial IS goal of twice the $V_T$ is widely accepted as a starting volume. A bedside IC may be less than that measured under laboratory conditions.

6. **C.** Review the mathematical process presented earlier in this chapter and in Chapter 4 for the calculation of IC.

7. **B.** It is widely accepted that an IS breath should be performed 10 times/hr while the patient is awake. Less often would be beneficial but not ideal; more often is probably not of any added benefit.

8. **D.** Tingling fingers and dizziness are signs of acute hyperventilation. Relaxing and breathing normally will restore the $CO_2$ level.

9. **A.** A pinched breathing tube is the simplest reason for the obstruction. No special flow resistance features exist on these units.

10. **C.** Normal vesicular breath sounds indicate normal lung expansion with no atelectasis.

11. **C.** Multiply the volume in 1 second by the number of seconds that the ball is elevated to calculate the inhaled volume.

12. **B.** Blowing into blow bottles significantly raises the lung pressure and can result in collapse of the airways. This will not help a COPD patient to breathe more effectively.

13. **D.** Because the patient is comfortable breathing at the current resistance level, it is reasonable to have him work a little harder by breathing through the next smallest hole.

# 8 Humidity and Aerosol Therapy

A review of the most recent Entry Level Examinations has shown an average of 7 questions (5% of the exam) that cover humidity and aerosol therapy.

## MODULE A
### Humidity and aerosol therapy

**1. Provide humidity and aerosol therapy to aid in the clearance of bronchopulmonary secretions** (NBRC code: IIIC3) [Difficulty: R, Ap]

Most patients receive supplemental humidity or aerosol delivered to their airways and lungs for one of two reasons. First, patients with excessive pulmonary secretions benefit from the inhalation of extra humidity or an aerosol to reduce the viscosity (thickness) of their secretions. This makes it easier for them to cough or to be suctioned out. Second, supplemental oxygen ($O_2$) from either the central delivery system or cylinders is absolutely dry. Adding humidity or aerosol to the $O_2$ prevents drying of the mucous membrane.

### a. Indications for humidity therapy
#### 1. Rehumidification of dry therapeutic medical gases in patients with normal upper airways

Body humidity is the water saturation condition of the gas in the lungs. Under normal conditions with air, it is 43.9 (44) mg/L absolute humidity and 46.90 (47) mm Hg at 37° C (98.6° F). In other words, air is always warmed to body temperature and saturated with water by the time it reaches the lungs. As can be seen in Table 8-1, both water content and vapor pressure in the lungs vary with the patient's temperature.

Humidity deficit is the difference between the body humidity conditions and the room air (or other gas) conditions. A humidity deficit is normal because the air must be warmed to body temperature and saturated by the time it reaches the lungs, and room conditions are rarely similar to those in the lung. The humidity deficit is eliminated through warming and humidifying of inhaled air by the respiratory passages.

The clinical practice guidelines of the American Association for Respiratory Care state that supplemental humidity is not needed for $O_2$ at flows of 4L/min or less. This includes nasal cannulas and some air-entrainment mask settings. As long as the patient has a normal upper airway and the hospital has a relative humidity (RH) of about 40%, the patient should be able to fully saturate the gas with no adverse effects. Some clinicians believe that *any* $O_2$ flow through a nasal cannula should be humidified to prevent the local mucosa from drying out. Usually, an unheated bubble-type humidifier is used to deliver about 40% RH at room temperature. The patient then is able to fully saturate the gas. All agree that dry $O_2$ at flows of greater than 4L/min by any device must be humidified.

#### 2. Elimination of the humidity deficit in a patient with a bypassed upper airway

Patients with bypassed upper airways *must* have the humidity deficit eliminated. Failure to do so will result in drying of the mucous membrane and mucus plugging. A heated humidifier is recommended and should be set to deliver gas at about 33° C ± 2° C to the patient to provide 80% to 100% RH in those temperature ranges.

#### 3. Reduction of airway resistance

Strong evidence exists that patients with exercise-induced and cold air–induced asthma are less likely to experience bronchospasm if they inhale warmed, humidified gas while exercising. The clinical goal in this case is to prevent an increase in airway resistance.

### b. Indications for aerosol therapy
#### 1. Rehumidification of dry therapeutic medical gases

Aerosol particles heated to body temperature can fully saturate the inhaled carrier gas through evaporation of some of the particles. This is indicated in patients who need the humidity *and* a medicinal aerosol. This way is not preferred for delivering just humidity to a patient, and it is possible to overhydrate the airway, especially in neonates, through long-term aerosol therapy. Aerosol particles can carry bacteria and other pathogens, whereas humidity (water vapor) alone cannot.

#### 2. Soothing of an irritated upper airway

Two generally accepted indications exist for delivery of a bland aerosol (sterile water or normal saline solution) to soothe an irritated upper airway: following extubation or laryngotracheobronchitis (LTB, or pediatric croup). Generally, a cool (room temperature) aerosol is delivered to reduce airway edema.

| TABLE 8-1 | Saturated Air Values for Absolute Humidity and Vapor Pressure Under Room and Body Temperature Ranges* | | |
|---|---|---|---|
| **Temperature** | | **Absolute Humidity (mg/L)** | **Vapor Pressure (mm Hg)** |
| **° C** | **° F** | | |
| 21 | 70 | 18.35 (18) | 18.62 (19) |
| 22 | 71.6 | 19.42 (19) | 19.79 (20) |
| 23 | 73 | 20.58 (21) | 21.02 (21) |
| 33 | 92 | 35.61 (36) | 37.59 (38) |
| 34 | 93 | 37.57 (38) | 39.75 (40) |
| 35 | 95 | 39.60 (40) | 42.02 (42) |
| 36 | 97 | 41.70 (42) | 44.40 (44) |
| 37† | 98.6 | 43.90 (44) | 46.90 (47) |
| 38 | 100 | 46.19 (46) | 49.51 (50) |
| 39 | 102 | 48.59 (49) | 52.26 (52) |
| 40 | 104 | 51.10 (51) | 55.13 (55) |
| 41 | 106 | 53.70 (54) | 58.14 (58) |

*The warmer the air is, the more water it can hold.
†So-called normal body temperature; it normally varies under different conditions.

| TABLE 8-2 | Aerosol Particle Sizes and Their Likely Deposition Points in the Airways and Lungs |
|---|---|
| **Location** | **MMAD* Particle Size (in μm)** |
| Nose or mouth to larynx | 10 and larger |
| Trachea to terminal bronchioles | 9–5 |
| Respiratory bronchioles to alveoli | 5–2 |
| Lung parenchyma (alveoli) | 1–3 |

MMAD, Mass median aerodynamic diameter.
*MMAD is defined as the aerosol diameter around which the mass is equally divided, that is, 50% of the aerosol mass is found in particles smaller than the MMAD, and 50% of the aerosol mass is found in particles larger than the MMAD.
*Note:* Some controversy exists over the size of the particles that deposit in the airways and lungs. This table lists what seems to be a majority opinion. Aerosol particle diameter sizes are listed in units of micrometers, which are one thousandth of a millimeter. As a point of clarification, most references list the symbol for a micrometer as μ; others use the international system unit of micrometer, which is symbolized as μm.

### 3. Delivery of medications to the airways and lungs

Respiratory therapists give many medications to patients, and these medications obviously must reach the target area. Table 8-2 gives the particle size of each medicinal aerosol and its most likely deposition area.

### 4. Increased clearance of secretions

Traditionally, many patients with a mild case of bronchitis were given breathing treatments with a bland aerosol to help them mobilize secretions. The aerosol was thought to add enough liquid to the secretions to enable the patient to cough them out. The patient, as it is now understood, can cough more effectively because the aerosol irritates the airway and the patient's own bronchial/submucosal glands pour out additional mucus. This reflex is mediated by the vagus nerve. This form of therapy is probably not indicated in most situations. It is clinically more effective to increase the patient's oral or intravenous fluids so that the bronchial/submucosal glands can produce secretions that are not thick.

### 5. Induce sputum production for a sputum specimen

Patients who have few, if any, secretions but from whom a sputum specimen is needed (e.g., patients with suspected tuberculosis or lung cancer) can have sputum production induced (see the mechanism of action previously described). Typically, the patient inhales an aerosol of hypertonic saline solution for about 5 to 10 min. Ultrasonic nebulizers are often used because they produce a dense mist of small particles.

### 2. Interview the patient to determine sputum production (NBRC code: IB4b) [Difficulty: R, Ap]

Find out from the patient approximately how much sputum is produced in a day. Also, find out if certain times of the day are more productive or less productive than others. Try to relate this to breathing treatments, medications, activities, meals, and allergies.

### 3. Observe the patient for changes in sputum characteristics (NBRC code: IIIE5) [Difficulty: R, Ap]

The patient's sputum characteristics (e.g., consistency, color, and smell) must be known if the effectiveness of humidity or aerosol therapy is to be assessed. Again, try to relate this to breathing treatments, medications, activities, meals, and allergies.

### 4. Assess the patient's overall cardiopulmonary status by auscultation to determine the presence of normal or abnormal breath sounds (NBRC code: IB3a) [Difficulty: R, Ap]

Review the discussion in Chapter 1, if necessary. If the patient is able to cough out secretions, abnormal breath sounds, such as crackles, should improve.

## MODULE B

### Humidity and aerosol generators and administrative devices

**1. Humidity delivered through small-bore tubing**

    **a. Bubble-type humidifiers**

        **1. Get the necessary equipment for the procedure (NBRC code: IIA3) [Difficulty: R, Ap]**

Bubble-type humidifiers are used on patients with a normal upper airway who need some supplemental humidity because of the dryness of medical $O_2$. These devices are not usually heated and, in fact, deliver gas cooled to below room temperature. They provide around 40% RH at the delivered gas temperature. The rest of the humidity has to be made up by the patient (Figs. 8-1 and 8-2). If clinically indicated, a wraparound type of heater can be added to raise the temperature of the delivered gas and reduce the patient's humidity deficit.

Three different types of these humidifiers are designed to add some humidity to dry $O_2$ delivered through small-bore tubing: traditional bubble humidifiers, jet humidifiers, and underwater jet humidifiers.

***Bubble humidifiers.*** Bubble humidifiers use a perforated capillary tube or porous diffusion head to break the

$O_2$ into small bubbles (see Fig. 8-2). This allows for greater surface area contact of the $O_2$ with the water and raises the RH by evaporation. The water level in the reservoir must be kept within the manufacturers' specifications and, if possible, as full as possible. The lower the water level, the lower the RH because less time exists for evaporation. The faster the $O_2$ flow, the lower the RH.

***Jet humidifiers.*** Jet humidifiers create an aerosol baffled out of the delivered gas flow. The RH is increased through

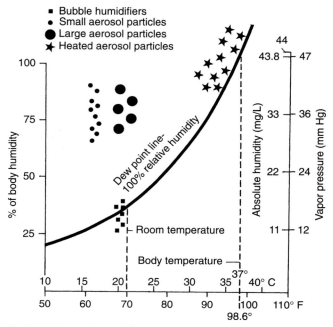

**Fig. 8-1** Comparison of humidity content by bubble-type humidifiers and various nebulizers.

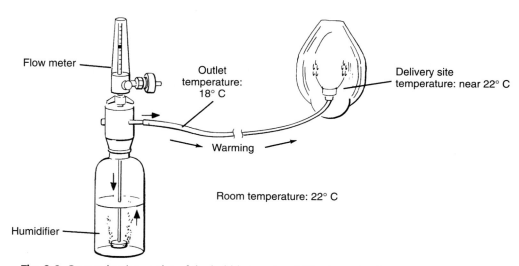

**Fig. 8-2** Oxygen leaving outlet of the bubble-type humidifier is cooler than room temperature because of evaporation. Some warming toward room temperature occurs as the oxygen travels through the tubing to the patient. *(From Scanlan CL: Humidity and aerosol therapy. In Scanlan CL, Spearman CB, Sheldon RL, editors: Egan's fundamentals of respiratory care, ed 5, St Louis, 1990, Mosby.)*

evaporation of some of the aerosol droplets. These units deliver a higher RH than is delivered by bubble humidifiers. They have the additional advantages of delivering the same RH at higher flow levels and as the water level drops.

***Underwater jet humidifiers.*** Underwater jet humidifiers create water vapor and an aerosol. The aerosol is not baffled out as it is in the jet humidifiers; therefore, these units deliver the highest RH. They can deliver the same humidity level at high gas flows and as the water level drops. Aerosol particles can carry pathogens, so strict infection control standards must be met to protect the patient. The water and humidifier must be changed at least every 24 hr. If the patient needs the highest-possible-delivered RH, a jet humidifier or underwater jet humidifier would be a better choice than a bubble type.

2. **Put the equipment together and make sure that it works properly (NBRC code: IIA3) [Difficulty: R, Ap]**
3. **Troubleshoot any problems with the equipment (NBRC code: IIA3) [Difficulty: R, Ap]**

Many simple bubble humidifiers come prepackaged with sterile water and can be used for many short-term patients (e.g., those in the recovery room) or for a single long-term patient. When the water runs low, they are discarded. Bubble and other types of humidifiers consist of a reservoir jar for the water and a diameter-index safety system (DISS) $O_2$ connector lid that screws on. Turn on the flowmeter, and make sure that $O_2$ flows through the delivery tube and bubbles into the water. Failure to bubble usually indicates that the lid and the jar are not screwed together tightly, or the delivery tube is plugged. If the tube cannot be cleared, it must be replaced.

Most of the newer bubble-type units have a pop-off type of high-pressure relief valve that is released if the pressure builds up to either 40 mm Hg or 2 psi. Pinch closed the small-bore tubing to build up pressure and test the pop-off valve. Feel for the gas to escape from the valve. Many valves whistle to signal a gas leak. Do not use a unit with a pop-off valve that does not open under pressure.

### b. Nasal cannula

As has been discussed earlier, current guidelines state that humidity does not need to be added to these devices if the flow is 4 L/min or less. However, some patients complain of nasal dryness and discomfort if the cannula's $O_2$ is not humidified. The physician and the practitioner may believe that the patient's discomfort warrants the addition of a bubble-type humidifier. Agreement exists on the addition of humidity to flows greater than 4 L/min. See Fig. 8-3 for a humidified nasal-cannula setup.

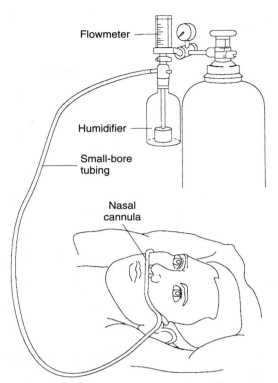

**Fig. 8-3** Adult wearing a nasal cannula that delivers oxygen humidified by a bubble-type humidifier. *(From Guidelines for disinfection of respiratory care equipment used in the home, Respir Care 33:801, 1988.)*

### c. Oxygen masks

As has been stated, the addition of humidity to any $O_2$ mask with an $O_2$ flow of 4 L/min or less is considered unnecessary. Humidity should be added to any mask with more than 4 L/min of $O_2$ added. This would include simple $O_2$ masks at higher flows, higher $O_2$ percentage air-entrainment masks, partial-rebreathing masks, and nonrebreathing masks.

## 2. Humidity delivered through large-bore tubing

Most patients who need delivery of humidity through large-bore tubing have had the upper airway bypassed by an endotracheal or tracheostomy tube; therefore, they cannot humidify inspired gas in the normal manner. In other cases, humidity is added because the patient is receiving dry medical $O_2$. Again, a heated humidifier is recommended for use with these patients. It should be set to deliver gas at between 31° C and 35° C to the patient and should be able to provide 80% to 100% RH in this temperature range. The following humidity- and aerosol-generating devices deliver the conditioned gas to the patient through large-bore (22-mm inner diameter [ID]) tubing.

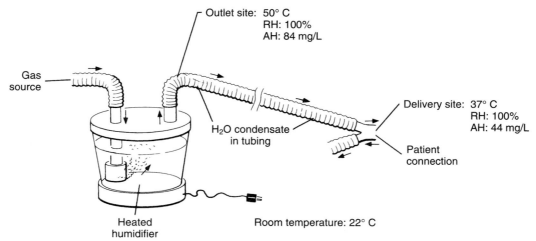

**Fig. 8-4** Gases leaving outlet of heated humidifier are hot and saturated with water vapor. As cooling occurs in the tubing, vapor condenses and absolute humidity *(AH)* decreases while relative humidity *(RH)* remains at 100% (saturated). Note that almost half of the original vapor is "lost" to condensate in this example. *(From Fink JB, Scanlan CL: Humidity and bland aerosol therapy. In Scanlan CL, Wilkins RL, Stoller JK, editors: Egan's fundamentals of respiratory care, ed 7, St Louis, 1999, Mosby.)*

### a. Large-volume humidifiers: cascade, wick, and passover types

#### 1. Get the necessary equipment for the procedure (NBRC code: IIA3) [Difficulty: R, Ap]

Cascade, wick, and passover-type humidifiers have an adjustable heater so that the water in the reservoir is at or greater than body temperature. This enables them to provide up to 100% of the patient's body humidity. With all of these units, the temperature of the inspired gas near the patient must be measured. The gas temperature is usually kept the same as the patient's or a few degrees cooler (Fig. 8-4).

The Bennett Cascade is a classic example of these types of humidifiers (Fig. 8-5). It was most commonly used with a mechanical ventilator but was also used with other types of systems for delivering humidity with or without oxygen. Its basic principle of operation is an efficient bubble-type humidifier. The inspiratory gas must flow through the water before evaporation can occur. A variety of similar devices are now on the market.

The wick-type heated humidifier employs a wick, often made of sponge or paper, to soak up water for evaporation. The water, wick, or both are heated so that 100% RH can be delivered. These units are also used with mechanical ventilators or other systems, including air-entrainment devices, because they have very little resistance to the gas flowing through them as evaporation occurs.

With passover-type humidifiers, the patient's gas simply passes over the surface of a reservoir of hot water. These are sometimes called "hot pots." By themselves, these units are probably the least effective at humidifying gas. When they are used on ventilators, other features such as copper mesh in a heated inspiratory tube are used to increase the surface area for evaporation.

#### 2. Put the equipment together and make sure it works properly (NBRC code: IIA3) [Difficulty: R, Ap]

#### 3. Troubleshoot any problems with the equipment (NBRC code: IIA3) [Difficulty: R, Ap]

Humidifiers must be properly assembled, especially when they are used to humidify a mechanical ventilator. Any loose connections result in an air leak and loss of tidal volume ($V_T$). Make sure that the water level is properly maintained.

Some cooling occurs as the heated gas passes through the large-bore tubing, which results in condensation that must be drained out. Placing a water trap in the lowest point of the tubing drains the water and helps keep the tubing clear. Remember to continue to look periodically for water puffing or sloshing back and forth in the tubing. Make sure that any condensate is drained out of the tubing and thrown away. Do not drain the condensate back into the water reservoir, because any microorganisms in the tubing or condensate could reproduce in the reservoir.

### b. Heat-moisture exchanger

#### 1. Get the necessary equipment for the procedure (NBRC code: IIA3) [Difficulty: R, Ap]

A heat-moisture exchanger (HME) contains a highly absorbent material that is warmed and moistened when a patient's exhaled breath passes through it. The patient's

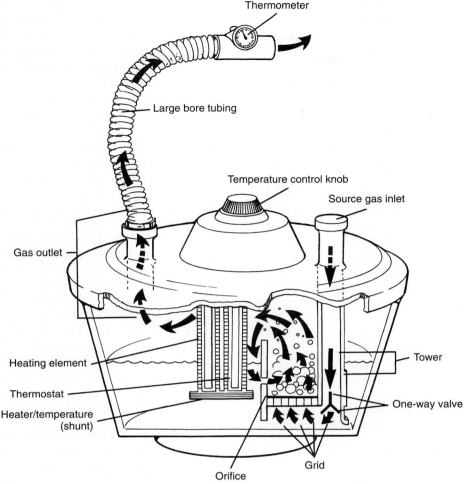

**Fig. 8-5** Cascade humidifier. *(From Scanlan CL: Humidity and aerosol therapy. In Scanlan CL, Spearman CB, Sheldon RL, editors: Egan's fundamentals of respiratory care, ed 5, St Louis, 1990, Mosby.)*

next inspiration is warmed and humidified by the HME. In effect, the patient is rebreathing his or her own exhaled water vapor. These units are not as efficient as the humidifiers described earlier and are not able to provide 100% of body humidity to a patient.

Many brands of HME exist, but only two main types have been documented. The first type is designed to be added to the outer part of a tracheostomy tube. A 15-mm ID opening can attach to the tube; the other end of the HME is open to room air. This type is small and convenient to use for many patients with a permanent tracheostomy; in addition, it improves a patient's mobility. The second type is used with patients who require mechanical ventilation. The patient end of the HME is a 15-mm ID opening that can attach to the endotracheal or tracheostomy tube; the other end of the HME has an opening that can be attached to the ventilator circuit. See Chapter 15 for greater detail.

**2. Put the equipment together and make sure it works properly (NBRC code: IIA3) [Difficulty: R, Ap]**

**3. Troubleshoot any problems with the equipment (NBRC code: IIA3) [Difficulty: R, Ap]**

HMEs typically come preassembled by the manufacturer. The 15-mm ID opening must be placed over the patient's endotracheal or tracheostomy tube. Secretions coughed into the HME can obstruct the flow of gas and thus make it difficult or impossible for the patient to breathe. The HME must be removed and discarded if it becomes obstructed, and it must be replaced by a new one. An HME should not be used with a patient known to cough out large amounts of secretions.

### 3. Nebulizers and related delivery systems
#### a. Ultrasonic nebulizers
##### 1. Get the necessary equipment for the procedure (NBRC code: IIA4) [Difficulty: R]

Ultrasonic units are often chosen for delivering bland solutions to the lower airways because of the small particle size and high output. Ultrasonic nebulizers work by converting electrical energy into high-frequency sound energy, which creates aerosol particles. The frequency is vital because it results in a stable aerosol with a mean particle size of about 3 μm in diameter. This is an ideal size for penetrating deeply into the lungs to the smallest airways. The only control on these units is for amplitude (power), and it controls the aerosol output. The range is usually up to 3 to 6 mL/min depending on the model. This output is greater than that possible with most pneumatic nebulizers. The aerosol can be carried to the patient via a built-in fan or by an outside $O_2$ source (Fig. 8-6). The warm aerosol that is created minimizes the patient's humidity deficit.

The ultrasonic nebulizer should not be chosen for upper airway aerosol deposition or for administering pharmacologically active medications such as bronchodilators, mucolytics, and antibiotics. These medications may not nebulize at the same rate as the saline diluent, which creates the risk that a very concentrated dose may be delivered at the end of treatment. Some medications may also be mechanically broken down by the high-frequency vibration and rendered useless.

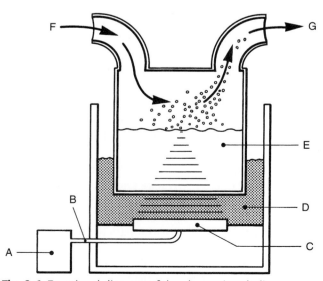

**Fig. 8-6** Functional diagram of the ultrasonic nebulizer. **A,** electric current generator; **B,** cable; **C,** piezoelectric crystal; **D,** couplant chamber; **E,** solution cup; **F,** carrier gas inlet; and **G,** aerosol outlet. *(From Barnes TA, editor: Core textbook of respiratory care practice, ed 2, St Louis, 1994, Mosby.)*

##### 2. Put the equipment together and make sure that it works properly (NBRC code: IIA4) [Difficulty: R]
##### 3. Troubleshoot any problems with the equipment (NBRC code: IIA4) [Difficulty: R]

Always follow the manufacturer's instructions when you are setting up the delivery system. Fig. 8-6 shows the common features, and Table 8-3 describes how to troubleshoot many common problems. Many clinical difficulties seem to involve keeping the proper fluid levels in the couplant chamber and the solution cup. If the sterile water in the couplant chamber is too low, the vibration cannot reach the solution cup, and no aerosol will be produced. If the saline level in the solution cup is either too low or too high, the vibrational energy will not focus properly on the surface of the saline solution, and no aerosol will be produced. Water should not be allowed to condense and fill low points in the large-bore tubing; if it does, ultrasonic particles will liquefy as the carrier gas is forced to pass through the condensate. The exiting gas would be humidified through evaporation but would carry no aerosol particles. If the carrier gas is $O_2$ blended with air through an air-entrainment system, any backpressure could result in an increase in the $O_2$ percentage and a decrease in the total flow. Remember to always measure the $O_2$ percentage near the patient.

#### b. Large-volume nebulizers
##### 1. Get the necessary equipment for the procedure (NBRC code: IIA4) [Difficulty: R]

All large-volume, pneumatically powered nebulizers share the common feature of having a liquid reservoir of at least 250 mL. They also typically entrain room air to increase the total gas flow. They share these common features:

a. All are powered by air or $O_2$ that is delivered through a flowmeter. As the gas flow drops, the aerosol output decreases.
b. All make use of Bernoulli's principle with a jet that is used to entrain liquid, room air, or both into the main gas flow.
c. All have a capillary tube that allows the liquid to flow *up* to the jet for nebulization. (Remember that with bubble-type humidifiers, $O_2$ flows *down* the capillary tube.)
d. All have a baffle against which the aerosol is sprayed to create a more uniform particle size.

Many, but not all, pneumatic nebulizers allow for a changeable inspired $O_2$ percentage. Provided that the jet is powered by $O_2$, the air-entrainment ports can be opened up to increase air entrainment (lowering the inspired $O_2$ percentage) or closed down to decrease air entrainment (raising the inspired $O_2$ percentage). The $O_2$ percentage usually can vary from 35% to 100%. Remember to always

| TABLE 8-3 | Ultrasonic Nebulizer Troubleshooting | |
|---|---|---|
| **Symptom** | **Possible Problem** | **Suggested Check** |
| Unit installed and connected as specified, but pilot light does not turn on when switch is turned to the "on" position | Electrical outlet defective<br>Circuit breaker tripped<br>Fuse blown | Check outlet with lamp or other appliance<br>Reset the circuit breaker, or change fuse on the power switch; if the circuit breaker continues to trip or the fuse blows again, service is needed |
| Unit installed and connected as specified; power pilot light turns on, normal ultrasonic activity visible in nebulizer chamber, but no aerosol output occurs | Nebulizer chamber contaminated | Wash nebulizer chamber; decontaminate |
| Unit installed and connected as specified; power pilot light turns on, but little ultrasonic activity is visible in the nebulizer chamber, and aerosol output is low (even when on the no. 10 power setting) | Couplant water excessively aerated<br>Nebulizer module and couplant water too cold<br>Diaphragm distorted, permitting air bubbles to interfere with proper transmission of vibrational energy into the nebulizer chamber | Wait for deaeration<br>Use warmer couplant water<br>Check to see that diaphragm is properly shaped and installed; be sure that the concave (recessed) side faces the interior of the chamber<br>Clean couplant compartment and replace couplant water |
| Same as symptom described previously but at a lower power setting | Power setting too low to start and establish nebulization | Turn output control knob to maximum power setting, then reduce to desired setting |
| Unit installed and connected as specified, and power pilot light turns on "Add couplant" light is on, and no ultrasonic activity is visible in the nebulizer chamber | Insufficient couplant water | Add water to the couplant compartment |
| Unit installed and connected as specified, and power pilot light turns on "Add couplant" light is off, but no ultrasonic activity is visible in the nebulizer chamber | Power supply overheated and its thermostatic control opened | The cooling air has been restricted, or cooling fins need cleaning The switch will reset when the equipment returns to room temperature |
| Liquid reservoir filled and properly connected to nebulizer chamber, but chamber does not fill (for continuous-feed system only) | Foreign material or air bubbles in feed tubes<br>Liquid level control in nebulizer chamber plugged with foreign material<br>Air leaks at tube connection or reservoir cap | Flush the system<br>Clean or flush the system<br>Tighten all connections by pushing tubes into fittings |

From Op't Holt T: Aerosol generators and humidifiers. In Barnes TA, editor: *Respiratory care practice*, Chicago, 1988, Mosby.

analyze the inspired $O_2$ percentage near the patient because both water in the aerosol tubing and back-pressure decrease the entrained air and raise the $O_2$ percentage.

2. **Put the equipment together and make sure that it works properly (NBRC code: IIA4) [Difficulty: R]**
3. **Troubleshoot any problems with the equipment (NBRC code: IIA4) [Difficulty: R]**

Most pneumatic nebulizers have an appearance that is similar to bubble-type humidifiers. Key components include a large reservoir jar and a top with a DISS $O_2$ con-

nector and a capillary tube to the jet. These units allow for variable $O_2$ percentages. Keep the capillary tube and jet clear of debris to keep the aerosol output from dropping. Keep the air-entrainment ports open so that proper gas mixing occurs and the desired $O_2$ percentage is provided (Fig. 8-7). Heating of the water, aerosol, or both is accomplished in one of the following ways:

a. A heated metal rod is immersed into the reservoir water through a port in the top of the nebulizer. A dial is used to control how hot the rod gets. Water temperature varies depending on how deep it is, so as the water level drops, the remaining water gets hotter. It is very important that the gas temperature near the patient be measured and that the water

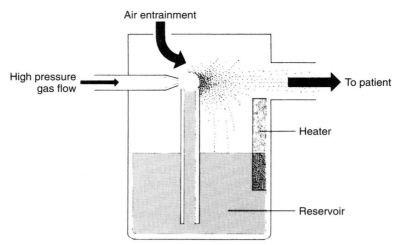

**Fig. 8-7** Large-volume, air-entrainment nebulizer. *(From Shapiro BA, Kacmarek RM, Cane RD, et al, editors: Clinical application of respiratory care, ed 4, St Louis, 1991, Mosby.)*

level be kept stable to prevent burning of the airway. The heated rod presents a risk of burns to a practitioner who accidentally touches it. It must be disinfected between patients and changed as often as the nebulizer is changed. Two other systems use variations on this idea of directly heating the water in the reservoir jar. The first heats the water as it passes through the capillary tube. The second type directly heats only a small amount of the reservoir water just before it is aerosolized. Each has the advantage of a short warm-up time compared with the heated metal rod systems. Some units have an external temperature probe for placement in the aerosol tubing. The probe acts as a servocontroller of the heating unit for better temperature regulation.

b. A flexible heater is wrapped around the outside of the reservoir. A dial is used to control how hot the heater gets. The water temperature increases as the water level drops. Monitor the gas temperature near the patient for safety purposes.

c. A clip-on heating base plate can be added to special reservoir jars with a metal plate. These are preferable to the previously mentioned types because they ensure a constant temperature to the aerosol as the water level drops.

Heating the water or aerosol reduces the patient's humidity deficit and is usually done if the secretions are thick. See Fig. 8-1 for the location of the aerosol particles and their relationship with the dew point and with the patient's body humidity.

## 4. Aerosol delivery systems

Large-bore tubing (also known as *aerosol tubing* or *corrugated tubing*) is needed to connect the aerosol generator with the patient. This tubing has a 22-mm ID.

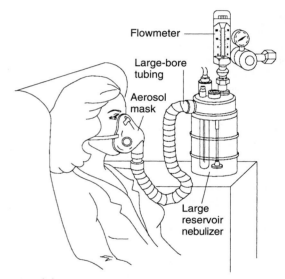

**Fig. 8-8** Adult wearing an aerosol mask who is receiving supplemental oxygen and aerosol from a heated large-volume nebulizer. *(From Guidelines for disinfection of respiratory care equipment used in the home, Respir Care 33:801, 1988.)*

### a. Aerosol masks

The aerosol mask looks similar to the simple $O_2$ mask, except that it has larger side ports for exhalation and a 22-mm outer diameter (OD) adapter for attachment of the large-bore tubing (Fig. 8-8). This is often considered to be a low-flow $O_2$ mask because the ports are open to room air; therefore, it is difficult to ensure that the patient receives the set $O_2$ percentage. If the flow is high enough that aerosol mist can be seen flowing out of the side ports during an inspiration, little room air is being inspired. Analyze the $O_2$ percentage inside the mask. Any of the previously mentioned humidity or aerosol devices can be used and powered by compressed air or $O_2$.

**b. Face tents**
**c. Tracheostomy masks/collars and Brigg's adapter/T-piece**

Face tents, tracheostomy masks and collars, and Brigg's adapter (T-piece) are discussed in Chapter 6. Any of the previously mentioned humidity or aerosol devices can be used with these and are powered by compressed air or $O_2$.

**d. Aerosol (mist) tents**
1. **Get the necessary equipment for the procedure** (NBRC code: IIA12) [Difficulty: R]
2. **Put the equipment together and make sure that it works properly** (NBRC code: IIA12) [Difficulty: R]
3. **Troubleshoot any problems with the equipment** (NBRC code: IIA12) [Difficulty: R]

Aerosol or mist tents are essentially like the $O_2$ tents discussed in Chapter 6. The main difference is that no supplemental $O_2$ is used because the patient does not need it. The top of the canopy then can be left open for better flow-through ventilation. At least 10 L/min of compressed air should still be run through the nebulizer to ensure that no $CO_2$ builds up. The nebulizer or ultrasonic system should be cared for as described earlier to ensure that enough aerosol is available to treat the condition.

Aerosol tents are sometimes used to treat upper respiratory tract problems such as laryngotracheobronchitis (LTB, or pediatric croup). A cool aerosol seems to be clinically preferred because it reduces airway edema. Never use so much aerosol that the child cannot be seen inside the tent. Also, be wary of fluid overloading in the young patient who is in the tent for a prolonged period.

**5. Medication delivery systems**
**a. Small-volume nebulizers**
1. **Get the necessary equipment for the procedure** (NBRC code: IIA4) [Difficulty: R]

A small-volume nebulizer (SVN) is designed to hold a relatively small volume of fluid (typically 3 to 5 mL) and to nebulize liquid medications such as bronchodilators, mucolytics, or antibiotics for inhalation. Either compressed air or $O_2$ can be used to generate the aerosol. These units operate under the same physical principles as the large-volume nebulizers described earlier.

Two different types of SVNs exist: mainstream and sidestream. *Mainstream nebulizers* are designed so that the main flow of gas to the patient comes through the aerosol as it is produced. A second high-pressure gas flow is used to power the jet to create the aerosol (Fig. 8-9). *Sidestream nebulizers* are designed so that the aerosol is produced from the main flow of gas and is supplemented by the jet's gas flow (Fig. 8-10). Many manufacturers produce disposable medication SVNs, typically sidestream, for intermittent positive-pressure breathing circuits or handheld circuits. Select the nebulizer that

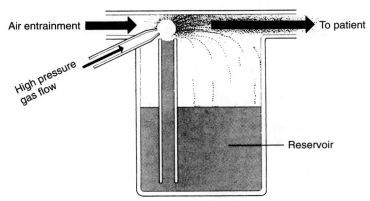

**Fig. 8-9** Mainstream-type small-volume nebulizer for medications. *(From Shapiro BA, Kacmarek RM, Cane RD, et al, editors: Clinical application of respiratory care, ed 4, St Louis, 1991, Mosby.)*

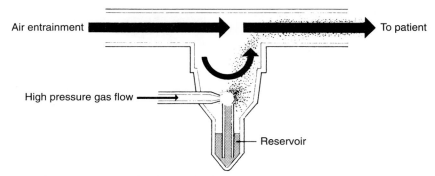

**Fig. 8-10** Sidestream-type small-volume nebulizer for medications. *(From Shapiro BA, Kacmarek RM, Cane RD, et al, editors: Clinical application of respiratory care, ed 4, St Louis, 1991, Mosby.)*

produces a particle size that matches the therapeutic target.

Fig. 8-11 shows a typical handheld nebulizer circuit. The nebulizer can be powered by either air or $O_2$. Flows of 4 to 6 L/min are typically used to nebulize 3 to 5 mL of medication in about 10 min. The nebulizer finger control allows the patient to power the nebulizer by covering the open hole in the "T." Uncovering the hole permits the gas to exit; thus, the medication is not nebulized and wasted. The reservoir tube serves to hold $O_2$ and medication for the next inspiration.

Practitioners face two possible risks when they use SVNs. First, any aerosolized medications that escape into the room air may be inhaled. It is possible that the practitioner, or anyone else nearby, may have an allergic or other adverse reaction. Second, nebulized secretions from the patient's airway and lungs may be inhaled, which may place the practitioner or others at risk for acquiring a pulmonary infection from the patient. Although actual problems like these rarely occur, they are possible. If either of these situations is a concern, an SVN with one-way valves and a downstream particle filter should be used. This filter will trap any exhaled aerosol droplets (Fig. 8-12). A filtered SVN is recommended when pentamidine isethionate is nebulized (NebuPent). It, or a similarly filtered SVN, could be used for any other antibiotic or medication that should not contaminate the room air.

2. **Put the equipment together and make sure that it works properly (NBRC code: IIA4) [Difficulty: R]**
3. **Troubleshoot any problems with the equipment (NBRC code: IIA4) [Difficulty: R]**

Most SVNs consist of a medication reservoir and a top piece that contains a capillary tube and a baffle. The top piece screws onto the reservoir and holds a mouthpiece and aerosol reservoir tube. Small-bore $O_2$ tubing connects

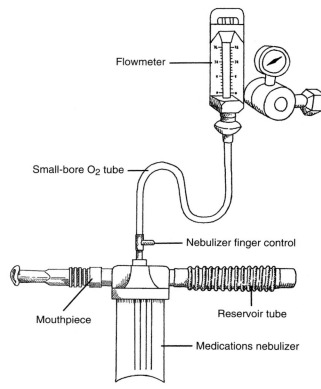

**Fig. 8-11** Handheld small-volume nebulizer, with added components, for medications. $O_2$, Oxygen. *(Adapted from Guidelines for disinfection of respiratory care equipment used in the home, Respir Care 33:801, 1988.)*

the SVN to the flowmeter. If an SVN fails to generate aerosol, make sure that the pieces are properly assembled and that the capillary tube is not plugged with debris. Sometimes, the capillary tube can be cleared by running it under water or pushing a needle through the channel. Make sure the liquid in the reservoir is at the proper depth (typically 3 to 5 mL). Do not use a nebulizer that does not generate an aerosol.

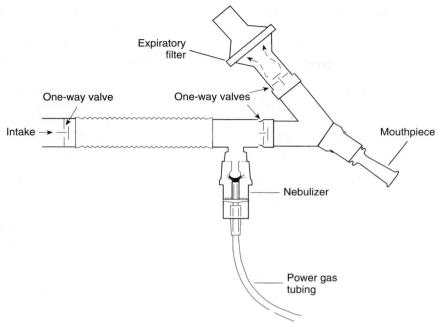

**Fig. 8-12** Diagram of the Respirgard II small-volume nebulizer system showing one-way valves and an expiratory filter to scavenge exhaust aerosol. *(From Rau JL Jr: Respiratory care pharmacology, ed 5, St Louis, 1998, Mosby.)*

**b. Metered dose inhalers**

1. **Get the necessary equipment for the procedure** (NBRC code: IIA22) [Difficulty: R]
2. **Put the equipment together and make sure that it works properly** (NBRC code: IIA22) [Difficulty: R]
3. **Troubleshoot any problems with the equipment** (NBRC code: IIA22) [Difficulty: R]

Metered dose inhalers (MDIs) are designed to dispense a premeasured amount of medication into the airway. Each activation increases the amount of medication taken by the patient. Available medications include sympathomimetic and anticholinergic bronchodilators, corticosteroid drugs, and an antibiotic (see Chapter 9 for details on the medications). All MDIs operate in the same way. They have several milliliters of medication and either a compressed chlorofluorocarbon (CFC) gas or hydrofluoroalkane (HFA) gas contained inside of a metal container with a built-in jet nozzle. Because of environmental concerns, CFC gas units will be replaced by HFA gas units by 2008.

Tipping the metering chamber over and back upright results in its filling with medication. A plastic actuator opens the jet when it is pressed into the container (Fig. 8-13). The patient can inhale the medication through the built-in mouthpiece. Also, adapters allow the medication

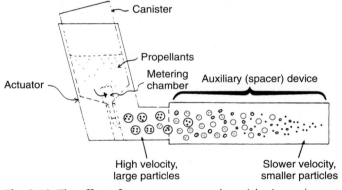

**Fig. 8-13** The effect of a spacer on aerosol particle size and velocity from a chlorofluorocarbon-powered metered dose inhaler. *(From Rau JL Jr: Respiratory care pharmacology, ed 5, St Louis, 1998, Mosby.)*

to be sprayed into a mechanical ventilator circuit or through a bronchoscopy adapter to an endotracheal tube. A specific amount of medication is nebulized with each actuation of the device.

Make sure, when you are assembling the MDI, that the medication canister nozzle fits into the jet of the actuator. Patients should be instructed to use warm, soapy water daily to wash out the actuator and keep open the jet channel.

### c. Spacer and holding chamber for a metered dose inhaler

1. **Get the necessary equipment for the procedure** (NBRC code: IIA22) [Difficulty: R]
2. **Put the equipment together and make sure that it works properly** (NBRC code: IIA22) [Difficulty: R]
3. **Troubleshoot any problems with the equipment** (NBRC code: IIA22) [Difficulty: R]

The addition of some sort of spacer or holding chamber between the actuator and the patient's mouth has been shown to increase the amount of inhaled medication. These devices slow down the aerosol so that less of it impacts on the back of the throat. This should result in fewer systemic adverse effects such as the risk of oral thrush (*Candidiasis* fungal infection) with an MDI-powered corticosteroid. Also, the patient with poor hand and breathing coordination wastes less medication.

A spacer is a simple, open extension tube that is placed between the actuator and the patient. Its main advantage over direct inhalation from the MDI mouthpiece is that the aerosol plume expands and slows down so that more medication is inhaled (see Fig. 8-13). The patient should be told to refrain from exhaling through the spacer because any remaining medication will be blown out and wasted. Some spacers are designed for use with a ventilator circuit when an MDI-based medication is to be given. A holding chamber holds the medication as does a spacer, but it also has valves. These valves prevent the medicine from being exhaled out and allow the patient to inhale several times to get more medication. This is especially helpful with children or small adults with small $V_T$s. Some holding chambers have a built-in whistle that sounds if the patient is inhaling too quickly (Fig. 8-14). Several types of spacers or holding chambers exist. Some

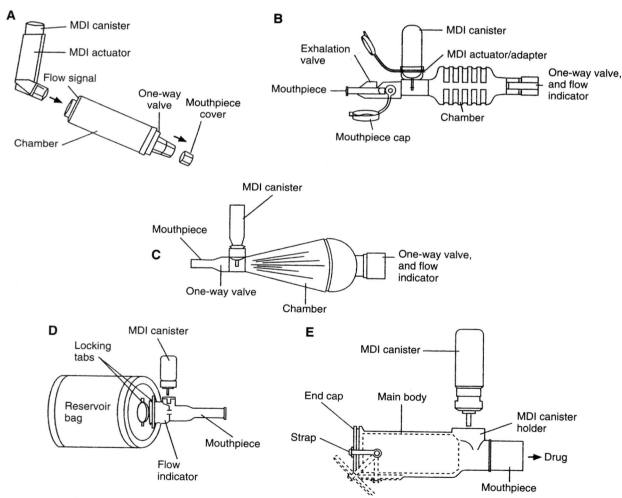

**Fig. 8-14** Five types of metered dose inhaler (MDI) spacers and holding chambers. **A,** AeroChamber; **B,** MediSpacer; **C,** Aerosol Cloud Enhancer; **D,** InspirEase; and **E,** OptiHaler. *(From Rau JL Jr: Respiratory care pharmacology, ed 5, St Louis, 1998, Mosby.)*

spacers are designed to fit with only one actuator, whereas others adapt to fit with any actuator. A facemask comes attached to some holding chambers so that pediatric patients or uncooperative adults can be given the medication.

Patients must be instructed to wash out the spacer or holding chamber on a daily basis. Warm, soapy water and a thorough rinsing are usually adequate for home use.

### d. Dry powder inhalers
1. **Get the necessary equipment for the procedure** (NBRC code: IIA23) [Difficulty: R]
2. **Put the equipment together and make sure that it works properly** (NBRC code: IIA23) [Difficulty: R]
3. **Troubleshoot any problems with the equipment** (NBRC code: IIA23) [Difficulty: R]

Dry powder inhalers (DPIs) dispense a dry medicinal powder into the patient's airways and lungs when inhaled. Relatively few drugs are currently available in the DPI form. The drug manufacturer sells both the medication and the dispenser to the patient. The first two DPI medicines discussed here are held in a plastic capsule until released. The device is designed to open the capsule and to allow the patient to inhale the medication (Fig. 8-15).

The Spinhaler is used to pierce the gelatin capsule that holds cromolyn sodium and dispense it into the patient's airway. As the patient inhales rapidly (a flow rate of at least 40–60 L/min is needed on any DPI), the plastic rotor blades spray the powder into the inhaled stream of air.

The patient should inhale as deeply as possible and should hold the breath for maximal deposition in the small airways. Care must be taken to hold the unit upright when the capsule is pierced and the powder is inhaled, or it may spill. Cromolyn sodium is used to prevent the onset of an asthma attack and is useless after an attack has begun.

The Rotahaler is designed to break in half a gelatin capsule that contains a powdered form of albuterol or beclomethasone. Care must be taken with the Rotahaler to hold it horizontally after the capsule has been broken, or the medication will spill out. A fast inhalation with a breath-hold is recommended to deliver the medication to the airways.

Multidose dispensers contain many doses of a medication within a drug reservoir (see Fig. 8-15). A single dose is loaded into the dispenser by the patient. A quick inhalation followed by a breath-hold is again needed. These dispensers are more convenient to use than are the single-dose units previously discussed. The following are currently available: Turbuhaler (terbutaline sulfate or budesonide), Rotadisk (albuterol or salmeterol), and Diskus (salmeterol). (See Chapter 9 for details on the medications.)

Practice is needed in the use of the Spinhaler and Rotahaler units. The two main pieces must be unscrewed so that the capsule can be placed in the holding chamber. With the Spinhaler, the plastic slide must be moved up and down once to pierce the capsule. With the Rotahaler, the mouthpiece is twisted around to break open the capsule. The medication is then forcefully inhaled. Unscrew both units to remove the empty capsule.

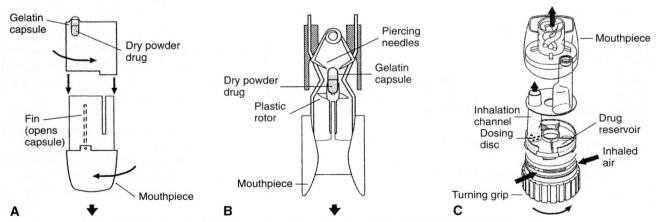

**Fig. 8-15** Three types of dry powder inhalers. The Rotahaler **(A)** and Spinhaler **(B)** need to have an individual medication capsule loaded for each inhalation. The Turbuhaler **(C)** has a drug reservoir that holds many doses of medication. *(From Rau JL Jr: Respiratory care pharmacology, ed 5, St Louis, 1998, Mosby.)*

## MODULE C
### Alter the patient's breathing pattern

### 1. Instruct the patient in proper breathing techniques (NBRC code: IIID1a) [Difficulty: R]

a. **Modify the patient's breathing pattern to properly deposit medication (NBRC code: IIIF2c1) [Difficulty: R, Ap]**

For medications to be properly deposited in either the upper or lower airway, the patient must breathe in the correct manner. Following are recommended breathing patterns.

#### 1. Upper airway deposition

Particles $10\,\mu m$ or larger are more likely to impact the upper airway (oropharynx, larynx, trachea, and mainstem bronchi) when the patient is coached to do the following:

a. Inhale at a normal or faster speed (the flow should be greater than 30 L/min)
b. Inhale a normal $V_T$
c. Breathe in a normal pattern

#### 2. Lower airway and alveolar deposition

Particles 2 to $5\,\mu m$ in size are more likely to deposit on the smaller airways (respiratory bronchioles) and in the alveoli when the patient is coached to do the following:

a. Inhale at a slow speed (the flow should be less than 30 L/min)
b. Inhale an inspiratory capacity (IC)
c. Hold the full breath for 10 sec, if possible, before exhaling

Obviously, not all patients can perform these techniques perfectly, but to the extent that they can, the medication is deposited where needed and the treatment is more effective.

## MODULE D
### Respiratory care plan

### 1. Analyze the available information to determine the patient's pathophysiologic state (NBRC code: IIIH1) [Difficulty: R, Ap, An]

a. **Auscultate the patient's chest and interpret changes in breath sounds (NBRC code: IIIE11) [Difficulty: R, Ap]**

The patient with many secretions should be helped by the addition of a bland aerosol or mucolytic medication and should be better able to clear them effectively. This should cause the patient to feel better and to have improved vital signs, oxygenation, breath sounds, and spirometry values. The use of a bland aerosol therapy can cause bron-

chospasm in some asthmatic patients. Patients with thick, dry secretions can have their airways occluded if aerosol therapy causes the secretions to take in water and swell. The patient must be able to cough out the thinned secretions, or suctioning equipment must be available to remove them.

### 2. Determine the appropriateness of the prescribed respiratory care plan and recommend modifications when indicated

a. **Recommend changes in the therapeutic plan if supportive data exist (NBRC code: IIIH4) [Difficulty: R, Ap]**

Changes in the patient's secretion volume and consistency may result in a change in the type of humidity and/or aerosol therapy needed. Be prepared to decrease humidity and/or aerosol therapy if the patient's secretions are decreased in volume and easy for the patient to cough out. In contrast, be prepared to increase humidity and/or aerosol therapy if the patient's secretions are thick and difficult to cough out.

#### 1. Change the type of equipment being used (NBRC code: IIIF2c2) [Difficulty: R, Ap]

Be prepared to change the type of humidity and aerosol delivery system from among those discussed in this chapter based on the patient's condition. Review the indications, contraindications, uses, and limitations of the various systems.

> **Exam Hint**
>
> The examination usually includes several questions that deal with making recommendations to change from one equipment item to another.

#### 2. Adjust the temperature of the aerosol (NBRC code: IIIF2c3) [Difficulty: R, Ap]

In general, a cool humidity or aerosol system is used with patients with the following conditions:

a. Pediatric croup
b. Upper airway irritation, such as after extubation or a bronchoscopy procedure

In general, a body temperature humidity or aerosol system is used with patients with the following conditions:

a. Bypassed upper airway (endotracheal or tracheostomy tube)
b. Thick secretions
c. Hypothermia
d. Maintenance of a neutral thermal environment for the neonate

3. **Change the output of aerosol by the equipment** (NBRC code: IIIF2c2) [Difficulty: R, Ap]

Neonates are sensitive to overhydration, so long-term aerosol therapy for them should be avoided or minimized. Adult patients with heart failure or pulmonary edema should also not be given long-term aerosol therapy. Instead, a cascade-type humidifier can be used.

The adult patient with thick secretions may be aided by long-term aerosol therapy of a dense mist, usually by an ultrasonic nebulizer at body temperature. Secretions are often liquefied and made easier to cough or suction out. The child with croup is usually given a dense mist of a cool bland aerosol in a mist tent. This therapy is usually needed for only a few days. Be wary of fluid overload if the mist is needed for a longer period.

b. **Stop the treatment or procedure if the patient has an adverse reaction to it** (NBRC code: IIIF1) [Difficulty: R, Ap, An]
c. **Discontinue treatment based on the patient's response** (NBRC code: IIIG1f) [Difficulty: R, Ap]

Based on the previous discussion, be prepared to stop a treatment or procedure if necessary. After further evaluation, it may be possible to continue again. However, if the patient has a serious adverse reaction, the treatment or procedure should be discontinued. Usually, this would be done after consultation with the patient's physician.

## BIBLIOGRAPHY

Adams DA: Humidity and aerosol therapy. In Wyka KA, Mathews PJ, Clark WF, editors: *Foundations of respiratory care*, Albany, 2002, Delmar.

American Association for Respiratory Care: Aerosol consensus statement, *Respir Care* 36:916, 1991.

American Association for Respiratory Care: Clinical practice guideline: Selection of aerosol delivery device, *Respir Care* 37:891, 1992.

American Association for Respiratory Care: Clinical practice guideline: Selection of aerosol delivery device for neonatal and pediatric patients, *Respir Care* 40:1325, 1995.

American Association for Respiratory Care: Clinical practice guideline: Bland aerosol administration, *Respir Care* 38:1196, 1993.

American Association for Respiratory Care: Clinical practice guideline: Bland aerosol administration—2003 revision & update, *Respir Care* 48:529, 2003.

American Association for Respiratory Care: Clinical practice guideline: Delivery of aerosols to the upper airway, *Respir Care* 39:803, 1994.

Barnes TA, editor: *Core textbook of respiratory care practice*, ed 2, St Louis, 1994, Mosby.

Branson RD, Hess DR, Chatburn RL, editors: *Respiratory care equipment*, ed 2, Philadelphia, 1999, Lippincott Williams & Wilkins.

Fink JB: Humidity. In Fink JB, Hunt GE, editors: *Clinical practice in respiratory care*, Philadelphia, 1999, Lippincott-Raven.

Fink JB: Humidity and bland aerosol therapy. In Wilkins RL, Stoller JK, Scanlan CL, editors: *Egan's fundamentals of respiratory care*, ed 8, St Louis, 2003, Mosby.

Fink JB, Dhand R: Aerosol drug therapy. In Fink JB, Hunt GE, editors: *Clinical practice in respiratory care*, Philadelphia, 1999, Lippincott-Raven.

Fink JB, Hess DR: Humidity and aerosol therapy. In Hess DR, MacIntyre NR, Mishoe SC, et al, editors: *Respiratory care principles & practices*, Philadelphia, 2002, WB Saunders.

Fink JB, Scanlan CL: Aerosol drug therapy. In Scanlan CL, Wilkins RL, Stoller JK, editors: *Egan's fundamentals of respiratory care*, ed 7, St Louis, 1999, Mosby.

Hess D: The delivery of aerosolized bronchodilator to mechanically ventilated intubated adult patients, *Respir Care* 35:399, 1990.

Hess D: Aerosol therapy. In Dantzker DR, MacIntyre NR, Bakow ED, editors: *Comprehensive respiratory care*, Philadelphia, 1995, WB Saunders.

Rau JL Jr: *Respiratory care pharmacology*, ed 5, St Louis, 1998, Mosby.

Shapiro BA, Kacmarek RM, Cane RD, et al, editors: *Clinical application of respiratory care*, ed 4, St Louis, 1991, Mosby.

Ward JJ, Hess D, Helmholz HF Jr: Humidity and aerosol therapy. In Burton GC, Hodgkin JE, Ward JJ, editors: *Respiratory care: a guide to clinical practice*, ed 4, Philadelphia, 1997, Lippincott-Raven.

Whitaker K: *Comprehensive perinatal & pediatric respiratory care*, ed 2, Albany, NY, 1997, Delmar.

White GC: *Equipment theory for respiratory care*, ed 3, Albany, NY, 1999, Delmar.

Wissing DR: Humidity and aerosol therapy. In Cairo JM, Pilbeam SP, editors: *Mosby's respiratory care equipment*, ed 7, St. Louis, 2004, Mosby.

## SELF-STUDY QUESTIONS

1. A 30-year-old patient has a face tent on for the delivery of a heated aerosol. Her secretions are still too thick to be easily coughed out. What would you recommend?
   A. Change to a mist tent.
   B. Change to a heated aerosol mask.
   C. Change to a simple $O_2$ mask.
   D. Change to a nonrebreather mask.

2. A comatose patient is intubated and is receiving 35% $O_2$ with aerosol through a T-piece (Briggs adapter). While watching the patient breathe, you notice that during each inspiration, the mist disappears from the downstream end of the T-piece. What would you recommend?
   A. Add 100 mL of aerosol tubing as a reservoir on the T-adapter.
   B. Change the $O_2$ to 30% and increase the flow.
   C. Change the $O_2$ to 40% and decrease the flow.
   D. Tell the patient not to breathe so deeply.

3. A 4-year-old patient with asthma is about to be discharged and needs to take an inhaled bronchodilator medication at home. What device would you recommend?
   A. MDI
   B. DPI
   C. DPI with holding chamber
   D. MDI with holding chamber

4. To help prepare a patient for a laryngoscopy procedure, the physician has ordered her to inhale nebulized lidocaine (Xylocaine). You would select a nebulizer that generates particles of what size?
   A. 1 to 3 μm
   B. 2 to 5 μm
   C. 5 to 7 μm
   D. 10 μm or larger

5. For an aerosolized medication to be primarily deposited in the larger airways, what breathing pattern would you recommend?
   I. Inhale a $V_T$.
   II. Inhale an IC.
   III. Inhale slowly.
   IV. Inhale at a normal speed.
   V. Breathe in a normal pattern.
   A. II and III
   B. I, IV, and V
   C. IV and V
   D. II and IV

6. A physician calls you to evaluate a 40-year-old patient with bronchitis and to make a recommendation for an aerosol delivery system. The patient's breath sounds indicate the presence of large airway secretions. Despite a good cough effort, the patient has difficulty in raising them. What would you recommend?
   A. Use a handheld nebulizer with 3 cc of normal saline every 4 hr.
   B. Place the patient into a mist tent.
   C. Start a continuous ultrasonic nebulizer to an aerosol mask.
   D. Start a cascade-type humidifier to an aerosol mask.

7. A patient's humidity deficit is going to be the *smallest* under which of the following conditions?
   A. Breathing in regular hospital room air at 72° F and 40% relative humidity
   B. Breathing in outside air at 80° F and 50% relative humidity
   C. Breathing in 6 L/min of $O_2$ through a nasal cannula running through an unheated bubble humidifier
   D. Breathing in 40% $O_2$ through a cascade-type humidifier at 95° F to an aerosol mask

8. An ultrasonic nebulizer would be recommended for aerosol therapy for the following reason:
   A. It delivers a wide variety of aerosol droplets.
   B. Its aerosol droplets are between 10 and 20 μm in diameter.
   C. It delivers a uniform aerosol droplet of about 3 μm in diameter.
   D. It can be used to nebulize bland aerosols and liquid medications into an aerosol.

9. Your patient has an endotracheal tube. Which of the following devices would be the *least* effective in reducing this patient's humidity deficit?
   A. Wick-type humidifier set at 35° C
   B. Cascade-type humidifier set at 35° C
   C. Unheated bubble-type humidifier
   D. Ultrasonic nebulizer

10. Your patient has a temperature of 98.6° F. To saturate the inhaled air, how much absolute humidity must be provided by the humidifier device?
    A. 37° C
    B. 47 mm Hg
    C. 760 mm Hg
    D. 44 mg/L

11. Your heated humidifier unit has a water reservoir temperature of 40° C. The humidified gas is traveling through large-bore tubing to the patient. Which of the following statements are true?
    I. Condensation will occur.
    II. The gas will warm and expand as it travels to the patient.
    III. The gas will remain saturated.
    IV. The relative humidity will decrease.
    V. The relative humidity will increase.
    A. I and III
    B. IV
    C. II and V
    D. I and IV

12. The pop-off valve is whistling on your patient's bubble humidifier to a 35% $O_2$, air-entrainment mask. What could be the problem?
    A. The reservoir jar is not screwed tightly into the top of the humidifier.
    B. The air-entrainment mask should be set at 28% $O_2$.
    C. The small-bore tubing is pinched.
    D. The air-entrainment mask should be set at 40% $O_2$.

13. Complications of bland aerosol therapy include all of the following EXCEPT:
    A. Increased humidity deficit
    B. Aerosol-induced bronchospasm
    C. Fluid overload in an infant
    D. Possible patient contamination if the reservoir water is infected

14. Your patient's air-entrainment nebulizer is not putting out as much aerosol as it was a short time ago. To correct the problem, you would check which of the following?
    I. Make sure that the water level is correct.
    II. Make sure that the one-way valve is patent.
    III. Make sure that the jet is patent.
    IV. Make sure that the $O_2$ can flow down the capillary tube.
    V. Make sure that the water can flow up the capillary tube.
    A. I and II
    B. I, III, and IV
    C. II and IV
    D. I, III, and V

15. Your patient has pneumonia and needs an inhaled antibiotic. What size particle generator would you recommend to treat the problem?
    A. 20 to 50 μm
    B. 10 to 20 μm
    C. 2 to 5 μm
    D. 1 to 3 μm

16. Your ultrasonic nebulizer has a flashing couplant indicator light. You notice that the output has decreased from what it was earlier. The most likely problem is
    A. Too much water in the solution cup
    B. Too much water in the couplant chamber
    C. Not enough water in the couplant chamber
    D. A loose electrical cable

17. You notice that water has collected at the low point of the large-bore tubing of your patient's heated aerosol system. The aerosol is "puffing" out of the end of the tubing. Your reaction should be to
    A. Add water to the reservoir jar
    B. Empty water from the reservoir jar
    C. Empty the water from the large-bore tubing into a wastewater jar
    D. Empty the water from the large-bore tubing into the reservoir jar so that it is not wasted

18. The physician wants a patient with a tracheostomy to inhale room air that is fully saturated at body temperature. The device that you select must be able to meet the following criteria:
    I. Deliver 40% relative humidity
    II. Deliver 100% relative humidity
    III. Provide 47 mm Hg vapor pressure
    IV. Provide 44 mm Hg vapor pressure
    V. Deliver 44 mg/L absolute humidity
    A. II and IV
    B. I, III, and V
    C. I and IV
    D. II, III, and V

19. It is best to coach your patient to breathe in the following pattern for particle deposition in smaller airways and alveoli:
    I. Inhale a $V_T$.
    II. Inhale rapidly.
    III. Inhale an IC.
    IV. Hold the breath for up to 10 sec before exhaling.
    V. Inhale at a slow speed.
    A. I and II
    B. III, IV, and V
    C. I and V
    D. I, II, and IV

## ANSWER KEY AND RATIONALE

1. **B.** A heated aerosol mask is the only option that provides aerosol that has been heated to reduce the humidity deficit. Mist tents are not used with adults. The other two masks are used with a bubble humidifier at room temperature.

2. **A.** Adding 100 mL of aerosol tubing as a reservoir will help to maintain the patient's inspired $O_2$ percentage. No clear reason exists for changing the patient's $O_2$ percentage by protocol, and no physician order exists to do so. Changing the flow will probably not stabilize the patient's $O_2$ percentage without the added reservoir tubing. A comatose patient will not follow instructions to "not breathe so deeply."

3. **D.** An MDI with holding chamber is the only practical way, from among those presented, to deliver this type of medication to a small child. A DPI necessitates an inspiratory flow that is too high for a small child. Holding chambers are not used with a DPI.

4. **D.** Upper (larger) airway deposition occurs with particles that are 10 µm or larger. Review Table 8-2.

5. **B.** Upper (larger) airway deposition is enhanced by $V_T$ breathing at a normal speed and in a normal pattern. A slow IC would increase the change of deposition in smaller airways.

6. **C.** An ultrasonic nebulizer generates the greatest quantity of aerosol particles from among the listed choices. An aerosol mask is appropriate for an adult. A handheld nebulizer used every 4 hr does not deliver enough aerosol fast enough to help the patient as the ultrasonic nebulizer would. A mist tent is not appropriate for an adult. A cascade-type humidifier does not deliver an aerosol that meets the patient's needs.

7. **D.** The cascade-type humidifier that is heated to near body temperature will provide almost 100% of the patient's body humidity needs. The other devices are all much cooler than body temperature and provide a lower humidity level.

8. **C.** The small, uniform droplet size produced by the ultrasonic unit is a reason for its use. It should not be used to nebulize a medication because vibrations of the ultrasonic unit may break down the drug.

9. **C.** An unheated bubble-type humidifier delivers humidity at room temperature or cooler. All of the other units deliver humidity or aerosol at a warmer temperature.

10. **D.** The absolute humidity of 44 mg/L is found in the airways of a person at normal body temperature. Review Table 8-1.

11. **A.** Condensation will occur because the saturated air is heated to above room temperature and will cool down as it goes through the tubing. The air will stay saturated with water vapor despite the cooling.

12. **C.** Backpressure on the humidifier will make the pop-off valve whistle. Pinched tubing could cause this. The delivered $O_2$ percentage does not affect the pop-off valve. If a leak occurs between the reservoir jar and the top of the humidifier, the gas will not leak out of the pop-off valve.

13. **A.** Humidity deficit will be decreased by aerosol therapy. Some patients will have bronchospasm after inhaling a bland aerosol. Infants can easily become fluid overloaded. Aerosol droplets are large enough to carry bacteria.

14. **D.** A nebulizer will fail because of too little water in the reservoir, a clogged jet, or a clogged capillary line to the reservoir. Air-entrainment nebulizers do not have any one-way valves. $O_2$ flows down a capillary tube in a bubble-type humidifier.

15. **D.** Particles in the 1- to 3-µm range will penetrate to the alveoli. All other sizes will impact on the airways. Review Table 8-2.

16. **C.** Low water level in the couplant chamber will cause the light to flash. No other indicators help with troubleshooting.

17. **C.** Wastewater should be emptied out of the tubing to prevent contamination. The water level in the reservoir jar has nothing to do with water in the tubing.

18. **D.** The three listed criteria all indicate that the patient's inhaled air is completely saturated with water vapor at body temperature. Review Table 8-1.

19. **B.** The best way for the patient to deposit an aerosol in small airways and alveoli is to slowly inhale an IC with a breath-hold when the lungs are full. A rapidly inhaled $V_T$ tends to deposit aerosol in the larger airways.

# 9 Pharmacology

A review of the most recent Entry Level Examinations has shown an average of 11 questions (8% of the exam) that cover pharmacology.

## MODULE A
### Recommend or administer medications

### 1. Bronchodilators
Bronchodilators are medications that are designed to relax the bronchial smooth muscles so that the airways dilate, airway resistance is reduced, and breathing is easier. The first two classes of medications in this group are widely given by respiratory therapists.

#### a. Inhaled adrenergic (sympathomimetic) agents
1. **Recommend their use** (NBRC code: IIIG4a) [Difficulty: R, Ap]
2. **Administer the prescribed medication** (NBRC code: IIIC3, IIID4a) [Difficulty: R, Ap]

This group of medications is often called *catecholamines, sympathomimetic amines, sympathomimetic bronchodilators,* or *beta-adrenergic bronchodilators.* They have the effect of stimulating the body's sympathetic nerves, which results in bronchodilation and other effects. Patients with asthma are most effectively treated with drugs from this group.

A brief review of the autonomic nervous system helps one to understand how these medications (and the following group of medications) work and which adverse effects may occur. The autonomic nervous system is not under voluntary control. It is an automatic system that is designed to regulate metabolism and the vital signs. This system is made up of two branches: the sympathetic nervous system and the parasympathetic nervous system. The lungs, heart, and most other organs are innervated by both branches. The blood vessels in the mucous membranes are innervated only by the sympathetic branch. The parasympathetic nervous system is usually dominant and keeps the body functioning normally. The sympathetic nervous system is an "emergency" system that is dominant during great stress (sometimes called the "fight or flight" system). Adrenaline (or epinephrine) is released by the adrenal glands in these emergencies. Adrenaline causes a number of effects, including one that many respiratory patients need: bronchodilation. The sympathetic nervous system has the following three types of receptors, which are located in different organs and are affected by adrenaline and related medications:

a. Alpha-1 receptors are located in the blood vessels of the mucous membranes (other tissues are not included in this discussion). Vasoconstriction results when alpha-1 receptors are stimulated.
b. Beta-1 receptors are located in the heart. Tachycardia, increased stroke volume, and possible arrhythmia result when beta-1 receptors are stimulated.
c. Beta-2 receptors are located in the airways. Bronchodilation results when beta-2 receptors are stimulated.

Aerosolized sympathomimetic bronchodilators are usually recommended under one of the three following situations:

***Acute bronchospasm with severe shortness of breath.*** This patient needs rapid relief. Recommend a fast-acting medication such as albuterol. Current asthma management guidelines list albuterol and similar medications as "rescue" agents. When the patient has recovered, a medication listed as a "controller" agent should be prescribed. Table 9-1 lists peak onset times and duration for various medications. Avoid drugs with unnecessary alpha-1 and beta-1 effects or long onset and peak times.

***Chronic but stable bronchospasm with moderate shortness of breath.*** These patients need a dependable medication of longer duration such as salmeterol or formoterol. These are considered to be "controller" agents with a long onset time and a duration of up to 12 hours. It is very important that the patient also have a prescription for a fast-acting drug in case of sudden bronchospasm. Several newer medications are available in both oral and aerosol preparations. When medications are taken in the evening, oral forms are especially helpful to help the patient get a good night's sleep. Table 9-1 lists information on administration methods, strengths, and dosages.

***Laryngeal edema or bleeding from a bronchoscopy biopsy site.*** The laryngeal edema problem requires the administration of a medication that reduces swelling of the mucous membrane of the larynx and epiglottis. If bleeding results from a biopsy performed during a bronchoscopy, the cut blood vessels must be made to constrict and clot. In both cases, racemic epinephrine (Micro-Nefrin, AsthmaNefrin) is the medication of choice

| TABLE 9-1 | Inhaled Adrenergic Bronchodilator Agents Currently Available in the United States | | | |
|---|---|---|---|---|
| **Drug** | **Brand Name** | **Receptor Preference** | **Adult Dosage** | **Time Course (Onset, Peak, Duration)** |
| Epinephrine | Adrenalin Cl | α, β | SVN: 1% solution (1:100), 0.25-0.5 ml (2.5-5.0 mg) qid<br>MDI: 0.2 mg/puff, puffs as ordered or needed | Onset: 3-5 min<br>Peak: 5-20 min<br>Duration: 1-3 hr |
| Racemic epinephrine | MicroNefrin, AsthmaNefrin, various | α, β | SVN: 2.25% solution, 0.25-0.5 ml (5.63-11.25 mg) qid | Onset: 3-5 min<br>Peak: 5-20 min<br>Duration: 0.5-2 hr |
| Isoproterenol | Isuprel, Isuprel Mistometer | β | SVN: 0.5% solution (1:200), 0.25-0.5 ml (1.25-2.5 mg) qid<br>MDI: 103 µg/puff, 2 puffs qid | Onset: 2-5 min<br>Peak: 5-30 min<br>Duration: 0.5-2 hr |
| Isoetharine | Isoetharine HCl | $\beta_2$ | SVN: 1% solution, 0.25-0.5 ml (2.5-5.0 mg) qid | Onset: 1-6 min<br>Peak: 15-60 min<br>Duration: 1-3 hr |
| Terbutaline | Brethaire | $\beta_2$ | MDI: 200 µg/puff, 2 puffs q4-6h<br><br>Tab: 2.5 or 5 mg, 5 mg q6h<br>Inj: 1 mg/ml, 0.25 mg SC | Onset: 5-30 min<br>Peak: 30-60 min<br>Duration: 3-6 hr |
| Metaproterenol | Alupent | $\beta_2$ | SVN: 5% solution, 0.3 ml (15 mg) tid, qid<br>MDI: 650 µg/puff, 2-3 puffs tid, qid<br>Tab: 10 or 20 mg, 20 mg tid, qid<br>Syrup: 10 mg/5 ml, 2 tsp tid, qid | Onset: 1-5 min<br>Peak: 60 min<br>Duration: 2-6 hr |
| Albuterol | Proventil, Proventil HFA, Ventolin | $\beta_2$ | SVN: 0.5% solution, 0.5 ml (2.5 mg) tid, qid<br>MDI: 90 µg/puff, 2 puffs tid, qid<br>DPI: 200 µg capsule, 1 capsule q4-6h<br>Tab: 2 mg, 4 mg tid, qid<br>Syrup: 2 mg/5 ml, 1-2 tsp tid, qid | Onset: 15 min<br>Peak: 30-60 min<br>Duration: 5-8 hr |
| Bitolterol | Tornalate | $\beta_2$ | SVN: 0.2% solution, 1.25 ml (2.5 mg) bid-qid<br>MDI: 370 µg/puff, 2 puffs q8h | Onset: 3-4 min<br>Peak: 30-60 min<br>Duration: 5-8 hr |
| Pirbuterol | Maxair | $\beta_2$ | MDI: 200 µg/puff, 2 puffs q4-6h | Onset: 5 min<br>Peak: 30 min<br>Duration: 5 hr |
| Lev albuterol | Xopenex | $\beta_2$ | SVN: 0.31 mg/3 ml tid; 0.63 mg/3 ml tid; or 1.25 mg/3 ml tid | Onset: 15 min<br>Peak: 30-60 min<br>Duration: 5-8 hr |
| | Xopenex HFA | | MDI: 45 µg/puff, 2 puffs q4-6h, ≥4 yr old | |
| Salmeterol | Serevent | $\beta_2$ | MDI: 25 µg/puff, 2 puffs bid<br><br>DPI: 50 µg/blister bid | Onset: 20 min<br>Peak: 3-5 hr<br>Duration: 12 hr |
| Formoterol | Foradil | $\beta_2$ | DPI: 12 µg/inhalation bid | Onset: 15 min<br>Peak: 30-60 min<br>Duration: 12 hr |

Modified from Rau JL Jr: Respiratory care pharmacology, ed 6, St. Louis, 2002, Mosby.
*DPI*, Dry powder inhaler; *MDI*, metered dose inhaler; *SVN*, small volume nebulizer.

because it stimulates alpha-1 receptors. This results in vasoconstriction of the mucosal and deeper blood vessels. Therefore, the laryngeal edema swelling is reduced and bleeding caused by the biopsy stops.

Most medications listed in this section are chemically derived from adrenaline. They are somewhat different in their structures so that the desired effects and adverse (unwanted) effects vary. Box 9-1 lists the adverse effects of the sympathomimetic bronchodilators. Clinically, the most dangerous of these adverse effects include palpitations, tachycardia, and hypertension.

---

**Exam Hint**

**R**ecommend a fast-onset medication (albuterol, Proventil or Ventolin) to treat a patient with acute bronchospasm. Recommend a long-duration medication (salmeterol, Serevent or formoterol, Foradil) to treat a patient with chronic bronchospasm. Recommend a vasoconstricting medication (racemic epinephrine, MicroNefrin or Asthma Nefrin) to treat airway edema or bleeding.

---

**BOX 9-1    Clinically Observed Adverse Effects of Sympathomimetic Aerosolized Bronchodilators From the Most Commonly Seen to the Least Commonly Seen**

- Tremor: gentle, uncontrollable, involuntary muscle shaking
- Palpitations and tachycardia: irregular heartbeats and fast heart rate
- Headache
- Increased blood pressure: possibly from both the alpha-1 effect on blood vessels and tachycardia
- Nervousness and irritability
- Dizziness
- Nausea
- Decreased $PaO_2$ level from a worsening of the ventilation/perfusion ratio

$PaO_2$, partial pressure of $O_2$ in arterial blood.

**b. Inhaled anticholinergic (parasympatholytic) agents**
   **1. Recommend their use** (NBRC code: IIIG4a) [Difficulty: R, Ap]
   **2. Administer the prescribed medication** (NBRC code: IIID4a, IIIC3) [Difficulty: R, Ap]

This group of medications works to promote bronchodilation by suppressing the action of the parasympathetic nervous system. This results in dominance of the sympathetic nervous system, which causes bronchial smooth muscle relaxation. The parasympatholytic (anticholinergic) group has been found to be more effective in helping patients with chronic obstructive pulmonary disease (COPD) (e.g., emphysema, chronic bronchitis) than in patients with asthma. However, it is often best to treat COPD and asthma patients with medications from both the sympathomimetic and parasympatholytic groups. Combivent combines a sympathomimetic and a parasympatholytic medication. See Table 9-2 for information on the parasympatholytic medications.

**c. Recommend a theophylline agent (NBRC code: IIIG4a) [Difficulty: R, Ap]**

The family of drugs called *xanthines* includes theophylline and caffeine. They have been used in a variety of situations. A theophylline agent (e.g., Aminophylline, Elixophyllin, or Theo-Dur) is sometimes taken to aid the breathing of a patient with status asthmaticus or moderate to severe COPD. Current guidelines indicate that theophylline agents should be given to these patients only if

---

**TABLE 9-2    Inhaled Anticholinergic Bronchodilator Agents**

| Drug | Brand Name | Adult Dosage | Time Course (Onset, Peak, Duration) |
|---|---|---|---|
| Ipratropium bromide | Atrovent | MDI: 18 μg/puff, 2 puffs qid<br>SVN: 0.02% solution (0.2 mg/ml), 500 μg tid, qid<br>Nasal spray: 0.03%, 0.06%; 2 sprays per nostril 2 to 4 times daily (dosage varies) | *Onset:* 15 min<br>*Peak:* 1–2 hr<br>*Duration:* 4–6 hr |
| Ipratropium bromide and albuterol | Combivent | MDI: ipratropium 18 μg/puff and albuterol 90 μg/puff, 2 puffs qid | *Onset:* 15 min<br>*Peak:* 1–2 hr<br>*Duration:* 4–6 hr |
| | DuoNeb | SVN: ipratropium 0.5 mg and albuterol 3.0 mg (equal to 2.5 mg albuterol base) | |
| Tiotropium bromide | Spiriva | DPI: 18 μg/inhalation, 1 inhalation daily | *Onset:* 30 min<br>*Peak:* 3 hr<br>*Duration:* 24 hr |

Modified from Rau JL Jr: Respiratory care pharmacology, ed 6, St. Louis, 2002, Mosby.
*DPI*, Dry powder inhaler; *MDI*, metered dose inhaler; *SVN*, small volume nebulizer.
A holding chamber is recommended with MDI administration to prevent accidental eye exposure.

optimal doses of inhaled bronchodilators and corticosteroid drugs have not managed the patient's problem. Then, intravenous theophylline ethylenediamine (Aminophylline) can be given. However, it should be used with caution. It is very difficult to regulate the proper serum level, and serious adverse effects have been noted.

Caffeine citrate (Cafcit) has been approved for oral or intravenous administration to a neonate with apnea of prematurity. It has been shown to stimulate the breathing of these neonates.

## 2. Antiinflammatory agents

### a. Recommend use of nonsteroidal antiinflammatory drugs (NBRC code: IIIG4b) [Difficulty: R, Ap]

Nonsteroidal antiinflammatory drugs (NSAIDs) comprise several different types of over-the-counter medications. None of these is as powerful an antiinflammatory as the corticosteroid drugs, but some offer other clinical benefits.

1. Acetylsalicylic acid (aspirin): antiinflammatory, mild analgesia, antipyretic, blocks platelet formation
2. Ibuprofen (Advil, Motrin): antiinflammatory, mild analgesia, antipyretic
3. Antihistamine (Claritin): antiinflammatory

### b. Inhaled corticosteroids

1. **Recommend use of corticosteroids (NBRC code: IIIG4b) [Difficulty: R, Ap]**
2. **Administer the prescribed medication (NBRC code: IIIC3, IIID4a) [Difficulty: R, Ap]**

Corticosteroids affect the respiratory system in two ways: they potentiate the effects of the sympathomimetic agents, and they stop the inflammatory response that occurs in the airways of asthmatic patients after exposure to an allergen. This prevents the development of mucosal edema. The patient with chronic airflow obstruction, such as mild asthma or asthmatic bronchitis, should be given inhaled corticosteroids. When these are used as directed, little systemic (bodily) absorption occurs. Table 9-3 shows specific strength and dosage information for the inhaled corticosteroids. The patient who is using any of these medications must gargle and rinse out his or her mouth after each use. If not, the patient runs the risk of developing a fungal infection of the mouth and throat.

The patient who is diagnosed with status asthmaticus should have systemic corticosteroids promptly given by the intravenous route. Examples of commonly used systemic corticosteroids include methylprednisolone (Medrol and Solu-Medrol), prednisone (Deltasone), prednisolone (Meticortelone and Delta-Cortef), cortisone (Cortone), and hydrocortisone (Cortef and Solu-Cortef). These drugs can be lifesavers if used properly. However, long-term use of large oral or IV doses can lead to serious systemic complications such as immunosuppression and adrenal gland insufficiency. If a patient has been taking systemic corticosteroids for an extended time, he or she should be gradually weaned off of them after an inhaled corticosteroid has been started. It is dangerous to suddenly stop an oral or intravenous corticosteroid that has been used for a prolonged time.

## 3. Nonsteroidal antiasthma agents

### a. Recommend the use of cromolyn sodium (NBRC code: IIIG4b) [Difficulty: R, Ap]

Cromolyn sodium (Intal) is indicated to prevent an asthma attack. It does this by coating the mast cells found in the airways, which protects them from rupture. Without cromolyn sodium, the mast cells of asthmatic patients would rupture when they are exposed to immunoglobin E (IgE) from allergen(s). This mast cell rupture would result in the spilling of leukotriene agents, histamine, and other chemical mediators that cause the bronchospasm, airway edema, and increased airway secretions of an asthma attack.

When cromolyn sodium, or nedrocromil sodium, is inhaled at least a week before exposure to the allergen, the asthmatic reaction is prevented or reduced. Cromolyn was first made available through a dry powder inhaler and is now available by metered dose inhaler or small-volume inhaler. Nedrocromil sodium (Tilade) is similar to cromolyn in its use and effects. It is available as a metered dose inhaler. See Table 9-4 for detailed information on both medications.

It is very important for the clinician to understand that both drugs are taken for prophylactic purposes to prevent an asthma attack. They are contraindicated *during* an asthma attack. A patient who is experiencing acute bronchospasm should be treated with a fast sympathomimetic bronchodilator, as was previously discussed.

### b. Recommend the use of leukotriene modifiers (NBRC code: IIIG4b [Difficulty: R, Ap]

Leukotrienes are chemicals found in mast cells that are released during an asthma attack. These released leukotriene chemicals stimulate bronchospasm, airway edema, and increased airway secretions. The leukotriene modifier medications work either to reduce the number of leukotriene chemicals that are released or to block the effects of leukotrienes on the airways. By doing this, the patient's asthma symptoms are reduced or eliminated. See Table 9-4 for detailed information on all four medications in this group.

As with cromolyn sodium, it is very important that the clinician understand that all of these drugs are taken for prophylactic purposes to prevent an asthma attack. They are contraindicated *during* an asthma attack. A patient who is experiencing acute bronchospasm should be

| TABLE 9-3 | Corticosteroids Available by Aerosol for Oral Inhalation* | |
|---|---|---|
| **Drug** | **Brand Name** | **Formulation and Dosage** |
| Beclomethasone dipropionate | Beclovent, Vanceril | MDI: 42 μg/puff<br>Adults: 2 puffs tid or qid<br>Children: 1–2 puffs tid or qid |
| | Vanceril 84 μg<br>Double Strength | MDI: 84 μg/puff<br>Adults and children ≥6 yr: 2 inhalations bid |
| Beclomethasone dipropionate HFA | QVAR | MDI: 40 μg/puff and 80 μg/puff<br>Adults ≥12 yr: 40 to 80 μg twice daily,† or 40 to 160 μg twice daily‡ |
| Triamcinolone acetonide | Azmacort | MDI: 100 μg/puff<br>Adults: 2 puffs tid or qid<br>Children: 1–2 puffs tid or qid |
| Flunisolide | AeroBid, AeroBid-M | MDI: 250 μg/puff<br>Adults: 2 puffs bid<br>Children: 2 puffs bid |
| Fluticasone propionate | Flovent | MDI: 44 μg/puff, 110 μg/puff, 220 μg/puff<br>Adults ≥12 yr: 88 μg bid,† 88–220 μg bid,‡ or 880 μg bid¶ |
| | Flovent Rotadisk | DPI: 50 μg, 100 μg, 250 μg<br>Adults: 100 μg bid,† 100–250 μg bid,‡ 1000 μg bid¶<br>Children 4–11 yr: 50 μg twice daily |
| Budesonide | Pulmicort Turbuhaler | DPI: 200 μg/actuation<br>Adults: 200–400 μg bid,† 200–400 μg bid,‡ 400–800 μg bid¶<br>Children ≥6 yr: 200 μg bid |
| | Pulmicort Respules | SVN: 0.25 mg/2 ml, 0.5 mg/2 ml<br>Children 1 to 8 yr: 0.5 mg total dose given once daily, or twice daily in divided doses†,‡; 1 mg given as 0.5 mg bid or once daily¶ |
| Fluticasone propionate/salmeterol | Advair Diskus | DPI: 100 μg fluticasone/50 μg salmeterol, 250 μg fluticasone/50 μg salmeterol, or 500 μg fluticasone/50 μg salmeterol<br>Adults and children ≥12 yr: 100 μg fluticasone/50 μg salmeterol, 1 inhalation twice daily, about 12 hours apart (starting dose if not currently on inhaled corticosteroids)<br>Maximum recommended dose is 500 μg fluticasone/50 μg salmeterol twice daily |

Modified from Rau JL Jr: Respiratory care pharmacology, ed 6, St. Louis, 2002, Mosby.
*Individual agents are discussed subsequently in a separate section. Detailed information on each agent should be obtained from manufacturers' drug insert.
†Recommended starting dose if on bronchodilators alone.
‡Recommended starting dose if on inhaled corticosteroids previously.
¶Recommended starting dose if on oral corticosteroids previously.

treated with a fast sympathomimetic bronchodilator, as has been discussed.

### 4. Mucolytics or proteolytic agents

**a. Recommend the use of mucolytics or proteolytic agents (NBRC code: IIIC3, IIIG4c) [Difficulty: R, Ap, An]**

**b. Administer the prescribed medication (NBRC code: IIIG4a) [Difficulty: R, Ap]**

Acetylcysteine (Mucomyst) is a mucolytic drug that has been widely used with patients who have thick (viscous) mucus or mucus plugs. Its bad odor (rotten eggs) may lead to nausea and vomiting in some patients. Of great

concern is the stimulation of bronchospasm in some asthmatic patients. Therefore, it is wise either to pretreat the patient with an aerosolized sympathomimetic bronchodilator or to mix one with the acetylcysteine before it is nebulized for the patient. Any fast-onset bronchodilator can be used in the usual dose. Mucomyst is usually administered by handheld nebulizer or intermittent positive-pressure breathing (IPPB). Most adult patients are given 3 to 5 mL of the 20% solution or 6 to 10 mL of the 10% solution. The 20% solution is often diluted with an equal volume of normal saline solution. Direct instillation of 1 to 2 mL of the drug into the trachea also helps to liquefy secretions. The manufacturer recommends that all

| TABLE 9-4 | Nonsteroidal Antiasthma Medications, with Brand and Generic Names, Formulations, and Usual Recommended Dosages* | |
| --- | --- | --- |
| **Drug** | **Brand Name** | **Formulation and Dosage** |
| **CROMOLYN-LIKE (MAST CELL STABILIZERS)** | | |
| Cromolyn sodium† | Intal | MDI: 800 µg/actuation |
| | | Adults and children ≥5 yr: 2 inhalations 4 times daily |
| | | SVN: 20 mg/amp or 20 mg/vial |
| | | Adults and children ≥2 yr: 20 mg inhaled 4 times daily |
| | Nasalcrom | Spray: 40 mg/ml (4%) |
| | | Adults and children ≥6 yr: 1 spray each nostril, 3-6 times daily every 4-6 hr |
| Nedocromil sodium | Tilade | MDI: 1.75 mg/actuation |
| | | Adults and children ≥12 yr: 2 inhalations 4 times daily |
| **ANTI-LEUKOTRIENES** | | |
| Zafirlukast | Accolate | Tablets: 20 mg |
| | | Adults and children ≥12 yr: 20 mg (1 tab) twice daily, without food |
| Montelukast | Singulair | Tablets: 10 mg, 4 mg, and 5 mg cherry-flavored chewable |
| | | Adults and children ≥15 yr: one 10 mg tab each evening |
| | | Children 6-14 yr: one 5 mg chewable tablet each evening |
| | | Children 2-5 years: one 4 mg chewable tablet each evening |
| Zileuton | Zyflo | Tablets: 600 mg |
| | | Adults and children ≥12 yr: one 600 mg tablet 4 times a day |
| Omalizumab | Xolair | Adults and children ≥12 years: subcutaneous injection every 4 weeks at 150 to 300 mg per dose; or subcutaneous injection every 2 weeks at 225, 300, or 375 mg per dose. Doses of more than 150 mg should be divided among more than one injection site. |

Modified from Rau JL Jr: Respiratory care pharmacology, ed 6, St. Louis, 2002, Mosby.
*Detailed prescribing information should be obtained from the manufacturer's package insert.
†Note: Cromolyn sodium is also available in an oral concentrate giving 100 mg in 5 ml (Gastrocrom), for treatment of systemic mastocytosis, and as an ophthalmic 4% solution (Opticrom, 40 mg/ml) for treatment of vernal keratoconjunctivitis.

| TABLE 9-5 | Mucoactive Agents Available for Aerosol Administration | | |
| --- | --- | --- | --- |
| **Drug** | **Brand Name** | **Adult Dosage** | **Use** |
| Acetylcysteine 10% | Mucomyst | SVN: 3-5 ml | Bronchitis; efficacy not proven |
| Acetylcysteine 20% | Mucosil-10 | | |
| Mucosil-20 | Mucomyst | | |
| Dornase alfa | Pulmozyme | SVN: 2.5 mg/ampule one ampule daily* | Cystic fibrosis |
| Aqueous aerosols: water, saline (0.45%, 0.9%, 5%-10%) | N/A | SVN: 3-5 ml | |
| | | SVN: 3-5 ml, as ordered | Sputum induction, secretion mobilization |
| | | USN: 3-5 ml, as ordered | |

From Rau JL Jr: Respiratory care pharmacology, ed 6, St. Louis, 2002, Mosby.
*Use recommended nebulizer system (see package insert).
*N/A*, Not applicable; *SVN*, small volume nebulizer; *USN*, ultrasonic nebulizer.

medication in a vial be used within 96 hr or discarded. It should be stored in the refrigerator. A slightly purple color is commonly seen after the vial has been opened, but the drug can still be used safely.

Dornase alpha (Pulmozyme; The NBRC refers to this drug as recombinant human deoxyribonuclease [RhDNAse].) is a proteolytic drug that has been approved for use in the treatment of patients with cystic fibrosis. It works by breaking up strands of DNA found in the secretions of patients with a pulmonary infection. Usually, a single daily dose of 2.5 mL of solution (containing 2.5 mg of dornase alpha) is inhaled by small-volume nebulizer (SVN). Store the drug in a refrigerator and protect it from strong light. It has no serious adverse effects. See Table 9-5 for detailed information on Mucomyst, Pulmozyme, and the saline solutions (discussed later).

## 5. Saline solutions

### a. Recommend the use of saline solutions (NBRC code: IIIG4c) [Difficulty: R, Ap]

### b. Administer the prescribed medication (NBRC code: IIIC3, IIIG4a) [Difficulty: R, Ap]

Various saline solutions (and sterile water) are known collectively as "bland" aerosols because they have no direct pharmacologic effect on the lungs and airways. When they are inhaled as an aerosol, however, a vagal nerve–mediated reflex causes the bronchial/submucosal glands to release additional watery secretions. Therefore, a saline aerosol is commonly used to help liquefy secretions and induce a patient to cough out sputum. See Table 9-5 and Box 9-2 for information on the various saline solutions.

---

### BOX 9-2    Saline Solutions Used as Mucolytics

**NORMAL SALINE SOLUTION, 0.9% SALINE**

- Direct instillation into the airway:
  Infants may be given about 1 mL several times before suctioning
  Adults may be given about 3-5 mL several times daily before suctioning
- Aerosol: most medication nebulizers hold 3-5 mL that is nebulized several times daily
- Miscellaneous:
  Usually is well tolerated because it is isotonic to the body
  Particle size is fairly stable as nebulized

**HYPOTONIC SALINE SOLUTION, 0.45% SALINE**

- Direct instillation into the airway: same as with normal saline solution
- Aerosol: same as with normal saline solution; many practitioners use this concentration in ultrasonic nebulizers
- Miscellaneous: particles tend to shrink because of evaporation, which results in smaller particles than those nebulized that are close to isotonic; effect is more likely to be noted in the smaller airways

**HYPERTONIC SALINE SOLUTION, 1.8%–20% SALINE**

- Aerosol: some practitioners use a large-reservoir nebulizer with a heater to generate the aerosol
  Hypertonic saline solution is most commonly used to induce a cough and sputum sample for cytology (lung cancer) or fungal or mycobacterial (tuberculosis) culture; it should not be used for a general bacterial culture because the high salt concentration inhibits the growth of most bacteria
- Miscellaneous:
  Particles tend to enlarge because of the absorption of water vapor, which results in larger particles than those nebulized that are close to isotonic; effect is more likely to be noted in the upper airway
  This concentration is the most likely to cause bronchospasm in asthmatic patients because it is the farthest from isotonic and, therefore, is the most irritating

---

## 6. Recommend the use of diuretic agents (NBRC code: IIIG4e) [Difficulty: R, Ap]

Diuretics are most commonly indicated in patients with edema or hypertension. Edema is usually a result of heart failure or fluid overload. Examples of diuretics used to treat these problems follow:

a. Furosemide (Lasix)
b. Ethacrynic acid (Edecrin)
c. Chlorothiazide (Diuril)

These are some of the most powerful diuretics in use. They produce a rapid increase in urine output and basically prevent the kidneys from retaining sodium so that water is excreted. An adverse effect of their use is a loss of potassium through the kidneys.

Another category of diuretic is used in patients who have increased intracranial pressure (ICP). Increased ICP is usually due to cerebral edema caused by a head injury. Examples of medications used to treat an increased ICP include the following:

a. Mannitol (Osmitrol)
b. Sterile urea (Ureaphil, Urevert)

These medications have a large molecular weight and, through osmosis, they "pull" fluid from the brain into the bloodstream. Therefore, they are sometimes called *osmotic diuretics*. The medication, after crossing into the kidney, prevents the reabsorption of water and increases urine output.

---

### Exam Hint

**A** patient who is receiving a drug such as Lasix must be given replacement potassium to avoid dangerous hypokalemia. Remember that the normal potassium level is 3.5 to 5.5 mEq/L.

---

## 7. Recommend the use of sedative agents (NBRC code: IIIG1b, IIIG4d) [Difficulty: R, Ap]

Sedatives are medications that affect the brain to induce calming in a patient who can be either simply anxious or very agitated and uncooperative. A patient would be given a sedative in the following situations: (1) When he or she is struggling against a necessary intubation or the mechanical ventilator, thus worsening his or her condition, (2) when he or she is displaying self-destructive behavior because of a drug reaction, and (3) before a medical procedure for so-called conscious sedation. Effects on the patient are dose related. Low to moderate doses calm the patient, and higher doses induce sleep. Three different groupings of these types of medications exist. The most widely used are the benzodiazepines because they have fewer adverse effects and fewer drug interactions and are less likely to cause addiction compared with the barbiturate drugs. Also, benzodiazepine agents can be pharmacologically reversed. Barbiturates are widely used during general anesthesia to rapidly induce sleep. Commonly used examples of the sedative agents include the following:

a. Benzodiazepine minor tranquilizers: midazolam (Versed), diazepam (Valium), chlordiazepoxide (Librium), alprazolam (Xanax), triazolam (Halcion), flurazepam (Dalmane)

b. Nonbarbiturate sedative-hypnotics: ethchlorvynol (Placidyl), meprobamate (Miltown), glutethimide (Doriden), chloral hydrate (Noctec)

c. Barbiturate sedative-hypnotics: pentobarbital sodium (Nembutal), secobarbital sodium (Seconal), phenobarbital (Luminol), thiopental sodium (Pentothal)

The benzodiazepine antagonist drug flumazenil (Romazicon) is indicated in the reversal of benzodiazepine agents such as Valium and Librium. Unconscious patients usually awaken quickly once the proper dose of Romazicon is given. Watch the patient for signs of seizure activity related to rapid reversal of the benzodiazepine medication. The patient should be observed for 2 hr in case resedation occurs. If so, Romazicon can be given again.

Analgesics are medications that control or block pain after injury or a surgical procedure. Morphine is indicated to control the pain of a myocardial infarction and to vasodilate the patient with pulmonary edema. Also, pain-relieving agents, when given in large enough doses, will sedate or induce sleep. The patient who is both in pain and agitated may be treated with a combination of an analgesic and a sedative (e.g., moderate doses of morphine and Valium). The two drugs potentiate each other. The physician may instead decide to give the patient only morphine at a larger dose. Examples of commonly used analgesics include the following:

a. Morphine sulfate (Duramorph), injection; (Oramorph SR), tablets

b. Codeine phosphate (methylmorphine)

c. Hydromorphone (Dilaudid)

d. Meperidine (Demerol)

e. Propoxyphene (Darvon)

Patients who are receiving sedatives or analgesics must be closely monitored. Each can cause respiratory center depression if given in great enough doses. The patient may hypoventilate and even experience apnea and death. Also, these agents (e.g., morphine) and other medications can become habit forming or addictive if they are used for a prolonged time.

The narcotic antagonist drug naloxone (Narcan) counteracts the effects of narcotic agents, such as morphine, heroin, and codeine. Narcan does *not* reverse benzodiazepine or barbiturate drugs. Remember that the patient who was given an accidental overdose of morphine to control pain will feel pain again when Narcan is given to reverse it.

## 8. Recommend the use of neuromuscular blocking agents (NBRC code: IIIG4b) [Difficulty: R, Ap]

Neuromuscular blocking agents are used to cause a pharmacologic paralysis. These medications block nerve transmission from reaching skeletal (voluntary) muscles; complete paralysis follows. They are most commonly used as part of balanced anesthesia before major thoracic or abdominal surgery. These drugs are also used in the intensive care unit to stop a patient from fighting against an intubation or to prevent the patient from struggling against the mechanical ventilator. All are given intravenously and act rapidly. Obviously, in all these cases, the patient stops breathing and must receive mechanical ventilation. Examples of commonly used neuromuscular blocking agents include the following:

a. Depolarizing blocker: succinylcholine chloride (Anectine, Quelicin)

b. Nondepolarizing blockers: pancuronium bromide (Pavulon) (preferred), vecuronium bromide (Norcuron), gallamine triethiodide (Flaxedil), atracurium besylate (Tracrium)

Nondepolarizing blockers (e.g., Pavulon) are preferred for their longer duration of action. Although all these agents induce complete paralysis of all voluntary muscles, they have little or no effect on the involuntary muscles or autonomic nervous system. Some patients may have a minor, passing change in heart rate and blood pressure. Remember that they are able to hear and feel pain, and are completely awake and alert to their surroundings. Care must be taken to sedate the patient for anxiety and give analgesics for pain. Talk to the patient normally and move the patient periodically to prevent pressure sores.

Nondepolarizing neuromuscular blocking agents can be reversed so that the patient can breathe and move again. These intravenous medications include neostigmine bromide (Prostigmin) (preferred) and edrophonium (Tensilon). It should be noted that these reversing agents cause an outpouring of oral and bronchial secretions. Atropine is given to prevent this. Reversing agents have no effect on the depolarizing neuromuscular blocker succinylcholine chloride. Patients given this drug usually regain movement within 15 min after the medication has been stopped.

---

**Exam Hint**

**E**xpect several questions that require the respiratory therapist to recommend the use of the medications discussed previously. Know the indications for these groups of medications and the main medications in each group.

**MODULE B**

**Drug dosage calculations (math review)**

### Exam Hint

The National Board for Respiratory Care (NBRC) examination content outline does not specifically list drug dosage calculations. However, previous entry-level examinations have included a calculation.

The problems are easier to solve by remembering the following:

a. One milliliter (1 mL) or 1 cubic centimeter (1 cc) of water = 1 gram (g) of mass

b. Most drug doses are listed in milligrams instead of grams. Convert grams to milligrams by moving the decimal point three places to the right (the same as multiplying by 1000). For example, 0.5 g equals 500 mg.

c. Know how to interconvert fractions, decimal fractions, and percentages. For example: 1:100 = 1/100 = 0.01 = 1%.

One common way to solve any drug dosage calculation is by creating a proportional problem. Drug concentration must be converted into a fractional form. The proportional problem can then be set up to solve for the unknown *amount of active ingredient*. For example:

1. How much active ingredient would be in 0.5 mL of Adrenalin?

A 1% (1:100) drug concentration means that there is 1 part of active ingredient in 100 parts of the solution, or 1 mL or 1 g of active ingredient in 100 mL or 100 g of the solution. This can be set up in the following proportion:

$$\frac{1\,mL\,active\,ingredient}{100\,mL\,total\,solution} =$$

$$\frac{unknown\,active\,ingredient\,or\,x}{0.5\,mL\,solution}(cross\text{-}multiply)$$

$100\,x = 0.5\,mL$ (divide both sides of the equation by 100)

$x = 0.005\,mL = 0.005\,g = 5\,mg$ of active ingredient

2. How much active ingredient would be in 0.25 mL of Alupent? (Alupent is 5.0% active ingredient)

A 5.0% drug concentration means that there are 5 parts of active ingredient in 100 parts of the solution, or 5 mL or 5 g of active ingredient in 100 mL or 100 g of the solution. This can be set up in the following proportion:

$$\frac{5\,mL\,active\,ingredient}{100\,mL\,total\,solution} =$$

$$\frac{unknown\,active\,ingredient\,or\,x}{0.25\,mL\,solution}(cross\text{-}multiply)$$

$100\,x = 1.25\,mL$ (divide both sides of the equation by 100)

$x = 0.0125\,mL = 0.0125\,g = 12.5\,mg$ of active ingredient

Thus, the *amount of active ingredient* can be calculated if the drug concentration is given in either a fractional or a percentage form.

The next two examples deal with calculating the *volume of medication solution* needed to deliver a desired amount of active ingredient. With these types, it is necessary to convert to consistent units, usually converting grams to milligrams.

3. How much 0.5% Proventil would be needed to give a patient 2.5 mg of active ingredient by SVN?

A 0.5% (1:200) drug concentration means that there is 1 part of active ingredient in 200 parts of the solution, or 1 mL or 1 g of active ingredient in 200 mL or 200 g of the solution. This converts to 1000 mg/200 mL. Set up the following proportion:

$$\frac{1000\,mg\,active\,ingredient}{200\,mL\,total\,solution}$$

$$= \frac{2.5\,mg}{x\,mL\,solution}(cross\text{-}multiply)$$

$$1000\,x = 500\,mL \left(\begin{array}{l}divide\,both\,sides\,of\\the\,equation\,by\,1000\end{array}\right)$$

$x = 0.5\,mL$ of Proventil should be given

4. How much 4.0% Xylocaine would be needed to give a patient 100 mg of active ingredient by handheld nebulizer before a bronchoscopy?

A 4.0% drug concentration means that there are 4 parts of active ingredient in 100 parts of the solution, or 4 mL or 4 g of active ingredient in 100 mL or 100 g of the solution. This converts to 4000 mg/100 mL. Set up the following proportion:

$$\frac{4000\,mg\,active\,ingredient}{100\,mL\,total\,solution}$$

$$= \frac{100\,mg}{x\,mL\,solution}(cross\text{-}multiply)$$

$$4000\,x = 10,000\,mL \left(\begin{array}{l}divide\,both\,sides\,of\\the\,equation\,by\,4000\end{array}\right)$$

$x = 2.5\,mL$ of Xylocaine should be given

Thus, the *volume of medication solution* needed to deliver a given amount of active ingredient can be calculated if the drug concentration is given in either a fractional or a percentage form.

## MODULE C
### Respiratory care plan

**1. Analyze the available information to determine the patient's pathophysiologic state (NBRC code: IIIH1) [Difficulty: R, Ap, An]**

The respiratory therapist should be able to determine if the patient is having cardiopulmonary problems. Review, if needed, information presented in Chapters 1, 3, 4, and 5 that deals with bedside assessment, blood gases, pulmonary function tests, and advanced cardiopulmonary monitoring.

**2. Participate in the development of the respiratory care plan (e.g., case management, development and application of protocols, disease management education) (NBRC code: ID2) [Difficulty: Ap]**

  **a. Determine the appropriateness of the prescribed therapy and goals for the patient's pathophysiologic state (NBRC code: IIIH3) [Difficulty: R, Ap, An]**

  **b. Recommend changes in the therapeutic plan if supportive data exist (NBRC code: IIIH4) [Difficulty: R, Ap]**

With many treatment protocols, the practitioner must count the patient's heart rate before, at least one time during, and after an aerosolized bronchodilator is given. This is needed because of the risk of tachycardia. It is generally acceptable to count for 30 sec and multiply by 2 to get a 1-min count. Record the various heart rates, and determine the heart rhythm as the pulse is measured. A stethoscope can be used to better determine an abnormality. Treatment is usually stopped if the patient's pulse increases by more than 20% from the initial level.

Listen for a reduction in wheezing after administration of an aerosolized bronchodilator as proof of an effectively reduced bronchospasm. If the patient were given an aerosolized bronchodilator for bronchospasm, spirometry results would be expected to move toward more normal values as the bronchospasm is reduced. The two most important bedside spirometry values to follow are the peak flow and forced expiratory volume in 1 sec. A 15% to 20% improvement in either one or both after inhalation of an aerosolized bronchodilator indicates that the medication works and the patient has reversible bronchospasm. A patient with stable asthma may be given a drug such as cromolyn sodium (Intal) or nedocromil sodium (Tilade) by inhalation to prevent a future asthma attack. Remember that these drugs are not to be used during an asthma attack. Listen for a reduction in airway secretions after a productive cough. The mucolytics should be helpful in making the secretions less thick.

If the patient's condition does not improve after administration of the prescribed medication, there may be another problem. A chest x-ray film might help to clarify the situation.

Most patients gladly speak of breathing easier after delivery of the proper medication. It is just as important to know when the patient does *not* feel any better. Possibly, the medication does not work, or the dose is insufficient. Stop a breathing treatment any time the patient appears to have had an allergic reaction to a medication. Tell the patient's physician about it, and ask for further orders.

**3. Make a recommendation to change the dosage or concentration of an aerosolized medication (NBRC code: IIIG2b) [Difficulty: R, Ap]**

  **a. Bronchodilators**

Make a recommendation to increase the amount of medication if the patient's bronchospasm is not reversed and no adverse effects are noted. Make a recommendation to decrease the amount of medication if the patient is having serious adverse effects such as tachycardia or palpitations.

  **b. Mucomyst or saline solutions**

Make a recommendation to increase the amount of medication if the patient's secretions are still too thick to cough out or suction and no adverse effects to the medication have been noted. Make a recommendation to decrease the amount of medication if the patient's secretions are watery enough for expectoration or suctioning, or if adverse effects to the drug (e.g., bronchospasm) are noted.

**4. Change the dilution of a medication used in aerosol therapy (NBRC code: IIIFc3) [Difficulty: R, Ap]**

Various saline solutions and sterile water are known collectively as *bland* aerosols because they have no direct pharmacologic effect on the lungs and airways. They are used to increase the volume of liquid in an SVN after the medication has been added. Most of these nebulizers work most efficiently when they hold about 3 to 5 mL of liquid. Usually, a normal saline solution (0.9% sodium chloride) is added.

Adding little or no saline to the medication results in inhalation by the patient of a very concentrated solution or inability of the nebulizer to function properly. The nebulizer will aerosolize the medication within a few minutes, and the patient should quickly feel the beneficial effects of the treatment. However, depending on the nature of the medication, the patient might find it to be irritating to the airway. Coughing or bronchospasm could result. Adverse effects (e.g., tachycardia) should be watched for with sympathomimetic agents because the medication enters the bloodstream so quickly.

The more saline is added, the less concentrated is the solution. The nebulizer will take longer to aerosolize the medication because of the added volume, and relief of symptoms will take longer. However, it will be less likely to irritate the airway. Adverse effects with sympathomimetic agents could be less severe because the drug is given over a longer period. However, remember that increasing the amount of saline causes no difference in the total amount of medication available in the nebulizer for the patient. Tachycardia or other adverse effects may still be observed if the total amount of medication is given.

Saline-only aerosol treatments, as for induced sputum, are more effective at higher concentrations of saline. See Box 9-2 for complete information on saline solutions.

## 5. Stop the treatment or procedure if the patient has an adverse reaction to it (NBRC code: IIIF1) [Difficulty: R, Ap, An]

As mentioned earlier, Box 9-1 lists the adverse effects most often seen with adrenergic (sympathomimetic) bronchodilators. The most serious problem is tachycardia. In some cases, patients may have cardiac arrhythmia. A common clinical guideline calls for treatment to be stopped if the patient's heart rate increases by more than 20% during treatment. The patient should be monitored for confirmation that the heart rate has slowed. Chart the information and notify the nurse.

> ### Exam Hint
> **E**xpect to see a question in which the decision has to be made to stop bronchodilator treatment because the patient's heart rate increases by more than 20% from baseline.

## 6. Respiratory care protocols
### a. Develop the outcomes of respiratory care protocols (NBRC code: IIIH6b) [Difficulty: R, Ap]

The respiratory therapist should be familiar with two widely used respiratory disease and medication protocols. Patients with asthma should be managed as described in "National Asthma Education and Prevention Program, Expert Panel Report II: *Guidelines for the diagnosis and management of asthma*." Patients with emphysema and chronic bronchitis should be managed as described in "Global Initiative for Chronic Obstructive Lung Disease (GOLD), Workshop Report: *Global strategy for the diagnosis, management, and prevention of COPD*." The bibliography provides complete publication information on these two documents.

Guidelines for asthma and COPD rank both conditions in four categories by severity of the patient's condition. Accordingly, medications are given on the basis of the severity ranking of the patient's condition.

### b. Monitor the outcomes of respiratory care protocols (NBRC code: IIIH7b) [Difficulty: R, Ap]

Both guidelines list key things that should be monitored for evaluation of patient success. Goals of therapy for the *asthma patient* include the following:
1. Minimal or no chronic symptoms day or night
2. Minimal or no episodes
3. No limitations on activities; no school/work missed
4. Peak expiratory flow ≥80% of personal best
5. Minimal use of inhaled short-acting beta-2 agonist medication (<1 per day)
6. No or minimal adverse effects from medications

Goals of therapy for the *COPD patient* include the following:
1. Prevent disease progression.
2. Relieve symptoms (e.g., dyspnea, cough, and fatigue).
3. Improve exercise tolerance.
4. Improve health status.
5. Prevent and treat complications.
6. Prevent and treat exacerbations.
7. Reduce mortality.

> ### Exam Hint
> **A** peak flow improvement of 15% or more after bronchodilator treatment shows that the medication is effective. See Chapter 4 for information on how to perform the calculation, if needed.

## 7. Discontinue treatment based on the patient's response (NBRC code: IIIG1f) [Difficulty: R, Ap]

The physician discontinues treatment for one of two reasons. First, the patient has recovered and no longer needs a medication. Some asthma patients may fully recover and no longer need any medication. However, it is more common that the right medications to control the condition are found, so that the patient does not need to use rescue medications. Patients with emphysema and/or chronic bronchitis (COPD) are likely to always need medications.

Second, the patient has a serious adverse reaction to the medication. As has been discussed, Box 9-1 lists adverse reactions to the adrenergic (sympathomimetic) bronchodilators. Repeated episodes of tachycardia and/or cardiac arrhythmia could lead to discontinuation of their use by the physician.

**BIBLIOGRAPHY**

Au JP, Ziment I: Drug therapy and dosage adjustment in asthma, *Respir Care* 31:415, 1986.

Bills GW, Soderberg RC: *Principles of pharmacology for respiratory care*, ed 2, Albany, NY, 1998, Delmar.

Carter C, Solberg C: Respiratory pharmacology. In Hess DR, MacIntyre NR, Mishoe SC, et al, editors: *Respiratory care: principles & practices*, Philadelphia, 2002, WB Saunders.

Colbert BJ, Mason BJ: *Cardiopulmonary drug guide*, Upper Saddle River, 2003, Prentice Hall.

Colbert BJ, Mason BJ: *Integrated cardiopulmonary pharmacology*, Upper Saddle River, 2002, Prentice Hall.

Cottrell GP, Surkin HB: *Pharmacology for respiratory care practitioners*, Philadelphia, 1995, FA Davis.

Global Initiative for Chronic Obstructive Lung Disease (GOLD), Workshop Report: *Global strategy for the diagnosis, management, and prevention of COPD*, Bethesda, MD, 2000, National Heart, Lung, and Blood Institute and the World Health Organization.

Hill F: *Delmar's respiratory care drug reference*, Albany, 1999, Delmar.

Howder CL: *Cardiopulmonary pharmacology: a handbook for respiratory practitioners and other allied health personnel*, ed 2, Baltimore, 1996, Williams & Wilkins.

Levine SR, McLaughlin AJ: *Pharmacology in respiratory care*, New York, 2001, McGraw-Hill.

Malmeister M: Pharmacology associated with respiratory care. In Fink JB, Hunt GE, editors: *Clinical practice in respiratory care*, Philadelphia, 1999, Lippincott-Raven.

McLaughlin AJ, Levine SR: *Respiratory care drug reference*, Gaithersburg, Md, 1997, Aspen.

National Asthma Education and Prevention Program, Expert Panel Report II: *Guidelines for the diagnosis and management of asthma*, Bethesda, MD, 1997, National Institutes of Health.

National Institutes of Health: *Practical guide for the diagnosis and management of asthma*, Washington, DC, October 1997, NIH, Pub. No. 97-4053.

*Physicians' desk reference*, ed 57, Montvale, NJ, 2003, Thomson PDR.

Rau JL: *Respiratory care pharmacology*, ed 6, St Louis, 2002, Mosby.

Rau JL: Airway pharmacology. In Wilkins RL, Stoller JK, Scanlan CL, editors: *Egan's fundamentals of respiratory care*, ed 8, St Louis, 2003, Mosby.

Tashkin DP: Dosing strategies for bronchodilator aerosol delivery, *Respir Care* 36:977, 1991.

Witek TJ, Schachter EN: *Pharmacology and therapeutics in respiratory care*, Philadelphia, 1994, WB Saunders.

Ziment I: Drugs used in respiratory care. In Burton GG, Hodgkin JE, Ward JJ, editors: *Respiratory care: a guide to clinical practice*, ed 4, Philadelphia, 1997, Lippincott-Raven.

## SELF-STUDY QUESTIONS

1. A patient with a fluid overload problem has been given a dose of furosemide (Lasix) intravenously. Following rapid diuresis in the patient, you note an arrhythmia that did not exist before the medication was given. What would you recommend?
   A. Check the patient's potassium level.
   B. Give more furosemide.
   C. Defibrillate the patient's heart.
   D. Give the patient epinephrine to reverse the allergic reaction to furosemide.

2. A 20-year-old asthmatic patient has received a standard dose of levalbuterol (Xopenex). Breath sounds reveal loud, bilateral wheezes. Over the course of the treatment, her heart rate changed from 98 to 105/minute. What would you recommend?
   A. Stop the treatment and notify the physician.
   B. Repeat the treatment and monitor the patient.
   C. Switch the medication to albuterol (Ventolin).
   D. Add theophylline (Aminophylline) to the intravenous line.

3. You are working in the emergency department when an automobile crash victim arrives by ambulance. She is conscious, screaming, and hysterical from the extreme pain of a broken lower leg. What would you recommend for sedation?
   A. Morphine sulfate (Duramorph)
   B. Ibuprofen (Advil)
   C. Succinylcholine chloride (Anectine)
   D. Ipratropium bromide (Atrovent)

4. An asthma patient is being taken off of her systemic corticosteroid. She will continue taking her aerosolized bronchodilator. The physician wants to know what you would recommend for an inhaled corticosteroid.
   A. Naloxone (Narcan)
   B. Neostigmine bromide (Prostigmin)
   C. Beclomethasone dipropionate (Vanceril)
   D. Methylprednisolone (Solu-Medrol)

5. Results of your patient's pulmonary function tests show that the peak expiratory flow rate increased the most when she inhaled an aerosolized sympathomimetic drug and an aerosolized parasympatholytic drug. The physician wants to know what you would recommend for the patient.
   A. Beclomethasone dipropionate (Vanceril)
   B. Ipratropium and albuterol (Combivent)
   C. Ipratropium bromide (Atrovent)
   D. Salmeterol (Serevent)

6. Your patient's airway was extubated 30 min ago. She is hoarse and complains of "tightness in my throat"; inspiratory stridor can be heard. The drug of choice for treating this problem is
   A. Racemic epinephrine (MicroNefrin)
   B. Acetylcysteine (Mucomyst)
   C. Isoproterenol (Isuprel)
   D. Isoetharine (Isoetharine HCl)

7. Your patient with COPD is coughing very hard to bring up viscous, thick mucus with plugs. What drug of choice would you recommend to treat this problem?
   A. Dopamine hydrochloride (Intropin)
   B. Acetylcysteine (Mucomyst)
   C. Cromolyn sodium (Intal)
   D. Dornase alpha (Pulmozyme)

8. You receive an order to administer 5 mL of Proventil (albuterol) by handheld nebulizer. You would proceed to
   A. Confirm that the order was written and give the treatment
   B. Have the shift supervisor give the treatment
   C. Call the physician to check on the medication dose
   D. Give 0.5 mL of medication because the physician probably meant to write that

9. You are working with a 10-year-old cystic fibrosis patient with a pulmonary infection and thick secretions. What would you recommend to help him cough out the secretions?
   A. 0.9% (normal) saline solution
   B. Instillation of acetylcysteine (Mucomyst) into his lungs
   C. Dornase alpha (Pulmozyme)
   D. 10% (hypertonic) saline solution

10. How much active ingredient would be found in 0.6 mL of 2.25% racemic epinephrine (MicroNefrin)?
    A. 26,700 mg
    B. 0.0267 mg
    C. 13.5 g
    D. 13.5 mg

11. You are administering an aerosolized bronchodilator to your patient. Her pretreatment pulse was 85 beats/min. You would stop the treatment if her pulse reached
    A. 90 beats/min
    B. 100 beats/min
    C. 110 beats/min
    D. 120 beats/min

12. Your patient is being given an aerosolized adrenergic (sympathomimetic) drug for the first time. What possible adverse effects of the medication should you watch for?
    I. Bradycardia
    II. Tremor
    III. Headache
    IV. Nervousness and irritability
    V. Tachycardia
    A. I and II
    B. III, IV, and V
    C. II, III, IV, and V
    D. II and IV

13. Your patient is being discharged and will receive aerosolized bronchodilator therapy at home. The best medication for this chronically sick but stable patient is
    A. Salmeterol (Serevent)
    B. Metaproterenol (Alupent)
    C. Isoetharine (Bronkosol)
    D. Albuterol (Ventolin)

14. Your patient has an order for an induced sputum sample to be analyzed for tuberculosis. The best medication for this is
    A. Dornase alpha (Pulmozyme)
    B. 10% saline solution
    C. 0.9% saline solution
    D. 0.45% saline solution

15. A patient, after finishing an aerosolized dose of Mucomyst, has breath sounds that reveal wheezing. These were not present at the start of treatment. What medication should be given before the Mucomyst treatment to prevent bronchospasm?
    A. Levalbuterol (Xopenex)
    B. Sterile water
    C. Salmeterol (Serevent)
    D. 0.9% saline solution

16. You are working the night shift when a 17-year-old patient with status asthmaticus is admitted through the emergency room. She has already been given Combivent and an inhaled corticosteroid medication. The intern on call asks for your recommendation on what additional medication to give the patient. You would recommend
    A. Formoterol (Foradil)
    B. Terbutaline (Brethaire)
    C. Albuterol (Proventil)
    D. Theophylline ethylenediamine (Aminophylline)

17. A 16-year-old patient has severe and chronic asthma. Her physician wishes to change her medications to prevent her from having asthma attacks. All of the following medications would be helpful EXCEPT
    A. Zileuton (Zyflo)
    B. Pirbuterol (Maxair)
    C. Cromolyn sodium (Intal)
    D. Zafirlukast (Accolate)

18. Your patient with COPD is being given a new inhaled adrenergic bronchodilator medication by small-volume nebulizer. Within 3 min, he complains of palpitations. His pulse was 85/minute before the treatment and is now 125/minute. What should you do?
    A. Change to a different medication for the next treatment.
    B. Discontinue the order.
    C. Stop the treatment and monitor the patient.
    D. Add more saline to dilute the medication for the next ordered treatment.

19. You have finished giving your 28-year-old patient with asthma an IPPB treatment with 0.5 mL of Alupent. You notice that her heart rate has increased 15% from before the treatment. Her breath sounds are now clear. What would you recommend to the physician for her next treatment?
    A. Give her 0.5 mL of isoproterenol (Isuprel).
    B. Discontinue her treatments altogether.
    C. Add more normal saline to the Alupent.
    D. Decrease the Alupent to 0.3 mL.
20. You are called to the recovery room to assist in the care of a patient who returned 2 hr ago from having a bowel resection. The patient is apneic and on a mechanical ventilator. Which medication(s) could be used to wean her from the machine?
    I. Flumazenil (Romazicon)
    II. Naloxone (Narcan)
    III. Dopamine (Intropin)
    IV. Succinylcholine chloride (Anectine)
    V. Diazepam (Valium)
    A. I and IV
    B. V
    C. II and III
    D. I and II
21. How much Alupent would it take to give the patient 20 mg of the active ingredient? Alupent contains 5% active ingredient.
    A. 1 mL
    B. 0.4 mL
    C. 40 mL
    D. 0.1 mL
22. A 10-year-old patient with status asthmaticus has been admitted to the hospital. The physician plans to start her on continuous nebulization of a fast-onset "rescue" inhaled bronchodilator medication. Which of the following would you recommend as part of her care plan?
    I. Admit her to the intensive care unit.
    II. Admit her to the pediatrics floor.
    III. She should be given salmeterol (Serevent).
    IV. She should be given levalbuterol (Xopenex).
    V. ECG monitoring should be done.
    VI. Pulse oximetry monitoring should be done.
    A. II, IV, and VI
    B. I, III, V, and VI
    C. II, IV, and VI
    D. I, IV, V, and VI

## ANSWER KEY AND RATIONALE

1. **A.** Lasix is a diuretic and is known to cause patients to urinate large amounts of potassium. The loss of potassium can result in cardiac arrhythmia. Giving more Lasix could worsen the loss of potassium. No indication is given that the patient has a life-threatening arrhythmia that needs to be defibrillated. No indication exists to give epinephrine.
2. **B.** Her continued wheezes justify more medication. The small increase in heart rate does not justify stopping the treatment. Vertolin will not be any more effective than Xopenex. Aminophylline is not indicated at this time. First, find out if more Xopenex causes bronchodilation.
3. **A.** Morphine is indicated to relieve severe, acute pain. In addition to controlling the pain, morphine will sedate the patient. Advil is not effective against severe pain. Anectine is a paralyzing medication. Atrovent is a parasympatholytic (anticholinergic) medication.
4. **C.** Vanceril is an inhaled corticosteroid that is widely used to treat asthma. Narcan is a reversing agent for morphine and related opium-based drugs. Prostigmin is a reversing agent for the nondepolarizing neuromuscular blocking agents. Solu-Medrol is a steroid taken by pill or intravenously for systemic effects.
5. **B.** Combivent combines a sympathomimetic and a parasympatholytic agent for effective bronchodilation. Vanceril is an inhaled corticosteroid medication. Atrovent is a parasympatholytic agent. Serevent is a long-duration sympathomimetic agent.
6. **A.** MicroNefrin will stimulate the alpha-receptors in the mucous membrane of the patient's airway to cause vasoconstriction and reduce edema. Mucomyst is a mucolytic. Isuprel and Bronkosol are sympathomimetic agents with no alpha-receptor effect.
7. **B.** Mucomyst is an effective mucolytic for most patients. Dopamine is a vasoconstrictor used to raise blood pressure. Intal is used to prevent an asthma attack. Pulmozyme is indicated in patients with cystic fibrosis who have pulmonary infection and thick secretions.
8. **C.** The physician should be called because 5 mL is too large a dose of Proventil. Any respiratory therapist should know not to give this large a dose even if the order is written. A respiratory therapist should not alter a written order from a physician or presume to know what a physician might want to do.

9. **C.** Pulmozyme is indicated in patients with cystic fibrosis who have pulmonary infection and thick secretions. Normal and hypertonic saline solutions are not the most effective options for liquefying secretions. Mucomyst effectively liquefies mucoid secretions but has no effect against purulent secretions with bacterial DNA. In addition, Mucomyst is not indicated for tracheal instillation in this patient.

10. **D.** Review the first two drug dosage calculations shown earlier to see how to set up this problem.

11. **C.** It is commonly accepted that an aerosolized bronchodilator treatment should be stopped if the patient's pulse increases by 20% or more (from 85 to 102 plus).

12. **C.** Tremor, headache, nervousness and irritability, and tachycardia are all known possible adverse effects.

13. **A.** Serevent is a long-duration medication indicated in stable patients with bronchospasm. The other medications are all sympathomimetic bronchodilators with a shorter duration of action.

14. **B.** Hypertonic (10%) saline is commonly used to induce a sputum sample in patients with tuberculosis. The other saline solutions will not be as effective. Pulmozyme is indicated in patients with cystic fibrosis who have purulent secretions.

15. **A.** Xopenex is a fast-acting sympathomimetic bronchodilator that should help to prevent a bronchospasm reaction from Mucomyst. Sterile water and normal saline are not bronchodilators and can cause bronchospasm in some asthmatic patients. Nembutal is a barbiturate.

16. **D.** Aminophylline is recognized as a medication that may be beneficial to a patient with status asthmaticus after inhaled bronchodilators and corticosteroids have been given. If a fast-onset sympathomimetic bronchodilator such as albuterol (in Combivent) has not been effective, it is doubtful if Proventil (more albuterol) or Brethaire would be effective. Foradil is an effective sympathomimetic bronchodilator that has too slow an onset for a patient who needs immediate help.

17. **B.** Pirbuterol (Maxair) is a fast-onset sympathomimetic bronchodilator. It may be used as a "rescue" inhaler during an asthma attack but is not used to prevent an asthma attack. Intal, Accolate, and Zyflo are all used as prophylactic agents to prevent an asthma attack. Intal stabilizes mast cells to prevent the release of leukotriene agents. Accolate and Zyflo block the effect of released leukotriene agents.

18. **C.** Treatment should be stopped because the patient's heart rate has increased by more than 20%. Monitor the patient's heart rate to find out if it returns to normal; chart the results. Only the physician can order a change in type of medication or medication amount. Only the physician can terminate treatment. Adding more saline to the medication will dilute the mixture but not reduce the amount of medication the patient receives. The same adverse reaction will probably happen again.

19. **D.** Decreasing the dose of Alupent is reasonable because it may be causing the patient's heart rate to increase. Adding saline will not reduce the total amount of medication that the patient will receive. Isuprel is more likely than Alupent to raise the patient's heart rate. No need exists to stop the treatment at this point based on this increase in her heart rate.

20. **D.** Romazicon reverses a barbiturate medication, and Narcan reverses a narcotic medication in the patient. Intropin is used to raise blood pressure. Anectine is a depolarizing neuromuscular blocking agent. Valium is a barbiturate.

21. **D.** Review the third and fourth drug dosage calculations shown earlier in the chapter to see how to set up this problem.

22. **D.** A patient in status asthmaticus should be admitted to the intensive care unit. She will be monitored more closely in the ICU than on the pediatric floor, and she will be cared for by personnel who are accustomed to critically ill patients. Xopenex is a fast-onset bronchodilator that is indicated for continuous nebulization. Continuous ECG monitoring should be performed to check on tachycardia or arrhythmia. Continuous pulse oximetry should be performed to check on oxygen level. Serevent is a slow-onset, long-duration bronchodilator that is indicated in stable patients with asthma.

# 10 Bronchopulmonary Hygiene Therapy

A review of the most recent Entry Level Examinations has shown an average of 3 questions (2% of the exam) that cover bronchopulmonary hygiene therapy issues.

## MODULE A
### Postural drainage therapy

Postural drainage therapy (PDT) is also known as chest physiotherapy, chest physical therapy, broncho-pulmonary drainage, postural drainage and percussion, and percussion and vibration.

1. **Recommend bronchopulmonary hygiene procedures** (NBRC code: IIIG1a) [Difficulty: R, Ap]
2. **Instruct and encourage bronchopulmonary hygiene techniques** (NBRC code: IIIC4) [R, Ap]

The American Association for Respiratory Care (AARC) clinical practice guideline on postural drainage therapy (1991) was used as the source of the following information. See Box 10-1 for indications for turning, postural drainage, percussion, and vibration. Contraindications are listed in Box 10-2, and recommended actions for a problem are listed in Box 10-3. Beyond the patient assessment issues listed in Box 10-4, the following should be evaluated to determine if PDT is needed:

  a. PDT is not indicated if an optimally hydrated patient is coughing out less than 25 mL/day with the procedure.

  b. A dehydrated patient should have apparently ineffective PDT continued for at least 24 hr after the patient has been rehydrated. The combination of rehydration and PDT may help to mobilize previously thick secretions.

  c. PDT is not indicated in a patient who produces more than 30 mL of secretions daily (if the PDT treatments do not increase the sputum production) because the patient is already able to effectively cough out the sputum.

3. **Perform postural drainage** (NBRC code: IIIC1a) [Difficulty: R, Ap]

Turning involves rotating the patient's body in the longitudinal (head-to-toe) axis to promote unilateral or bilateral lung expansion. Patients can be turned from their back to one side, from side to side, or from one side to back to the other side, depending on their needs. The bed may be moved to any head-up or head-down position according to what the patient needs and tolerates. Patients should be turned every 1 to 2 hr as tolerated. The patient can turn himself or herself, can be turned by a

---

**BOX 10-1**    **Indications for Turning, Postural Drainage, and Percussion and Vibration**

**TURNING**
- Patient is unable to change his or her body position (e.g., the patient has a cerebral injury or neuromuscular disease, is being mechanically ventilated, or has been medicated to cause sedation or paralysis)
- Atelectasis or the potential for its development
- Hypoxemia associated with a particular position; if one-sided lung disease is present, the patient is typically turned so that the affected lung is superior
- Patient with an artificial airway

**POSTURAL DRAINAGE**
- Mobilize retained secretions so that they can be coughed or suctioned out; patient has difficulty coughing out secretions but produces more than 25–30 mL/day; evidence or indications that a patient with an artificial airway has retained secretions
- Atelectasis that is known or is believed to be caused by mucus plugging
- Patient diagnosed with cystic fibrosis, bronchiectasis, or cavitating lung disease
- Foreign body in an airway
- Removal of aspirated foreign body or stomach contents

**PERCUSSION AND VIBRATION**
- Patient receiving postural drainage who has a large volume of thick sputum; this suggests that external manipulation of the thorax would assist gravity in its movement toward a more central airway

Based on information found in American Association for Respiratory Care: Clinical practice guidelines: postural drainage therapy, Respir Care 36:1418, 1991.

---

**BOX 10-2   Contraindications of Turning/Postural Drainage and Percussion and Vibration**

**TURNING/POSTURAL DRAINAGE***

All positions are contraindicated for patients with the following:

1. Unstabilized head or neck injury, or both (absolute)
2. Active hemorrhage and hemodynamic instability (absolute)
3. ICP greater than 20 mm Hg
4. Recent spinal surgery, such as a laminectomy, or acute spinal injury
5. Active hemoptysis
6. Empyema
7. Bronchopleural fistula
8. Pulmonary edema as a result of congestive heart failure
9. Large pleural effusions
10. Advanced age, anxiety, or confusion and intolerance of position changes
11. Fractured rib(s) with or without flail chest
12. Healing tissue or surgical wound

Trendelenburg position is contraindicated in patients with the following:

1. ICP greater than 20 mm Hg
2. Sensitivity to increased ICP (e.g., neurosurgery, cerebral aneurysms, eye surgery)
3. Uncontrolled hypertension
4. Distended abdomen
5. Esophageal surgery
6. Recent gross hemoptysis (especially if associated with lung cancer that was recently treated surgically or by radiation therapy)
7. Uncontrolled airway if at risk for aspiration (recent meal or tube feeding); many authors regard less than 1 hr after eating as a contraindication

Reverse Trendelenburg position is contraindicated in patients who

1. Are hypotensive
2. Are receiving a vasoactive medication

**PERCUSSION AND VIBRATIONS**

1. All of the previously listed contraindications
2. Subcutaneous emphysema (several authors list an untreated pneumothorax as an absolute contraindication)
3. Spinal anesthesia or recent epidural spinal infusion for pain control
4. Recent thoracic skin grafts or skin flaps
5. Thoracic burns, open wounds, or skin infections
6. Recently placed transvenous or subcutaneous pacemaker (especially true if a mechanical percussor/vibrator is to be used)
7. Suspicion of pulmonary tuberculosis
8. Lung contusion
9. Bronchospasm
10. Osteomyelitis of the ribs
11. Osteoporosis
12. Clotting disorder (coagulopathy)
13. Complaints of chest wall pain

In addition, a number of authors have listed the following as contraindications to percussion and vibration:

1. Not over bare skin
2. Not over buttons, zippers, folded clothes, or seams of clothing
3. Not over female breast tissue
4. Not over the spine, sternum, or kidneys
5. Not over an area with a known lung tumor

ICP, Intracranial pressure.

* These are relative contraindications except those marked as absolute.

Based on information found in American Association for Respiratory Care: Clinical practice guidelines: postural drainage therapy, Respir Care 36:1418, 1991.

---

caregiver, or can be placed in a bed that is motorized and programmed to change positions in a set pattern.

Postural drainage (bronchopulmonary drainage) is performed to clear secretions or prevent the accumulation of secretions. The patient is positioned so that the bronchus of a particular segment is as vertical as possible. Gravity pulls the secretions toward a major bronchus or the trachea; secretions are then either coughed or suctioned out.

The anatomy of the pulmonary lobes with their segments and respective bronchi should be reviewed (Fig. 10-1). Note that each segment, along with its bronchus, adjoins the right or left mainstem bronchus at a particular angle. This critical angle determines the positioning that must be used to drain the various segments. Obviously, putting the patient in the wrong position does nothing to drain the desired segment. Auscultation, palpation, and percussion of the chest should guide the practitioner in learning where the secretions are.

Individual segments should be drained when the physician's order specifies this, or when the practitioner determines that secretions are present. Individual segments are generally drained for 3 to 15 min. Drainage may need to be provided for a longer period in special situations. Postural drainage and external manipulation of the patient's thorax (percussion and vibration) can be very strenuous or contraindicated in some patients. Watch for hypoxemia or an increase in dyspnea. If the patient normally has supplemental $O_2$, it should be provided throughout the drainage positions. Some patients need supplemental $O_2$ only when they are in certain positions, and it must be made available to them.

Coughing should be encouraged after each segment has been drained. The patient should not cough in a

---

### BOX 10-3 Hazards/Complications, With Recommended Actions, and Limitations of Postural Drainage and Percussion and Vibration

**HAZARDS/COMPLICATIONS**

- *Hypoxemia.* The patient known to be hypoxic or prone to hypoxemia during the procedure should be given a higher inspired $O_2$ percentage. Give 100% $O_2$ to any patient who becomes hypoxic during the procedure. Stop treatment, return the patient to the original resting position, make sure ventilation is adequate, and consult with the physician before continuing.
- *Increased intracranial pressure or acute hypotension during the procedure.* If either of these happens, stop the treatment, return the patient to the original resting position, and consult with the physician before you continue.
- *Pulmonary hemorrhage.* If this happens, stop treatment, return the patient to the original resting position, and call the physician immediately. Give the patient supplemental $O_2$ and keep an open airway until the physician responds.
- *Pain or injury to the patient's muscles, ribs, or spine.* Stop the therapy that seems to be causing the problem. Carefully move the patient to a more comfortable position and call the physician before you continue.
- *Vomiting and aspiration.* Stop treatment, apply suction as needed to clear the airway, give supplemental $O_2$, maintain a patent airway, return the patient to the original resting position, and call the physician immediately.
- *Bronchospasm.* If this happens, stop treatment, return the patient to the original resting position, and give or increase the supplemental $O_2$ while you call the physician. Give the patient any aerosolized bronchodilators that have been ordered by the physician.
- *Arrhythmia.* If this happens, stop treatment, return the patient to the original resting position, and give or increase supplemental $O_2$ while you call the physician.

**LIMITATIONS**

- Be careful to give postural drainage therapy only to those patients who would benefit from it. Do not rely on past experiences with other patients when you judge current situations.
- Patients with ineffective coughs may be unable to clear the airways as well as desired.
- Critically ill patients are difficult to position optimally.

Based on information found in American Association for Respiratory Care: Clinical practice guidelines: postural drainage therapy, Respir Care 36:1418, 1991.

head-down position, however, because of the risk of increased intracranial pressure. Have the patient sit up to cough vigorously.

### 1. Pulmonary drainage positions
*Lower lobes*
a. Posterior basal segment (Fig. 10-2)
   1. The patient lies face-down on the bed. A pillow is placed beneath the hips.

---

### BOX 10-4 Assessment of the Patient's Needs for Postural Drainage Therapy (PDT)*

- Excessive production of sputum
- Ineffectiveness of cough
- Patient history of PDT that was helpful in treating past problem (e.g., bronchiectasis, cystic fibrosis, lung abscess)
- Abnormal breath sounds (e.g., decreased breath sounds, crackles, or rhonchi, suggesting airway secretions)
- Change in the patient's vital signs
- Abnormal chest x-ray film finding consistent with infiltrates, atelectasis, or mucus plugging

Based on information found in American Association for Respiratory Care: Clinical practice guidelines: postural drainage therapy, Respir Care 36:1418, 1991.
*These problems should be assessed *together* to evaluate the patient's need for PDT. Not all patients experience all of these problems. The seriousness of these problems should be assessed by the clinician in determining which patients will benefit from PDT.

   2. The foot of the bed is elevated 18 inches or 30 degrees.
   3. If ordered, percussion or vibration is performed over the lower ribs near the spine on either or both sides, depending on whether one or both segments are to be drained. Note the shaded areas in Fig. 10-2.
b. Lateral basal segment (Fig. 10-3)
   1. The patient is placed in a position from which the right lateral basal segment can be drained. The left lateral basal segment is drained when the patient is placed the same way on the opposite side.
   2. The patient lies one-fourth turn up from the face-down position. A pillow may be placed in front of the patient for support or between the knees for comfort.
   3. The foot of the bed is elevated 18 inches or 30 degrees.
   4. If ordered, percussion or vibration is performed over the posterolateral areas of the lower ribs. See the shaded areas in Fig. 10-3.
c. Anterior basal segment (Fig. 10-4)
   1. The patient is shown in a position that drains the left anterior basal segment. (*Note:* This combined segment is the anatomic equivalent of the medial basal segment and the anterior basal segment of the right lung.) The right anterior basal and medial basal segments are drained when the patient is placed the same way on the opposite side.
   2. The patient lies straight up on his or her side. Pillows may be used in front of or behind (or both) the patient for positioning, or between the knees for comfort.

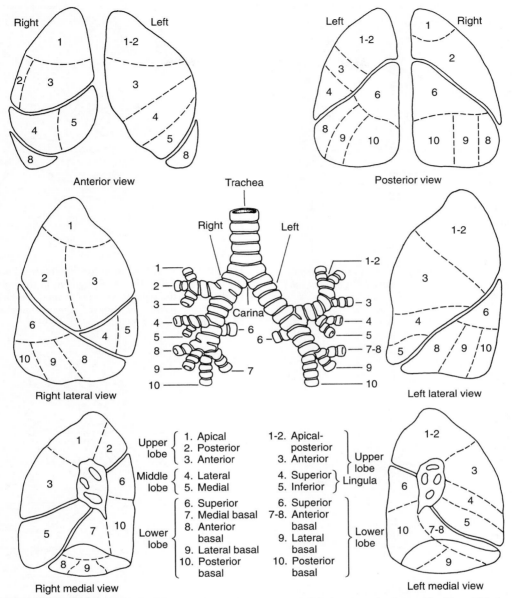

**Fig. 10-1** Names and locations of the lung segments and their respective bronchi. *(From Shibel EM, Moser KM, editors: Respiratory emergencies, St Louis, 1977, Mosby.)*

3. The foot of the bed is elevated 18 inches or 30 degrees.
4. If ordered, percussion or vibration is performed over the lower ribs below the axilla. See the shaded areas in Fig. 10-4.

d. Superior segment (Fig. 10-5)
   1. The patient lies face-down on the bed. A pillow is placed beneath the hips.
   2. The bed is flat.
   3. If ordered, percussion or vibration is performed over the middle of the back below the scapula on either one or both sides of the spine, depending on whether one or both segments are to be drained. See the shaded areas in Fig. 10-5.

***Right middle lobe and left lingula***

a. Right lateral and medial segments (Fig. 10-6)
   1. The same position is used to drain both segments.
   2. The patient lies one-fourth turn up from the back-down position. A pillow may be placed in back of the patient for support or between the flexed knees for comfort.
   3. The foot of the bed is elevated 14 inches or 15 degrees.

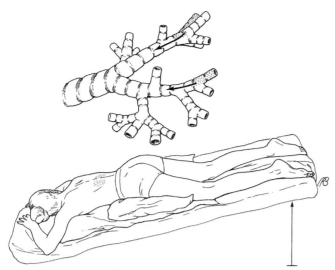

**Fig. 10-2** Drainage position for the posterior basal segments of both lower lobes. *(From Eubanks DH, Bone RC: Comprehensive respiratory care, ed 2, St Louis, 1990, Mosby.)*

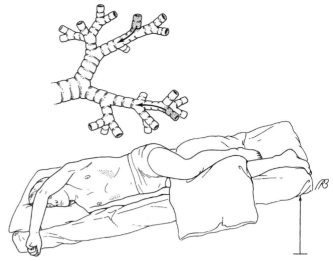

**Fig. 10-4** Drainage position for the anterior basal segment of the left lower lobe. The same segment in the right lung would be drained if the patient were positioned similarly on the left side. *(From Eubanks DH, Bone RC: Comprehensive respiratory care, ed 2, St Louis, 1990, Mosby.)*

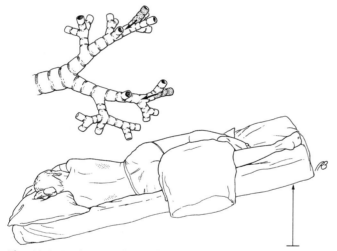

**Fig. 10-3** Drainage position for the lateral basal segment of the right lower lobe. The same segment in the left lung would be drained if the patient were positioned similarly on the right side. *(From Eubanks DH, Bone RC: Comprehensive respiratory care, ed 2, St Louis, 1990, Mosby.)*

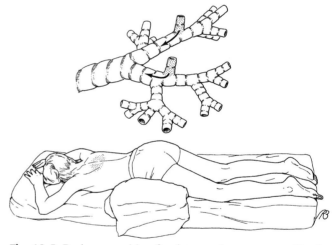

**Fig. 10-5** Drainage position for the superior segments of both lower lobes. *(From Eubanks DH, Bone RC: Comprehensive respiratory care, ed 2, St Louis, 1990, Mosby.)*

4. If ordered, percussion or vibration is performed below the right nipple area in a male patient. See the shaded area in Fig. 10-6. Percussion and vibration may not be possible with a female patient.

b. Left superior and inferior lingula segments (Fig. 10-7)

1. The same position is used to drain both segments.

2. The patient lies one-fourth turn up from the back-down position. A pillow may be placed in the back of the patient for support or between the flexed knees for comfort.

3. The foot of the bed is elevated 14 inches or 15 degrees.

4. If ordered, percussion or vibration is performed below the left nipple area in a male patient. See the shaded area in Fig. 10-7. Percussion and vibration may not be possible with a female patient.

***Upper lobes***

a. Posterior segment (Fig. 10-8)

1. The patient leans forward 30 degrees. This can occur over the back of a chair (as shown in Fig.

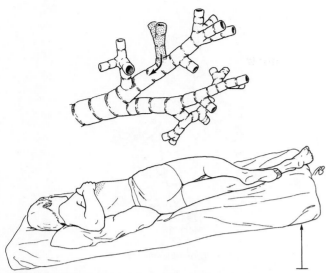

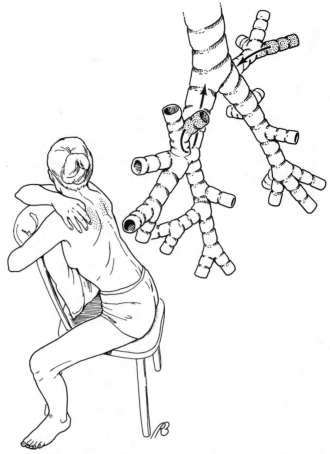

**Fig. 10-6** Drainage position for the lateral and medial segments of the right middle lobe. *(From Eubanks DH, Bone RC: Comprehensive respiratory care, ed 2, St Louis, 1990, Mosby.)*

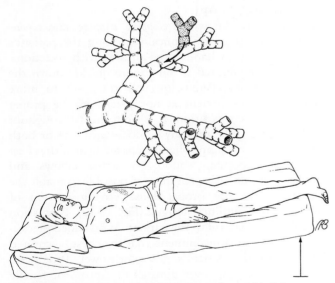

**Fig. 10-7** Drainage position for the superior and inferior segments of the lingula. *(From Eubanks DH, Bone RC: Comprehensive respiratory care, ed 2, St Louis, 1990, Mosby.)*

**Fig. 10-8** Drainage position for the posterior segments of both upper lobes. *(From Eubanks DH, Bone RC: Comprehensive respiratory care, ed 2, St Louis, 1990, Mosby.)*

10-8) or in bed. A pillow can be used for leaning against or for supporting the chest.

2. If ordered, percussion or vibration is performed over the upper portion of the back on either or both sides of the spine, depending on whether one or both segments are being drained. See the shaded areas in Fig. 10-8.

b. Apical segment (Fig. 10-9)
  1. The patient leans backward 30 degrees. This can occur in bed (as shown in Fig. 10-9) or in a chair.

A pillow can be leaned against for support of the lower portion of the back.

2. If ordered, percussion or vibration is performed between the clavicle and the top of the scapula on either one or both sides, depending on whether one or both segments are being drained. See the shaded areas in Fig. 10-9.

c. Anterior segment (Fig. 10-10)
  1. The patient lies supine in bed with a pillow placed under the knees. This enables the abdominal muscles to relax so that the patient can breathe more easily.
  2. If ordered, percussion or vibration is performed between the clavicle and the nipple of a male patient on either one or both sides, depending on whether one or both segments are being drained. See the shaded areas in Fig. 10-10. Percussion and vibration may not be possible on a female patient.

Some authors may list slightly different positions or several additional positions. The most commonly

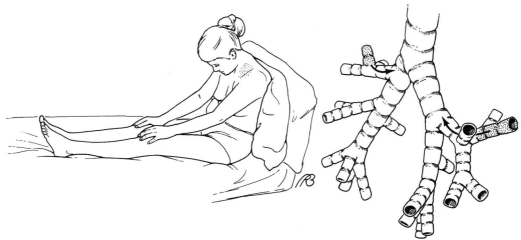

**Fig. 10-9** Drainage position for the apical segments of both upper lobes. *(From Eubanks DH, Bone RC: Comprehensive respiratory care, ed 2, St Louis, 1990, Mosby.)*

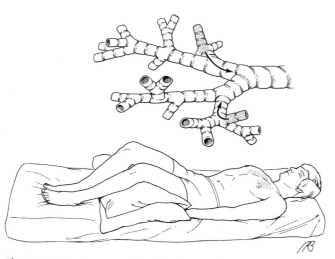

**Fig. 10-10** Drainage position for the anterior segments of both upper lobes. *(From Eubanks DH, Bone RC: Comprehensive respiratory care, ed 2, St Louis, 1990, Mosby.)*

accepted postural drainage positions have been presented. Postural drainage positions recommended for the infant are basically the same as in the adult. Positioning can be accomplished more easily with the use of pillows. Fig. 10-11 shows various segmental drainage positions.

### Exam Hint

The examination usually includes at least one question that involves knowing the correct position to drain a particular lobe. The lower lobes are usually tested.

### 4. Perform percussion (NBRC code: IIIC1a) [Difficulty: R, Ap]

Percussion (also known as *clapping, cupping,* and *tapotement*) is the act of rhythmically striking the patient's chest with cupped hands over an area with secretions. Secretions are vibrated to flow more quickly down the vertical bronchus. Percussion will not work to move secretions if the patient is not placed in the proper postural drainage position. It is performed throughout the breathing cycle and can be done with one or both hands. A properly cupped hand traps air against the chest and causes a popping sound. The wrists, elbows, and shoulders should be kept as loose as possible to enable the practitioner to use proper loose waving motion of the hand and minimize fatigue (Fig. 10-12). Percussion should not be painful to the patient. As an added precaution, most authors recommend that the chest be covered lightly with the patient's gown or towel. Percussion should not be done over buttons or zippers or female breast tissue.

Percussion is recommended for 5 min or longer in each position. Some patients, however, may not tolerate this length of treatment; 1 min seems to be the shortest time for some therapeutic benefit. No agreement exists on the ideal rate of percussion. The practitioner must vary the rate, depending on how the patient feels and what seems to produce the best clearance of secretions.

Infants can be percussed by placement of the index, middle, and ring fingers together into a kind of three-sided tent. This enables the practitioner to percuss a small area of the chest wall. Mechanical percussors/vibrators and other devices may be used to supplement manual percussion and are discussed later in this chapter.

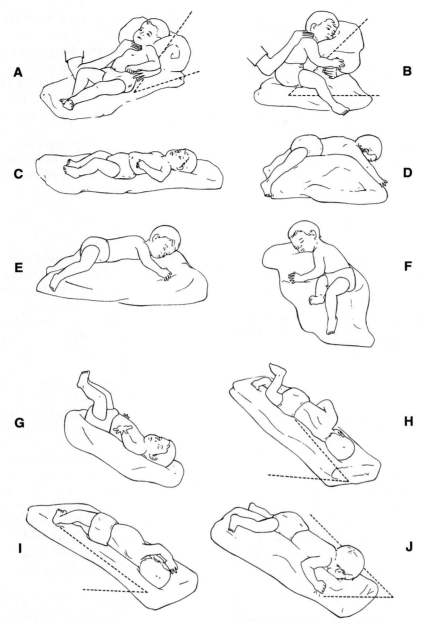

**Fig. 10-11** Drainage positions in infants. **A,** Apical segment of upper lobes. **B,** Posterior segments of upper lobes. **C,** Anterior segments of upper lobes. **D–F,** Superior segments of lower lobes. **G** and **H,** Anterior basal segments of both lower lobes (**H** on right and left sides). **I,** Segments of the right middle lobe and lingula (shown). **J,** Posterior basal segments of the lower lobes. *(From Crane LD: Physical therapy for the neonate with respiratory disease. In Irwin S, Tecklin JS, editors: Cardiopulmonary physical therapy, ed 3, St Louis, 1995, Mosby.)*

## 5. Perform vibration (NBRC code: IIIC1a) [Difficulty: R, Ap]

Vibration is the gentle, rapid shaking of the chest wall directly over the lung segment that is being drained. It may be performed alone or with percussion. The practitioner places his or her hands side by side if the chest area is large enough, or one on the other for a smaller chest area. The elbows are locked with the arms straight (Fig.

10-13). The patient's chest is gently but effectively shaken during exhalation. The patient should exhale at least the complete tidal volume ($V_T$) as the chest wall is vibrated. Blowing out the expiratory reserve volume should help to clear out more secretions. A vibration rate of 200/min (about 3/sec) has been recommended as ideal for helping to move secretions. The literature differs as to how the patient should exhale during the procedure. Both

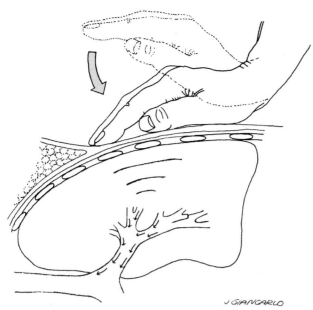

**Fig. 10-12** Movement of the cupped hand at the wrist during chest percussion. *(From Shapiro BA, Kacmarek RM, Cane RD, et al: Clinical application of respiratory care, ed 4, St Louis, 1991, Mosby.)*

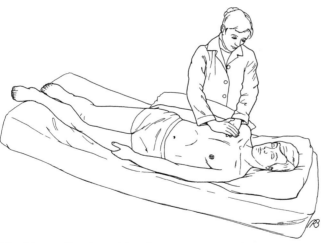

**Fig. 10-13** Vibration of the chest during postural drainage therapy. *(From Eubanks DH, Bone RC: Comprehensive respiratory care, ed 2, St Louis, 1990, Mosby.)*

breathing out slowly through pursed lips and breathing out forcefully through an open mouth have been recommended. A pursed-lip exhalation pattern seems reasonable if the patient has a problem with bronchospasm and air trapping. A patient without this problem should exhale forcefully because this helps to clear more secretions. Vibration should be performed for several expiratory efforts or until it is no longer effective in helping to mobilize secretions.

## 6. Modify the postural drainage therapy (NBRC code: IIIF2e) [Difficulty: R, Ap]

### a. Change the length of treatment time

Lung segments should generally be drained for 3 to 15 min. If the patient is tolerating the position and secretions are still being cleared, the position can be held longer. Stop treatment if the patient is showing any signs of intolerance.

Total time for the procedure is recommended to be no longer than 30 to 40 min because the patient may become exhausted by the various position changes. If so, the practitioner must select the worst segments to be drained first. Several drainage sessions may be needed to get to all of the involved segments.

### b. Change the treatment techniques used

Be prepared to modify the postural drainage, percussion, and vibration procedures, depending on how the patient tolerates them. For example,

1. Some patients cannot tolerate certain positions, especially head-down, because of pain, shortness of breath (SOB), hypoxemia, or elevated blood pressure.
2. Percussion rate, pressure, and hand position may need to be modified, depending on the patient's tolerance, chest size, and secretion clearance.
3. It may not be possible to percuss or vibrate female patients in the right middle lobe and left lingular positions because of breast tissue.
4. Hypoxemia should be prevented with supplemental $O_2$ in those patients who need it. Pulse oximetry could be performed before and during the procedure to monitor the patient's $O_2$ saturation.
5. Cardiac patients should have heart rate, heart rhythm, and blood pressure monitored. Check heart rate before the procedure and with each position change.
6. Postoperative or trauma patients may not tolerate certain positions or percussion or vibration because of pain.
7. Patients with copious secretions that cannot be coughed out (e.g., those who are not alert or those who have a tracheostomy) should not be put in a compromising situation. Suctioning equipment must be made available.
8. Very obese patients may not tolerate any head-down positions because of increased SOB.

### c. Organize the sequence of drainage positions and treatment techniques

Differences of opinion exist as to the sequence in which the segments should be drained. Some authors prefer an apices-to-bases approach, whereas others lean toward a bases-to-apices pattern. It makes sense to take an apices-to-bases approach for a first treatment when all lobes are to be drained. This pattern gives the patient time to get used to the whole procedure. It may also be safer because the practitioner can evaluate the patient through a sequence of positions that progresses from the least to the most stressful.

If the patient can tolerate all positions without any difficulties, and the lower lobes are the worst in terms of secretions, drain the lower lobes first. If time permits, work up through the middle lobe and lingula to the upper lobes.

### d. Change the postural drainage therapy position based on the patient's response

During treatment, the patient's secretions may be more effectively drained if he or she is repositioned from what would seem to be the ideal angle. The patient's airway anatomy may be different from what is expected. Patients with chronic lung disease such as cystic fibrosis or bronchiectasis often know what positions and angles are best for draining their lungs. Follow their advice if it produces good results.

Some patients cannot tolerate being properly placed because their underlying lung or heart disease is aggravated by the unnatural body position. This is most commonly seen in head-down positions used to drain the lower lobes. Watch for signs of hypoxemia and SOB. The patient may have to be put in a better tolerated but less desirable position. As long as some downward angle to the bronchus exists, mucus will drain. Each patient must be evaluated on an individual basis.

### 7. Stop the treatment if the patient has an adverse reaction to it (NBRC code: IIIF1) [Difficulty: R, Ap, An]

Be prepared to stop treatment if the patient has an adverse reaction. Often this results when a patient is placed into a head-down position. Review Box 10-3 for hazards and complications of postural drainage, percussion, and vibration.

> ### Exam Hint
>
> **B**e prepared to stop treatment if the patient becomes short of breath, becomes hypoxic, develops a headache or dizziness, or needs to cough.

### 8. Postural drainage therapy equipment: percussors and vibrators

#### a. Get the necessary equipment for the procedure (NBRC code: IIA14) [Difficulty: R]

The terms *percussor* and *vibrator* are sometimes used interchangeably. Several manufacturers produce either

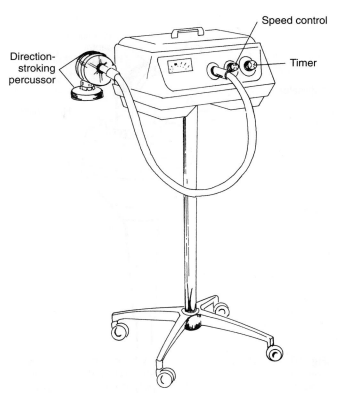

**Fig. 10-14** An electrically powered mechanical percussor/vibrator. *(From Eubanks DH, Bone RC: Comprehensive respiratory care, ed 2, St Louis, 1990, Mosby.)*

electrically or pneumatically powered percussors/vibrators. Some are large enough to be wheeled into the patient's room (Fig. 10-14). Obviously, electrically powered units need a standard electrical outlet for power, and pneumatically powered units need to be plugged into a 50-psi $O_2$ or air source.

Battery-powered pediatric units must be small to accurately focus on the very small target area of the infant's chest. Some practitioners find that an electric toothbrush with padded bristles works very well. Manual percussion of infants can be aided by the use of soft rubber palm cups that are available in several pediatric sizes.

#### b. Put the equipment together and make sure that it works properly (NBRC code: IIA14) [Difficulty: R]

Because various devices are powered by wall electrical output, 50-psi source gas, or batteries, you should check the power source if the device fails to work. Some units have different patient applicators and connectors. These must be fastened properly so that the vibrating action does not cause them to loosen or fall off. For example, the Vibramatic has several patient applicators that must be screwed into the percussion adapter, which is then screwed into the ring adapter (Fig. 10-15).

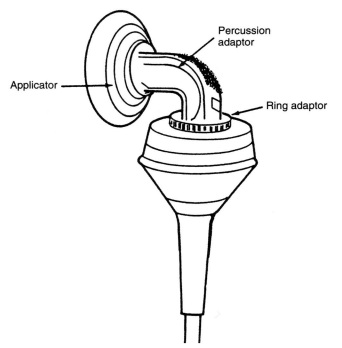

**Fig. 10-15** Right-angle adapter for Vibramatic chest percussor. The percussion adapter must be tightly screwed into the ring adapter, and the various patient applicators must be tightly screwed into the percussion adapter. *(Courtesy of General Physiotherapy, Inc., St Louis, Mo.)*

Some electrically powered units use a rubber belt and different-sized wheels to change gears and produce several vibration rates. Others electrically vary the motor speed to change the vibration rate. Some pneumatically driven units can have their percussion force and rate adjusted.

### c. Troubleshoot any problems with the equipment (NBRC code: IIA14) [Difficulty: R]

Pneumatically powered units would suddenly fail if the high-pressure hose to the wall gas outlet or the $O_2$ tank were to become disconnected. Electrically powered units would fail if the electrical cord should be unplugged or the batteries depleted.

## MODULE B
### Positive expiratory pressure therapy

### 1. Alter the treatment duration and positive expiratory pressure (PEP) therapy techniques as needed (NBRC code: IIIF2e) [Difficulty: R, Ap]

Positive expiratory pressure (PEP) therapy involves having a spontaneously breathing patient exhale against a fixed-orifice resistor to create expiratory pressures between 10 and 20 cm $H_2O$. This therapy is also called *PEP mask therapy* because many pediatric patients use a facemask to deliver the pressure to the airways. Box 10-5 lists indica-

---

- To reduce air trapping in patients with emphysema, bronchitis, and asthma
- To prevent or reverse atelectasis
- To help mobilize retained secretions in patients older than 4 years of age who have cystic fibrosis, chronic bronchitis, bronchiectasis, or bronchiolitis obliterans
- To maximize the delivery of aerosolized medications, such as bronchodilators, to patients receiving bronchial hygiene therapy

---

**BOX 10-6   Relative Contraindications to Positive Expiratory Pressure Therapy**

- Untreated pneumothorax
- Intracranial pressure greater than 20 mm Hg
- Active hemoptysis
- Recent trauma or surgery to the skull, face, mouth, or esophagus
- Patient with asthma attack or acute worsening of chronic obstructive pulmonary disease who cannot tolerate increased work of breathing
- Acute sinusitis or epistaxis
- Tympanic membrane rupture or other known or suspected middle ear pathology
- Nausea

---

tions for PEP therapy. In patients with air trapping because of small-airways disease, PEP therapy acts similarly to pursed-lips breathing to keep the small airways from collapsing. This allows the trapped alveolar gas to be more completely exhaled. Patients with atelectasis or who are at risk for developing atelectasis respond well to PEP therapy. PEP seems to push air through pores of Kohn from open alveoli into adjacent areas of atelectasis to force the alveoli open. Other indications are discussed in the following sections.

Box 10-6 lists relative contraindications to PEP therapy. There are no absolute contraindications. Box 10-7 lists hazards or complications of PEP therapy. These should be weighed against benefits to the patient when the recommendation is made to start PEP therapy. Other considerations include the patient's history of pulmonary disease and the response to postural drainage therapy, ineffective cough to clear retained secretions, and breath sounds and chest radiograph findings of secretions.

PEP therapy has proved effective in helping patients with chronic, copious amounts of secretions, primarily children 4 years of age or older with cystic fibrosis. It also helps patients with chronic bronchitis, bronchiectasis, or bronchiolitis obliterans. Clinical evidence indicates that PEP dilates the small airways so that air is able to get past obstructing secretions. This fills the alveoli and on expiration tends to force secretions into the larger airways for coughing or suctioning out. See Fig. 10-16 for an example of a PEP therapy system.

PEP therapy also seems to increase the effectiveness of inhaled aerosolized bronchodilators. Some PEP systems can be joined with a small-volume nebulizer (SVN) (Fig. 10-17). Slowed exhalation during PEP breathing should promote better deposition of medication in the small airways.

The patient must be old enough to understand instructions and must be able to perform the procedure. Box 10-8 lists the steps to be followed in performing a proper PEP therapy treatment. Be prepared to adjust the expiratory resistance to meet the clinical goal of PEP therapy. Initially, the pressure or resistance to exhalation should be kept low. As training continues, the resistance or pressure the patient breathes against can be increased. Goals are to maintain a PEP of 10 to 20 cm $H_2O$ with an inspiratory:

expiratory (I:E) ratio of about 1:3. If the pressure is too high or the expiratory time too long, the patient will likely become fatigued. If the orifice is too large, the pressure will not be high enough to be of any benefit. The patient will probably become tired if the total treatment time lasts longer than 20 min.

## 2. Coordinate the sequence of therapies to modify bronchial hygiene (NBRC code: IIIF2e) [Difficulty: R, Ap]

Coordinate PEP therapy with effective "huff" cough techniques, PDT, or aerosolized medication delivery. As listed in Box 10-8, PEP breaths should be alternated with huff

---

**BOX 10-7** **Hazards or Complications of Positive Expiratory Pressure Therapy**

- Pulmonary barotrauma
- Increased intracranial pressure
- Myocardial ischemia or decreased venous return to the heart
- Increased work of breathing
- Air swallowing that can lead to vomiting
- Discomfort from mask or skin breakdown from mask pressure
- Claustrophobia

---

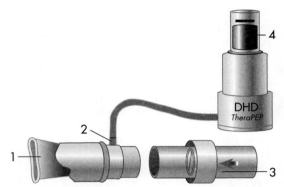

**Fig. 10-16** Drawing of the DHD TheraPEP device. 1, Patient mouthpiece. 2, Hose to connect the mouthpiece to the pressure generator. 3, One-way inlet valve for inspiration. 4, Pressure generator through which the patient exhales to create positive expiratory pressure. *(From Myslinski MJ, Scanlan CL: Bronchial hygiene therapy. In Wilkins RL, Stoller JK, Scanlan CL, editors: Egan's fundamentals of respiratory care, ed 8, St Louis, 2003, Mosby.)*

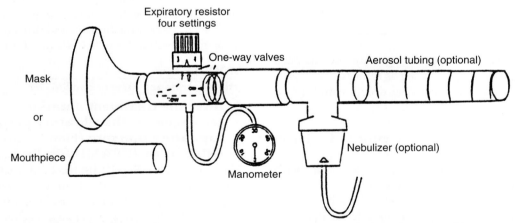

**Fig. 10-17** Positive expiratory pressure (PEP) mask components. The basic PEP assembly necessitates a transparent mask or mouthpiece, an expiratory resistor (this shows the Resistex), and a pressure manometer with connecting oxygen tubing. If a nebulized medication is added, the following are also needed: a small-volume nebulizer with T-piece, oxygen tubing to flowmeter, and large-bore tubing for an aerosol reservoir. *(From Malmeister MJ, Fink JB, Hoffman GL, et al: Positive-expiratory-pressure mask therapy: theoretical and practical considerations and a review of the literature, Respir Care 36:1218, 1991.)*

---

### BOX 10-8   Steps in Performing Positive Expiratory Pressure (PEP) Therapy

1. Put the equipment together as shown in Figs. 10-16 or 10-17.
2. Have the conscious patient sit up straight, rest elbows on a table, and hold the PEP mask comfortably but tightly over the nose and mouth. The patient may use a mouthpiece and noseclips if preferred.
3. The patient should inhale a deeper-than-normal breath, but not to total lung capacity, by using the diaphragm. The unconscious patient will inhale only a tidal volume breath.
4. The conscious patient should exhale to functional residual capacity fast enough to generate 10 to 20 cm $H_2O$ in the manometer. Have the patient look at the pressure manometer to judge how fast to exhale. The unconscious patient will exhale passively but will still benefit from the increased baseline pressure.
5. The patient should have an expiratory time that is about three times longer than the inspiratory time (an inspiratory:expiratory ratio of 1:2 to 1:4 is acceptable). The clinician can accomplish this by changing the expiratory resistor and/or having the patient change the force of exhalation.
6. Between 10 and 20 proper PEP breaths should be performed.
7. The patient should now perform two or three "huff"-type coughing efforts to raise secretions.
8. Repeat steps 2 to 7 between four and eight times (for about 10-20 min) for a full PEP treatment.

Patients in the intensive care unit can perform PEP therapy as often as every hour or as rarely as every 6 hr. They should be reevaluated for treatment effectiveness every 24 hr.

Patients in the acute care or home care setting can perform PEP therapy between two and four times each day. The acute care patient should be reevaluated every 72 hr; the home care patient can be evaluated at longer intervals or when a change in pulmonary status occurs.

---

coughs to clear secretions. Huff coughs are not full, deep coughs; rather, they are performed as follows:

a. Have the patient inhale a slow, deep breath but not to total lung capacity (TLC).
b. Hold in the breath for 1 to 3 sec.
c. Perform several quick, forced exhalations with an open epiglottis.
d. Small children may be taught to say "huff" with each quick exhalation. It may also help to have the young patient perform a "chicken breath" by flapping his or her arms against the sides of the chest during exhalation.

PDT may be used before or after PEP therapy, or it may be alternated with PEP therapy, to help in the removal of secretions. Likewise, aerosolized medications may be inhaled before or simultaneously with PEP therapy. Bronchodilators and mucolytic agents should be very helpful when used with PEP therapy to mobilize secretions. Evaluate sputum for quantity, color, odor, and thickness.

### 3. Stop the treatment if the patient has an adverse reaction to it (NBRC code: IIIF1) [Difficulty: R, Ap, An]

During treatment, ask the patient if he or she feels dyspnea, pain, or chest discomfort. Also, monitor the patient's breath sounds, blood pressure, heart rate, and breathing pattern and rate. Monitor oxygenation by assessing pulse oximetry, mental clarity, and skin color. Be prepared to stop treatment if necessary. Review the contraindications listed in Box 10-6 and the hazards listed in Box 10-7.

### 4. Positive expiratory pressure therapy equipment
   a. **Get the necessary equipment for the procedure (NBRC code: IIA15) [Difficulty: R, Ap]**
   b. **Put the equipment together and make sure that it works properly (NBRC code: IIA15) [Difficulty: R, Ap]**
   c. **Troubleshoot any problems with the equipment (NBRC code: IIA15) [Difficulty: R, Ap]**

As shown in Figs. 10-16 and 10-17, component pieces must be gathered and properly put together. Make sure that all connections are airtight. If a leak is present, the desired PEP goal will not be reached or maintained. In addition, an air leak may be felt or a high-pitched sound may be heard. If a small-volume nebulizer (SVN) is added for aerosolizing medications, ensure that it works properly. Connect the SVN into the system as shown in Fig. 10-17. Add the medication and run a flow of $O_2$ or air through the nebulizer at 4 to 6 L/min (as is customary).

## MODULE C
### High-frequency airway oscillation

### 1. Alter the treatment duration and technique for the vibratory positive expiratory pressure (Flutter valve) devices (NBRC code: IIIF2e) [Difficulty: R, Ap]

The Flutter valve (Fig. 10-18) has been used with patients with cystic fibrosis to help them loosen their secretions. High-frequency oscillations of backpressure on the airway caused by the fluttering steel ball are believed to help dislodge viscous secretions.

Because of the simplicity of this device, both small children and adults can be instructed in its use. The patient is taught to take a deeper-than-usual breath, hold the flutter valve with the cap up, and blow out through the mouthpiece. The exhaled breath pushes the

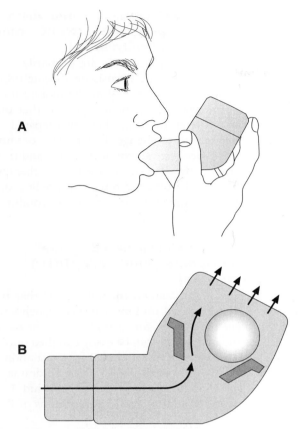

**Fig. 10-18 A,** Patient correctly holding the Flutter valve for an exhalation. **B,** Cross-sectional drawing of the Flutter valve showing how the steel ball is lifted by the patient's exhaled tidal volume. When the ball drops back down, the backpressure is transmitted to the airways. *(From Fink JB, Hess DR: Secretion clearance techniques. In Hess DR, MacIntyre NR, Mishoe SC, et al, editors: Respiratory care principles & practice, Philadelphia, 2002, WB Saunders.)*

ball up in the bowl, air briefly escapes, and the ball falls back down again. When the ball falls back, greater pressure is exerted against the patient's airway. Airway pressure generated during the exhalation varies from 10 to 25 cm $H_2O$, depending on how fast the patient blows out. The rate at which the ball flutters up and down is about 15 Hz (hertz or cycles/sec) and varies with the angle of the bowl.

**2. Coordinate the sequence of therapies to modify bronchial hygiene** (NBRC code: IIIF2e) [Difficulty: R, Ap]

If inhaled bronchodilator or mucolytic medications are ordered for the patient, these should be taken before the flutter valve treatment is undertaken. Typically, the patient repeats the Flutter valve maneuver for 10 to 20 breaths. The patient should then perform two or three huff-type coughs. The cycle of Flutter valve exhalations and huff coughs is repeated four to eight times.

Total treatment time should not be longer than 20 minutes.

**3. Stop the treatment if the patient has an adverse reaction to it** (NBRC code: IIIF1) [Difficulty: R, Ap, An]

It is unlikely that a patient will have an adverse reaction that results from use of the Flutter valve. However, it is possible that some patients will not like the feeling of increased pressure in the lungs. In this case, it may be best to stop the treatment and switch to another method of secretion management.

**4. Vibratory positive expiratory pressure (Flutter) mucus clearance device equipment**
   **a. Get the necessary equipment for the procedure** (NBRC code: IIA16) [Difficulty: R, Ap]
   **b. Put the equipment together and make sure that it works properly** (NBRC code: IIA16) [Difficulty: R, Ap]
   **c. Troubleshoot any problems with the equipment** (NBRC code: IIA16) [Difficulty: R, Ap]

The Flutter valve is a pipe-shaped device with a steel ball that nests loosely inside the bowl. A perforated cap over the bowl keeps the ball from falling out but lets exhaled air escape. Make sure that these are properly assembled as shown in Fig. 10-18. If the ball does not move loosely, it may be stuck because of secretions. In this case, unscrew the cap, take out the ball, and clean out the secretions. Once reassembled, the ball should move loosely within the bowl.

## MODULE D
### Respiratory care plan

**1. Analyze the available information to determine the patient's pathophysiologic state** (NBRC code: IIIH1) [Difficulty: R, Ap, An]

The patient's breath sounds should be auscultated before the treatment is begun to determine which segments are normal or have secretions. Auscultate each segment after treatment and after the patient has coughed. Listen for air moving into formerly silent areas or areas that are cleared of secretions.

Make a recommendation for a chest x-ray examination to find specific areas for PDT. A white shadow on a chest x-ray film over what should be normal lung may indicate areas of atelectasis or infiltrates that can be targeted for treatment. Chest x-ray examinations should be repeated to look for an improvement in the lungs. The resolution may be slow or dramatic, depending on the original problem and how it responds to the various treatments used on it.

**2. Observe the patient for changes in sputum production** (NBRC code: IIIE5) [Difficulty: R, Ap]

See the previous discussion or Chapter 1 as needed.

**3. Auscultate the patient's breath sounds and interpret any changes** (NBRC code: IIIE11) [Difficulty: R, Ap]

See the previous discussion or Chapter 1 as needed.

**4. Determine the appropriateness of the respiratory care plan and recommend modifications when indicated**

**a. Review the interdisciplinary patient and family care plan** (NBRC code: IIIH2b) [Difficulty: R, Ap]

**b. Review the planned therapy to establish the therapeutic plan** (NBRC code: IIIH2a) [Difficulty: R, Ap]

**c. Determine the appropriateness of the prescribed therapy and goals for the patient's pathophysiologic state** (NBRC code: IIIH3) [Difficulty: R, Ap, An]

**d. Recommend changes in the therapeutic plan if supportive data exist** (NBRC code: IIIH4) [Difficulty: R, Ap]

The AARC clinical practice guideline (1991) recommends that the following be evaluated to determine if postural drainage therapy is needed:

1. PDT is usually not indicated if an optimally hydrated patient is coughing out less than 25 mL/day with the procedure.

2. A dehydrated patient should have apparently ineffective PDT continued for at least 24 hr after the patient has been rehydrated. The combination of rehydration and PDT may help to mobilize previously thick secretions.

3. PDT is not indicated in a patient who produces more than 30 mL of secretions/day if the treatments do not increase sputum production. The patient is already able to effectively cough out the sputum.

For any of the previously discussed procedures, be prepared to measure the patient's blood pressure, heart rate, and respiratory rate before, during, and after a change in therapy. Minor changes (less than 20%) can be expected. The patient's oxygenation should improve as secretions and mucus plugs are removed and atelectatic areas open. The patient's breath sounds should be auscultated before and after any treatment procedure. Listen for air moving into formerly silent areas and for secretions that are being cleared.

Ask the patient how he or she feels before, during, and after the treatment. PDT should not be performed for at least 1 hr after a patient has eaten to minimize the chances of nausea from the head-down positions.

**e. Conduct patient education and disease management programs** (NBRC code: IIIG2a, IIIA1) [Difficulty: R, Ap]

The previously discussed procedures are primarily used with patients who have cystic fibrosis or chronic bronchitis. All have been shown to help in the mobilization of secretions. However, each patient may find that one procedure works better than another. Be prepared to make recommendations to change the type of procedure and how each procedure is conducted. In addition, other respiratory care procedures (e.g., $O_2$ therapy) and inhaled bronchodilators and mucolytic medications may have to be modified as the patient's condition warrants.

**5. Discontinue treatment based on the patient's response** (NBRC code: IIIG1f) [Difficulty: R, Ap]

Review the previous discussion for indications that the patient has recovered and no longer needs bronchopulmonary hygiene procedures, for example, when the secretions have decreased and/or can be easily coughed out by the patient. Review Boxes 10-2 and 10-3 for contraindications and hazards/complications of postural drainage, percussion, and vibration. Review Boxes 10-6 and 10-7 for contraindications and hazards/complications of PEP therapy.

## BIBLIOGRAPHY

American Association for Respiratory Care: Clinical practice guideline: directed cough, *Respir Care* 38:495, 1993.

American Association for Respiratory Care: Clinical practice guideline: postural drainage therapy, *Respir Care* 36:1418, 1991.

American Association for Respiratory Care: Clinical practice guideline: use of positive airway pressure adjuncts to bronchial hygiene therapy, *Respir Care* 38:516, 1993.

Branson RD, Hess DR, Chatburn RL: *Respiratory care equipment*, ed 2, Philadelphia, 1999, Lippincott Williams & Wilkins.

Cairo JM: Lung expansion devices. In Cairo JM, Pilbeam SP, editors: *Mosby's respiratory care equipment*, ed 7, St Louis, 2004, Mosby.

Campbell TC, Ferguson N, McKinlay RGC: The use of a simple self-administered method of positive expiratory pressure (PEP) in chest physiotherapy after abdominal surgery, *Physiotherapy* 72:498, 1986.

Eid N, Buchheit J, Neuling M, et al: Chest physiotherapy in review, *Respir Care* 36:270, 1991.

Eubanks DH, Bone RC: *Comprehensive respiratory care*, ed 2, St Louis, 1990, Mosby.

Fink JB: Bronchial hygiene therapy and lung expansion. In Fink JB, Hunt GE, editors: *Clinical practice in respiratory care*, Philadelphia, 1999, Lippincott-Raven.

Fink JB: Volume expansion therapy. In Burton GC, Hodgkin JE, Ward JJ, editors: *Respiratory care: a guide to clinical practice*, ed 4, Philadelphia, 1997, Lippincott-Raven.

Fink JB, Hess DR: Secretion clearance techniques. In Hess DR, MacIntyre NR, Mishoe SC, et al, editors: *Respiratory care principles & practice*, Philadelphia, 2002, WB Saunders.

Frownfelter DL: Chest physical therapy and airway care. In Barnes TA, editor: *Core textbook of respiratory care practice*, ed 2, St Louis, 1994, Mosby.

Hess DR, Branson RD: Chest physiotherapy, incentive spirometry, intermittent positive-pressure breathing, secretion clearance, and inspiratory muscle training. In Branson RD, Hess DR, Chatburn RL, editors: *Respiratory care equipment*, ed 2, Philadelphia, 1999, Lippincott Williams & Wilkins.

Hill KV: Bronchial hygiene therapy. In Aloan CA, Hill TV, editors: *Respiratory care of the newborn and child*, ed 2, Philadelphia, 1997, Lippincott-Raven.

Hoffman GL, Cohen NH: Positive expiratory pressure therapy, *NBRC Horizons* 19:1, 1993.

Johnson NT, Pierson DJ: The spectrum of pulmonary atelectasis: pathophysiology, diagnosis, and therapy, *Respir Care* 31(11): 1107, 1986.

Malmeister MJ, Fink JB, Hoffman GL: Positive-expiratory-pressure mask therapy: theoretical and practical considerations and a review of the literature, *Respir Care* 36:1218, 1991.

Myslinski MJ, Scanlan CL: Bronchial hygiene therapy. In Wilkins RL, Stoller JK, Scanlan CL, editors: *Egan's fundamentals of respiratory care*, ed 8, St Louis, 2003, Mosby.

Oberwaldner PT, Evans JC, Zach MS: Forced expirations against a variable resistance: a new chest physiotherapy method in cystic fibrosis, *Pediatr Pulmonol* 2:358, 1986.

Rutkowski JA: Pulmonary hygiene and chest physical therapy. In Wyka KA, Mathews PJ, Clark WF, editors: *Foundations of Respiratory Care*, Albany, 2002, Delmar.

Scott AA, Koff PB: Airway care and chest physiotherapy. In Koff PB, Eitzman D, Neu J, editors: *Neonatal and pediatric respiratory care*, ed 2, St Louis, 1993, Mosby.

Shapiro BA, Kacmarek RM, Cane RD, et al, editors: *Clinical application of respiratory care*, ed 4, St. Louis, 1991, Mosby.

Sobush DC, Hilling L, Southorn PA: Bronchial hygiene therapy. In Burton GC, Hodgkin JE, Ward JJ, editors: *Respiratory care: a guide to clinical practice*, ed 4, Philadelphia, 1997, Lippincott-Raven.

White GC: *Equipment theory for respiratory care*, ed 3, Albany, NY, 1999, Delmar.

Wojciechowski WV: Incentive spirometers, secretion evacuation devices, and inspiratory muscle training devices. In Barnes TA, editor: *Core textbook of respiratory care practice*, ed 2, St Louis, 1994, Mosby.

## SELF-STUDY QUESTIONS

1. A 15-year-old patient with cystic fibrosis has copious amounts of secretions. She cannot tolerate PDT because she gets a headache when tipped head-down. Aerosolized bronchodilators and mucolytic agents are ordered every 4 hr by SVN. What else would you recommend?
   A. Add incentive spirometry.
   B. Give the aerosolized medications by IPPB therapy.
   C. Add PEP therapy.
   D. Modify the PDT positions so that the head is not lower than the patient's body.

2. To get the best patient results, manual percussion should be performed with
   I. The hand cupped
   II. A tight, fixed-wrist position
   III. The elbows relaxed
   IV. The hand flat
   V. The wrist relaxed
   A. III, IV, and V
   B. II, III, and IV
   C. II and IV
   D. I, III, and V

3. How should vibration be done as part of PDT?
   I. On inspiration
   II. At a rate of 20 to 30 cycles/sec
   III. On expiration
   IV. At a rate of 3 cycles/sec
   V. Throughout the breathing cycle
   A. II and IV
   B. I and IV
   C. III and IV
   D. IV and V

4. When a patient's chart is reviewed, it is important to look for contraindications to PDT. They would include all of the following EXCEPT:
   A. Increased intracranial pressure in a patient with a recent head injury
   B. Recent stroke
   C. Small vital capacity in a bedridden patient
   D. The patient has just eaten

5. A stroke patient has been admitted and is in a coma and unable to care for himself. The physician is concerned that he may develop atelectasis and pneumonia. What would you recommend to help prevent these problems?
   A. Regular turning from side to side
   B. PEP therapy
   C. IPPB
   D. CPAP

6. You receive an order to perform postural drainage, percussion, and vibration on a patient. No segments are specified. On reviewing the chest x-ray film, you notice infiltrates in the lower right lung field. You would proceed to treat the following segments:
    I. Apical
    II. Lateral basal
    III. Superior
    IV. Medial
    V. Posterior basal
    A. II and V
    B. III, IV, and V
    C. I and IV
    D. II, III, and V

7. For drainage of the superior and inferior lingular segments, the patient should be positioned
    I. With the foot of the bed elevated 14 inches
    II. One-fourth turn up from the front-down position on the bed
    III. One-fourth turn up from the back-down position on the bed
    IV. With the foot of the bed elevated 30 degrees
    V. Flat on his or her back
    A. I and III
    B. IV and V
    C. I and II
    D. I and V

8. All of the following are contraindications to percussion and vibration EXCEPT:
    A. Performing the procedure over the kidneys
    B. Mobilizing large amounts of secretions
    C. Performing the procedure over bare skin
    D. Performing the procedure over or near a surgical site

9. A patient is positioned on her left side with the foot of the bed raised 18 inches. She would be draining which lung segment?
    A. Anterior basal
    B. Superior
    C. Lateral and medial lingular
    D. Posterior basal

10. Your patient has been ordered to start PEP therapy. During the initial instruction and patient practice, you notice that the pressure is 25 cm $H_2O$ and the patient's I : E ratio is 1 : 5. You would proceed to
    A. Adjust the PEP device to have the patient exhale through a larger hole
    B. Have the patient continue but coach him to exhale faster
    C. Adjust the PEP device to have the patient exhale through a smaller hole
    D. Add a bronchodilator medication to the PEP device

11. When you are reviewing a patient's chart, it is important to look for indications for postural drainage. These would include all of the following EXCEPT:
    A. A patient with bronchiectasis and retained secretions
    B. A patient with cystic fibrosis who has retained secretions
    C. Draining of an empyema
    D. Removal of an aspirated foreign body

12. You receive an order to perform postural drainage, percussion, and vibration on a 23-year-old female patient. The lateral and medial segments of the right middle lobe are among those that need to be treated. You would proceed to
    A. Drain, percuss, and vibrate the segments
    B. Drain and vibrate the segments
    C. Drain but not percuss or vibrate those segments
    D. Drain and use a mechanical percussor

13. You are working with a patient who begins to cough up blood after being positioned for drainage of the superior segment of the left lower lobe. Percussion was provided with a mechanical device. After the patient has coughed out 50 mL of blood, you would recommend the following as the best action:
    A. Continue the treatment because the patient has not lost a great deal of blood.
    B. Continue the treatment on only the upper and middle lobes.
    C. Discontinue the treatment, sit the patient up, and call the physician.
    D. Continue the treatment with manual percussion only.

14. A patient with bilateral pneumonia is positioned for drainage of the lateral and medial segments of her right middle lobe. After 5 min in this position, the patient complains of SOB. The electrocardiogram shows the patient to be having premature ventricular contractions. The most likely cause of this is
    A. Hypoxemia
    B. A full stomach that is causing vagal stimulation
    C. Increased intracranial pressure
    D. Increased venous return to the heart

15. You are using a pneumatically powered mechanical percussor on a patient receiving PDT. The unit is powered by an E-cylinder of $O_2$ because piped-in $O_2$ is unavailable. After a few minutes of operation, you notice that the percussor begins to slow down and then stops. What would you do?
    A. Switch to an electrically powered percussor.
    B. Make sure the cylinder is completely turned on.
    C. Check the unit's batteries.
    D. Check the electrical cord.

16. PDT (with percussion and vibration) has been performed for 5 days on a cooperative patient with bronchiectasis. During that time, he has been treated with antibiotics and well fed and hydrated. He has produced a total of 20 mL of sputum during the past 24 hr. What would you recommend?
    A. Continue the current treatment program for 48 hr and evaluate the patient again.
    B. Add ultrasonic nebulizer treatments to the PDT to better liquefy the secretions.
    C. Add nasotracheal suctioning to the PDT to remove the secretions.
    D. Discontinue the PDT and follow the patient's progress.

## ANSWER KEY AND RATIONALE

1. **C.** PEP therapy has been shown to help in mobilizing secretions. In addition, some PEP units can be coupled with an SVN to more efficiently deliver the medication. Incentive spirometry does not help with secretion mobilization or medication delivery. IPPB *may* help with medication delivery if the patient cannot properly perform the SVN treatment. However, no indication of this problem exists. The benefits of improperly positioning a patient for PDT are questionable.

2. **D.** Manual percussion should be performed with a cupped hand and relaxed wrist and elbow joints.

3. **C.** Vibration should be performed only on expiration. Most people cannot vibrate at a faster rate than about 3 cycles/second.

4. **C.** There is no reason that a bedridden patient with a small vital capacity cannot have PDT. Head-down positions place a patient with a recent stroke or known increased intracranial pressure at risk for further brain damage. A patient who has just eaten should not be placed in a head-down position because of the risk of vomiting.

5. **A.** Regular turning is an easy and inexpensive way for the patient to alter his breathing pattern and to move the $V_T$ into different lung segments. This helps to prevent atelectasis. IPPB may be needed, but only after regular turning has been shown to be ineffective. CPAP is not indicated for the treatment of simple atelectasis from inactivity.

6. **D.** The lateral basal, superior, and posterior basal segments are all located in the right lower lobe where the infiltrates are located. The apical segment is located in the upper lobe, and the medial segment is located in the middle lobe. Review Fig. 10-1.

7. **A.** Review Fig. 10-7 and the related discussion for this position.

8. **B.** All references indicate that percussion and vibration are beneficial in mobilizing large quantities of secretions. Review Box 10-2 for contraindications for percussion and vibration.

9. **A.** Review Fig. 10-4 and the related discussion for the position recommended to drain the anterior basal segment of the right lower lobe.

10. **A.** When the patient exhales through a larger hole, the pressure should decrease and the expiratory time should shorten. Review Box 10-8 for the steps to be followed in the PEP therapy procedure. Having the patient exhale faster or exhale through a smaller hole increases the pressure and expiratory time. A bronchodilator medication has not been ordered for the patient.

11. **C.** Because an empyema is a collection of pus in the pleural cavity, it cannot be drained through postural drainage. The other options are all indications for postural drainage. See Box 10-1 for the indications.

12. **C.** Neither manual nor mechanical percussion or vibration should be performed over female breast tissue.

13. **C.** Hemoptysis indicates pulmonary trauma. The treatment should be stopped and the physician notified. No further treatment should be done until after the patient is assessed, and it is found safe to proceed with the treatment.

14. **A.** Hypoxemia is the only possibility for the problem from among those listed. A full stomach does not cause vagal stimulation that results in PVCs. The patient's symptoms of SOB and PVCs do not correspond with increased intracranial pressure or increased venous return to the heart.

15. **A.** Switching to an electrically powered percussor is the only workable option from among those provided. A pneumatically powered percussor does not have batteries or an electrical cord. The way that the percussor gradually lost function indicates that the tank ran out of compressed $O_2$ with which to run the unit.

16. **D.** According to the AARC clinical practice guideline (1991), PDT should be discontinued because the patient is able to cough out the secretions with no other assistance. Continuing the treatment and adding procedures is not necessary and may add to the patient's costs.

# 11 Cardiac Monitoring and Cardiopulmonary Resuscitation

A review of the most recent Entry Level Examinations has shown an average of 6 questions (4% of the exam) that cover cardiac monitoring and CPR issues.

## MODULE A
### Cardiac monitoring

1. **Electrocardiography equipment**
   a. **Cardiac electrodes**
      1. **Get the necessary equipment for the procedure** (NBRC code: IIA19) [Difficulty: R, Ap]
      2. **Put the equipment together and make sure that it works properly** (NBRC code: IIA19) [Difficulty: R]

Cardiac electrodes, or leads, pick up the electrical signal from a heart contraction and conduct it to the electrocardiograph (ECG) machine. Several different types of cardiac electrodes are distinguished by their placement on the patient and how long they are used.

The first type is used for hours or days for basic rhythm monitoring or Holter monitoring. They are usually called *chest leads*, *precordial leads*, or *chest electrodes* and consist of four parts: (1) a conducting wire coated with an electrically neutral plastic, (2) an adapter at one end of the wire that plugs into the ECG machine, (3) a different adapter at the opposite end of the wire that attaches to a patient electrode, and (4) the patient electrode (Fig. 11-1). Conducting jelly is added to the surface of the electrode to reduce the skin's resistance to the heart's electrical signal. An adhesive ring holds the electrode tightly to the skin. The conducting wire snaps or clips onto the back of the electrode. Typically, three chest leads are used for rhythm monitoring. Holter monitoring, discussed later in this chapter, involves the use of long-term chest leads and limb leads.

The second type of cardiac electrode is often used for only a few minutes during a diagnostic ECG. Two sets of electrodes are used for different placements. Limb leads come as a group of four, with one for each limb (Fig. 11-2). Chest leads come in a group of six and are placed on the chest in the positions shown in Fig. 11-3. Long-term chest leads need to be used for a Holter monitor. A conducting and adhesive jelly is used to reduce the skin's resistance and hold the lead in place. The limb leads are longer and may need to be held in place by a rubber strap. With all types of cardiac leads, bad skin contact, dried conducting jelly, or a disconnected wire causes a distorted or absent electrical signal.

3. **Troubleshoot any problems with the equipment** (NBRC code: IIA19) [Difficulty: R]

Clinical experience is important in the performance of a diagnostic ECG. Improper placement of the chest or limb leads can easily result in a misleading ECG tracing and a misdiagnosis. For example, reversing the arm leads causes the QRS to be reversed in lead I. Technical errors in grounding the patient and not keeping the patient still during the ECG also result in useless tracings because of electrical interference and an unstable baseline.

   b. **Electrocardiograph**
      1. **Get the necessary equipment for the procedure** (NBRC code: IIA19) [Difficulty: R]
      2. **Put the equipment together and make sure that it works properly** (NBRC code: IIA19) [Difficulty: R]

*Twelve-lead ECG test for diagnostic purposes.* A 12-lead test requires an ECG machine that is capable of receiving electrical input from the four limb leads and the six chest leads (see Figs. 11-2 and 11-3). The operator can manually select the combinations needed to get the 12 different combinations for a 12-lead ECG tracing, or they can be selected automatically. The various ECG combinations are printed out on ECG paper. Modern units also store the patient's information on a self-contained computer.

*Basic bedside rhythm monitoring.* A bedside rhythm monitoring unit usually receives input from only three or four chest leads (see Fig. 11-1). This collective electrical signal is sent to an oscilloscope (video display terminal) for a real-time display of the patient's rhythm. Electrocardiographs have several additional features. They continuously display the patient's heart rate, and they offer the feature of high and low heart rate alarm settings that can be set. If the high or low setting is reached, an audible and

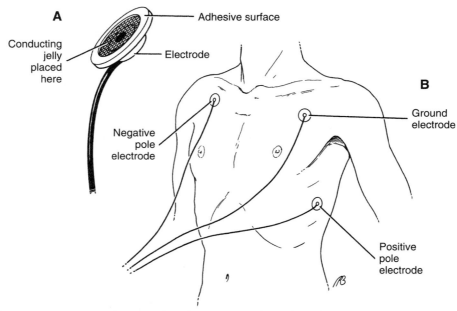

**Fig. 11-1 A,** Features of a prepackaged monitoring electrode or lead. **B,** Standard chest electrode placements for lead II monitoring. This causes the traditional ECG waveform with upright P, QRS, and T waves. (*Note:* The electrodes are often labeled as right arm instead of negative pole, left arm instead of ground electrode, and left leg instead of positive electrode.) (*From Eubanks DH, Bone RC: Comprehensive respiratory care, ed 2, St Louis, 1990, Mosby.*)

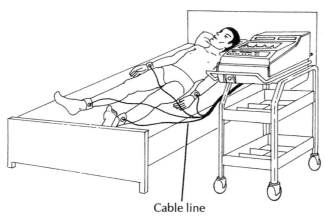

**Fig. 11-2** Limb electrodes or leads properly placed on all four of the patient's limbs. Make sure that the right leg lead is placed on the right leg, the right arm lead is placed on the right arm, and so forth. The electrode cables are then plugged into the electrocardiograph (ECG) machine to record the ECG tracings. (*From Eubanks DH, Bone RC: Comprehensive respiratory care, ed 2, St Louis, 1990, Mosby.*)

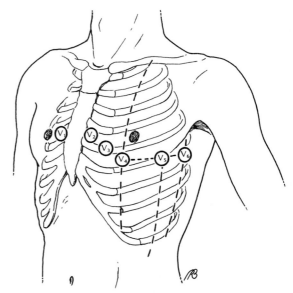

**Fig. 11-3** Proper placement of the six chest leads. (See Table 11-1 for location descriptions.) (*From Eubanks DH, Bone RC: Comprehensive respiratory care, ed 2, St Louis, 1990, Mosby.*)

visual alarm is triggered. The patient's heart rhythm can be recorded on ECG paper manually by pushing of a "record" button, or automatically when an alarm setting is reached. These units are often mounted at the patient's bedside in the intensive care unit.

***Cardiopulmonary resuscitation cart.*** A cardiopulmonary resuscitation (CPR) "crash" cart has an electrocardio-

graph mounted on it with the additional feature that it is connected to the defibrillator. This allows for synchronous defibrillation (cardioversion). It has other features as well that are similar to those of bedside rhythm monitoring units. Portable versions of these units, which are used when the patient must be transported, operate on

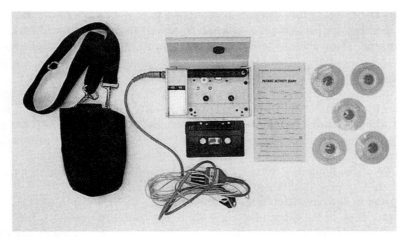

**Fig. 11-4** Holter monitoring system for ambulatory electrocardiography. *(From Pagana K, Pagana TJ: Mosby's manual of diagnostic and laboratory tests, St Louis, 1998, Mosby.)*

batteries when they are unplugged from the wall electrical outlet.

***Holter monitoring.*** Holter monitoring involves recording a patient's complete ECG for 1 to 3 days through the use of a portable, battery-powered monitor. In addition, the patient keeps a diary of any episodes of symptoms such as chest pain or dyspnea. The whole system includes the recording device, magnetic tape to record the patient's ECG, a set of chest leads (and limb leads if needed), a carrying bag for the recording device, and a patient activity diary (Fig. 11-4).

### 3. Troubleshoot any problems with the equipment (NBRC code: IIA19) [Difficulty: R]

Successful ECG monitoring necessitates that the correct electrodes be chosen, put together properly, attached to the patient as indicated, and connected to the needed electrocardiograph machine. Any errors cause a distorted or absent electrical signal. Recheck all patient electrodes and wire connections if a problem is seen.

## 2. Perform an electrocardiogram (NBRC code: IB7a) [Difficulty: R]

An electrocardiogram (ECG or EKG) test is indicated if the patient is suspected of having cardiac problems. Symptoms such as syncope, angina pectoris, sudden crushing chest pain, shortness of breath (SOB), or unstable heart rate and blood pressure point to a heart problem. An ECG test is indicated to document the nature of the cardiac problem or to rule out the heart as a source of the symptoms.

A patient who has been admitted for a suspected myocardial infarction (MI) or another serious cardiac condition probably has had an ECG test performed. Review the interpretation report to find out if a cardiac problem exists. If the patient did have an MI, he or she will have

| TABLE 11-1 | Standard Electrocardiogram Leads | | |
|---|---|---|---|
| | **Leads** | **Positive electrode** | **Negative electrode** |
| Bipolar | I | Left arm | and Right arm |
| | II | Left leg | and Right arm |
| | III | Left leg | and Left arm |
| Unipolar | aV$_R$ | Right arm | |
| | aV$_L$ | Left arm | Central |
| | aV$_F$ | Left leg | terminal* |
| Precordial | V$_1$ | Right of sternum in 4th intercostal space (4th ICS) | |
| | V$_2$ | Left of sternum in 4th ICS | Central terminal* |
| | V$_3$ | Midway between V$_2$ and V$_4$ | |
| | V$_4$ | Midclavicular line in 5th ICS | |
| | V$_5$ | Midway between V$_4$ and V$_6$ | |
| | V$_6$ | Lateral chest in 5th ICS | |

From Phillips RE, Feeney MK: The cardiac rhythms: a systematic approach to interpretation, ed 3, Philadelphia, 1990, WB Saunders. *ICS,* Intercostal space.
*The *central terminal* is a combination of electrode potentials that produces a summation effect. This serves as the single negative or *indifferent* electrode. The specific combination of electrodes for each lead is automatically determined in the lead selector switch.

had a series of ECG tests performed to follow its progress and patient response to treatment.

In any of these situations, a 12-lead ECG must be performed to determine the patient's cardiac diagnosis. This test involves the use of an electrocardiograph with heat-sensitive ECG recording paper, four limb leads, and six chest leads (see Figs. 11-2 and 11-3). Table 11-1 describes the locations of the leads and the positive and negative electrode combinations that are used to record the heart's electrical signal through the 12 different leads. Each lead records the heart's electrical activity from a unique position in relation to the heart. These 12 leads give the physician a three-dimensional impression of how the cardiac conduction system and myocardium are functioning. Abnormal functioning can be diagnosed. Review the normal anatomy and physiology of the heart and its conduction system if necessary.

Holter monitoring is done to diagnose noncritical patients with a suspected cardiac problem. Because the patient will be mobile for at least a day, the limb leads are placed on the upper and lower chest areas. Chest leads are placed normally. A tight undershirt or netlike dressing should be worn to keep the leads in place. The patient cannot bathe while the leads are on.

Emergency ECG monitoring is done on any patient with a serious cardiopulmonary problem. If the possibility exists that the patient will experience serious changes in heart rate or rhythm, he or she should be continuously monitored. In this case, bedside rhythm monitoring should be used. The unit should have an oscilloscope for viewing the rhythm and additional features for counting the heart rate, setting high and low heart rate alarms, and recording the rhythm on standard ECG paper for a permanent record.

The most common chest electrode pattern used for rhythm monitoring is called *lead II*. The three chest electrodes are placed as shown in Fig. 11-1, *B*. The negative (right arm or RA) electrode is on the right upper chest. The positive (left leg or LL) electrode is placed on the left lateral chest. The ground (left arm or LA) electrode is placed on the left upper chest. With this electrode configuration, known as Einthoven's triangle, the heart's electrical signal is followed as it flows from the right atrium to the left ventricle. This results in a so-called normal ECG tracing with upright P, R, and T waves. (See Module D for examples of normal and abnormal ECG tracings.)

## MODULE B
### Cardiopulmonary resuscitation equipment

### 1. Manual resuscitator (bag-valve)

#### a. Get the necessary equipment for the procedure (NBRC code: IIA5) [Difficulty: R, Ap]

The first consideration in the decision about which manual resuscitator to select is the size of the patient. Although the volume of the reservoir bag and the tidal volume ($V_T$) expelled from it vary among the types of bags, three basic sizes exist. An infant or newborn unit typically has a reservoir bag volume of about 250 mL. A pediatric unit usually has a reservoir bag volume of about 250 to 500 mL. An adult unit typically has a reservoir bag volume of 1500 to 2000 mL. In addition to all of these reusable units, a number of disposable units are thrown away after one patient use. They also come in comparable infant, pediatric, and adult reservoir bag volumes. The standard bag connector fits the 15-mm adapter on any endotracheal tube (see Fig. 12-18).

If the patient has not had an endotracheal tube inserted, a patient mask must be connected to the resuscitation bag (Fig. 11-5). These masks are available in a variety of styles in newborn, pediatric, and adult sizes to fit the patient's face. The standard bag connector fits into the mask. When the facemask is attached, some practitioners refer to the entire unit as a bag-valve-mask (or BVM), as shown in Fig. 11-5.

Any resuscitation bag should deliver 100% $O_2$ at the flow rate recommended by the manufacturer (usually no more than 15 L/min). An $O_2$ reservoir system must be added to the basic unit for this percentage to be achieved. The valve to the patient must be clearable within 20 sec if it becomes fouled by vomitus, sputum, or blood. Neonatal and pediatric units must have a pressure-release (pop-off) valve that opens at 40 cm $H_2O$ pressure. The pressure may be adjustable. If an adult unit has a pressure-release valve, it must have an override system that is easy to operate.

#### b. Put the equipment together and make sure that it works properly (NBRC code: IIA5) [Difficulty: R, Ap]

Fig. 11-5 shows line drawings of a complete set of Laerdal infant, pediatric, and adult manual resuscitators. The following steps should be taken when the function of a manual resuscitator is evaluated:

1. Squeeze and release the bag to see if the non-rebreathing valve and air/$O_2$ reservoir intake valve open and close properly.
2. Feel the air as it leaves the outlet port of the non-rebreathing valve when the bag is squeezed.
3. Occlude the outlet port and squeeze the bag. No gas should leak out; if present, the pop-off valve should open at the correct pressure.
4. The facemask should fit onto the 22-mm outer diameter (OD) fitting, and its cushion should be properly inflated.

#### c. Toubleshoot any problems with the equipment (NBRC code: IIA5) [Difficulty: R, Ap]

Check for a reversed or improperly seated one-way valve if the gas does not enter or exit the unit as it should. In clinical use, mucus, vomitus, and blood can foul the non-rebreathing valve system and must be cleared within 20 sec. Do this by disconnecting the unit from the patient, aiming the adapter into a neutral area, and squeezing the bag to blow out the obstruction. Replace a unit that cannot be promptly cleared.

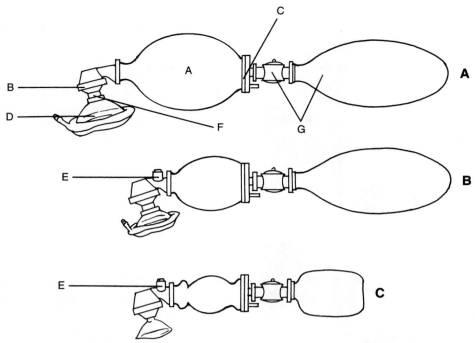

**Fig. 11-5 A,** Adult Laerdal resuscitator; **B,** Pediatric Laerdal resuscitator; **C,** Infant Laerdal resuscitator. These features are found on all modern units: *A,* Self-filling reservoir bag; *B,* Exhalation valve that does not jam at an oxygen flow of 15 L/min or in subfreezing temperatures (it must be clearable of debris within 20 sec); *C,* Intake valve for addition of room air or supplemental O₂ into the reservoir bag; *D,* Transparent mask that easily conforms to the patient's face; *E,* Pressure-relief (pop-off) valve set to open at 40 cm H₂O; *F,* Standard 15-mm inner diameter/22-mm outer diameter connector for the endotracheal tube or facemask; *G,* Oxygen enrichment/reservoir system. In addition, some units have an adjustable positive end-expiratory valve (not shown) attached to the exhalation valve. *(From Eubanks DH, Bone RC: Comprehensive respiratory care, ed 2, St Louis, 1990, Mosby.)*

## 2. Mouth-to-valve mask resuscitator

### a. Get the necessary equipment for the procedure (NBRC code: IIA5) [Difficulty: R, Ap]

The following considerations are important when the best device for the victim is selected:

a. The mask must fit the victim's face to prevent air leaks. Infant, child, and adult sizes should be available.

b. The mouthpiece should be designed to fit only one way into the mask. Some units include a short length of aerosol tubing between the mouthpiece and the mask for greater flexibility.

c. The one-way (nonrebreathing) valve should be designed to ensure that all of the rescuer's breath is directed into the victim and the victim's exhaled breath is vented to room air rather than back at the rescuer. Some units include a bacteria filter in the one-way valve between the rescuer and the victim.

d. It should be possible to add supplemental O₂ through a T-piece or a nipple on the mask. This is important for hospital or ambulance use. If a T-piece is added, it must be designed to easily fit between the mouthpiece and the facemask. An O₂ administration nipple should have a cap over it when it is not in use to prevent leakage of the delivered breath.

### b. Put the equipment together and make sure that it works properly (NBRC code: IIA5) [Difficulty: R, Ap]

Mouth-to-valve mask resuscitators are relatively simple devices. Most have only two or three pieces: facemask, mouthpiece with a one-way valve, and possibly an O₂ T-piece (Fig. 11-6). The "male" and "female" connections are designed to fit together in only one way. When they are properly assembled, no air leaks should occur when breath is delivered to the victim.

### c. Troubleshoot any problems with the equipment (NBRC code: IIA5) [Difficulty: R, Ap]

If the breath cannot be delivered, check the one-way valve to make sure that it has not been put together backward. Reverse it, if necessary, and ventilate the victim's airway.

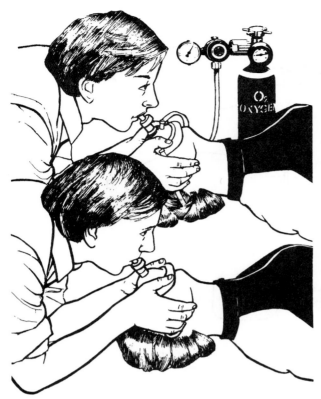

**Fig. 11-6** Proper positioning for use of a mouth-to-valve mask resuscitator. The top rescuer has added supplemental oxygen to the device. The bottom rescuer is ventilating without the use of added oxygen. *(Courtesy of Laerdal Medical Corporation, Wappingers Falls, NY.)*

Keep the $O_2$ nipple on the mask or the T-piece capped off if not in use. Air will leak out during the delivered breath if the cap is left off the nipple.

---

**Exam Hint**

**U**sually, an examination question is included that deals with a malfunctioning resuscitation bag or mouth-to-valve resuscitator. Know how to identify the problem (you are bagging and the patient's chest is not rising) and how to fix it.

---

**Exam Hint**

**A** patient should have an endotracheal tube placed as soon as possible during a CPR attempt. Then, a manual resuscitation bag should be attached to it for ventilation. If the patient is not intubated, either a mask and manual resuscitator or a mouth-to-mask resuscitator can be used for ventilation. A gas-powered pneumatic (demand-valve) resuscitator should not be used.

---

## MODULE C
### Perform cardiopulmonary resuscitation (CPR) and related functions

In 2000, the American Heart Association released revised CPR guidelines that differentiated between what the lay public would be taught to do and what healthcare providers would do during a resuscitation attempt. The following discussion on CPR efforts summarizes a healthcare provider's activities. See the Bibliography listing at the end of this chapter for references that provide the full guidelines.

### 1. Basic cardiac life support (NBRC code: III I1a) [Difficulty: R, Ap]

The key steps for basic cardiac life support (BCLS) include the following:

#### a. Establish that the patient is unresponsive and needs cardiopulmonary resuscitation

Observing a patient who *appears* to be dead does not prove that the patient needs CPR. Clinical death must be proved before CPR is begun. Adults should be tapped or gently shaken while the rescuer shouts, "Are you okay?" Infants should have the bottoms of their feet gently slapped while the rescuer shouts, "Wake up!" The rescuer can also clap his or her hands together loudly to wake a sleeping infant. CPR should never be started on a person who does not need it.

#### b. Call out for help

Call out for help if the victim does not respond to any attempts at arousal. The second rescuer should be told to call in the cardiac arrest team. Many hospitals have a cardiac arrest button in each patient's room. If this is the case, the first rescuer can push the button while calling out for help. Dial 911 if the victim is found at home.

#### c. Open the airway

The head-tilt/chin-lift maneuver is the procedure of choice for opening the airway of all victims except for those with a known or suspected cervical (neck) spine injury. The victim is gently positioned on his or her back. In an adult, the head is firmly pushed back with one hand, and the jaw is pulled upward with the fingers of the other hand (Fig. 11-7). In an infant, it is not necessary to tilt the head back beyond a neutral position. Children may need to have the head pushed back slightly beyond neutral.

The jaw-thrust maneuver is the procedure of choice for opening the airway of all victims with a known or suspected cervical spine injury. The rescuer's elbows are rested on the ground, and the hands are placed on either side of the victim's jaw. Lifting of the jaw usually opens

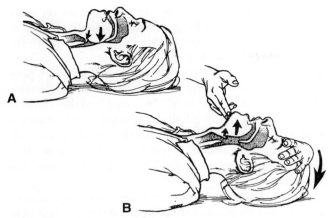

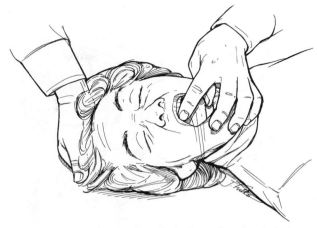

**Fig. 11-7** Opening the adult airway. **A,** Airway obstruction produced by the tongue and epiglottis. **B,** Relief by head-tilt/chin-lift method. *(From Standards and guidelines for cardiopulmonary resuscitation [CPR] and emergency cardiac care [ECC], JAMA 268:2186, 1992.)*

**Fig. 11-9** The cross-finger method of opening the victim's mouth to look for an obstruction. *(From Watson MA: Cardiopulmonary resuscitation. In Barnes TA, editor: Respiratory care practice, Chicago, 1988, Mosby.)*

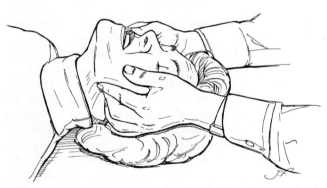

**Fig. 11-8** Opening the adult airway by the jaw-thrust method. *(From Watson MA: Cardiopulmonary resuscitation. In Barnes TA, editor: Respiratory care practice, Chicago, 1988, Mosby.)*

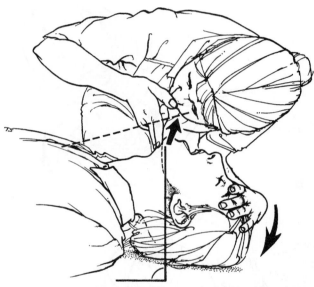

**Fig. 11-10** Determining breathlessness by looking, listening, and feeling. *(From Standards and guidelines for cardiopulmonary resuscitation [CPR] and emergency cardiac care [ECC], JAMA 268:2187, 1992.)*

the airway and eliminates the need to tilt the head back. Fig. 11-8 shows the adult maneuver.

Any obstruction visible in the mouth or throat should be removed. The cross-finger technique can be used to open the mouth wide enough so that a finger or suction device can be inserted to remove a blockage (Fig. 11-9). An oral airway should be used only in an unconscious patient to keep the tongue from falling back and blocking the airway.

### d. Determine that the patient is not breathing

The rescuer places his or her face close to the victim's to *look* for rising and falling of the chest, to *listen* for air movement, and to *feel* any air movement caused by the victim's breathing (Fig. 11-10). This should be done to ensure that the patient is really apneic and is not just breathing slowly. The entire procedure should not take longer than 10 seconds.

### e. Ventilate the patient
#### 1. Mouth-to-mouth breathing

The first rescuer should begin mouth-to-mouth breathing as soon as possible if the victim does not breathe spontaneously once the airway has been opened. An effective seal must be made between the rescuer and the victim regardless of the victim's age. The adult victim's nose must be pinched closed; often, the infant's nosed can be blocked by the cheek of the rescuer. Both the nose and the mouth of an infant can be covered by the mouth of the rescuer. Alternative methods of ventilation include mouth to nose and mouth to stoma (Fig. 11-11).

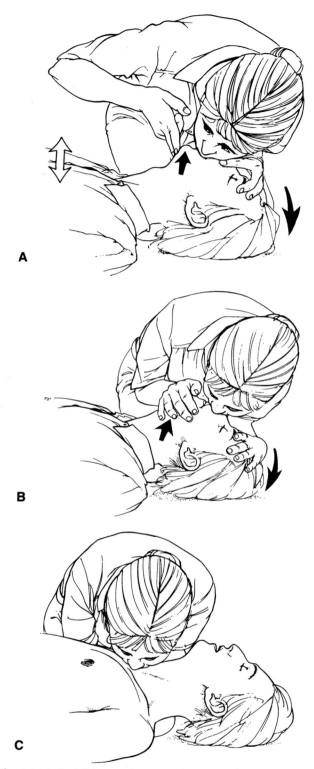

**Fig. 11-11 A,** Adult mouth-to-mouth, **B,** mouth-to-nose, and, **C,** mouth-to-stoma ventilation. *(From Standards and guidelines for cardiopulmonary resuscitation [CPR] and emergency cardiac care [ECC], JAMA 268:2188, 1992.)*

In an adult, two breaths large enough to raise the victim's chest should be given. An adequate volume of 700 mL, and up to 1000 mL, may be given. Blow into the victim's mouth for 2 seconds to ensure that a large enough volume is given without the need for much pressure. Keeping the ventilating pressure as low as possible minimizes the risk that air will be forced into the stomach. Ensure that the victim exhales completely by watching the chest fall and feeling the air escape against your cheek. Rescue breathing should be performed at a rate of 10 to 12 times/min (every 4 to 5 sec) if the victim has a pulse but is apneic.

In a child, two breaths large enough to raise the victim's chest should be given; the volume is obviously less than that needed in an adult. All of the same considerations apply as in the adult. Rescue breathing should be performed at a rate of 20 times/min (every 3 sec) in an infant and a child. A newly born infant should be ventilated at a rate of 30/min.

If the victim's airway cannot be ventilated, reposition the head and attempt to ventilate again. Failure to ventilate a second time means that the victim has an obstructed airway. The following steps should be taken:

### Unconscious adult obstructed airway maneuvers
a. Position: Position the victim on his or her back.
b. Heimlich maneuver: Perform the Heimlich maneuver several times, if needed, by kneeling astride the victim and placing the heel of one hand midline on the abdomen, slightly above the navel but well below the xiphoid process. The other hand is placed on top, and both are quickly thrust upward toward the chest (Fig. 11-12). The markedly obese or obviously pregnant victim can be given chest thrusts. The rescuer's hands should be placed on the lower half of the sternum, as with cardiac compressions. Several compressions should be performed slowly but similarly to a cardiac compression.
c. Finger sweep: Attempt to clear out any foreign body with a finger sweep. First, grasp the victim's tongue and jaw between your thumb and fingers, and lift the jaw open. Next, insert the index finger of the other hand along the inside of the victim's cheek and down the back of the throat to hook and remove the obstruction (e.g., food, gum, dentures).

### Unconscious child (1 year old and older) obstructed airway maneuvers
a. Position: Same as the adult position previously described.
b. Heimlich maneuver: Same as the adult maneuver previously described but with up to five thrusts performed if needed. Chest thrusts are not used.
c. Finger sweep: Same as the adult sweep except that the index finger is inserted only when a foreign body has been observed. Blindly inserting the index finger may push a foreign body farther down the throat.

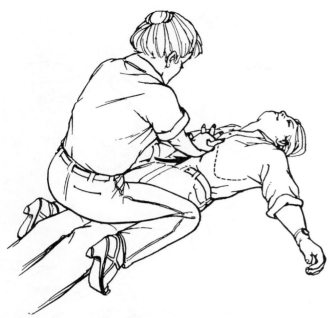

**Fig. 11-12** Administering the Heimlich maneuver to an unconscious adult victim of an airway obstruction. *(From Standards and guidelines for cardiopulmonary resuscitation [CPR] and emergency cardiac care [ECC], JAMA 268:2193, 1992.)*

***Unconscious infant obstructed airway maneuver***

a. Position: The infant is straddled over one forearm of the rescuer. His or her jaw and head are held by the hand. The infant's head should be positioned lower than the body. Five firm back blows are delivered between the shoulder blades with the heel of the rescuer's other hand (Fig. 11-13).

b. Heimlich maneuver: The infant is sandwiched by the rescuer's other arm, and the head and body are supported and turned to a supine position. The head should remain lower than the body. Five chest thrusts are performed in the same location and manner as cardiac compressions but at a slower rate. Steps **a** and **b** can be performed by placing the infant on the rescuer's lap.

c. Finger sweep: Same as the finger sweep in the unconscious child, mentioned previously.

## 2. Manual resuscitator (bag-valve)

A manual resuscitator that delivers 100% oxygen should be used during hospital-based CPR as soon as one becomes available. The resuscitation mask must be held to the face to prevent air leaks during forced inspiration (Fig. 11-14). An assistant can hold the mask tightly to the face so that the rescuer who is pumping the resuscitation bag can use both hands. This has been shown to produce a larger $V_T$. If the victim's airway contains an endotracheal or tracheostomy tube, the valve adapter fits directly over the tube adapter. Rescue breathing would continue with

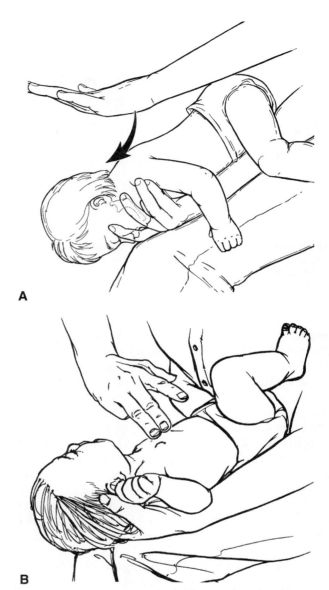

**Fig. 11-13** Administering **A,** back blows and **B,** chest thrusts to an infant victim of an obstructed airway. *(From Standards and guidelines for cardiopulmonary resuscitation [CPR] and emergency cardiac care [ECC], JAMA 268:2258, 1992.)*

the previously mentioned considerations for volume and rate. After an adult victim has had an endotracheal tube placed, the tidal volume goal is 400 to 600 mL (6–7 mL/Kg) over 1 to 2 seconds.

## 3. Mouth-to-valve mask ventilation

A mouth-to-valve mask device (or *pocket mask*) combines a resuscitation mask with a one-way valve mouthpiece. It is used to ventilate an apneic patient rather than to perform mouth-to-mouth breathing. Concerns about protecting the rescuer from patient infection such as acquired immunodeficiency syndrome and hepatitis have led to their widespread acceptance. As shown in Fig. 11-6, the

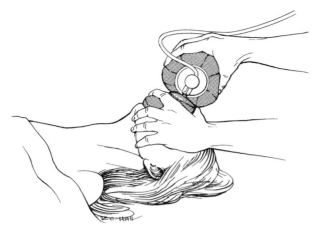

**Fig. 11-14** Ventilation of an adult with a manual resuscitation bag and mask. Note the tube that brings oxygen into the bag. *(From Eubanks DH, Bone RC: Comprehensive respiratory care, ed 2, St Louis, 1990, Mosby.)*

patient's neck is hyperextended, the mask is applied over the mouth and nose for an airtight seal, and the rescuer breathes into the mouthpiece. The rescuer is best positioned at the victim's head so that the chest can be seen to rise with each delivered breath. The one-way valve is designed so that the victim's exhaled gas is vented out to the room air. Some units have a nipple adapter so that supplemental $O_2$ can be added to the delivered breath. Simply attach $O_2$ tubing between the nipple and the $O_2$ flowmeter, and turn the flowmeter on to the manufacturer's recommended flow. When this is done with an adult victim, the tidal volume goal is 400 to 600 mL (6–7 mL/Kg) over 1 to 2 seconds. These devices should be replaced with a manual resuscitator as soon as possible.

### f. Add supplemental oxygen (NBRC code: IIIF2d1) [Difficulty: R, Ap]

The victim should be given 100% $O_2$ as soon as possible. No contraindication exists for giving pure $O_2$ during a resuscitation effort. This can be done easily if a manual resuscitator is used to ventilate the victim. All modern units have the capability of giving 100% $O_2$ if the $O_2$ flow is high enough and an oxygen reservoir is added.

### g. Determine pulselessness

The carotid pulse is sought in all victims except children younger than 1 year by gently feeling with two or three fingers in the groove between the larynx and the sternocleidomastoid muscle on either side of the neck (Fig. 11-15). Check to be sure that the victim is pulseless and is not just bradycardiac. In addition, check for other signs of circulation such as spontaneous breathing, coughing, and movement. The entire procedure should not take longer than 10 seconds. In an infant younger than 1 year, you should feel the pulse in the brachial artery because the

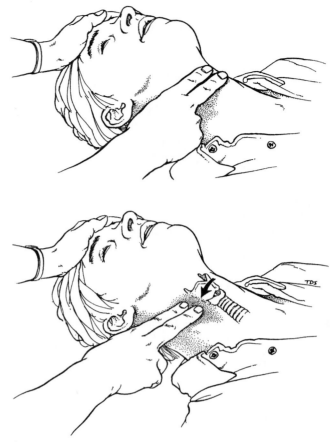

**Fig. 11-15** Determining pulselessness by checking the carotid pulse of an adult. *(From Standards and guidelines for cardiopulmonary resuscitation [CPR] and emergency cardiac care [ECC], JAMA 268:2189, 1992.)*

carotid artery is difficult to find in such young children with short, chubby necks.

The femoral pulse can be used as an alternative site in all victims, although it is limited to victims in the hospital who are wearing few clothes. Once the CPR team has arrived and two-person CPR is begun, the femoral pulse may be the one that is most accessible for monitoring the pulse and assessing the effectiveness of chest compressions.

### h. Perform external chest compressions

The absence of a pulse confirms cardiac arrest. Blood must be pumped by external chest compressions of the heart. The victim must be placed supine on a hard surface. A CPR backboard is placed behind a victim in bed.

In adults, large children, or children older than 8 years of age, the heel of the rescuer's hand is placed over the lower half of the sternum. You can find the sternum by placing the middle finger of one hand in the notch where the ribs meet the sternum, placing the index finger next to it, and placing the other hand next to the finger. The

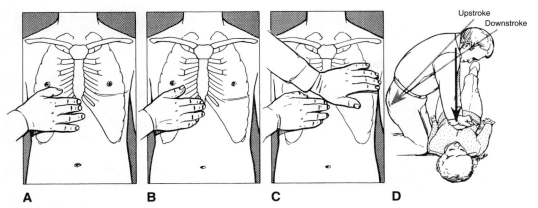

**Fig. 11-16** Cardiac compression of an adult. **A,** Locate tip of xyphoid process. **B,** Place two fingertips at xyphoid process. **C,** Place palm of other hand on sternum next to fingers. **D,** Arm and body positions for cardiac compression. *(From Barnes TA, editor: Respiratory care practice, Chicago, 1988, Mosby.)*

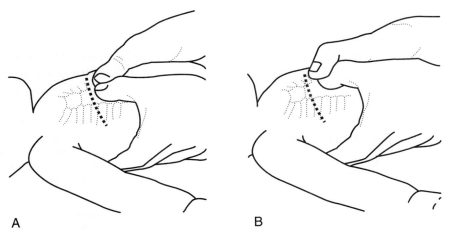

**Fig. 11-17** The preferred way to provide chest compressions on a newly born neonate is called two thumbs–encircling hands. This method is best when one rescuer can provide chest compressions and another can ventilate the patient. **A,** Side-by-side thumb placement for most newborns. **B,** Overlapping thumbs for very small newborns. *(From Aloan CA, Hill TV, editors: Respiratory care of the newborn and child, ed 2, Philadelphia, 1997, Lippincott-Raven.)*

first hand is placed over it, the elbows are locked, and the shoulders are placed directly over the hands. This creates the most efficient pumping action (Fig. 11-16). The rescuer pivots from the hips, with half the time spent pumping down and half the time releasing pressure. The hands should always touch the victim's chest. The sternum must be compressed 4 to 5 cm (1.5 to 2 in) in an average adult at a rate of 100 compressions/min for an actual rate of >80/min.

In a child 8 years of age or younger, the hands are positioned as in the adult. The child's sternum must be compressed with *one* hand to a depth of 2.5 to 3.8 cm (1 to 1.5 in). Half the time should be spent on compression and half the time on relaxation. The rate should be

100 compressions/min for a rate of >80 compressions/min between ventilations.

In newly born infants and older infants, the preferred method of chest compression is called *the two thumb–encircling hands technique* (Fig. 11-17). This methods works best when a second rescuer can ventilate the infant. It is also acceptable to compress with two or three fingers placed over the middle of the sternum one fingerwidth below an imaginary line drawn between the nipples (Fig. 11-18). This method is easier to perform when one rescuer must provide both ventilations and compressions. In either case, the child's sternum must be compressed to a depth of 1.3 to 2.5 cm (0.5 to 1 in). Half the time should be spent on compression and half the time on relaxation. A newly

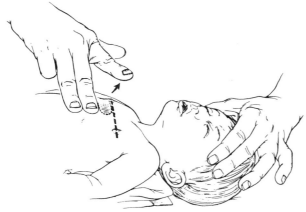

**Fig. 11-18** An alternate way to provide chest compressions to an infant uses two or three fingers over the midchest. Note the proper way to identify the finger positions. This method is preferred when there is only one rescuer who must be positioned at the side of the victim. *(From Standards and guidelines for cardiopulmonary resuscitation [CPR] and emergency cardiac care [ECC], JAMA 268:2256, 1992.)*

born infant should be given compressions at a rate of at least 120 compressions/min for an actual rate of 90/min to be achieved.

The steps for one- and two-person CPR follow:

Note: Review the most recent CPR guidelines for updates on the following procedures.

### 1. Adult one-rescuer cardiopulmonary resuscitation

a. Assess the victim's need for CPR.
b. Call out for help.
c. Open the airway.
d. Assess the victim's lack of breathing.
e. Give two rescue breaths.
f. Assess the victim's lack of a pulse.
g. Perform 15 chest compressions at a rate of 100 compressions/min to get an actual rate of >80/min. Count them out as "one and, two and, three and . . ."
h. Reopen the airway, and give two breaths of 2-seconds' duration each.
i. Repeat this cycle (15:2) four times.
j. Check the victim's carotid pulse for <10 sec. If it has not returned, give two breaths and continue with compressions.
k. If the pulse has returned, check for the return of breathing. If breathing has not returned, give 12 breaths/min.
l. If CPR is continued, check for the return of a heartbeat and breathing every few minutes.

### 2. Adult two-rescuer cardiopulmonary resuscitation

a. Perform steps **a** to **f** as previously described for adult one-rescuer CPR.

b. The first rescuer performs five chest compressions at a rate of 100 compressions/min to achieve a rate of >80/min. He or she counts them out as "one and, two and, three and . . . ."
c. The second rescuer gives two breaths during a pause between sets of compressions.
d. Repeat this cycle (15:2) several times.
e. The second rescuer calls for a pause of <10 seconds after 1 minute and checks for the return of pulse or breathing.
f. Provide breathing, circulation, or both as needed. If CPR is continued, check for the return of a heartbeat and breathing every few minutes.
g. After the victim has had an endotracheal tube placed, the compressions:ventilations ratio changes to 5:1. A manual resuscitator with 100% oxygen is also used to ventilate the victim.
h. Switch positions whenever one rescuer becomes tired. Make the switch at the end of a cycle, check the victim for a return of pulse or breathing, and continue as needed.

### 3. Infant and child one- and two-rescuer cardiopulmonary resuscitation

a. Perform steps **a** to **f** as previously described for adult one-rescuer CPR.
b. For either infants or children, a rescuer performs sets of five chest compressions. These are delivered at a rate of at least 100 compressions/min for delivery of at least 80 compressions/min between ventilations. Count them out as "one and, two and, three and . . . ."
c. One breath is given during a pause between sets of compressions.
d. Repeat this pattern (5:1) for about 1 min (20 cycles).
e. Pause for <10 sec to check for the return of a pulse or breathing.
f. Provide breathing or circulation as needed. If CPR is continued, check for the return of a heartbeat and breathing every few minutes.
g. Switch positions whenever one rescuer becomes tired. Make the switch at the end of a cycle, check the victim for a return of pulse or breathing, and continue as needed.

> **Exam Hint**
>
> **P**ast examinations have focused on adult BCLS procedures. Expect about two questions.

### 2. Advanced cardiac life support (NBRC code: III I1b) [Difficulty: R, Ap]

It is beyond the scope of this text to present advanced cardiac life support (ACLS) in detail. The following items relate to ACLS procedures that are important in the advanced care of adult, pediatric, or neonatal patients.

### a. Endotracheal intubation

Oral endotracheal intubation is usually performed as soon as possible during a CPR attempt. See Chapter 12 for a complete discussion of endotracheal tubes, intubation equipment, and the process of performing intubation. If an endotracheal tube cannot be inserted, continue with manual resuscitation (bag-valve) or mouth-to-valve resuscitation with oxygen. A laryngeal mask airway may be inserted to protect the airway.

### b. Make the recommendation to defibrillate the patient

Defibrillation must be performed as soon as possible if the patient has either of the following arrhythmias: ventricular fibrillation or ventricular tachycardia when the patient is pulseless, unresponsive, hypotensive, or in pulmonary edema. Current standards in the hospital require that the patient can be defibrillated <4 min after CPR is started. The electrical shock sends a specific amount of direct electrical current through the patient's chest wall and heart. This stimulates the entire cardiac muscle and electrical system so that the source of an abnormal signal is suppressed. The sinoatrial node then usually takes over as the normal pacemaker. Box 17-1 lists the electrical power levels recommended in defibrillation and cardioversion.

Cardioversion (synchronized defibrillation) should be performed under the following circumstances: atrial flutter, paroxysmal atrial tachycardia, atrial fibrillation, and ventricular tachycardia unless the patient is pulseless, unresponsive, hypotensive, or in pulmonary edema. A more complete discussion of cardioversion is presented in Chapter 17.

### c. Make a recommendation for an arterial blood gas measurement (NBRC code: IB9) [Difficulty: R, Ap]

Blood for arterial blood gas (ABG) determination is usually drawn in any hospital-based CPR effort. This should not be done at the expense of time that should be spent in starting effective ventilations and chest compressions or defibrillating the heart. Blood gas values reveal important information about the patient's oxygenation and whether the patient is acidotic. Changes in ventilation efforts and medications such as bicarbonate are based on information obtained from the ABGs.

The femoral site is usually the best from which to draw in a CPR situation because it is the largest artery and is easiest to hit. It is also far enough from the chest that this does not interfere with chest compression efforts.

### d. Recommend medications during an emergency

Current guidelines list several clinical scenarios in which emergency medications should be administered. Frequently seen situations are listed here. See the full set of ACLS pharmacology guidelines (2001) for recommended doses.

*Bradycardia or asystole.* An adult with bradycardia is usually given an intravenous dose of atropine. It blocks the cholinergic (parasympathetic) nervous system so that the patient's heart rate increases. If this does not work, the patient is given an intravenous dose of epinephrine. This drug directly stimulates the adrenergic (sympathetic) nervous system to raise the heart rate. When a newborn is being resuscitated, epinephrine is given if the heart rate is <60/min after 30 seconds of adequate ventilations. Epinephrine is especially indicated in a newborn with asystole.

*Premature ventricular contraction (PVC).* Lidocaine (Xylocaine) is usually given when a patient has PVCs or ventricular tachycardia (VT) that results in hemodynamic instability. It may also be given to a patient who has ventricular fibrillation or pulseless VT after defibrillation and administration of epinephrine.

*Ventricular fibrillation (VF).* If the patient does not respond to defibrillation attempts, intravenous epinephrine should be given. It should also be given every 3 to 5 min thereafter, if the patient has not converted to normal sinus rhythm. Vasopressin may be administered intravenously, one time only, as a substitute medication for epinephrine.

*Sodium bicarbonate.* According to recent guidelines, bicarbonate (sodium bicarbonate) should be used, if at all, only after all other CPR procedures have been performed. Bicarbonate may then be used if a diagnosis has been made and the patient has a preexisting metabolic acidosis, hyperkalemia, or tricyclic or phenobarbital overdose. Bicarbonate may also be beneficial if the patient has been in prolonged arrest, or if CPR has been performed for an extended time.

Bicarbonate should be given initially at a dose of 1 mEq/kg. If available from ABGs, use the calculated base deficit or bicarbonate concentration as a guideline for giving additional bicarbonate. Do not completely correct the base deficit to avoid accidentally making the patient alkalotic.

> **Exam Hint**
>
> **E**pinephrine is used during bradycardia, asystole, and ventricular fibrillation because it increases the heart rate, the pumping of the heart (stroke volume), and vasoconstriction to raise blood pressure. In addition, it is a bronchodilator.

### e. Recommend the instillation of medications through the endotracheal tube during an emergency situation

Cardiac medications should be instilled down the endotracheal tube when a resuscitation attempt is under way and the patient does not have a functional central or peripheral intravenous (IV) line. Lidocaine, epinephrine, and atropine may be instilled into all patients. In addition, naloxone may be given to newly born patients. Adults should be given a dose 2 to 2.5 times the normal IV amount. The medication(s) should be diluted by adding 10 mL of normal saline or distilled water.

### f. Instill the ordered medication down the endotracheal tube

The following steps for instillation are recommended:
1. Disconnect the manual resuscitator from the endotracheal tube and stop the chest compressions.
2. Pass a suction catheter or feeding tube past the distal tip of the endotracheal tube.
3. Quickly inject the drug solution down the catheter.
4. Withdraw the suction catheter.
5. Reconnect the manual resuscitator to the endotracheal tube, and give the patient several deep breaths. This helps to force the medication down to the alveolar level or causes aerosolization for faster absorption.
6. Resume chest compressions and ventilation.

### g. Observe the size of the patient's pupils and their reaction to light

Normally, the pupils constrict when a light is shined into them. The pupils dilate within 30 to 40 sec after cardiac arrest and do not constrict normally when the brain is hypoxic. If CPR is being done properly to deliver $O_2$ to the brain, the pupils should constrict normally. Fixed (nonreactive) and dilated pupils is an ominous sign. Even if the heart can be restarted, the brain has probably suffered irreversible damage.

Several conditions exist in which the pupils will not react as expected. The pupils remain constricted if the victim has received morphine sulfate or other opiates. The pupils dilate if the victim has received atropine, quinidine, or epinephrine. Hypothermia also causes the pupils to dilate.

### h. Recommend capnography to evaluate the adequacy of resuscitation

The general discussion of capnography is presented in Chapter 5. If quickly available, capnography can be used to help confirm that the endotracheal tube is properly located in the trachea. It is also helpful if the patient is being transported, or the endotracheal tube is being repositioned. The presence of exhaled carbon dioxide ($CO_2$) confirms that the tube is properly positioned in the trachea. In addition, clinical evidence shows that monitoring the exhaled $CO_2$ level during a CPR attempt is helpful in evaluating the patient's response. In general, if chest compressions and assisted ventilation are effective, $CO_2$ will be removed from the tissues and circulated to the lungs for exhalation. If CPR efforts are ineffective, little exhaled $CO_2$ will be measured.

### 3. Pediatric advanced life support (NBRC code: III I1c) [Difficulty: R, Ap]

The general steps and procedures related to pediatric advanced life support (PALS) are covered in this chapter. Also review Chapters 12 and 9 as needed.

### 4. Neonatal resuscitation program (NBRC code: III I1d) [Difficulty: R, Ap]

A neonatal resuscitation program (NRP) provides training in resuscitating a newborn at birth in the delivery room. In addition to the basic and advanced CPR steps discussed in this chapter and Chapters 9 and 12, the person trained in NRP is prepared to perform the following:
a. Dry the newborn and keep it warm.
b. Suction the airway to remove amniotic fluid or meconium.
c. Be prepared to provide manual resuscitation (bag-valve) if spontaneous ventilations do not result in a heart rate <100/min. The assisted ventilation rate is 30/min.
d. Provide chest compressions if the heart rate is absent or <60/min despite assisted ventilation for 30 sec. A rate of compressions of 120/min is needed to achieve an actual rate of 90/min. The ratio of compressions to ventilations is 3:1.

It is beyond the scope of this text to cover all aspects of ACLS, PALS, and NRP training. The Bibliography listed at the end of this chapter lists helpful resources.

> **Exam Hint**
>
> **H**istorically, the NBRC has focused its CPR examination questions on BCLS, life-threatening arrhythmia recognition, intubation, and defibrillation. However, every opportunity should be made to learn advanced CPR procedures.

## MODULE D
### Respiratory care plan

### 1. Analyze the available information to determine the patient's pathophysiologic state (NBRC code: IIIH1) [Difficulty: R, Ap, An]

### 2. Determine the appropriateness of the prescribed therapy and goals for the patient's pathophysiologic state (NBRC code: IIIH3) [Difficulty: R, Ap, An]

It is critically important that the respiratory therapist be able to recognize the need to start CPR procedures. This

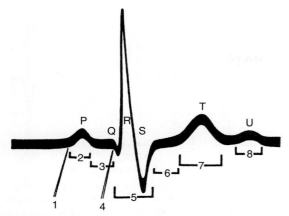

**Fig. 11-19** Sequence of electrical events of the cardiac cycle during normal sinus rhythm. (See Table 11-2 for the description of each event.) *(From Phillips RE, Feeney MK: The cardiac rhythms: a systematic approach to interpretation, ed 3, Philadelphia, 1990, WB Saunders.)*

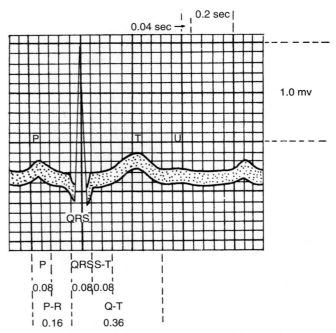

**Fig. 11-20** Timing of the electrical events of the cardiac cycle during normal sinus rhythm. *(From Scanlan CL, Sheldon RL: Egan's fundamentals of respiratory care, ed 5, St Louis, 1990, Mosby.)*

chapter's discussion should provide helpful preparation for this possibility. Airway management is discussed in Chapter 12. The following discussion focuses on cardiac arrhythmias and their treatment.

It is beyond the scope of this text to discuss all of the possible cardiac arrhythmias. Instead, the focus is on the most life-threatening arrhythmias because knowledge of these has been tested on past National Board for Respiratory Care (NBRC) examinations. First, normal sinus rhythm should be reviewed.

**Normal sinus rhythm.** The normal cardiac rhythm, which is usually called *normal sinus rhythm* (NSR), must be understood so that it can be distinguished from abnormal rhythm. NSR has these characteristics:

1. Heart rate between 60 and 100 beats/min while at rest
2. Rhythm that varies by no more than ±10% between QRS complexes
3. P wave before every QRS complex and upright in lead II
4. A QRS complex that follows every P wave
5. Proper timing of the components of the ECG rhythm

Sequential electrical events of the NSR are detailed in Fig. 11-19 and Table 11-2. Fig. 11-20 shows normal timing of the components of the normal ECG tracing.

**Abnormal cardiac rhythms.** The following list of abnormal cardiac rhythms (usually called *arrhythmias* or *dysrhythmias*) includes the most dangerous ones that are commonly encountered in clinical practice. Each of the following cardiac irregularities is defined, exemplified, described, discussed in terms of clinical significance, and accompanied by a treatment description.

a. Premature ventricular contraction

A premature ventricular contraction (PVC) is an abnormal, fast contraction of the ventricles that originates from

| TABLE 11-2 | Electrophysiologic Events Represented by the Electrocardiogram | |
|---|---|
| **Sequential electrical events of the cardiac cycle** | **Electrocardiographic representation** |
| 1. Impulse from the sinus node | Not visible |
| 2. Depolarization of the atria | P wave |
| 3. Depolarization of the atrioventricular node | Isoelectric |
| 4. Depolarization of the atria | Usually obscured by the QRS complex |
| 5. Depolarization of the ventricles | QRS complex |
|   a. Intraventricular septum | Initial portion |
|   b. Right and left ventricles | Central and terminal portions |
| 6. Quiescent state of the ventricles immediately after depolarization | ST segment: isoelectric |
| 7. Repolarization of the ventricles | T wave |
| 8. Afterpotentials following repolarization of the ventricles | U wave |

From Phillips RE, Feeney MK: *The cardiac rhythms: a systematic approach to interpretation*, ed 3, Philadelphia, 1990, WB Saunders.

a focus below the atrioventricular (A-V) node within a ventricular wall (Fig. 11-21). This is usually a sign of a diseased or hypoxic ventricle. Pathologic causes include atherosclerotic heart disease and MI. An example of an isolated PVC is shown in Fig. 11-22; it has the following traits:

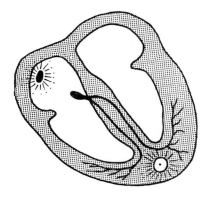

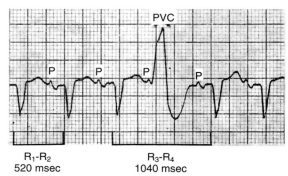

R₁-R₂
520 msec

R₃-R₄
1040 msec

**Fig. 11-22** Premature ventricular contractions (PVCs) cause a fully compensatory pause. Note that the interval between the two sinus beats that surround the PVC (R₃ and R₄ in this case) is exactly two times the normal interval between the sinus beats R₁ and R₂. Notice that the P waves come on time, except that the third P wave is interrupted by the PVC and therefore does not conduct normally through the atrioventricular junction. The next (fourth) P wave also comes on time. The fact that the sinus node continues to pace despite the PVC results in a fully compensatory pause. *(From Goldberger AL, Goldberger E: Clinical electrocardiography, ed 5, St Louis, 1994, Mosby.)*

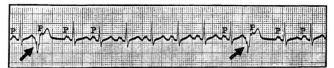

**Fig. 11-21** Premature ventricular contraction *(arrows)* is detected when an impulse is propagated from a ventricular focus before the next normal beat is due. The QRS complex is commonly widened and is not preceded by a P wave. A longer than usual (compensatory) pause follows. Retrograde activation of the atria may occur following a premature contraction, or the normal sinus P waves may continue. The sinus P waves following the PVC are blocked because of conduction system refractoriness. *(From Stein E: Clinical electrocardiography: a self-study course, Philadelphia, 1987, Lea & Febiger.)*

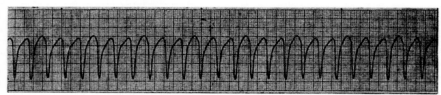

**Fig. 11-23** Example of an electrocardiogram showing ventricular tachycardia. If this arrhythmia is not treated promptly, it will deteriorate into ventricular flutter or ventricular fibrillation. *(From Kacmarek RM, Mack CW, Dimas S: The essentials of respiratory care, ed 3, St Louis, 1990, Mosby.)*

1. It is premature and happens before the normal heartbeat.
2. No P wave exists.
3. The QRS complex looks bizarre and is more than 0.12 sec wide.
4. The T wave is inverted.
5. Usually, a fully compensatory pause occurs before the next normal heartbeat.

A single PVC is not dangerous unless it originates during the T wave, when the heart is especially vulnerable to electrical stimulation. The PVC could then cause ventricular fibrillation. Patients with PVCs should be watched more closely and probably should be treated when their PVCs are seen at a more frequent rate than one in ten beats, occur in groups of two or three, or manifest in multiple configurations. For example, two different-looking PVCs indicates that two different ventricular foci are firing prematurely. Bigeminy occurs when every second beat is a PVC; trigeminy occurs when every third beat is a PVC. Dangerous PVCs must be treated rapidly. Lidocaine (Xylocaine) is given intravenously if the heart rate is faster than 60 beats/min. If this does not work, procainamide hydrochloride (Pronestyl) is added.

   b. Ventricular tachycardia

Ventricular tachycardia (VT or V tach) is a serious consequence of untreated PVCs (Fig. 11-23). VT is defined as a series of three or more consecutive PVCs. Runs of VT may be fairly short or prolonged. The rate counted during VT is 110 to 250 beats/min. Cardiac output falls dramatically during this arrhythmia. If the patient has a stable blood

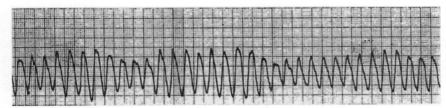

**Fig. 11-24** Example of an electrocardiogram showing ventricular flutter. If this arrhythmia is not treated promptly, it will deteriorate into ventricular fibrillation. *(From Kacmarek RM, Mack CW, Dimas S: The essentials of respiratory care, ed 3, St Louis, 1990, Mosby.)*

pressure, VT is treated by an antiarrhythmic such as lidocaine. Synchronized cardioversion is needed if the lidocaine is ineffective. If the VT is sustained and the patient is unresponsive, pulseless, or hypotensive, or has pulmonary edema, unsynchronous cardioversion is necessary. If left untreated, VT usually progresses to either ventricular flutter (Fig. 11-24) or ventricular fibrillation (VF or V fib). Ventricular flutter looks similar to VT on the ECG except that the rate is usually faster and the rhythm is less regular. Treatment is the same as for VT and, if left untreated, VT will progress to VF. Both of these arrhythmias originate from a single fast ventricular focus, as shown in Fig. 11-21.

c. Ventricular fibrillation

VF is caused when multiple, fast ventricular foci are firing (Fig. 11-25 shows the electrical pathways). When several ventricular foci are firing in an uncoordinated manner, the rhythm is chaotic and has no pattern (Fig. 11-26). There is virtually no cardiac output, and the patient is pulseless and has no blood pressure. This is a true medical emergency, and, if it is not treated immediately, brain death will occur within minutes. CPR must be started to provide $O_2$ to the brain. The treatment of choice for VF is defibrillation given as quickly as possible (within 5 min). No attempt is made to synchronize the electrical shock. Fig. 11-27 shows the usual position of the defibrillator paddles. Rapid defibrillation and CPR are the patient's only hope for a return to normal sinus rhythm and recovery.

d. Ventricular asystole

Ventricular asystole (or *asystole*) occurs when no cardiac electrical signal and no myocardial activity exist. The ECG tracing shows a flat line that indicates that no cardiac electrical activity exists. The presence of this arrhythmia is ominous. When seen after a full attempt at CPR, it indicates a nonfunctioning heart. The patient will almost assuredly die. Some physicians may elect to defibrillate the patient in asystole to attempt to generate some sort of rhythm. Because of the dire consequences of asystole, it is wise to double-check all the equipment to ensure that no technical error exists. This includes the ECG leads or defibrillator paddles used to check the rhythm, all electrical connections, and the ECG monitor.

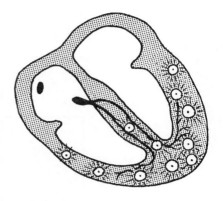

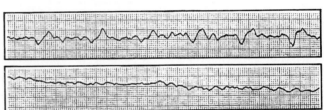

**Fig. 11-25** Multiple disorganized contractions of the ventricles characterize ventricular fibrillation and represent cardiac arrest. It may be of sudden onset or may follow ventricular premature contractions, ventricular tachycardia, or ventricular flutter. The two ECG strips show course (*on top*) and fine (*on bottom*) ventricular fibrillation. *(From Stein E: Clinical electrocardiography: a self-study course, Philadelphia, 1987, Lea & Febiger.)*

**Exam Hint**

Expect to see at least one ECG strip as part of an exam question. It could depict normal sinus rhythm that requires no treatment. However, it is usually a serious arrhythmia such as premature ventricular contractions (PVCs), ventricular tachycardia (VT or Vtach), or ventricular fibrillation (VF or Vfib). These require immediate treatment.

If the ECG tracing shows ventricular fibrillation or ventricular tachycardia without a pulse, know that the arrhythmia is life threatening and that CPR and defibrillation are necessary.

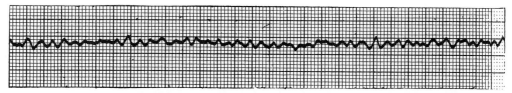

**Fig. 11-26** Ventricular fibrillation. Note that no rhythm can be seen on the tracing. *(From Goldberger AL, Goldberger E: Clinical electrocardiography, ed 4, St Louis, 1995, Mosby.)*

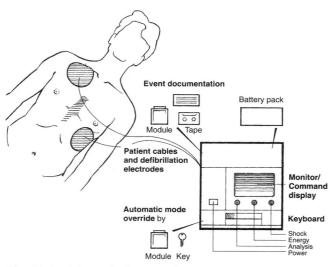

**Fig. 11-27** Schematic drawing of automated external defibrillator and its attachment to the patient. *(Modified from Cummins RO: Advanced cardiac life support, Dallas, 1994, American Heart Association.)*

### 3. Discontinue treatment based on the patient's response (NBRC code: IIIG1f) [Difficulty: R, Ap]

BCLS, ACLS, PALS, and NRP are all CPR-related protocols. CPR should be started, adjusted, and terminated based on these protocols and the patient's recovery.

The practitioner should make a recommendation to the physician to stop a procedure that is being performed as an adjunct to CPR, if the patient is suffering an adverse reaction to it. For example, bag and mask ventilation may force air into the stomach; recommend endotracheal intubation. Always notify the physician of any change in the patient's condition, or if a complication to any CPR-related procedure occurs.

### 4. Participate in intrahospital patient transport (NBRC code: IIIHI2a) [Difficulty: R, Ap]

Be prepared to perform all of the respiratory care practices and procedures to be performed during patient transport that have been described in this and other textbooks. It is extremely important that all equipment and supplies be accounted for before the patient leaves the hospital. Make sure that all equipment is working properly. Calculate the duration of the oxygen cylinders at the expected liter flow. Make sure that batteries and light bulbs work and that spares are available.

If mechanical ventilation will be needed, bring a unit that is lightweight and portable, has solid state circuitry, and can be powered by both alternating current (AC) and direct current (DC) from a battery. Check the expected duration of the battery. If the ventilator will be used for helicopter or unpressurized cabin fixed-wing aircraft, it must be able to deliver a synchronized intermittent mandatory ventilation (SIMV) mode through a demand valve rather than a reservoir system. The ventilator controls should not be affected by changes in atmospheric pressure during ascent and landing.

> **Exam Hint**
>
> **O**ne question often arises that deals with the effects of increased altitude when one is flying in an unpressurized helicopter or airplane. Remember that as altitude increases, barometric pressure ($P_B$) decreases.
>
> Decreased barometric pressure directly leads to a decrease in the alveolar pressure of oxygen. This causes the patient's arterial oxygen pressure to drop and can lead to hypoxemia. In addition, as barometric pressure decreases at increased altitude, gases within the patient (stomach, intestine, pneumothorax, and lung) expand. Also, the air in the endotracheal tube cuff expands, and the set tidal volume increases. This requires adjustments in the ventilator settings. Later, when the aircraft descends to land, increasing barometric pressure results in a decrease in the tidal volume and in the patient's internal gas volumes. Be prepared to adjust the ventilator again.

### 5. Participate in disaster management (NBRC code: IIIHI2b) [Difficulty: R, Ap]

Respiratory therapists are an important group of health care professionals who take part in disaster planning. Be prepared to perform any and all respiratory care practices and procedures listed in this book or in other respiratory care textbooks.

## BIBLIOGRAPHY

Abedin Z, Conner RP: *12-Lead ECG interpretation: the self-assessment approach*, Philadelphia, 1989, WB Saunders.

Aloan CA, Hill TV, editors: *Respiratory care of the newborn and child*, ed 2, Philadelphia, 1997, Lippincott-Raven.

American Association for Respiratory Care: Clinical practice guideline: resuscitation in acute care hospitals, *Respir Care* 38:1179, 1993.

American Association for Respiratory Care: Clinical practice guideline: defibrillation during resuscitation, *Respir Care* 40:744, 1995.

American Association for Respiratory Care: Clinical practice guideline: management of airway emergencies, *Respir Care* 40:749, 1995.

American Heart Association: *ACLS provider manual*, Dallas, 2001, American Heart Association.

American Heart Association in collaboration with International Liaison Committee on Resuscitation: Guidelines 2000 for cardiopulmonary resuscitation and emergency cardiac care: international consensus on science, *Circulation* 102:suppl I, 2000.

American Heart Association: *PALS provider manual*, Dallas, 2002, American Heart Association.

Barnes TA, editor: *Core textbook of respiratory care practice*, ed 2, St Louis, 1994, Mosby.

Barnes TA, Boudin KM: Cardiopulmonary resuscitation. In Burton GG, Hodgkin JE, Ward JJ, editors: *Respiratory care: a guide to clinical practice*, ed 4, Philadelphia, 1997, Lippincott-Raven Publishers.

Barnes TA, Hess DR: Cardiopulmonary resuscitation. In Hess DR, MacIntyre NR, Mishoe SC, editors: *Respiratory care principles & practice*, Philadelphia, 2002, WB Saunders.

Barnhart SL, Czervinske MP: *Perinatal and pediatric respiratory care*, Philadelphia, 1995, WB Saunders.

Branson RD, Hess DR, Chatburn RL, editors: *Respiratory care equipment*, ed 2, Philadelphia, 1999, Lippincott Williams & Wilkins.

Burton GC, Hodgkin JE, Ward JJ, editors: *Respiratory care: a guide to clinical practice*, ed 4, Philadelphia, 1997, Lippincott-Raven.

Butler HH: How to read an ECG, *RN* 36:35, 1973.

Butler HH: How to read an ECG, *RN* 36:49, 1973.

Butler HH: How to read an ECG, *RN* 36:50, 1973.

Cairo JM, Pilbeam SP: *Mosby's respiratory care equipment*, ed 6, St Louis, 1999, Mosby.

Davis D: *Differential diagnosis of arrhythmias*, Philadelphia, 1991, WB Saunders.

Durbin CG: Airway management. In Cairo JM, Pilbeam SP: *Mosby's respiratory care equipment*, ed 7, St Louis, 2004, Mosby.

Eubanks DH, Bone RC: *Comprehensive respiratory care*, ed 2, St Louis, 1990, Mosby.

Fink JB, Hunt GE, editors: *Clinical practice in respiratory care*, Philadelphia, 1999, Lippincott-Raven.

Fluck RR: Emergency medicine. In Wyka KA, Mathews PJ, Clark WF, editors: *Foundations of respiratory care*, Albany, 2002, Delmar.

Goldberger AL, Goldberger E: *Clinical electrocardiography*, St Louis, 1981, Mosby.

Harwood R: *Exam review and study guide for perinatal/pediatric respiratory care*, Philadelphia, 1999, FA Davis.

Hess D, Goff G, Johnson K: The effect of hand size, resuscitator brand, and use of two hands on volumes delivered during adult bag-valve ventilation, *Respir Care* 34:805, 1989.

Kacmarek RM, Mack CW, Dimas S: *The essentials of respiratory care*, ed 3, St Louis, 1990, Mosby.

Madama VC: Safe mouth-to-mouth resuscitation requires adjunct equipment, caution, *Occup Health Saf* 60:56, 1991.

Marriott HJL: *Practical electrocardiography*, ed 7, Baltimore, 1983, Williams & Wilkins.

Marshak AB: Emergency life support. In Wilkins RL, Stoller JK, Scanlan CL, editors: *Egan's fundamentals of respiratory therapy*, ed 8, St Louis, 2003, Mosby.

Pagana K, Pagana TJ: *Mosby's manual of diagnostic and laboratory tests*, St Louis, 1998, Mosby.

Patel JM, McGowan SG, Moody LA: *Arrhythmias: detection, treatment, and cardiac drugs*, Philadelphia, 1989, WB Saunders.

Phillips RE, Feeney MK: *The cardiac rhythms: a systematic approach to interpretation*, ed 3, Philadelphia, 1990, WB Saunders.

Shapiro BA, Kacmarek RM, Cane RD, et al, editors: *Clinical application of respiratory care*, ed 4, St Louis, 1991, Mosby.

Stein E: *Clinical electrocardiography: a self-study course*, Philadelphia, 1987, Lea & Febiger.

Sweetwood HM: *Clinical electrocardiography for nurses*, Rockville, Md, 1983, Aspen Systems.

Whitaker K: *Comprehensive perinatal & pediatric respiratory care*, ed 2, Albany, 1997, Delmar.

White GC: *Equipment theory for respiratory care*, ed 3, Albany, NY, 1999, Delmar.

## SELF-STUDY QUESTIONS

1. A completely compensatory pause is seen after which type of heartbeat?
   A. Normal sinus rhythm
   B. PVC
   C. Paroxysmal atrial tachycardia
   D. VT

2. All the following are acceptable ways to ventilate a patient during CPR EXCEPT:
   A. Endotracheal tube
   B. Pneumatic (demand-valve) resuscitator
   C. Mouth-to-valve resuscitator
   D. Manual resuscitator.

3. A patient comes into the emergency room appearing ashen gray and complaining of sudden, severe pain beneath his sternum and shortness of breath. He says this began after he exercised vigorously for 45 min. After putting an $O_2$ mask on the patient, what should you do?
   A. Start ECG monitoring.
   B. Recommend that he begin a supervised exercise program at the hospital.
   C. Perform a peak flow test to check on exercise-induced asthma.
   D. Immediately draw an ABG sample.

4. The nurse calls you into a patient's room. You notice from the ECG monitor that the patient is in ventricular tachycardia. You cannot find a carotid pulse, and the nurse says that he cannot find a blood pressure. What would you recommend?
   A. Check the other arm for a blood pressure.
   B. Defibrillate the patient.
   C. Intubate the patient and start her on a ventilator.
   D. Initiate synchronized cardioversion of the patient.

5. Counting from the left, the first and sixth rhythms on the ECG strip shown below (top) represent
   A. Atrial flutter
   B. Second-degree heart block
   C. Unifocal PVCs
   D. Multifocal PVCs

6. A 65-year-old patient has been successfully resuscitated in the emergency room after suffering an MI. He is still unstable with frequent PVCs. He needs to be transported to the cardiac care unit for management. Which of the following would be most important for monitoring him during the transportation?
   A. Pulse oximeter
   B. Portable capnography unit
   C. Portable ECG machine with defibrillator
   D. 12-lead ECG unit to record any arrhythmias

7. You are performing chest compressions during a resuscitation attempt while another therapist is manually ventilating the intubated patient. The nurse and physician are both unable to start an IV line to give medications. What would you recommend?
   A. Instill the medications down the endotracheal tube.
   B. Keep trying new sites from which to start the IV line.
   C. Nebulize the medications.
   D. Give the medications by subcutaneous injection.

8. You are doing $O_2$ rounds on patients in the coronary care unit. You notice that the patient whose 28% Venturi mask you are checking is unresponsive to your questions. Looking up, you see the ECG rhythm strip shown below (bottom). What would you recommend as a first reaction?
   A. Check the calibration on the ECG machine.
   B. Replace the ECG leads.
   C. Increase the $O_2$ percentage because the patient is hypoxic.
   D. Defibrillate the patient.

Figure for question 5:

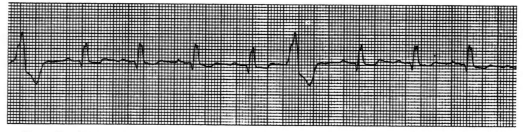

(From Patel JM, McGowan SG, Moody LA: *Arrhythmias: detection, treatment, and cardiac drugs,* Philadelphia, 1989, WB Saunders.)

Figure for question 8:

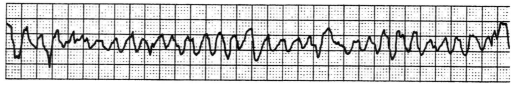

(From Patel JM, McGowan SG, Moody LA: *Arrhythmias: detection, treatment, and cardiac drugs,* Philadelphia, 1989, WB Saunders.)

9. You notice during a diagnostic ECG that the QRS complex is inverted on lead II. What would most likely cause this?
   A. The electrodes are attached properly.
   B. The leg electrodes are reversed.
   C. The arm electrodes are reversed.
   D. The unit is out of calibration.

10. You enter a patient's room to check on her nasal cannula. She is slumped over in her chair and appears cyanotic. Your first reaction would be to
    A. Open the airway
    B. Determine whether the patient is responsive
    C. Begin mouth-to-mouth ventilation
    D. Check for a pulse

11. You are working in the emergency department when an automobile accident victim is brought in. You suspect that the driver has a cervical spine injury. What is the best way to open the airway?
    A. Tracheostomy
    B. Head-tilt/chin-lift maneuver
    C. Jaw-thrust maneuver
    D. Nasal intubation

12. To determine breathlessness, it is best to
    I. Feel for air movement with your cheek by the victim's mouth
    II. Feel the chest rise and fall with your hand
    III. Listen for air movement with your ear by the victim's mouth
    IV. Look at the victim's chest for a rising and falling movement
    V. Look at the victim's face for nasal flaring
    A. I and II
    B. III and V
    C. I, III, and IV
    D. IV and V

13. The best way to determine pulselessness in a 10-month-old infant is by checking
    A. Brachial pulse for 5 to 10 sec
    B. Carotid pulse for 3 to 5 sec
    C. Femoral pulse for 3 to 5 sec
    D. Brachial pulse for 3 to 5 sec

14. While doing $O_2$ equipment rounds, you come upon a cyanotic patient who is not breathing. As you reposition the patient and hyperextend his neck, you notice that he has open lip ulcers. What would be the best way to ventilate this patient?
    A. Perform mouth-to-mouth ventilation.
    B. Use a mouth-to-valve device stored in the room for this purpose.
    C. Run to the CPR crash cart and get a manual resuscitation bag and mask.
    D. Wait for the anesthesiologist to intubate the patient's airway, then use a manual resuscitation bag.

15. When two health care workers are performing CPR on an intubated adult, what chest compression:ventilation ratio should be used?
    A. 5:2
    B. 5:1
    C. 15:2
    D. 1:5

16. To ensure that a manual ventilator is ready for use, you would
    I. Make sure that no gas escapes through the outlet port when it is closed off and the bag is squeezed
    II. Squeeze the bag and make sure that the air/$O_2$ reservoir intake valve closes properly
    III. Squeeze the bag and make sure the nonrebreathing valve opens properly
    IV. Feel air leave the outlet port when the bag is squeezed
    V. Squeeze the bag and make sure that the air/$O_2$ reservoir intake valve opens properly
    A. I, II, III, and IV
    B. I, II, and V
    C. IV and V
    D. II and III

17. Blood for an ABG measurement needs to be drawn during a CPR attempt. Which site would you recommend for this?
    A. Carotid
    B. Radial
    C. Brachial
    D. Femoral

## ANSWER KEY AND RATIONALE

1. **B.** See Fig. 11-22 for a tracing and explanation of a PVC.

2. **B.** Current CPR guidelines state that effective ventilation can be achieved by an endotracheal tube, mouth-to-valve resuscitator, and/or manual resuscitator. A pneumatic (demand-valve) resuscitator is not recommended for use because it is difficult to control the delivered tidal volume and air tends to be forced into the patient's stomach.

3. **A.** The patient's signs and symptoms could indicate a cardiac problem, so ECG monitoring is justified. An exercise program is not indicated in this situation and could be dangerous for the patient. A peak flow test is not indicated now and would not help with the diagnosis of exercise-induce asthma. It is best to wait at least 10 min after putting $O_2$ on a patient before drawing an ABG sample to check on the patient's $O_2$ level.

4. **B.** Defibrillation is indicated if the patient has VT and is without pulse or blood pressure. The patient should then be evaluated for full CPR efforts. The other options would delay effective treatment.

5. **C.** See Fig. 11-22 for a tracing of a PVC and explanation. *Unifocal* means that all of the PVCs originate from a single area. *Multifocal* means that PVCs originate from more than one area.

6. **C.** A portable defibrillator must be with the patient in case it is needed. The other items are useful for monitoring but offer no way to treat a life-threatening arrhythmia.

7. **A.** Direct instillation into the patient's airways and lungs offers the fastest way to administer the medications when an IV line is not available.

8. **D.** Defibrillation should be performed as quickly as possible when a patient is in VF. Fig. 11-26 shows another example. All of the other options delay effective treatment.

9. **C.** Reversing the arm electrodes results in the heart's electrical signal being received by the ECG machine in the opposite direction of normal. This results in reversal of the ECG signal.

10. **B.** The first step in a suspected CPR situation is to assess the patient. CPR should be performed only when needed.

11. **C.** The jaw-thrust maneuver should be a safe way to open the airway of a patient with a known or suspected cervical spine injury. The patient's head should not be tilted back because of the possibility of spine injury. Nasal intubation and tracheostomy should be performed, if needed, only after the jaw-thrust maneuver is tried.

12. **C.** "Look, listen, and feel" for air movement to determine breathlessness. Feeling with a hand for chest movement is helpful. However, both hands should be used to hyperextend and support the patient's neck and head.

13. **A.** A 5- to 10-sec check of the brachial pulse should be done to determine pulselessness because an infant's pulse is more difficult to check at the carotid or femoral sites.

14. **B.** A mouth-to-valve device allows for quick ventilations without risk to the rescuer from the patient. Mouth-to-mouth ventilation should be avoided if possible in this situation. The other options would unnecessarily delay ventilations.

15. **B.** Review the BCLS guidelines in this chapter.

16. **A.** All are correct except that the air/$O_2$ intake valve should not open when the resuscitation bag is squeezed. This allows the gas to escape rather than be directed to the patient.

17. **D.** The femoral site is recommended because it is a large artery that should be relatively easy to hit and is away from the patient's chest during compressions.

# 12 Airway Management

A review of the most recent Entry Level Examinations has shown an average of 9 questions (7% of the exam) that cover airway management issues.

## MODULE A

### Care for artificial airways and equipment to maintain a patent airway

### 1. Recommend the insertion of an artificial airway or a change of the type of artificial airway (NBRC code: IIIG1c) [Difficulty: R, Ap]

An artificial airway is indicated in any patient who cannot protect his or her airway. The patient could be at risk for upper airway obstruction that results from the tongue falling back, may have facial trauma or surgery, may be at risk for vomiting and aspirating, or may need mechanical ventilation for assisted breathing. A number of possible airways are available; select the best one according to the patient's needs.

An oropharyngeal airway is used in an unconscious patient who is at risk for airway obstruction caused by his or her tongue or for seizure activity. It prevents the tongue from being bitten during a seizure. It should not be used in a conscious patient because it may cause gagging. (See additional discussion and illustrations later in this chapter.)

A nasopharyngeal airway is used to keep the tongue from blocking the airway when an oropharyngeal airway cannot be used. This would occur with conscious patients or those with oral trauma or surgery. It is also used as a guide for passage of a catheter for tracheal suctioning. (See additional discussion and illustrations later in this chapter.)

An endotracheal tube is indicated when a patent airway is required for endotracheal suctioning or mechanical ventilation. Aspiration is also prevented when the cuff is inflated. An oral endotracheal tube is indicated in most emergency situations because it is faster and easier to place than a nasal endotracheal tube. A nasal endotracheal tube is indicated when the patient has oral trauma or when a cervical spine injury prevents the neck from being hyperextended for placement of the oral tube. (See additional discussion and illustrations later in this chapter.)

A tracheostomy tube is indicated for long-term airway management or when facial trauma or surgery prevents the use of an oral or nasal endotracheal tube. This tube also provides a patent airway for suctioning and mechanical ventilation and prevents aspiration. In addition, it is more comfortable than an endotracheal tube, and it allows the patient to eat and drink. So-called "talking" tracheostomy tubes permit the patient to vocalize with the aid of an additional source of airflow through the vocal cords. (See additional discussion and illustrations later in this chapter.)

A laryngeal mask airway (LMA) is used by an anesthesiologist as a way to ventilate an anesthetized patient without placement of an endotracheal tube (Fig. 12-1). The LMA is available in six sizes for insertion into patients ranging in weight from a small child to an adult. The distal end has a cuff that surrounds and seals the larynx when it is inflated. The proximal end of the attached tube has a standard adapter for ventilation with a manual resuscitator or an anesthesia machine. The LMA does not absolutely protect against aspiration, and tidal volume gas can leak if mechanical ventilation pressures greater than 20 cm water are needed.

> **Exam Hint**
>
> The NBRC commonly asks questions about which airway would be appropriate in a given patient care situation.

### 2. Properly position the patient to maintain a patent airway and minimize hypoxemia (NBRC code: IIIB1) [Difficulty: R, Ap]

Positioning of the head to open the airway is discussed in Chapter 11. Use the head-tilt/chin-lift maneuver to hyperextend the neck of an adult, and slightly extend the neck of a child to open the airway. A small pad can be placed behind the neck and head to put the patient in the "sniff position." Always keep the head in line with the body. If the patient has a known or suspected cervical spine injury, the neck cannot be hyperextended. Instead, open the airway with the jaw-thrust maneuver. Keep the head in line with the body.

The patient may be supine during the airway opening procedures just mentioned. Frequently, however, the patient is positioned with the head and body elevated. An unconscious patient is less likely to vomit and aspirate in

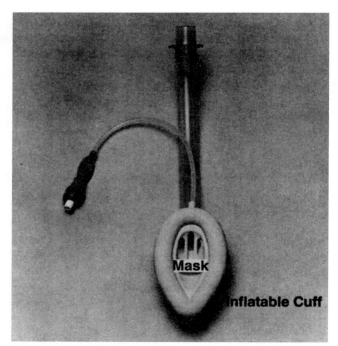

Fig. 12-1 Laryngeal mask airway (LMA). It features an inflatable mask that creates a seal around the patient's larynx. The proximal end of the tube can be connected to a resuscitation bag, anesthesia machine, or mechanical ventilator. *(From Intavent International SA, Henley-on-Thames, England.)*

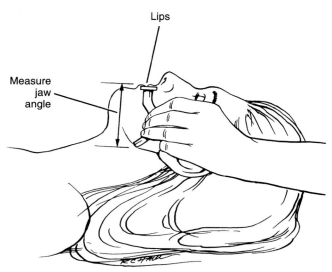

Fig. 12-2 Procedure for measuring the proper size of the oropharyngeal airway. *(From Eubanks DH, Bone RC: Comprehensive respiratory care, ed 2, St Louis, 1990, Mosby.)*

either Fowler's or semi-Fowler's position. The combination of either of these body positions with the head and neck hyperextended into the sniff position should keep the airway open, minimize the risk of aspiration of vomitus, and reduce the patient's work of breathing (WOB). This should help to minimize hypoxemia.

### 3. Humidify an artificial airway (NBRC code: IIIB5b) [Difficulty: R]

Patients with an endotracheal or tracheostomy tube in place should ideally be provided 100% relative humidity at body temperature. If not, secretions in the airway may dry and cause mucus plugs. Patients with an oropharyngeal or nasopharyngeal airway may also be given supplemental humidity through a simple aerosol mask to help prevent drying of secretions. See Chapter 8 for a complete discussion of humidity and aerosol therapy and administrative devices.

### 4. Oropharyngeal airways
#### a. Get the necessary equipment (NBRC code: IIA7a) [Difficulty: R]

The oropharyngeal airway (or *bite block*) is made of plastic that is hard enough to withstand any patient's biting force. This airway is indicated in two situations: First, in an unconscious, supine patient who is experiencing upper airway obstruction because the tongue is falling back and blocking the oropharynx; second, in a patient who is unconscious and biting down hard when having a seizure. This can cause injury to the patient or pinch off an oral endotracheal tube if one is present.

A properly sized and placed oropharyngeal airway lifts the tongue forward from the posterior portion of the oropharynx to keep a patent airway and make suctioning oral secretions easier. An oropharyngeal airway is poorly tolerated in a conscious patient and can cause gagging and even vomiting. Oropharyngeal airways come in a variety of sizes from infant to adult. The proper size is found by holding it against the patient's face with the flange against the lips. The end of the airway should reach the angle of the jaw (Fig. 12-2). Too large an airway can block the oropharynx by extending past the tongue; too small an airway can push the tongue back into the oropharynx rather than pulling the tongue forward as it should. Fig. 12-3 shows a properly placed and sized oropharyngeal airway.

A number of manufacturers make oropharyngeal airways, which fall into two basic types: hollow center and I-beam (Fig. 12-4).

#### 1. Hollow center

Hollow center oropharyngeal airways have an oval or rectangular shape in cross section and are hollow in the center. A suction catheter can be placed easily through the hollow center to the back of the throat to clear out secretions. Some types have an outer tube that can be attached by a practitioner to provide a mouthpiece for rescue breathing. If rescue breathing must be performed, it is probably more effective to ventilate with a mask and manual resuscitator when one becomes available.

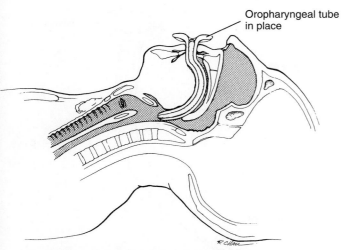

Oropharyngeal tube in place

**Fig. 12-3** Cross section through the head showing the proper position of an oropharyngeal airway. *(From Eubanks DH, Bone RC: Comprehensive respiratory care, ed 2, St Louis, 1990, Mosby.)*

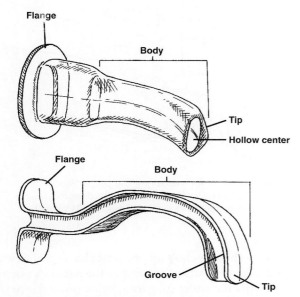

**Fig. 12-4** Close-ups of hollow center and I-beam types of oropharyngeal airways.

### 2. I-Beam

I-beam oropharyngeal airways are shaped like an I-beam in cross section. A suction catheter can be guided easily along the groove on either side of the I-beam to the back of the throat to clear out secretions.

#### b. Put the equipment together and make sure that it works properly (NBRC code: IIA7a) [Difficulty: R]

Most oropharyngeal airways are single units with nothing to assemble. Some hollow center types have an attachable outer part. The outer part is snapped onto the oropha-

ryngeal airway when the practitioner needs to perform rescue breathing. It has a wide flange so that the lips can be covered and sealed to prevent a leak.

#### c. Troubleshoot any problems with the equipment (NBRC code: IIA7a) [Difficulty: R]

Make sure that the channel in the hollow center type is patent. If a unit is plugged by secretions, blood, or foreign debris, the patient cannot breathe through the opening, and a suction catheter cannot be passed through. Remove an airway through which the patient cannot breathe.

#### d. Insert the correct oropharyngeal airway (NBRC code: IIIB2) [Difficulty: R, Ap]

Two methods are widely used to insert an oropharyngeal airway.

##### 1. First method

a. Open the patient's mouth with the cross-finger technique. Insert the airway backward into the patient's mouth until it reaches the palate. Some authors recommend inserting it past the uvula.

b. Twist the airway 180 degrees, and insert it the rest of the way until the tongue is supported by the curved body.

c. The flange should rest at the lips (Fig. 12-5).

##### 2. Second method

a. Open the patient's mouth with the cross-finger technique. Insert the airway into the mouth with the curved body rotated toward a cheek.

b. Twist the airway 90 degrees, and insert it the rest of the way so that the tongue is supported by the curved body.

c. The flange should rest at the lips.

### 5. Nasopharyngeal airways

#### a. Get the necessary equipment (NBRC code: IIA7a) [Difficulty: R]

Nasopharyngeal airways (also known as *nasal airways, nasal trumpets,* or *nasal stints*) are made of a relatively soft and pliable plastic or rubber. This material decreases the chances that the delicate mucous membranes of the nose and nasopharynx will be damaged. A nasopharyngeal airway is often used in a supine patient to ensure a patent airway by pushing the tongue forward off of the posterior portion of the oropharynx. The nasopharyngeal airway is probably not as effective as the oropharyngeal airway in keeping the tongue forward. However, an advantage of the nasopharyngeal airway is that it is better tolerated in a semiconscious or alert patient than an oropharyngeal airway. Nasopharyngeal airways are also commonly used to provide a secure channel through which a suction catheter or bronchoscope can be passed. The nasopharyn-

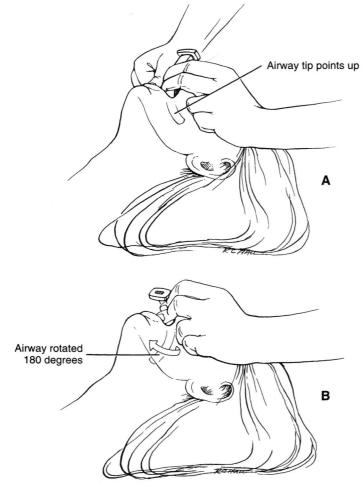

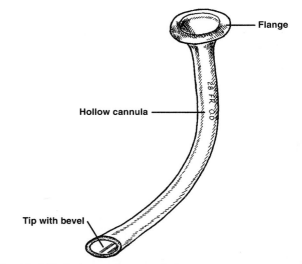

**Fig. 12-6** Typical nasopharyngeal airway.

**Fig. 12-5** One procedure for inserting an oropharyngeal airway. **A,** Airway is placed with the tip pointing toward the palate. **B,** Airway is rotated 180 degrees to support the tongue. *(From Eubanks DH, Bone RC: Comprehensive respiratory care, ed 2, St Louis, 1990, Mosby.)*

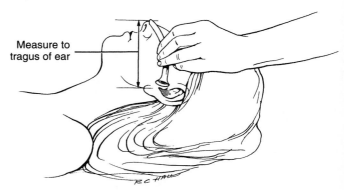

**Fig. 12-7** Procedure for measuring the proper size of the nasopharyngeal airway. *(From Eubanks DH, Bone RC: Comprehensive respiratory care, ed 2, St Louis, 1990, Mosby.)*

geal airway protects the patient's mucous membranes from the trauma of repeatedly passed catheters. A nasopharyngeal airway can be used in a patient with trauma to the jaw or seizures with a tightly closed jaw. In these cases, an oropharyngeal airway cannot be used. The nasopharyngeal airway can be passed into the patient's oropharynx to push the tongue forward and maintain an airway.

Several manufacturers make the two basic types of nasopharyngeal airways: the *blunt tip* and the *beveled tip.* The beveled tip types come with right-sided and left-sided cut bevels. If possible, get the airway with the bevel cut that opens toward the patient's oropharynx (toward the nasal septum). For instance, if the airway is going to be inserted into the left naris, the bevel should be cut on the right side of the tube to open to the patient's oropharynx. If the tube is being inserted into the right naris, the bevel should be cut on the left side of the tube.

Fig. 12-6 shows a close-up of a nasopharyngeal airway. All have a flange that fits up close to the patient's nostril. This prevents the entire tube from being pushed into the patient. All have a cannula with a channel through which breathing or suctioning can occur. Nasopharyngeal airways are available in a variety of sizes for adults. They can be properly sized by measuring from the tip of the nose to the tragus of the ear and adding 2 to 3 cm (Fig. 12-7).

**b. Put the equipment together and make sure that it works properly (NBRC code: IIA7a) [Difficulty: R]**
**c. Troubleshoot any problems with the equipment (NBRC code: IIA7a) [Difficulty: R]**

All nasopharyngeal airways are made up of a single piece with nothing to assemble. Make sure the tube is not plugged by dried secretions, blood, or foreign debris. If the tube is plugged, the patient cannot breathe through it and a suction catheter cannot be passed through it. Remove a plugged nasopharyngeal airway.

**d. Insert the correct nasopharyngeal airway (NBRC code: IIIB2) [Difficulty: R, Ap]**

The following steps are used for nasopharyngeal airway insertion:

1. Select the most patent nostril. Check the patient's chart for a history of a broken nose, deviated septum, or current head cold. Interview the conscious patient to see whether one nostril is more open than the other. Place a finger in front of the patient's nostrils to feel which one has greater airflow. Avoid forcing the airway into a nostril and nasal passage that can be damaged by the procedure.
2. Lubricate the properly sized airway with a sterile, water-soluble lubricant (e.g., K-Y Jelly). Place the lubricant on a sterile, 4 × 4-inch gauze pad, and smear it over the length of the airway.
3. Tell the patient what to expect during the procedure.
4. Gently place the airway into the nostril. It should be directed straight back parallel to the hard palate. Stop and try a different angle if resistance is felt. Do not force the airway. Try the other nostril if necessary.
5. Check the placement by looking into the patient's mouth with a flashlight and tongue depressor. A properly placed nasopharyngeal airway can be seen in the oropharynx extending behind the tongue (Figs. 12-8 and 12-9).
6. Secure the airway by sticking a safety pin through the flange and taping the pin to the bridge of the patient's nose or cheek (see Fig. 12-8). This prevents accidental pulling out or pushing in the airway.
7. Rotate the airway to the other nostril, if possible, on a regular basis. This prevents ulceration of the mucous membrane. Some authors recommend rotation at least every 48 hr, whereas others recommend rotation at much shorter intervals.

## 6. Tracheostomy tubes
### a. Get the necessary equipment (NBRC code: IIA7c) [Difficulty: R, Ap]

The tracheostomy tube offers the same uses as the endotracheal tube, such as maintaining a secure airway, providing a direct suctioning route to the lungs, preventing aspiration, and ensuring a safe route by which mechanical ventilation can be provided. In addition, it is placed in the patient who has an upper airway obstruction or facial trauma, thus making intubation impossible. A tracheostomy tube is often placed in a patient who requires long-term mechanical ventilation or who needs a perma-

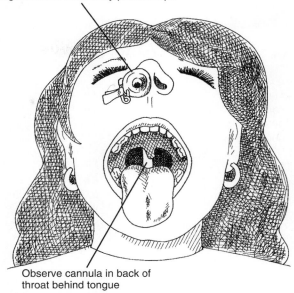

**Fig. 12-8** Proper position of the nasopharyngeal airway behind the tongue can be determined by looking into the mouth. The tube is secured by a safety pin that is placed through the flange taped to the cheek.

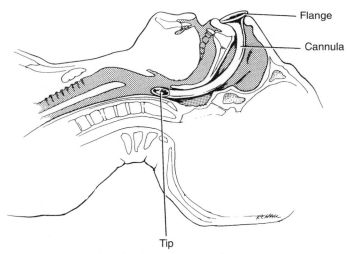

**Fig. 12-9** Cross section of the head showing the proper position of the nasopharyngeal airway. *(From Ellis PD, Billings DM: Cardiopulmonary resuscitation: procedures for basic and advanced life support, St Louis, 1980, Mosby.)*

nent artificial airway. In the long term, a tracheostomy is considered more comfortable than an endotracheal tube, even though it necessitates a surgical procedure. An additional advantage of a tracheostomy tube over an endotracheal tube is the ability of the patient to eat and drink.

Tracheostomy tubes come in a variety of sizes for patients of all ages from neonates to adults. Table 12-1

| Age | ID (mm) | Approximate OD (mm) | Fr Size (OD) |
|---|---|---|---|
| **TABLE 12-1** Endotracheal and Tracheostomy Tube Sizes Based on Patient Age* | | | |
| **NEWBORN** | | | |
| <1000 g | 2.5 | 4.0 | 12 |
| 1000–2000 g | 3.0 | 5.0 | 14 |
| 2000–3000 g | 3.5 | 5.5 | 16–18 |
| 3000 g to 6 mo old | 3.5–4.0 | | |
| **PEDIATRIC** | | | |
| 18 mo | 4.0 | 6.0 | 18 |
| 3 yr | 4.5 | 6.5 | 20 |
| 5 yr | 5.0 | 7.0 | 22 |
| 6 yr | 5.5 | 8.0 | 24 |
| 8 yr | 6.0 | 9.0 | 26 |
| **ADULT** | | | |
| 16 yr | 7.0 | 10.0 | 30 |
| Normal-sized woman | 7.5–8.0 | 11.0 | 32–34 |
| Normal-sized man | 8.0–8.5 | 12.0 | 34–36 |
| Large adult | 9.0–10.0 | 13.0–14.0 | 38–42 |

*Fr*, French; *ID*, Internal diameter; *OD*, outer diameter.
*Two notes: First, it is important to always use the largest tube that can be placed into the patient without causing any harm during the intubation. This is because the larger the ID of the tube, the less airway resistance it causes. Be prepared to insert a tube that is one size larger or smaller than anticipated based on individual variances. Second, the mathematical relationship between the OD in millimeters and Fr size can be easily calculated. The Fr size is determined by multiplying the OD in millimeters by 3. The OD in millimeters is found by dividing the Fr size by 3.

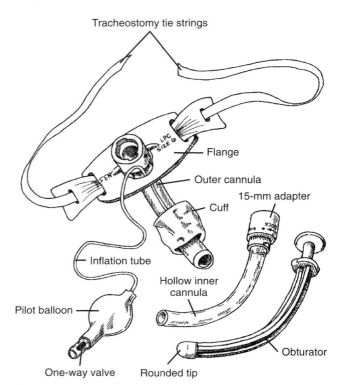

**Fig. 12-10** Typical tracheostomy tube with its component parts and features.

shows tracheostomy tube sizes for patients according to age. Most modern tracheostomy tubes are constructed of a hard polyvinyl chloride plastic and have a high-volume, low-pressure cuff. Some specialty tubes are made of silver, rubber, or latex. The older silver tubes have a removable cuff. Specific information on three types of tubes follows.

### b. Put the equipment together and make sure that it works properly (NBRC code: IIA7c) [Difficulty: R, Ap]

Following are commonly seen examples of tracheostomy tube styles:

### 1. Standard tracheostomy tube

Most patients have a standard tracheostomy tube that is placed after the tracheostomy procedure. Refer to Fig. 12-10 for these features of a typical tracheostomy tube:

a. The cannula is the airway through which the patient breathes. The proximal end is outside of the patient's stoma and is attached to an adjustable flange. The angle of the flange can be adjusted so that the distal end of the cannula fits properly into

the patient's trachea. Soft, cloth tracheostomy tie strings are tied to the ends of the flange. The loose ends are tied behind the patient's neck to hold the tube in place. The distal end of the cannula has a small area imbedded with radiopaque material. As with an endotracheal tube, this allows the end of the cannula to be seen on a chest x-ray film. The cuff is a high residual volume, low pressure type. Air is put into and taken out of the cuff by an inflation tube with a pilot balloon and one-way valve.

b. The obturator is slid into the outer cannula's opening before it is inserted into the patient's stoma. The obturator has a rounded end that protrudes from the end of the cannula. This prevents tissue trauma during the insertion. The obturator is removed as soon as the cannula is in place.

c. An inner cannula is slid into the outer cannula's opening and is locked into place with a clockwise twist. This completes the airway. The proximal end has a standard 15-mm outer diameter (OD) adapter so that all respiratory care equipment fits onto it. The distal end is flush with the end of the outer cannula. Some practitioners say that the inner cannula should be periodically removed and cleansed so that secretions do not build up. Other practitioners say this is unnecessary if the airway is properly humidified and suctioning is performed as needed.

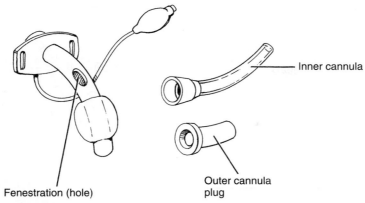

**Fig. 12-11** Fenestrated tracheostomy tube with its component parts and features. *(From Eubanks DH, Bone RC: Comprehensive respiratory care, ed 2, St Louis, 1990, Mosby.)*

### 2. Fenestrated tracheostomy tube

This tube is often placed in a patient who can breathe spontaneously and who is being considered for complete removal of the tracheostomy tube. If the patient does well with this tube, it can probably be removed safely. If the patient has difficulty, the plug can be removed, the inner cannula can be replaced, and the patient's airway can be suctioned or mechanically ventilated.

Refer to Fig. 12-11 when reviewing these features of the fenestrated tracheostomy tube:

a. The outer cannula has an opening called the *fenestration* (Dutch for "window"). The rest of the cannula, cuff, inflation tube, and flange are the same as previously discussed.

b. The inner cannula functions as described previously. When the inner cannula is in place, the tube functions as the standard model does.

c. The outer cannula plug is used to prevent the patient from breathing through the proximal end of the tube. The plug does not cover the fenestration; therefore, the patient is able to breathe through the upper airway. The patient can now talk and cough up any secretions.

### c. Troubleshoot any problems with the equipment (NBRC code: IIA7c) [Difficulty: R, Ap]

Most tubes have cuffs that must be inflated before they are into the patient to make sure that the cuff is sealed and the one-way valve does not leak. Do not use a tube with a leaking cuff or one-way valve. Make sure that the obturator, inner cannula, and plug all fit properly into the outer cannula. All should easily snap into place and should be easily removable. Check this before you insert the tube into the patient.

Secretions or foreign matter can plug the lumen of the cannula. Suction to remove any obstruction. If the catheter cannot be inserted beyond the tube and the patient is having respiratory distress, the tube will have to be removed and replaced. A mucus plug or cuff that has herniated or slipped over the end of the tube can cause this.

### d. Troubleshoot any problems with a speaking tracheostomy tube (NBRC code: IIA25) [Difficulty: R, Ap]

Refer to Fig. 12-12 when you review these features of the speaking tracheostomy tube:

a. The cannula is the standard type except that an additional tube has been added to carry a compressed gas through a hole in the back of the cannula. This gas flows up through the vocal cords and allows the patient to speak. The voice is not as strong as it normally is, but it is still a great help to the patient's psychological well-being. The patient can be mechanically ventilated and suctioned, and can eat and drink as usual.

b. A Y-connector is added to the compressed gas tube. Usually, about 4 to 6 L/min of compressed air or oxygen ($O_2$) is set by a flowmeter to run to the Y. Closing off the other opening in the Y with a finger diverts the gas into the patient's larynx for speaking. A little experimentation with flows can help the patient find the flow that works best for speaking. If the patient cannot speak at all, check that the gas is turned on and the tubing is properly connected.

### 7. Tracheostomy buttons
### a. Get the necessary equipment (NBRC code: IIA7c) [Difficulty: R, Ap]

A tracheostomy button is a hard plastic tube that is placed into the patient's stoma to keep it open after the tracheostomy tube has been removed. The patient is able to eat, talk, and cough normally. Yet, in case the patient has difficulty or needs a breathing treatment, the airway can be reestablished quickly. In general, patient sizes for

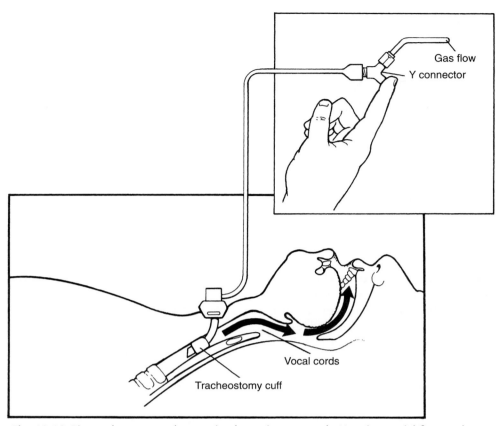

**Fig. 12-12** Pitt tracheostomy tube permits the patient to speak. Note its special feature that directs an outside gas flow past the vocal cords. *(From Scanlan CL, Simmons KF: Airway management. In Scanlan CL, Wilkins RL, Stoller JK, editors: Egan's fundamentals of respiratory care, ed 7, St Louis, 1990, Mosby.)*

tracheostomy buttons match those for tracheostomy tubes listed in Table 12-1. Information follows on the two types of buttons.

### b. Put the equipment together and make sure that it works properly (NBRC code: IIA7c) [Difficulty: R, Ap]

Refer to Fig. 12-13 when you review these features of the tracheostomy button:

1. The hollow outer cannula has a slightly flared proximal end, which keeps it from slipping all the way into the patient. The distal end is flanged and split into several flexible "grippers."

2. A closure plug fits into the outer cannula and snaps into the flexible grippers on the end of the outer cannula. This seals the button so that the patient breathes through the upper airway.

3. A hollow inner cannula can be inserted into the outer cannula instead of the plug. This inner cannula has a standard 15-mm OD so that a Briggs adapter or other respiratory care equipment can be attached if needed. The patient can also be suctioned.

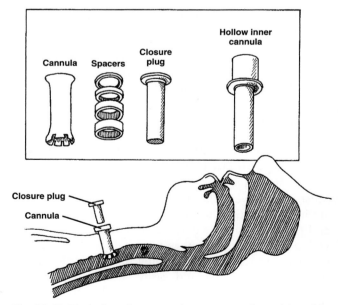

**Fig. 12-13** Typical tracheostomy button properly positioned in a patient. The insert shows its component parts.

4. Spacers of various widths are used to ensure that the inner cannula is placed into the patient to the right depth. The end of the tube should enter the trachea but not obstruct it. See Fig. 12-13 for the proper position.

### c. Troubleshoot any problems with the equipment (NBRC code: IIA7c) [Difficulty: R, Ap]

Make sure that all component pieces of the tracheostomy buttons fit together properly and can be easily disconnected if necessary. The cannula must be kept clear of secretions, blood, and foreign debris. A suction catheter should be passable through the hollow opening in the cannula. If the button is obstructed and the patient is having trouble breathing through his or her upper airway, the button should be removed and replaced with another or with a tracheostomy tube.

### d. Troubleshoot any problems with a speaking tracheostomy button/valve (NBRC code: IIA25) [Difficulty: R, Ap]

Special tracheostomy buttons are used with patients who are not able to breathe in through their upper airway but may breathe out through it. This enables the patient to speak. Kistner and Passey-Muir are two common types. Refer to Fig. 12-14 when you review these features of the Kistner tracheostomy tube:

a. The hollow plastic cannula keeps the stoma open. The distal end is flanged so that it is not likely to be pulled out of the trachea accidentally.
b. The proximal end of the cannula is capped with a one-way valve, which allows the patient to breathe in room air or an $O_2$- or aerosol-enriched gas source.

Expiration occurs through the upper airway. The patient can talk, eat, and cough normally.

### 8. Intubation equipment: laryngoscope and blades

#### a. Get the necessary equipment (NBRC code: IIA7d) [Difficulty: R, Ap]

The laryngoscope is made up of two basic parts: a handle and a blade. The most commonly seen handle is made of stainless steel; some newer units are made of plastic. The handle contains two C batteries to power the light source in the blade. All handles have a common base with a hooking bar so that the blades can be attached (Figs. 12-15 and 12-16).

Blades are available in a variety of sizes from pediatric to adult. They all have a common hook for snapping and locking in place on the handle. The stainless steel handles use stainless steel blades; the newer plastic handles use plastic blades. The two different sets of handles and blades are not interchangeable. Blades come in two different shapes: Miller blades are straight, and MacIntosh blades

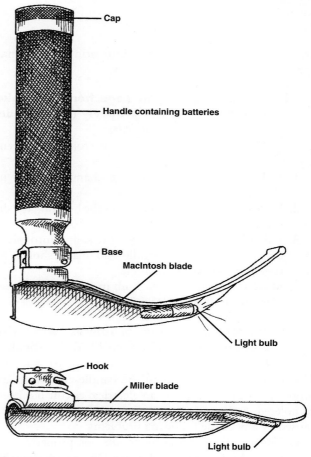

**Fig. 12-15** Laryngoscope handle with a MacIntosh (curved) blade attached *(top)* and a Miller (straight) blade *(bottom)*. Note the component parts and features.

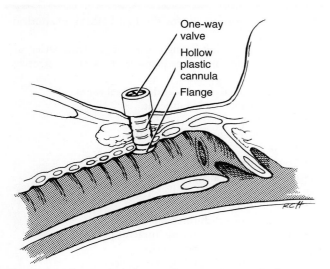

**Fig. 12-14** Kistner tracheostomy button. *(From Eubanks DH, Bone RC: Comprehensive respiratory care, ed 2, St Louis, 1990, Mosby.)*

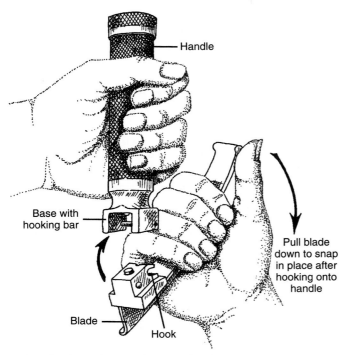

Handle

Base with hooking bar

Pull blade down to snap in place after hooking onto handle

Blade

Hook

**Fig. 12-16** Motions used to attach a laryngoscope to a handle.

are curved (see Fig. 12-15). The intubating person may specify a specific blade style and size.

### b. Put the equipment together and make sure that it works properly (NBRC code: IIA7d) [Difficulty: R, Ap]

See Fig. 12-16 for the steps you should follow in fastening the blade to the handle.

1. Hold the handle in the left hand and the blade in the right hand.
2. Place the hook on the blade over the hooking bar on the base of the handle.
3. Pull the blade down so that it snaps into place on the handle. The handle and blade should fit together at a 90-degree angle.
4. Make sure that the light bulb in the stainless steel blade is tight.

### c. Troubleshoot any problems with the equipment (NBRC code: IIA7d) [Difficulty: R, Ap]

The light source shines when the handle and blade are properly connected because an electrical circuit has been completed. Failure of the light source to shine could be caused by any of the following problems:

a. The handle and the blade are not properly connected and snapped into place. Disconnect them by performing the opposite motions, and reconnect them properly.

b. You have cross-connected stainless steel and plastic components. Stainless steel handles go only with stainless steel blades, and plastic handles go only with plastic blades.

c. The batteries are low as shown by the bulb's failing to glow or glowing yellow instead of white. Unscrew the cap from the handle. Replace the old batteries with two new C batteries. When reassembled, the bulb should glow white.

d. The batteries are not placed properly. It does not matter if a positive or a negative pole touches the base of the handle. Be sure that a positive pole touches a negative pole or vice versa so that electrical current will flow properly. When reassembled, the bulb should glow white.

e. The light bulb in the stainless steel blade is loose or defective. Tighten the light bulb by turning it clockwise. It should light up if it was just loose. Unscrew and throw away a defective light bulb, and replace it with a light bulb of the same size. When reassembled, the bulb should glow white. The newer plastic laryngoscopes use a fiberoptic bundle as the light source; no light bulb is involved, so no tightening or replacing is necessary.

Besides the laryngoscope handle and blades, some additional items (Box 12-1) are typically needed to ensure a smooth, safe intubation procedure.

---

### Exam Hint

**K**now how to troubleshoot and fix a malfunctioning laryngoscope and blade.

---

### BOX 12-1   Equipment for Oral and Nasal Intubation

- Pediatric and adult laryngoscope handles with batteries
- Straight and curved pediatric and adult laryngoscope blades
- Variety of nasal and oral endotracheal tubes
- Water-soluble, sterile lubricant
- Metal stylet
- Magill forceps for nasal intubation
- Hemostat
- Tongue depressors
- Oropharyngeal airways
- Bite block
- Nasopharyngeal airways
- 10-mL syringe with three-way stopcock
- Manometer for measuring intracuff pressure
- Tape or tube-restraining device
- Yankauer or other oral suction device
- Sterile suction catheter for tracheal suctioning
- Stethoscope for listening to breath sounds

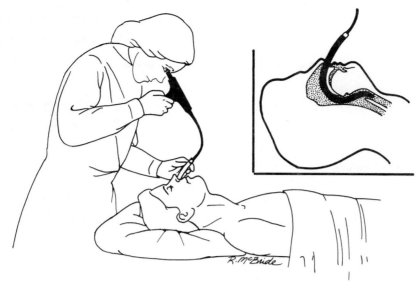

**Fig. 12-17** A fiberoptic laryngoscope that is being used to insert an endotracheal tube through the nasal passage. *(From Scanlan C, Simmons K: Airway management. In Scanlan CL, Wilkins RL, Stoller JK, editors: Egan's fundamentals of respiratory care, ed 7, St Louis, 1999, Mosby.)*

### 9. Intubation equipment: fiberoptic devices

**a. Get the necessary equipment (NBRC code: IIA7d) [Difficulty: R, Ap]**

A physician may use a fiberoptic laryngoscope (Fig. 12-17) or bronchoscope (see Fig. 17-3) to visualize the larynx and trachea during a difficult intubation. Either one can be used during a nasal or oral endotracheal intubation procedure.

**b. Put the equipment together and make sure that it works properly (NBRC code: IIA7d) [Difficulty: R, Ap]**

**c. Troubleshoot any problems with the equipment (NBRC code: IIA7d) [Difficulty: R, Ap]**

Review the discussion on bronchoscopy in Chapter 17 for details on the equipment. The fiberoptic tube should be lubricated so that it will easily slide through the lumen of the endotracheal tube (see Fig. 12-17). After the physician has confirmed that the distal end of the fiberoptic tube has entered the trachea, the endotracheal tube is gently pushed into the trachea. The fiberoptic tube is then withdrawn, the cuff is inflated, and the endotracheal tube is secured. If the endotracheal tube will not slide into the patient's trachea, it is too large, or not enough lubricant has been placed on the fiberoptic tube. It may be necessary to withdraw it, correct the problem, and start over again.

### 10. Oral and nasal endotracheal tubes

**a. Get the necessary equipment (NBRC code: IIA7b) [Difficulty: R, Ap]**

An endotracheal tube is the best emergency device for maintaining a secure airway. It also provides a direct suctioning route to the lungs and prevents aspiration. Mechanical ventilation can easily be provided through it. An endotracheal tube is meant to be a temporary airway; however, it can be kept in patients for weeks if necessary. Virtually all endotracheal tubes used clinically are made of pliable plastic. Always select a tube with a large residual volume, low pressure cuff, unless a specific opposing reason exists. For the most part, oral and nasal endotracheal tubes can be used interchangeably. In a side-by-side comparison, a nasal endotracheal tube is longer and more curved than an oral endotracheal tube. The greater curve of the nasal tube should result in less pressure on the nasal mucosa. An anesthesiologist would request a nasal tube if he or she were going to place it by the nasal route. Oral tubes are used in most patients.

Tubes are available in sizes from 4 mm OD through 14 mm OD, so that patients of all ages and sizes can be intubated. OD size increments are 0.5 mm. The outer wall of the tube varies from 0.5 to 1 mm. This results in reduction in the inner diameter (ID) of the tube by about 1 to 2 mm. Table 12-1 lists the approximate ID of an endotracheal tube that is placed into a patient according to his or her age. The size of an endotracheal tube (or tracheostomy tube) is commonly referred to by its inner diameter. Once the tube has been properly placed into the patient, the excess tube (beyond 3 to 4 cm past the teeth) should be

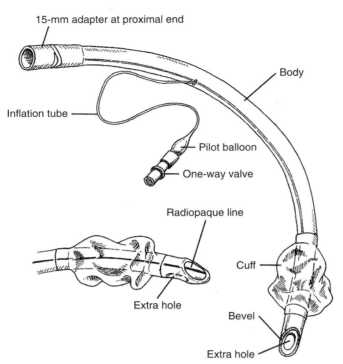

**Fig. 12-18** Typical, modern endotracheal tube with its component parts. The insert shows the important features found at the distal end of the tube.

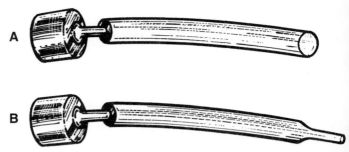

**Fig. 12-19** Comparison of the two different types of pediatric endotracheal tubes. **A,** This tube is made by several manufacturers and has a uniform diameter. **B,** This tube is made by Cole and features a narrowing of the distal tip to pass through the vocal cords. Note that neither has a cuff. *(From Burgess WR, Chernick V: Respiratory therapy in newborn infants and children, ed 2, New York, 1986, Thieme.)*

cut off. This reduces airway resistance and mechanical dead space.

Most endotracheal tubes have the standard features shown in Fig. 12-18. A number of specialty endotracheal tubes are in limited use. They all share the same characteristics except for some special feature. These tubes are needed in specific patient care situations.

### 1. Pediatric endotracheal tubes

Pediatric endotracheal tubes come in two basic types. One type has a constant diameter. During intubation, the tube should be inserted until the black mark (about 2 cm from the tip) is at the vocal cords. The second type has a relatively wide proximal part to the body that narrows at the distal end. This design allows the smaller diameter tip to be passed through the vocal cords but prevents the wide "shoulder" from passing into the trachea. Both types of tube end with a single opening with a bevel cut (Fig. 12-19). Neither type has a cuff on any tube that is 2 to 3 mm ID or smaller.

### 2. Armored tubes

Armored tubes have a steel spring coiled through them. An advantage of armored tubes over regular ones is that they do not collapse if the patient should bite down. Furthermore, the tube may be pre-bent for shape and does not kink as a plastic tube might.

### 3. Preformed tubes

Preformed tubes have been pre-shaped for better patient comfort or security. One style has a forward bend so that the tube can be taped to the chin. A pediatric tube with a bend for taping it to the forehead also exists.

### 4. Guidable (trigger) tubes

Guidable trigger tubes have a wire imbedded within the tube wall. When the ring at the proximal end is pulled, the distal tip is flexed up to shorten the radius of the curve. This allows direction of the tube into the anterior trachea. Guidable trigger tubes make it easier for the clinician to intubate a patient with an anterior larynx or to perform a blind nasal intubation.

### 5. Double-lumen endotracheal tubes

Double-lumen endotracheal tubes allow independent lung ventilation. A double-lumen tube is also used during special procedures with one lung such as bronchoscopy, bronchoalveolar lavage, lobectomy, and pneumonectomy. The other lung may be mechanically ventilated so that the patient's blood gas values can be maintained (Fig. 12-20). An adapter can be added to join the two proximal ends of the channels so that a single ventilator can be used to ventilate both lungs. The Carlens tube is used to preferentially intubate the left bronchus. The White tube is used to preferentially intubate the right bronchus (Fig. 12-21). Robertshaw makes tubes for either right or left bronchial intubation.

Several limitations are inherent in all double-lumen tubes. First, they can be used only on adults because the smallest size is 8 mm OD. Second, the small ID of the two lumina results in high airway resistance. Third, a much smaller than normal suction catheter must be used for removal of any tracheal secretions.

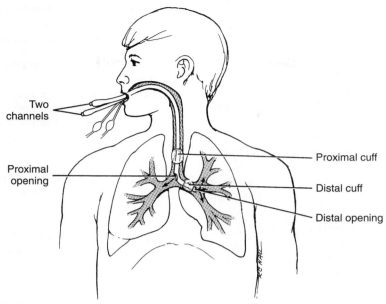

**Fig. 12-20** A double-lumen endotracheal tube properly positioned in the patient so that both lungs can be independently ventilated and suctioned, or so that special procedures can be performed. *(From Eubanks DH, Bone RC: Comprehensive respiratory care, ed 2, St Louis, 1990, Mosby.)*

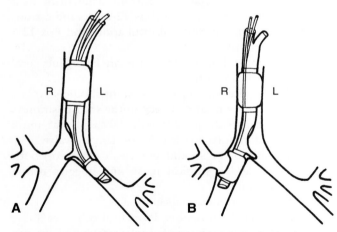

**Fig. 12-21** Two types of double-lumen endotracheal tubes. **A,** Carlens tube; its distal tube enters the left mainstem bronchus. **B,** White tube; its distal tube enters the right mainstem bronchus. Note how both tubes have a cuff that seals the trachea and a cuff that seals a bronchus. Each has its own inflation tube, pilot balloon, and one-way valve. *(From Miller RD, editor: Anesthesia, New York, 1981, Churchill Livingstone.)*

### Exam Hint

**K**now the proper sizes of the endotracheal or tracheostomy tube that is used for an adult male or female and an infant.

## b. Put the equipment together and make sure that it works properly (NBRC code: IIA7b) [Difficulty: R, Ap]

Refer to Fig. 12-18 for these components of a standard endotracheal tube:

1. The hollow curved body is the main part of the tube. Through it, the patient can breathe or a suction catheter can be placed. Printing on the side shows the OD and ID. Make sure that the central channel is not plugged by dried secretions, blood, or foreign debris.

2. The proximal end is left outside of the patient's nose or mouth. An adapter with a 15-mm-OD equipment connector is inserted into the tube. The other end of the adapter narrows and is individually sized to fit snugly into the ID of the endotracheal tube. Adapters cannot be cross-fitted to different sizes of endotracheal tubes.

3. The distal end is inserted into the patient's trachea. The tip is cut with either a right- or a left-sided bevel. The bevel cut creates an oval-shaped opening that is less likely to become plugged with secretions compared with a round opening. An extra hole (the Murphy eye) is cut into the tube on the opposite side of the bevel.

4. A line of radiopaque material is imbedded in the tube from the tip back to the cuff. This is important because it is seen as a white line on the chest x-ray film to show where the tip of the tube is located in the trachea (see the insert in Fig. 12-18).

5. A cuff (balloon) is located a few centimeters back from the tip of the tube. It is blown up with air to seal the trachea so that mechanical ventilation can be performed and aspiration prevented. Most modern tubes have a large residual volume, low pressure cuff. *Note:* All tubes with a 5-mm or greater OD have cuffs. Smaller neonatal and pediatric tubes are available with or without a cuff.

6. A cuff-filling inflation tube is connected about halfway down the tube. The proximal end is left out of the patient's mouth, and the distal end goes to the cuff so that it can be inflated and deflated. A pilot balloon that inflates and deflates with the cuff is found in the middle of the capillary tube or is connected with the one-way valve at the distal end. The one-way valve has an end that connects to any syringe. When the syringe is disconnected, the one-way valve seals to prevent the air in the cuff from escaping.

7. With a double-lumen endotracheal tube, each lumen has its own 15-mm adapter, cuff, one-way valve, pilot balloon, and inflation tube to inflate the cuff. As with traditional endotracheal tubes, both cuffs should be test-inflated. They should hold the air without a leak and then be easily deflated. One additional piece of equipment can be used with a double-lumen tube: A plastic Y can be used to connect the proximal ends of both tubes. This is done by removal of both 15-mm adapters and insertion of one branch of the Y into each of the proximal ends of the tubes. The open end of the Y has a 15-mm adapter so that it can be connected to a ventilator or $O_2$ source.

### c. Troubleshoot any problems with the equipment (NBRC code: IIA7b) [Difficulty: R, Ap]

Cuff(s) should be inflated and the syringe disconnected from the one-way valve before the tube is placed in the patient to make sure the system works properly. The cuff(s) should hold the air. Do not use any tube with a leaking cuff or one-way valve. Deflate the cuff before you place the tube into the patient.

## MODULE B

### Perform endotracheal intubation (NBRC code: IB7l) [Difficulty: R, Ap]

Oral endotracheal intubation is the recommended procedure for securing the airway during an emergency such as a cardiopulmonary resuscitation (CPR) attempt. In uncomplicated cases, the patient can be quickly intubated with an apneic period of no longer than 20 sec. It is recommended that this procedure should be performed by a team of two respiratory therapists. It is difficult, if not impossible, for a single therapist to perform this impor-

---

### BOX 12-2   Indications and Contraindications for Oral Endotracheal Intubation

**GENERAL INDICATIONS FOR ENDOTRACHEAL INTUBATION**
Provide a secure, patent airway
Provide a route for mechanical ventilation
Prevent aspiration of stomach or mouth contents
Provide a route for suctioning the lungs
Use general anesthesia

**INDICATIONS FOR ORAL INTUBATION**
Fastest, easiest method by which to secure the airway
Simpler, less invasive method cannot ensure an open airway

**CONTRAINDICATIONS FOR ORAL INTUBATION**
Cervical spine injury such that the patient's neck cannot be hyperextended
Lower facial injury
Oral surgery

---

tant task without placing the patient at great risk. Usually, the therapist who intubates is considered the leader, and another therapist acts as the assistant. Therapists must feel comfortable in both roles. Box 12-2 lists indications and contraindications for oral intubation, and Box 12-3 lists complications.

Perform the following steps for an emergency oral endotracheal intubation:

1. Prepare the patient. The assistant should
   a. Place the head and neck in the sniff position
   b. Ventilate the patient with 100% $O_2$ by facemask and manual resuscitator or demand valve

2. The intubator should put clean gloves on both hands and a surgical mask and goggles before proceeding.

3. Prepare the endotracheal tube.
   a. Select the proper endotracheal tube (see Table 12-1 for recommended tube sizes based on age). If time permits, the next smaller and larger tube size should also be selected.
   b. Inflate the cuff with a 10- or 20-mL syringe. Remove the syringe from the one-way valve. Make sure that it can hold the air and can then deflate the cuff completely.
   c. Lubricate the distal few centimeters of the endotracheal tube with a water-soluble lubricant.
   d. Lubricate a stylet with the sterile water-soluble lubricant. Place the stylet into the tube so that the natural curve of the tube is maintained. The tip of the stylet should not go past the end of the tube (Fig. 12-22). Some practitioners may prefer not to use a stylet. Many believe that the stylet offers the advantage of being able to bend

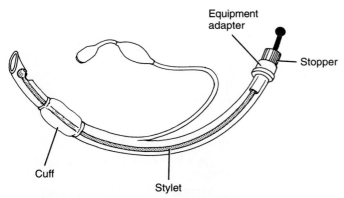

**Fig. 12-22** Stylet with stopper properly placed in a standard endotracheal tube to maintain its curved shape. *(From Eubanks DH, Bone RC: Comprehensive respiratory care, ed 2, St Louis, 1990, Mosby.)*

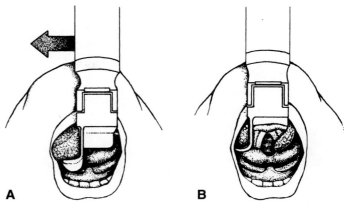

**Fig. 12-23** Proper placement of the laryngoscope blade for moving the patient's tongue. **A,** Proper placement of the laryngoscope blade to the right of the patient's tongue to move it to the left. This should give a clear view of the glottis. **B,** Tongue partially obstructs the view if it is not moved to the left. *(From Shapiro BA, Harrison RA, Kacmarek RM, et al: Clinical application of respiratory care, ed 4, St Louis, 1991, Mosby.)*

## BOX 12-3 Complications of Endotracheal Intubation

### GENERAL COMPLICATIONS
- Reflex laryngospasm
- Perforation of the esophagus or pharynx
- Esophageal intubation
- Bronchial intubation
- Reflex bradycardia
- Tachycardia or other arrhythmias from hypoxemia
- Hypotension
- Bronchospasm
- Aspiration of tooth, blood, gastric contents, or laryngoscope bulb
- Laceration of pharynx or larynx
- Nosocomial infection
- Vocal cord injury
- Laryngeal or tracheal injury from the tube or excessive cuff pressure

### COMPLICATIONS OF THE ORAL ROUTE
- Cervical spine injury
- Tooth trauma from pulling back of the blade
- Eye trauma from the handle or the operator's hand

### COMPLICATIONS AFTER EXTUBATION
- Reflex laryngospasm
- Aspiration of stomach contents or oral secretions
- Sore throat
- Hoarseness
- Laryngeal edema (postintubation croup)

to match the patient's anatomy if a second attempt is needed.

4. Prepare the laryngoscope and blade.
   a. Select a laryngoscope handle.
   b. Select a laryngoscope blade. The blades are available in several sizes from pediatric to adult.

There are two main classes of blades: straight and curved (see Fig. 12-15). Straight blades (e.g., Miller) are designed to lift the epiglottis to expose the tracheal opening. Curved blades (e.g., MacIntosh) are designed to fit into the vallecula (between the base of the tongue and the epiglottis). As the blade is lifted, the epiglottis is raised and the tracheal opening can be seen. Personal experience and training lead the practitioner to select between the two styles.
   c. Attach the blade to the handle (see Fig. 12-16). Make sure that the light bulb shines brightly.

5. The intubator should tell the assistant to stop ventilating the patient and stand clear so that an intubation can be attempted. The assistant should check his or her watch to silently count 20 sec. The intubator should be told when 20 sec has passed so that the patient can be reventilated if the intubation is difficult.

6. Open the victim's mouth as widely as possible without using force. Remove any dentures or foreign material. Suction out any saliva, blood, or vomitus.

7. Grasp the laryngoscope handle in the left hand. Carefully advance the blade between the teeth or gums along the right side of the mouth. Move the tongue to the left of the mouth to allow a clear view of the oropharynx (Fig. 12-23). Advance the blade along the base of the tongue until the epiglottis is seen.

8. With *a straight blade*, you should
   a. Advance the blade so that it barely passes the epiglottis

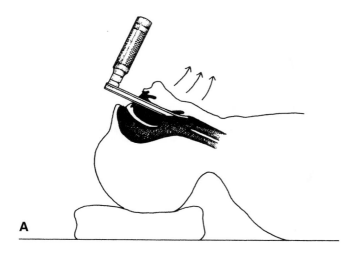

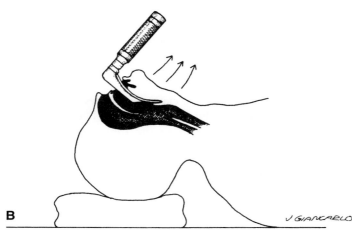

**Fig. 12-24** Proper use of the laryngoscope blade to expose the larynx by lifting the glottic structures. Note how the lifting occurs at a 45-degree angle toward the patient's chest. *Never* pull back on the blade against the teeth. **A,** Straight blade is used to lift the epiglottis to expose the trachea. **B,** Curved blade is used to lift the soft tissues of the vallecula to expose the trachea. *(From Shapiro BA, Harrison RA, Kacmarek RM, et al: Clinical application of respiratory care, ed 4, St Louis, 1991, Mosby.)*

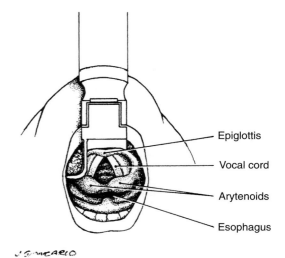

**Fig. 12-25** Major anatomic features that will be seen when the epiglottis is lifted. The opening to the trachea can be seen between the vocal cords. *(From Shapiro BA, Harrison RA, Kacmarek RM, et al: Clinical application of respiratory care, ed 4, St Louis, 1991, Mosby.)*

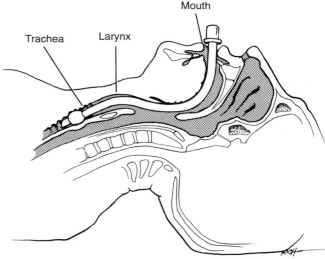

**Fig. 12-26** Oral endotracheal tube properly positioned within the trachea. *(From Eubanks DH, Bone RC: Comprehensive respiratory care, ed 2, St Louis, 1990, Mosby.)*

   b. The blade must not be advanced too far, or it will enter the esophagus or trachea.
   With a *curved blade,*
   a. Advance the blade tip into the vallecula
   b. Lift the blade tip into this space
9. With either blade, lift the laryngoscope handle and blade toward the patient's chest at a 45-degree angle (Fig. 12-24). The straight blade lifts the epiglottis. The curved blade lifts the soft tissues of the vallecula, and the epiglottis lifts with them. Do *not* pull back on the patient's upper teeth. If necessary, you should tell the assistant to put downward pressure on the patient's larynx.
10. The vocal cords and glottis should be seen clearly (Fig. 12-25).

11. The assistant should place the endotracheal tube into the intubator's right hand.
12. Place the tube into the patient's mouth and trachea. In adults, the proximal end of the cuff should be placed 3 to 4 cm past the vocal cords (Fig. 12-26). In children younger than 6 months who have an uncuffed endotracheal tube, the end of the tube should be placed about 1 cm past the vocal cords.
13. Hold the tube in place.

14. Withdraw the laryngoscope blade.
15. Tell the assistant to inflate the cuff. Place about 10 mL of air into the cuff (of an adult's tube) so that some resistance can be felt. The cuff pressure can be measured and adjusted later.
16. Pull out the stylet (if used).
17. The assistant should ventilate the patient with the manual resuscitator bag or a demand valve.
18. Listen to both lung fields in the upper lobes and bases. Bilateral breath sounds should be heard.
19. If the breath sounds are equal and bilateral, the assistant can secure the tube in place with tape or a tube holder. If the breath sounds are unequal or absent on one side, the tube has been placed into a bronchus (usually the right mainstem). The cuff should be deflated and the tube then withdrawn 1 to 2 cm in the adult (less in a child). The cuff should be reinflated and breath sounds listened to again. When the breath sounds are equal, the tube can be secured.
20. If no breath sounds are heard, you should listen over the stomach area. If air is heard bubbling into the stomach, the tube has been placed into the esophagus. Immediately remove the tube. Ventilate the patient, and prepare to attempt reintubation with a new endotracheal tube.

The practitioner should perform only those procedures for which he or she has been trained. If the patient cannot be intubated with the standard equipment and procedure, an anesthesiologist or trained physician should be called. Be prepared to assist as necessary.

## MODULE C

### Ensure that the artificial airway has been properly placed and is maintained

### 1. Auscultate the patient's breath sounds and interpret any changes (NBRC code: IB3a) [Difficulty: R, Ap]

Respiratory efforts without breath sounds indicate that a complete obstruction exists in the patient's airway. Inspiratory or expiratory stridor or wheezing would indicate that a partial obstruction exists in the patient's airway. Listen for stridor over the larynx and wheezing over the major airways. Restoration of the normal airway should result in the return of normal breath sounds over all areas of both lung fields (unless another, unrelated problem exists).

It is especially important to check for bilateral breath sounds after an endotracheal tube has been placed. If the tube has been inserted too far, it will usually enter the right mainstem bronchus because it comes off of the trachea at a less acute angle than does the left mainstem bronchus. No breath sounds would be heard over the left lung field. If both lung fields cannot be auscultated, you should listen at least to the right apical area. This one site

can be checked because the segmental bronchus to the right upper lobe comes off of the right mainstem bronchus in such a way that if the right mainstem bronchus is intubated, the upper lobe segmental bronchus will be blocked (see Fig. 10-1).

### 2. Exhaled carbon dioxide detector

#### a. Get the necessary equipment (NBRC code: IIA7d) [Difficulty: R, Ap]

An exhaled carbon dioxide ($CO_2$) detector can be placed on an endotracheal tube to monitor proper placement of the endotracheal tube. This is often done if a patient is being transported and the tube becomes dislodged. A disposable unit such as the Easy Cap end-tidal $CO_2$ detector could be selected (Fig. 12-27). The Easy Cap comes in a neonatal/pediatric size for infants smaller than 15 kg and a standard size for larger children and adults. Its $CO_2$ indicator changes color from dark purple to yellow when $CO_2$ is exhaled through it. Another choice is the MiniCAP III $CO_2$ detector. It is a reusable, battery-powered item that has a mainstream type of infrared $CO_2$ detector. Its light-emitting diode signals the presence of $CO_2$ with each exhalation. A capnograph should be selected if a more accurate $CO_2$ reading is necessary. Its general function and the interpretation of capnography tracings are discussed in Chapter 5.

#### b. Put the equipment together and make sure that it works properly (NBRC code: IIA7d) [Difficulty: R, Ap]

The Easy Cap comes as a single unit within a sealed foil container. Before you use it, you should match the initial purple color of the indicator with the purple color labeled CHECK on the product dome. Do *not* use an Easy Cap

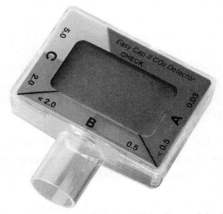

**Fig. 12-27** Easy Cap $CO_2$ detector. This disposable device comes in adult and pediatric sizes and is used to detect exhaled carbon dioxide. Color change from dark purple to yellow indicates exhaled carbon dioxide and confirms tracheal placement of the endotracheal tube or effective efforts at cardiopulmonary resuscitation. *(From Nellcor, Hayward, Calif.)*

unit with a color that is different from or darker than that on the product dome. Remove both caps from the patient and circuit connector ports. The Easy Cap is then attached to the patient's endotracheal tube by its 15-mm-ID connector port. The Easy Cap's 15-mm-OD circuit end is connected to the manual resuscitator to ventilate the patient. If a heat and moisture exchanger is used, it should be placed between the patient's endotracheal tube and the Easy Cap and manual resuscitator. The Easy Cap should not be used with a heated humidifier or nebulizer because too much humidity affects its accuracy.

The MiniCAP III has a disposable adapter that connects the mainstream $CO_2$ detector to the patient's endotracheal tube. The adapter has a 15-mm-ID end for attachment to the endotracheal tube and a 15-mm-OD end to which the manual resuscitator can be attached. Assembly and operation of a capnograph are discussed in Chapter 5.

### c. Troubleshoot any problems with the equipment (NBRC code: IIA7d) [Difficulty: R, Ap]

Because Easy Cap comes as a self-contained single-piece unit, there is nothing to repair. The following items can contaminate the Easy Cap and cause a patchy yellow or white discoloration of the indicator: stomach contents, mucus, pulmonary edema fluid, and intratracheal epinephrine. If the color does not change with the breathing cycle, and the unit should be discarded. The caps over the two connector ports must be removed so the Easy Cap can be attached to the endotracheal tube and manual resuscitator. The 15-mm-ID patient connector port fits only over the endotracheal tube adapter; the 15-mm-OD circuit connector port fits only into the manual resuscitator or demand-valve adapter. The adapter is the only removable part in the MiniCAP III; it fits in only one direction into the $CO_2$ detection unit. The other end of the adapter fits only into a manual resuscitator outlet. Troubleshooting with a capnograph is discussed in Chapter 5.

Some limitations exist with an Easy Cap $CO_2$ detector. It should not be used with mouth-to-mouth resuscitation, to detect right mainstem bronchus intubation, to detect hypercarbia, or to determine the placement of an esophageal obturator airway.

### 3. View the upper airway or chest x-ray film to see the position of the endotracheal or tracheostomy tube (NBRC code: IA5, IB6a) [Difficulty: R]

A chest x-ray film should always be taken to confirm the location of a newly placed endotracheal or tracheostomy tube. The chest x-ray film should be repeated if a significant change has occurred in the patient's condition, or if the tube has been pulled back or pushed more deeply into the trachea. If needed, an upper airway x-ray film can be taken to look for a foreign body or to check the position of the tracheostomy tube.

All modern endotracheal and tracheostomy tubes contain a strip of radiopaque material near the distal tip of the tube. This is easily noticed as the white line seen on the chest x-ray film and confirms the location of the tip of the tube in the airway (see Fig. 12-18). The ideal location of the tip of the endotracheal tube is the middle third of the trachea. When the tube is positioned properly, it is less likely that the tip will be pushed into the carina when the patient bends his or her head forward or that the cuff will hit the vocal cords when the patient's head is bent back. Both endotracheal and tracheostomy tubes should be positioned midline within the trachea. They should not be twisted laterally because the tip can damage the tracheal wall.

### 4. Identify the placement of the endotracheal tube by any available means (NBRC code: IIIB3) [Difficulty: R, Ap, An]

In addition to the methods described here, the endotracheal tube can often be palpated in an infant as it is being inserted through the larynx. This is because the laryngeal structures are so pliable. When the tube can be felt as it is inserted through the larynx, it is properly located within the trachea. When the tube cannot be palpated through the larynx, it has probably been inserted into the esophagus. It is more difficult to use this technique with confidence in adults because their laryngeal structures are stiffer than those of children.

---

**Exam Hint**

**B**e prepared to assess the proper placement of the endotracheal tube by palpation of the neck, auscultation of breath sounds, detection of exhaled $CO_2$, or viewing of the tube on a chest x-ray film.

---

### 5. Ensure that the endotracheal or tracheostomy tube stays properly positioned (NBRC code: IIIF2f1) [Difficulty: R, Ap, An]

The endotracheal tube body has centimeter marks placed on it, starting at the distal end and finishing at the proximal end. Check and record the centimeter mark at the patient's teeth or gums. The average adult's distance from the midtrachea to the teeth is about 23 to 25 cm. The practitioner can tell if the tube has been accidentally pulled out a bit or pushed farther into the patient by looking at the current centimeter mark. When the tube is intentionally adjusted, the new centimeter mark should be checked and recorded.

A wide variety of handmade and manufactured devices are available for use in securing the endotracheal tube in

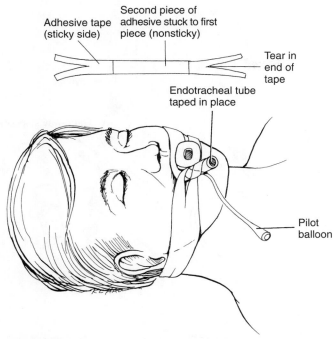

Adhesive tape (sticky side)

Second piece of adhesive stuck to first piece (nonsticky)

Tear in end of tape

Endotracheal tube taped in place

Pilot balloon

**Fig. 12-28** Taping the endotracheal tube to secure it in the airway. *(From Eubanks DH, Bone RC: Comprehensive respiratory care, ed 2, St Louis, 1990, Mosby.)*

the correct position. Fig. 12-28 shows an inexpensive way to make a tube holder from adhesive tape. This method has the advantage of being flexible when the patient moves. Tincture of benzoin can be applied to the patient's cheeks to hold the tape more securely without tearing the skin. When the patient is unconscious, an oropharyngeal airway may be used. When the patient is unconscious and has a history of seizures, one *should* be used.

The manufactured tube holders are made of plastic with cloth ties and usually include a built-in bite block. Make sure it is sized properly to the patient's mouth. Too large a bite block can injure the tongue, lips, and mouth. Watch for a gag reflex. This type of holder is useful in the patient who is prone to seizures.

## 6. Change the position of the endotracheal or tracheostomy tube (NBRC code: IIIF2f1) [Difficulty: R, Ap. An]

As has been mentioned earlier, an endotracheal tube is ideally located within the middle third of the trachea. Check the chest x-ray film for positioning. If the tube is too high within the trachea, it may be pulled up through the vocal cords if the patient's head is hyperextended. An air leak likely would be heard at the larynx if the patient is using a mechanical ventilator. In this case, the cuff should be deflated and the tube inserted more deeply into the trachea.

Conversely, if the tip of the tube is inserted too deeply into the trachea, it may be pushed into a mainstem

bronchus if the patient's head is moved toward the chest. In this situation, no breath sounds are heard in the opposite lung (usually on the left). This problem would require that the cuff should be deflated and the tube pulled up into the middle third of the trachea. In either case, the cuff should be reinflated after the tube has been repositioned. A chest x-ray film should be taken to confirm the tube's position after it has been moved.

A tracheostomy tube should be positioned so that the flange is snug against the base of the neck and the outer cannula is within the trachea. If the cuff is pulled out too far, it likely will be seen at the stoma. An air leak may be heard or secretions may be seen to bubble out of the stoma. Correct the problem by deflating the cuff, inserting the tube so that the flange is against the base of the neck, and reinflating the cuff.

> **Exam Hint**
>
> Usually, a question is included that deals with the understanding that the lack of breath sounds over the left lung indicates that the endotracheal tube has been placed into the right mainstem bronchus. The tube needs to be withdrawn to the trachea.

## 7. Monitor endotracheal and tracheostomy tube cuff pressure (NBRC code: IIIE10) [Difficulty: R, Ap]
   **a. Get the needed cuff pressure manometer (NBRC code: IIA17) [Difficulty: R]**
   **b. Put the equipment together and ensure that it works properly (NBRC code: IIA17) [Difficulty: R]**

A cuff pressure manometer measures the air pressure within an endotracheal or tracheostomy tube cuff. When a tracheal tube is first inserted, the volume of air injected into the cuff should be measured and charted. After that is done, if more air is inserted or any air is removed from the cuff, it should be measured and recorded on the chart. A number of manufactured units are available for measuring cuff pressure. The Cufflator, for example, consists of a pressure gauge that is calibrated in centimeters of water, a hand-pumped reservoir, an internal one-way valve, a pressure-release valve, and an adapter that fits into the one-way valve on the cuff-inflating tube (Fig. 12-29). A three-way stopcock can be added to the one-way valve adapter to prepressurize the system before the adapter is attached to the patient's one-way valve on the cuff-inflating tube. The pressure in the cuff can be measured as air is added with the hand pump or as air is removed with the pressure-release valve. The volume of air that is added or removed cannot be measured.

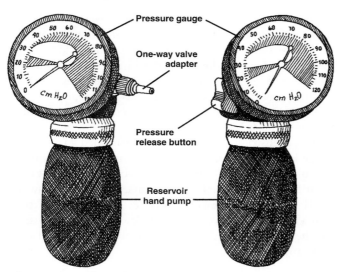

Fig. 12-29 Cufflator device used to measure cuff pressure with its component parts.

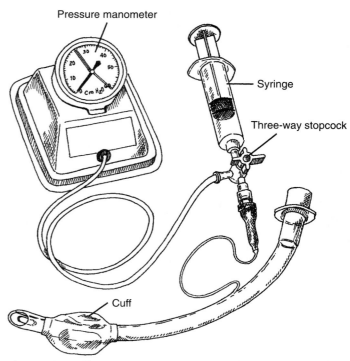

Fig. 12-30 Cuff measuring device made from a pressure manometer, three-way stopcock, and 10-mL syringe.

A second system, although also commercially available, can be "home made." It consists of a 5- to 10-mL syringe, a three-way stopcock, and a pressure gauge (either millimeters of mercury or centimeters of water). The syringe and pressure gauge are attached to two of the ports on the stopcock. The third port on the stopcock is connected to the one-way valve on the cuff-inflating tube. When the stopcock handle is opened to all three ports, pressure throughout the system and the cuff is the same. Air can be added or removed with the syringe. The pressure gauge shows the system and cuff pressure as the air volume is adjusted (Fig. 12-30). One advantage of this system over the Cufflator is that the volume of air that is added or subtracted can be measured. This system can also be pre-pressurized so that its pressure matches the pressure anticipated in the cuff.

### c. Troubleshoot any problems with the equipment (NBRC code: IIA17) [Difficulty: R]

With any of these systems, connections must be kept airtight. An air leak is noticeable as the pressure drops unexpectedly. Tighten the connections to create a seal so that the pressure is maintained.

## 8. Keep an endotracheal or tracheostomy tube cuff properly inflated

### a. Determine tracheal tube cuff volume and pressure (NBRC code: IB7k) [Difficulty: R]

All of the adult and larger pediatric endotracheal and tracheostomy tubes have a cuff that is used for sealing the airway. Most brands of modern tubes have cuffs that have been designed with a relatively large reservoir volume that fills at a relatively low pressure. The soft, flexible balloon seals the airway with a large surface area that conforms to the shape of the trachea. The cuff can be inflated and safe cuff pressure maintained in two slightly different ways. Both methods can be used only with patients who are on a positive-pressure ventilator.

### 1. Minimal leak

The purpose is to find the cuff pressure that results in a *small leak* at the cuff when the patient's airway pressure is greatest. The following steps are used in the procedure:

a. Connect the cuff pressure–measuring device (see earlier discussion) to the one-way valve on the cuff-inflating tube.

b. Listen with a stethoscope over the patient's larynx.

c. Inflate or deflate the cuff as necessary while you listen for an air leak.

d. Stop changing the air volume when a minimal leak is heard at peak airway pressure in the breathing cycle. The tidal volume should still be delivered except for this minor leak.

e. Note the cuff pressure where the minimal leak was heard. Note the cuff volume, if possible.

f. Disconnect the cuff pressure–measuring device.

g. Volume and pressure may need to be added to the cuff if the leak gets worse when the peak airway pressure increases.

## 2. Minimal occluding volume

The purpose is to find the cuff pressure that results in *no leak* at the cuff when the patient's airway pressure is greatest. The following steps are used in the procedure:

a. Connect the cuff pressure–measuring device (see earlier discussion) to the one-way valve on the cuff-inflating tube.

b. Listen with a stethoscope over the patient's larynx.

c. Inflate or deflate the cuff as necessary while you listen for an air leak.

d. Stop changing the air volume when no leak is heard at peak airway pressure in the breathing cycle.

e. Note the cuff pressure where the seal was heard. Note the cuff volume, if possible.

f. Disconnect the cuff pressure–measuring device.

g. Volume and pressure may need to be added to the cuff if a leak results when peak airway pressure increases.

It must be reinforced that this discussion relates only to those tubes that must be actively filled with air and that have variable intracuff pressures. Several manufacturers have developed endotracheal and tracheostomy tubes with built-in cuff-pressure limitations. Follow the manufacturer's guidelines when you inflate these cuffs. This discussion would not be complete without mention of the recent manufacture of systems designed to raise the cuff pressure to match peak airway pressure of a patient who is using a mechanical ventilator. A tube connects the inspiratory circuit to the one-way valve on the cuff-inflating tube. As a positive-pressure breath is delivered, pressure in the circuit is also applied to the patient's cuff. No loss of tidal volume should occur. When the patient exhales and airway pressure drops to normal, cuff pressure also drops back to its normal level.

### b. Maintain tracheal tube cuff volume and pressure (NBRC code: IIIB5a) [Difficulty: R, Ap]

Cuff pressure should be monitored at least every 8 hr, or whenever air is taken out of or put into the cuff.

### c. Interpret the tracheal tube cuff volume and pressure (NBRC code: IB8h) [Difficulty: R, Ap]

All manufacturers (except Kamen-Wilkinson) have designed cuffs that must be actively filled with air by way of a one-way valve and syringe. These cuffs have greater-than-atmospheric pressure within them. That pressure is placed against the wall of the trachea. The greater the pressure on the wall of the trachea, the greater is the disruption of normal lymphatic and blood flow. Shapiro and associates (1991) state that the following effects are noted at these cuff pressures in a patient with a normal blood pressure (120/80 mm Hg):

1. Lymphatic flow blockage occurs at pressures greater than 5 mm Hg (8 cm $H_2O$). Edema of the tracheal mucosa results.

2. Capillary blood flow blockage occurs at pressures greater than 18 mm Hg (24 cm $H_2O$). Venous (and lymphatic) drainage stops as a result.

3. Arterial blood flow blockage occurs at pressures greater than 30 mm Hg (42 cm $H_2O$). Arterial (and lymphatic and capillary) flow stops as a result.

In general, the clinical goal is to keep the cuff pressure as low as possible to ensure that circulation through the tracheal wall is normal. According to Shapiro and associates (1991), keeping the cuff pressure at no greater than 15 mm Hg (21 cm $H_2O$) seems reasonable. This holds true for all normotensive patients. Hypertensive patients may be able to tolerate higher cuff pressures compared with normotensive patients before blood flow to the tracheal tissues is stopped. Hypotensive patients suffer from loss of blood flow to the tracheal wall at lower cuff pressures than those previously listed.

### d. Inflate and deflate the cuff as indicated (NBRC code: IIIH2f4) [Difficulty: R, Ap]

The cuff must be inflated in a spontaneously breathing patient to prevent the aspiration of oral secretions into the lungs. In general, the pressure should be kept at about 15 mm Hg (21 cm $H_2O$), as has been discussed earlier. A higher cuff pressure may be necessary in a mechanically ventilated patient. However, Shapiro and associates (1991) recommend that if the cuff pressure must be greater than 20 mm Hg (25 cm water), the endotracheal or tracheostomy tube is too small. Ideally, the tube should be replaced with a larger one. However, some patients are too unstable to tolerate reintubation of their airways, and cuff pressure must simply be increased temporarily.

A cuff pressure that is greater than the patient's mucosa capillary pressure clearly prevents the flow of blood through the area covered by the cuff. Tissue ischemia (hypoxia) results. If the ischemia is severe enough, tissue necrosis will follow. The higher the cuff pressure and the longer the high cuff pressure is maintained, the greater is the likelihood of tissue necrosis. If the necrosis is circumferential (all the way around) to the trachea, tracheal stenosis will likely occur. Tracheal stenosis occurs when the diameter of the trachea is narrowed because of scar tissue buildup after the normal mucosa and underlying tissues have died. The patient's airway is permanently narrowed and, if serious, this must be surgically corrected. Another severe complication of high cuff pressures and tracheal necrosis is the development of a tracheoesophageal fistula. This is an opening between the trachea and esophagus. This is more likely to occur when the patient also has a nasogastric tube in place. The fistula permits food to pass into the airway and lungs, causing pneumonia. Mechanical ventilation is more difficult to perform because of air leak from the lungs to the esophagus. Surgical repair of the fistula is required.

## MODULE C
### Change a tracheal tube

### 1. Change the endotracheal tube (NBRC code: IIIH2f1) [Difficulty: R, Ap, An]

Usually, a patient's endotracheal tube is replaced for one of two reasons. First, the tube should be changed if it is too small and the cuff must be overfilled to seal the airway. Excessive pressure results in damage to the tracheal wall, as has been discussed.

Second, the tube should be replaced if the cuff is leaking or ruptured and the airway cannot be sealed. The patient may be reintubated by the procedure described earlier, or a tube-changing stylet may be used (Fig. 12-31). The stylet is a hollow, flexible, plastic tube that can be bent and holds its shape. It has a center mark and 1-cm markings that count out to each end to help guide the clinician to the proper depth for inserting the replacement endotracheal tube. It can be used on an endotracheal tube that is at least 7.5 mm OD. The procedure for changing the endotracheal tube with a tube-changing stylet includes the following:

a. Obtain the needed equipment: replacement endotracheal tube and one that is a size smaller, 10-mL syringe to inflate the cuff, sterile gloves, goggles, and sterile, water-soluble lubricant. Make sure the cuff inflates and deflates properly.

b. Tell the patient what to expect during the procedure. Put on the gloves and goggles.

c. Remove the patient's $O_2$ equipment.

d. Suction secretions from the patient's trachea and oral pharynx.

e. Reoxygenate and ventilate the patient.

f. Place some lubricant on the outside of the stylet.

g. Remove the $O_2$ equipment and pass the stylet through the endotracheal tube into the patient's trachea.

h. Insert it to about the same depth as that marked on the distal end of the endotracheal tube. For example, if the distal end of the endotracheal tube is 22 cm, insert the tube changer to 22 cm.

i. Deflate the cuff on the endotracheal tube.

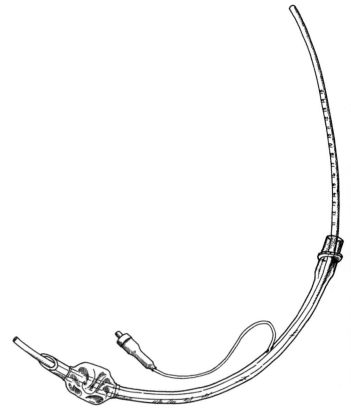

**Fig. 12-31** An endotracheal tube changer (guide) inserted through an endotracheal tube. The JEM 400 unit can be inserted through a tube that is 7.5 mm outer diameter or larger. The tube changer is used to aid in the replacement of an esophageal obturator airway or a defective endotracheal tube with a functional endotracheal tube. *(Reference Heffner JE: Managing difficult intubations in critically ill patients, Respir Management 19:3, 1989.)*

j. While you hold the distal tip of the tube changer in place, pull the defective endotracheal tube over it and out of the patient.

k. Advance the new endotracheal tube over the stylet. Hold the distal end of the stylet and push the new tube into the patient to the same depth mark on the stylet as is on the old tube.

l. Hold the endotracheal tube in place and remove the stylet.

m. Ensure that the tube has been placed into the trachea to the proper depth by listening for bilateral breath sounds.

n. Inflate the cuff to a safe pressure.

o. Secure the tube in place and note the depth marking at the patient's teeth or gums.

p. Obtain a chest x-ray film.

A defective one-way valve or severed cuff-inflating tube may not necessarily lead to a reintubation. It often can be bypassed by slipping a small-diameter needle (usually about 21-gauge) into the inflating tube, attaching a three-

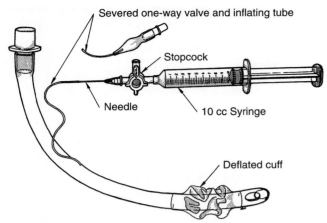

**Fig. 12-32** An emergency system for inflating the cuff when the one-way valve and inflating tube are severed. *(From Sills JR: An emergency cuff inflation technique, Respir Care 31:199, 1986.)*

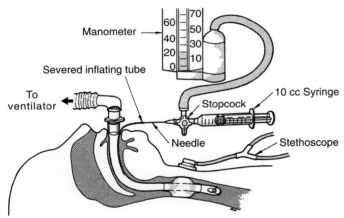

**Fig. 12-33** Measuring intracuff pressure as the cuff is reinflated with an emergency system. The stethoscope is used to listen for the presence of a leak at the larynx. *(From Sills JR: An emergency cuff inflation technique, Respir Care 31:199, 1986.)*

way stopcock to the hub of the needle, and screwing a 10-cc syringe into one of the stopcock ports (Fig. 12-32). Cuff pressure can be measured by a pressure manometer that is attached to the other port on the stopcock. Air can be added by the 10-cc syringe and the pressure measured simultaneously (Fig. 12-33). A commercially available system exists for bypassing a severed cuff-inflating tube.

## 2. Change the tracheostomy tube (NBRC code: IIIH2f1, IIIB4) [Difficulty: R, Ap, An]

Similar to an endotracheal tube, a tracheostomy tube may have to be changed because of a ruptured cuff or because of another problem. In addition, patients with a permanent tracheostomy have the tube changed on a routine schedule as part of the tracheostomy care. These two different situations are discussed separately.

### a. Emergency tube change

Several situations can cause the clinical emergency of obstruction, such as the cuff being herniated over the end of the tube, a mucus plug blocking the lumen, or the end of the tube being forced into the tracheal tissues. Unfortunately, these problems cannot be seen from the outside. If the patient is in acute respiratory distress and an obstruction is suspected, attempt to pass a suction catheter. Failure to pass it beyond the end of the tube confirms the obstruction. A rapid clinical decision about the best action must be made. The tube should be removed if the obstruction is complete and the patient cannot breathe. A spontaneously breathing patient continues to breathe through the stoma. An apneic patient must be temporarily ventilated with mouth-to-stoma breaths. As rapidly and carefully as possible, another tracheostomy tube should be inserted. This usually results in a patent airway. If loose tracheal mucosa is blocking the airway, an endotracheal tube will have to be inserted past the tissue and more deeply into the trachea. Call the physician as soon as possible so that the patient's condition can be evaluated.

### b. Routine tube change

It is important to avoid changing the tube, if possible, until several days after a fresh tracheostomy procedure has been done. This allows time for the stoma site to form granulomatous tissue as it begins to heal. The site is then less likely to bleed as the tube is changed. The tracheostomy tube is usually changed as part of the tracheostomy wound care procedure. Following are typical steps involved in changing the tracheostomy tube:

1. Gather the necessary equipment: new tracheostomy tube of the same size and the next size smaller, its 15-mm adapter, its obturator, tracheostomy tie strings to secure the tube in the patient (see Fig. 12-10), a sterile 4 × 4-inch gauze pad, sterile scissors, a 10-mL syringe to inflate the cuff, sterile water-soluble lubricant, sterile gloves, and goggles. Make sure that the cuff inflates and deflates properly.
2. Put on the gloves and goggles.
3. While maintaining sterile technique, make sure the obturator easily fits into and comes out of the tracheostomy tube.
4. Cut a slit in the center of the gauze pad.
5. Apply some sterile, water-soluble lubricant to the tip of the tracheostomy tube.
6. Tell the patient what to expect during the procedure.
7. Remove the $O_2$ or aerosol from the patient.
8. Suction the patient's trachea. Reoxygenate the patient.
9. Untie the tracheostomy strings.
10. Deflate the cuff.

11. Remove the 4 × 4-inch gauze pad.
12. Remove the tracheostomy tube by pulling it in a curved motion toward the patient's chest.
13. Inspect the tracheostomy opening for signs of infection, such as redness, pus, or swelling. Report signs of infection to the nurse or physician.
14. Carefully insert the new tracheostomy tube with obturator into the stoma. The motion should be opposite that used to remove the original tube. Make sure not to force the tube into the tissues of the trachea.
15. Remove the obturator and insert the 15-mm adapter. Lock it into place.
16. Give the patient $O_2$ or aerosol as before.
17. Inflate the cuff to a safe pressure.
18. Listen for bilateral breath sounds.
19. Slide the new 4 × 4-inch gauze pad around the tube so that the slit fits around it.
20. Tie the tracheostomy tie strings behind the patient's neck.

### 3. Perform tracheostomy care (NBRC code: IIIF2f5) [Difficulty: R, Ap]

Routine tracheostomy care includes the previous steps without removal of the tracheostomy tube. It is done to inspect the stoma for possible signs of infection, clean the stoma site, apply a topical antiobiotic, and replace the 4 × 4-inch gauze pad.

## MODULE D

### Extubate the patient (NBRC code: IIIB6) [Difficulty: R, Ap]

Extubation should be performed only by trained personnel and under proper conditions to ensure the patient's safety. Box 12-4 lists complications that can occur after extubation.

### 1. Endotracheal tube

Steps that are generally recommended in extubation include the following:
a. Evaluate the patient's cardiopulmonary status. The reason(s) that the tube is placed should be corrected. The most recent blood gas results should be acceptable. Tracheal secretions should be minimal and not too thick to be coughed out by the patient. Bedside spirometry results should show an acceptable tidal volume, vital capacity, and maximal inspiratory pressure.
b. Inform the patient about the removal of the tube and necessary follow-up care.
c. The patient's inspired $O_2$ percentage may be kept the same or increased before the extubation. If increased, this should be done at least 5 to 10 min before the tube is removed.

---

**BOX 12-4   Complications After Extubation**

**ENDOTRACHEAL TUBE REMOVAL**
Laryngospasm
Regurgitation and aspiration of stomach contents
Aspiration of saliva
Sore throat
Dysphagia
Postintubation laryngeal edema (croup)
Hoarseness from vocal cord edema or paralysis

**TRACHEOSTOMY TUBE REMOVAL**
Difficult tube removal from a tight stoma
Granuloma or scar at the stoma
Unhealed, open stoma

**CUFF-RELATED COMPLICATIONS**
Granuloma
Tracheomalacia
Tracheal stenosis
Tracheal web formation
Tracheoesophageal fistula
Arterial fistula

---

d. Suction the trachea until all secretions are removed.
e. Suction the oral pharynx to remove all saliva. Be prepared to suction out additional oral secretions and mucus after extubation.
f. In rapid succession:
   1. Give a deep sigh breath.
   2. Deflate the cuff. Cut the inflation tube to the cuff to ensure its collapse.
   3. Pull out the tube when the lungs are full.
Alternatively, in rapid succession:
   1. Give a deep sigh breath.
   2. Place a suction catheter through the tube into the trachea. This works best with a self-contained catheter and sheath system.
   3. Deflate the cuff. Cut the inflation tube to the cuff to ensure its collapse.
   4. Pull out the tube when the lungs are full.
   5. Apply suction as the tube is withdrawn.
g. Have the patient cough vigorously to remove any secretions.
h. Apply a cool, bland aerosol by facemask with the previous amount of $O_2$.
i. Monitor and evaluate the patient every 30 min for several hours. Encourage deep breathing and coughing. Check vital signs. Measure pulse oximetry or arterial blood gases (ABGs) after 20 min. Listen to the breath sounds and larynx.

**2. Tracheostomy tube**

a. Follow steps **a** to **g** from the previous list.

b. Depending on the physician's order, do one of the following:

1. Apply a bland aerosol by tracheostomy mask to the stoma site with the previous amount of $O_2$.

2. Cover the stoma site with a sterile $4 \times 4$ dressing, and tape it into place. Apply a bland aerosol by facemask with the previous amount of $O_2$.

3. Monitor and evaluate the patient every 30 min for several hours. Encourage deep breathing and coughing. Check vital signs and breath sounds. Measure pulse oximetry or ABGs after 20 min. Be prepared to reintubate the patient if necessary.

4. Routine stoma care on each shift to ensure healing usually includes the following:

aa. Remove the dressing. Inspect the stoma for signs of infection such as pus, redness, and swelling.

bb. Clean the stoma site with hydrogen peroxide on a sterile gauze pad.

cc. Apply antibiotic ointment to the stoma site.

dd. Reapply a sterile dressing.

## MODULE E
### Respiratory care plan

**1. Analyze available information to determine the patient's pathophysiologic state (NBRC code: IIIH1) [Difficulty: R, Ap, An]**

Be able to recognize an airway obstruction problem in a patient and to recommend or place the proper airway device to correct the problem. A chest x-ray film should always be taken to confirm the location of a newly placed endotracheal or tracheostomy tube. All modern endotracheal and tracheostomy tubes contain a strip of radiopaque material near the distal tip of the tube. This is easily noticed as the white line seen on the chest x-ray and confirms the location of the tip of the tube in the airway (see Fig. 12-18). The chest x-ray examination should be repeated if a significant change has occurred in the patient's condition, or if the tube has been pulled back or pushed more deeply into the trachea. The chest x-ray film also shows a pneumothorax related to the tracheostomy procedure or other pulmonary conditions.

**2. Recommend changes in the therapeutic plan if supportive data exist (NBRC code: IIIH4) [Difficulty: R, Ap]**

Indications or uses for the various airways are listed with the information provided by the manufacturer on that airway. In general, the airway should be removed when it is no longer needed. Typically, an oropharyngeal airway should be removed from a patient who has regained consciousness. A nasopharyngeal airway should be removed if the patient no longer needs it as an airway or for a suctioning route. Endotracheal and tracheostomy tubes can be removed when the patient is no longer in danger of aspiration or does not need mechanical ventilation, a suctioning route, or a permanent artificial airway.

Effective communication is important for good patient care. The conscious patient with an endotracheal tube or tracheostomy is unable to speak. Alternative ways to communicate must be provided, such as alphabet boards and picture boards for pointing, as well as pencil and paper for notes. Head nods and lip reading are often used. Questions must be worded in such a way that they can be answered with a "yes" or a "no." Avoid questions that require a lengthy written answer unless the patient seems ready and willing to provide it.

Predictions about how a patient will react to the placement of an artificial airway or its prolonged need are impossible. Some patients react with relief and relax when the WOB is reduced. Others may become angry at the limitations imposed on them. Still others may become depressed. Be prepared to deal with these reactions or changes in the patient's emotional response to this very stressful situation.

**3. Initiate suctioning of artificial airways (NBRC code: IIIF2f3) [Difficulty: R, Ap]**

Be prepared to suction a patient's endotracheal or tracheostomy tube, as needed, to remove secretions. The procedure is described in Chapter 13.

**a. Discontinue treatment based on the patient's response (NBRC code: IIIG1f) [Difficulty: R, Ap]**

Be prepared to discontinue the use of a particular airway and initiate the use of another, as needed. The indications for each type of airway have been presented earlier in the chapter.

### BIBLIOGRAPHY

American Association for Respiratory Care: Clinical practice guideline: management of airway emergencies, *Respir Care* 40:749, 1995.

American Association for Respiratory Care: Clinical practice guideline: removal of the endotracheal tube, *Respir Care* 44:85, 1999.

American Heart Association, Emergency Cardiac Care Committee and Subcommittees: Guidelines for cardiopulmonary resuscitation and emergency cardiac care: adult advanced cardiac life support, *JAMA* 268:2199, 1992.

Durbin CG, Artificial airways. In Cairo JM, Pilbeam SP, editors: *Mosby's respiratory care equipment*, ed 7, St Louis, 2004, Mosby.

Eubanks DH, Bone RC: *Comprehensive respiratory care*, ed 2, St Louis, 1990, Mosby.

Frownfelter DL: Chest physical therapy and airway care. In Barnes TA, editor: *Core textbook of respiratory care practice*, ed 2, St Louis, 1994, Mosby.

Gorback MS: Airway management. In Dantzker DR, MacIntyre NR, Bakow ED, editors: *Comprehensive respiratory care*, Philadelphia, 1995, WB Saunders.

Heffner JE: Managing difficult intubations in critically ill patients, *Respir Management* 19:53, 1989.

Hess DR, Branson RD: Airway and suction equipment. In Branson RD, Hess DR, Chatburn RL, editors: *Respiratory care equipment*, ed 2, Philadelphia, 1999, Lippincott Williams & Wilkins.

JEM 400 Endotracheal Tube Changer (Guide), product literature, Instrumentation Industries Inc, Bethel Park, Penn.

Kovac AL: Dilemmas and controversies in intubation, *Respir Management* 21:77, 1991.

Levitzky MG, Cairo JM, Hall SM: *Introduction to respiratory care*, Philadelphia, 1990, WB Saunders.

Lewis RM: Airway care. In Fink JB, Hunt GE, editors: *Clinical practice in respiratory care*, Philadelphia, 1999, Lippincott-Raven.

May RA, Bortner PL: Airway management. In Hess DR, MacIntyre NR, Mishoe SC, et al, editors: *Respiratory Care Principles & Practice*, Philadelphia, 2002, WB Saunders.

McIntyre D: Airway management. In Wyka KA, Mathews PJ, Clark WF, editors: *Foundations of respiratory care*, Albany, 2002, Delmar.

Plevak DJ, Ward JJ: Airway management. In Burton GC, Hodgkin JE, Ward JJ, editors: *Respiratory care: a guide to clinical practice*, ed 4, Philadelphia, 1997, Lippincott-Raven.

PressureEasy Cuff Pressure Controller, ReviveEasy PtL Airway, and Endotracheal/Trach Tube Pilot Tube Repair Kit, product literature, Respironics, Monroeville, Penn.

Roth P: Airway care. In Aloan CA, Hill TV, editors: *Respiratory care of the newborn and child*, ed 2, Philadelphia, 1997, Lippincott-Raven.

Scanlan C, Simmons K: Airway management. In Scanlan CL, Wilkins RL, Stoller JK, editors: *Egan's fundamentals of respiratory care*, ed 7, St Louis, 1999, Mosby.

Shapiro BA, Kacmarek RM, Cane RD, et al, editors: *Clinical application of respiratory care*, ed 4, St Louis, 1991, Mosby.

Sills JR: An emergency cuff inflation technique, *Respir Care* 31:199, 1986.

Simmons KF, Scanlan CL: Airway management. In Wilkins RL, Stoller JK, Scanlan CL, editors: *Egan's fundamentals of respiratory care*, ed 8, St Louis, 2003, Mosby.

Whitaker K: *Comprehensive perinatal & pediatric respiratory care*, ed 2, Albany, NY, 1997, Delmar.

White GC: *Equipment theory for respiratory care*, ed 3, Albany, NY, 1999, Delmar.

## SELF-STUDY QUESTIONS

1. You are preparing a stainless steel–type laryngoscope handle and blade for an anesthesiologist. The light does not shine. Which of the following would you do to fix the problem?
   I. Get a smaller blade to fit the handle.
   II. Get a larger blade to fit the handle.
   III. Tighten the light bulb.
   IV. Replace the handle with a plastic one.
   V. Check the batteries and replace them if necessary.
   A. I and IV
   B. II
   C. III and V
   D. IV

2. An oropharyngeal airway would be indicated under which of the following conditions?
   I. Maintaining an airway before performing a tracheostomy
   II. When seizure activity is expected or present
   III. An unconscious patient is lying supine with a soft-tissue upper airway obstruction
   IV. Stabilizing the mouth in a patient with a traumatic jaw injury
   V. An orally intubated patient is biting the tube
   A. III and V
   B. IV and V
   C. I and IV
   D. II, III, and V

3. You have just assisted with the intubation of an adult patient. To minimize the risk of soft-tissue injury to the trachea, what is the highest endotracheal tube cuff pressure that should be kept?
   A. Less than 30 mm Hg in a hypertensive patient
   B. Less than 20 cm $H_2O$ in a normotensive patient
   C. Greater than 20 mm Hg in a hypertensive patient
   D. Greater than 30 cm $H_2O$ in a hypertensive patient

4. During a CPR attempt, a pediatric patient has had an oral endotracheal tube placed. To ensure that the endotracheal tube is placed properly, you would recommend all of the following EXCEPT:
   A. Listen to the right upper lobe if the left lung field is inaccessible.
   B. Listen for bilateral lung sounds.
   C. Have a lateral neck x-ray film taken.
   D. Have a chest x-ray film taken.

5. While checking the tracheostomy tube cuff pressure on a patient in the recovery room, you find that the pressure is 33 mm Hg. This cuff pressure will likely cause which of the following?
   I. Loss of capillary flow through the tracheal soft tissues
   II. Loss of lymphatic flow through the tracheal soft tissues
   III. Tracheal wall damage
   IV. Protection of the vocal cords from damage caused by the tracheostomy tube
   V. Loss of venous flow through the tracheal soft tissues
   A. I, II, III, and V
   B. II and IV
   C. V
   D. I and II

6. While assisting with a CPR attempt, the anesthesiologist asks you to get a properly sized endotracheal tube so that the patient's airway can be quickly intubated. The patient is an average-sized man. What would you get?
   A. A 7.0-mm-ID oral endotracheal tube
   B. A 10.0-mm-ID nasal endotracheal tube
   C. An 8.0-mm-ID nasal endotracheal tube
   D. An 8.0-mm-ID oral endotracheal tube

7. You have just measured a tracheostomy tube's cuff pressure with a blood pressure–type mercury manometer. The pressure was 17 mm Hg. What would you recommend?
   A. Leaving the cuff pressure as it is and charting the measured value
   B. Increasing the cuff pressure to 20 mm Hg
   C. Rechecking the cuff pressure with a Cufflator device
   D. Replacing the tube with a larger one

8. A 45-year-old female patient is brought into the emergency room from an automobile accident. She has facial trauma, including a broken nose and jaw. Because of heavy bleeding into her mouth, she is having difficulty breathing. Which of the following would you recommend to ensure a safe, effective airway?
   A. Place an oral airway.
   B. Place a tracheostomy tube.
   C. Place a nasopharyngeal airway.
   D. Place a nasal endotracheal tube.

9. While working in the neonatal intensive care unit, you are called to assist in the care of a newborn. The neonatologist asks you to get the proper endotracheal tube size for a premature newborn. What size tube would you get?
   A. 1.5 mm ID
   B. 2.5 mm ID
   C. 3.5 mm ID
   D. 4.0 mm ID

10. Immediate complications of an oral intubation include all of the following EXCEPT:
    A. Tooth trauma
    B. Esophageal intubation
    C. Tracheoesophageal fistula
    D. Bronchial intubation

11. You are going to assist in the ambulance transport of a 25-year-old patient. The patient has an oral endotracheal tube, and you are going to manually ventilate him during the trip. Which of the following would you choose to help you be sure that the endotracheal tube stays properly placed within the trachea?
    A. Pulse oximeter
    B. Capnograph
    C. Disposable exhaled-$CO_2$ detector
    D. Electrocardiogram

12. All of the following should be monitored after a patient returns from having a tracheostomy tube placed EXCEPT:
    A. Cuff pressure
    B. Bowel sounds
    C. Bilateral breath sounds
    D. Excessive bleeding

13. Auscultation of a recently intubated patient in respiratory failure reveals absent breath sounds on the left side of the chest. The most likely cause of this finding is
    A. Placement of the endotracheal tube in the right mainstem bronchus
    B. Placement of the endotracheal tube in the left mainstem bronchus
    C. Placement of the endotracheal tube in the esophagus
    D. A pneumothorax on the right side

14. While working the night shift, you are called to intubate an apneic patient. Which of the following would you need for an emergency oral intubation?
    I. Laryngoscope handle
    II. Stylet
    III. Proper laryngoscope blade
    IV. 10-mL syringe
    V. Magill forceps
    A. I and II
    B. I, II, and V
    C. I, II, III, and IV
    D. II, IV, and V

15. You are assisting with the extubation of an adult patient. At what point in the procedure should the tube be removed?
    A. At the end of a peak inspiratory effort
    B. At the end of a normal exhalation
    C. At the start of a peak inspiratory effort
    D. During a forced vital capacity effort
16. A tracheostomy patient has just returned from a series of x-ray procedures. Suddenly, she develops respiratory distress and cannot breathe. Your attempt to pass a suction catheter through the tracheostomy tube does not work. You should proceed to
    A. Attempt to pass a smaller suction catheter
    B. Remove the tracheostomy tube
    C. Attempt to ventilate the patient with a manual resuscitator
    D. Insert an endotracheal tube
17. Indications for oral intubation include all the following EXCEPT:
    A. The patient requires mechanical ventilation
    B. The patient has a cervical spine injury
    C. The patient requires frequent tracheal suctioning
    D. The patient is at risk for vomiting and aspirating

18. Your patient is an 18-year-old woman who was found unconscious from a drug overdose. She has severe atelectasis of the left lung caused by lying on her left side for 2 days. Her right lung is normal. She is going to require mechanical ventilation to open the atelectatic areas. What endotracheal tube would you suggest should be used to properly treat the abnormal lung?
    A. Double-lumen
    B. Standard
    C. Fenestrated tracheostomy tube
    D. Armored
19. Your patient has epilepsy and has been having unpredictable seizure activity. What oral endotracheal tube would you suggest should be used to provide a secure airway?
    A. Double-lumen
    B. Preformed
    C. Armored
    D. Guidable

## ANSWER KEY AND RATIONALE

1. **C.** Common problems with intubation equipment include a loose or burned-out light bulb in the laryngoscope blade or depleted batteries in the handle. Changing the blade for one that is larger or smaller than appropriate would make the intubation procedure more difficult and dangerous. A plastic handle cannot be used with a stainless steel blade.

2. **D.** An oropharyngeal airway is indicated to open the airway of an unconscious patient, protect the airway of a patient with seizures, and prevent an oral endotracheal tube from being bitten. A patient with a tracheostomy does not need an oral airway because he or she is not breathing through the mouth. An oropharyngeal airway probably should not be inserted into the mouth of a patient with a traumatic jaw injury because of the risk that further injury could occur.

3. **B.** A cuff pressure of 20 cm $H_2O$ should be safe for a patient with a normal blood pressure. A cuff pressure of 20 mm Hg/30 cm $H_2O$ is likely to place the patient at risk for damage to the mucous membrane of the trachea.

4. **C.** A lateral neck x-ray film provides less useful information on proper placement of the endotracheal tube than is provided by a chest x-ray film. The presence of bilateral or at least right upper lobe breath sounds indicates proper tube placement.

5. **A.** A cuff pressure of 33 mm Hg is likely to cut off blood and lymphatic flow to the tracheal soft tissues. This pressure does nothing to protect the vocal cords. In addition, the tracheostomy tube does not pass between the vocal cords.

6. **D.** An 8.0-mm-ID oral endotracheal tube is appropriate for an adult. Review Table 12-1 for tube sizes. Also, the oral tube is more appropriate than a nasal tube in an emergency situation.

7. **A.** A cuff pressure of 17 mm Hg should be safe. No need exists to increase the pressure or replace the tube.

8. **B.** A tracheostomy tube is indicated in a patient with trauma to the nose and mouth and an upper airway obstruction. All of the other airway devices would pass through the upper airway.

9. **B.** A 2.5-mm-ID tube would be most appropriate. Review Table 12-1.

10. **C.** A tracheoesophageal fistula is a risk related to high cuff pressure; it would take several days to develop. The other complications would happen during placement of the tube.

11. **C.** A disposable exhaled-$CO_2$ detector would be easy to use and would give an immediate indication if the tube were removed from the trachea. A capnography device is expensive and is not designed for easy use in a transport situation. Pulse oximetry will give information on $O_2$ saturation, not on $CO_2$ removal from the lungs. An ECG will not give immediate feedback on the patient's condition related to the tube. If the patient were to be accidentally extubated, both the pulse oximeter and the ECG devices would eventually give information indicating that the patient is in trouble. However, this information is not specific to the patient who has been extubated.

12. **B.** Bowel sounds should not be affected by the placement of a tracheostomy tube. It is highly unlikely that the tracheostomy tube would be accidentally placed into the esophagus, which can happen during the placement of an endotracheal tube. All other items should be monitored.

13. **A.** Placement of the endotracheal tube into the right mainstem bronchus would result in the absence of breath sounds over the left lung. Placement of the tube into the left mainstem bronchus would result in the absence of breath sounds over the right lung. Placement of the tube into the esophagus would result in the absence of breath sounds over both lungs. A right pneumothorax could result in absent breath sounds over the right lung, not over the left lung.

14. **C.** Everything listed except the Magill forceps would be needed. Review Box 12-1.

15. **A.** A patient should be extubated when the lungs are full so that a full coughing effort can follow and clear out any secretions in the airways. All of the other options would result in less volume in the patient's lungs.

16. **B.** The tracheostomy tube should be removed quickly if there is evidence that the tube is blocked. In addition, the tracheotomy tube should be replaced with a new one so that a secure airway is maintained.

17. **B.** A patient with a cervical spine injury should *not* have his or her neck hyperextended as is needed during an oral intubation procedure. See Box 12-2.

18. **A.** A double-lumen tube is indicated because she can receive independent lung ventilation through it. This mode of ventilation would allow her lung with atelectasis to be ventilated differently than her normal lung. None of the other tubes offers this option.

19. **C.** An armored tube would prevent her from biting and collapsing the tube during a seizure. None of the other tubes offers this security.

# 13 Suctioning the Airway

A review of the most recent Entry Level Examinations has shown an average of 4 questions (3% of the exam) that cover suctioning procedures.

## MODULE A

### Suctioning devices

### 1. Oropharyngeal suction devices

#### a. Get the necessary equipment for the procedure (NBRC code: IIA8) [Difficulty: R]

Oropharyngeal suctioning is considered to be a clean (not sterile) procedure. The suctioning device is packaged sterile but may be used more than once. The widely used Yankauer suction catheter is made of hard plastic and has an angled catheter that reaches into the back of the mouth. The tip of the catheter may have one large opening or several medium-sized openings. The openings are large enough to permit easy suctioning of saliva, food, or vomit. Some handles include a thumb-control valve so that suction can be applied to the tip only when it is wanted. Covering the opening with a thumb creates a vacuum at the tip for suctioning the patient's mouth (Fig. 13-1). The Yankauer may be discarded when no longer needed, or it may be sterilized for use with another patient.

A flexible plastic or rubber catheter can also be used. It should be of the largest diameter possible to reduce the chance that it could become plugged. The opening at the catheter tip should be cut straight across (perpendicular) instead of at an angle. No side openings should exist (Fig. 13-2). The catheter is discarded when it is no longer needed.

#### b. Put the equipment together and make sure that it works properly (NBRC code: IIA8) [Difficulty: R]

The catheters just mentioned are single pieces with nothing to assemble. They must be attached to a vacuum source by a length of soft rubber tubing. With clean gloves on both hands, attach the Yankauer catheter or plastic or rubber catheter to the vacuum tubing. The vacuum must be applied to the tip of the catheter to remove oral secretions. Check for a vacuum at the tip by any of the following methods:

1. Listen for the sound of air being drawn into the tip.
2. Put the tip into a container of sterile water. Close the thumb-control opening. The water must be drawn up the catheter.

3. Place a clean-gloved hand over the tip if water is unavailable. Close the thumb control opening. The glove should be attracted to the catheter.

#### c. Troubleshoot any problems with the equipment (NBRC code: IIA8) [Difficulty: R]

Failure to have a vacuum at the catheter tip can mean any of the following:

1. The vacuum is not turned on. Check the following:
   a. Some centralized vacuum systems have a single dial that turns the system off and on and sets the vacuum level. Other centralized vacuum systems have an on/off switch and a dial for setting the vacuum level.
   b. Free-standing vacuum systems must be plugged into a working electrical outlet. The on/off switch must be turned on. Simpler systems have a preset vacuum level, but variable vacuum levels can be set with a dial in the more sophisticated systems.
2. The system is not sealed, so the vacuum is lost to the atmosphere. Check the following:
   a. Make sure that the rubber vacuum tubing fits tightly over the connectors on both the catheter and the vacuum system.
   b. Make sure that the catheter and vacuum tubing are not cracked or cut. Replace any defective Yankauer, plastic, or rubber catheter or vacuum tubing.
   c. Close the thumb control if it has been left open.
   d. Check the central or free-standing vacuum system to ensure that the secretion collection bottle is sealed properly.
3. The system is blocked, and no vacuum can get through to the tip. Check the following:
   a. Check for a pinch in the vacuum tubing or soft catheter.
   b. Check for a blockage in the catheter or vacuum tubing. Try to suction some sterile water to clear the blockage into the secretion collection bottle. Replace the catheter, vacuum tubing, or both if the blockage cannot be cleared.
   c. Empty out a full collection bottle.

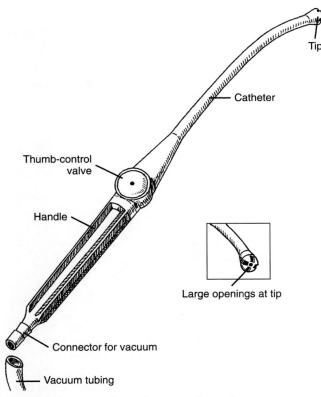

Tip

Catheter

Thumb-control valve

Handle

Large openings at tip

Connector for vacuum

Vacuum tubing

**Fig. 13-1** Features of a Yankauer suction catheter.

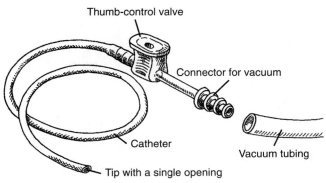

Thumb-control valve

Connector for vacuum

Catheter

Vacuum tubing

Tip with a single opening

**Fig. 13-2** Features of a suction catheter with a cross-cut tip.

## 2. Suction catheters

Suctioning catheters, which are packaged sterile and individually, remove secretions and foreign material from the trachea. The outer diameter (OD) of the catheter is recommended to be no more than one-half the inner diameter (ID) of the airway through which it is passing. This guideline minimizes obstruction to the airway and lets the patient breathe around the catheter.

| TABLE 13-1 | Recommended Suction Catheter French Sizes for the Various Endotracheal and Tracheostomy Tube Sizes* | |
|---|---|---|
| Age | ID of tube sizes (mm) | Suction catheter size (Fr) |
| **NEWBORN** | | |
| <1000 g | 2.5 | 5 |
| 1000–2000 g | 3.0 | 6 |
| 2000–3000 g | 3.5 | 8 |
| 3000 g to 6 mo old | 3.5–4.0 | 8 |
| **PEDIATRIC** | | |
| 18 mo | 4.0 | 8 |
| 3 yr | 4.5 | 8 |
| 5 yr | 5.0 | 10 |
| 6 yr | 5.5 | 10 |
| 8 yr | 6.0 | 10 |
| **ADULT** | | |
| 16 yr | 7.0 | 10 |
| Normal-sized woman | 7.5–8.0 | 12 |
| Normal-sized man | 8.0–8.5 | 14 |
| Large adult | 9.0–10.0 | 16 |

ID, Inner diameter.

*Note: It is recommended that a suction catheter with an outer diameter no more than one-half the ID of the endotracheal tube should be used.

### Exam Hint

**R**emember that the diameter of the suction catheter should be no more than one-half the ID of the endotracheal tube. This is often tested on the examination.

Table 13-1 gives the recommended suction catheter sizes for various endotracheal or tracheostomy tubes. The practitioner can also easily compare the relative size of the tube and the suction catheter at the bedside before suctioning. Suction catheters are sized by the French (Fr) scale of their OD. Endotracheal and tracheostomy tubes are sized by ID and OD in millimeters and often by ID in French (review Table 12-1).

***Catheter size calculation (math review).*** The following formula and example show how the OD of any suction catheter can be calculated so the clinician can know the endotracheal or tracheostomy tube with which it may be used. Because each French (Fr) unit is about 0.33 mm, the OD in millimeters of a suction catheter can be found by multiplying the French size by 0.33. For example, calculate the OD of a 12 Fr suction catheter as follows:

$$12 Fr \times 0.33 = 3.96 (about 4.0) mm OD of the catheter$$

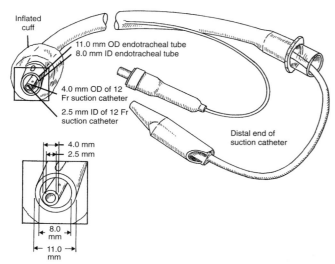

**Fig. 13-3** No. 12 Fr suction catheter inside of an 8.0-mm-inner diameter (ID) endotracheal tube. The outer diameter of the catheter should be no more than one-half the ID of the tube so that the patient can still breathe around it.

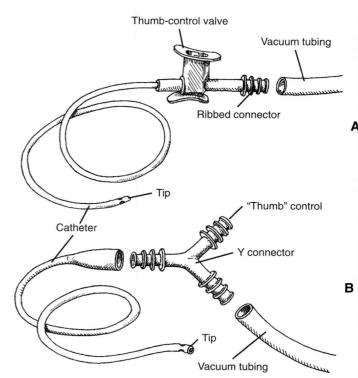

**Fig. 13-4** Features of two types of suction catheters with angle-cut tips and side holes. **A,** Suction catheter with its own thumb-control valve. **B,** Suction catheter needing a thumb-control valve constructed from a Y-connector.

It is also possible to estimate the maximum French size suction catheter for the inner diameter of an endotracheal or tracheostomy tube. Use this formula:

$$\frac{\text{Inner diameter (ID) of endotracheal tube} \times 3}{2}$$
$$= \text{maximum diameter (French size)}$$

Example for a size 8.0 (ID) endotracheal or tracheostomy tube:

$$\frac{8.0 \times 3}{2} = \frac{24}{2} = 12 \text{Fr suction catheter}$$

Therefore, a 12 Fr suction catheter could be used on an 8.0-mm-ID endotracheal tube. Fig. 13-3 shows the relative sizes of this endotracheal tube and catheter.

Knowing the ID of a suction catheter can also be clinically useful because this relates to the maximum particle size that can pass through it. The following formula can be used to interconvert from French to millimeters:

$$mm = \frac{Fr - 2}{4}$$

### EXAMPLE

What is the ID (in mm) of a 12 Fr suction catheter?

$$mm = \frac{12 - 2}{4}$$
$$mm = \frac{10}{4}$$
$$mm = 2.5 \,(\text{see Fig. 13-3})$$

### a. Get the necessary catheter for an open airway suctioning procedure (NBRC code: IIA8) [Difficulty: R]

Open airway suctioning refers here to the process whereby the patient spontaneously breathes room air after being disconnected from the source of supplemental oxygen ($O_2$). This happens to the patient with a normal upper airway when the $O_2$ mask is removed for nasotracheal suctioning. It also happens when the patient with an endotracheal or tracheostomy tube has the aerosol T-piece (Briggs adapter) or ventilator circuit removed for suctioning purposes.

These types of catheters have been in use for many years. Fig. 13-4 shows the two basic types. Closing the thumb control allows the vacuum to be selectively applied to the secretions when desired (Fig. 13-5). The tips of the catheters can vary greatly because considerable effort has been spent trying to develop a catheter tip that most effectively removes secretions without damaging the tracheal mucosa. Fig. 13-6 shows some of the catheter tips that have been developed to minimize mucosal damage. Note that all tips feature at least one opening in the catheter that is back from the opening at the tip. Compare this with the single-end opening found on the oral suction catheter (see Fig. 13-2). Side openings are designed to

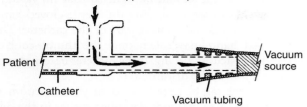

An open thumb-control valve lets room air enter
so that no vacuum is applied to the patient

Patient

Catheter

Vacuum tubing

Vacuum
source

**Fig. 13-5** Close-up of a thumb-control valve showing how
room air is drawn into the vacuum tubing when the valve is left
open. Closing the valve applies vacuum to the catheter tip to
suction secretions.

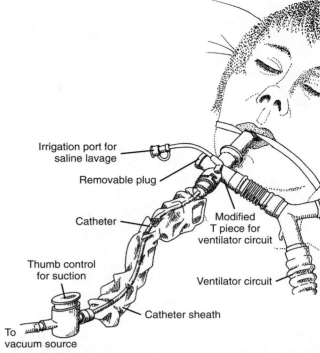

Irrigation port for
saline lavage

Removable plug

Catheter

Thumb control
for suction

To
vacuum source

Modified
T piece for
ventilator circuit

Ventilator circuit

Catheter sheath

**Fig. 13-7** Self-contained catheter and sheath suctioning system
for closed airway suctioning. *(Based on the Kimberly Clark/Ballard
Trach Care closed endotracheal suction device.)*

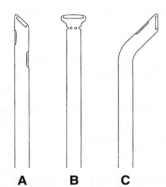

A      B      C

**Fig. 13-6** Close-up of the ends of three different suction
catheters. **A,** Catheter with a bevel cut of the tip with two
offset side holes. **B,** Catheter with a ring tip with several side
holes around it. **C,** A Coudé (curved-tip) catheter, which may
help in guiding it into either the left or the right mainstem
bronchus. *(From Rarey KP, Youtsey JW: Respiratory patient care,
Englewood Cliffs, NJ, 1981, Prentice-Hall.)*

prevent application of the vacuum to the tip when it
makes contact with the mucosa.

Note in Figs. 13-4 and 13-6 that most catheters are
straight throughout their length. All of these catheters
tend to enter the right mainstem bronchus during deep
suctioning because its angle off of the trachea is less acute
compared with the left mainstem bronchus. As a result, it
is difficult, if not impossible, for any of these catheters to
suction the left mainstem bronchus. The Coudé catheter
has been designed with an angled tip to better enable
guidance into the left (or right) mainstem bronchus (see
Fig. 13-6, **C**). When these catheters are used, the direction
of the thumb-control valve can help determine the angle
of the bent tip.

Use of traditional types of catheters during open
airway suctioning always results in some level of hypoxemia. The use of a relatively new type of suction catheter
may help to alleviate this problem. The insufflating
suction catheter is designed to alternatively provide $O_2$
through the catheter or vacuum for suctioning. The
thumb control end of the catheter is modified with two

male-type tubing connectors and a way to switch the
lumen of the catheter between them. The thumb control
is set so that the $O_2$ is directed through the catheter and
into the patient as the catheter is advanced. After the
catheter has been placed deeply into the trachea for suctioning, the thumb control is switched from $O_2$ delivery
to suction application.

### b. Get the necessary catheter for a closed airway suctioning procedure (NBRC code: IIIA8) [Difficulty: R]

Closed airway suctioning refers here to suctioning that is
done when the patient remains connected to the original
source of $O_2$. This may be done through a special aerosol
T-adapter or, more commonly, with the patient receiving
mechanical ventilation. Spontaneously breathing patients
are less likely to suffer hypoxemia with closed airway suctioning because they can continue to inhale the prescribed
$O_2$ percentage.

In closed airway suctioning systems, a flexible, clear
plastic sheath covers the catheter to maintain its sterility
(Fig. 13-7). Gloves are not needed by the practitioner.
Because self-contained systems can be reused, they offer a
financial advantage over the traditional catheter-and-
gloves suctioning method in patients who need frequent
suctioning. These closed system suction catheters come

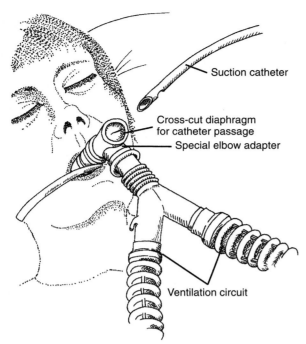

**Fig. 13-8** Features and placement of a special elbow adapter for closed airway suctioning without loss of tidal volume or pressure during mechanical ventilation.

with either the traditional straight tip or the Coudé tip for selective bronchial suctioning.

Another device that is used to create a sealed system for endotracheal tube suctioning consists of an elbow adapter with an inner plastic sleeve or diaphragm. As the traditional catheter is inserted into the opening on the elbow adapter, the sleeve or diaphragm conforms to the catheter and prevents an air leak (Fig. 13-8). This ensures that the ventilator-delivered volumes and pressures are not decreased.

### c. Put the suctioning equipment together and make sure that it works properly (NBRC code: IIA8) [Difficulty: R]

Refer to Fig. 13-4 to see the attachment of an open airway suction catheter to the vacuum tubing. Fig. 13-7 shows the attachment of a closed airway suction catheter to the vacuum tubing. The other end of the vacuum tubing is attached to the vacuum regulator system.

With open airway suctioning, only a hand covered by a sterile glove can touch the area of the catheter that enters the patient's trachea. The practitioner's other hand should also be gloved. A clean glove is acceptable because it does not touch the part of the catheter that enters the patient's trachea.

While holding the body of the catheter and the thumb-control valve and vacuum connector with the sterile-gloved hand and the vacuum tubing with the clean-gloved

hand, slip the vacuum tubing over the catheter's vacuum connector. The seal should be tight so that no vacuum leak occurs. From now on, only the sterile-gloved hand may touch the patient contact part of the catheter. The clean-gloved hand may touch only the thumb-control valve and the vacuum tubing. If the catheter becomes contaminated, it must be discarded.

The catheter can be tested for patency and vacuum at the tip by the three methods described earlier in the discussion of oropharyngeal suction devices. Note that only a *sterile* glove may be touched against the tip of the suction catheter to check for a vacuum.

Gloves are not needed by the practitioner when a self-contained catheter is used for closed airway suctioning because the sheath covers the catheter to prevent contamination.

> **Exam Hint**
>
> **R**emember that endotracheal suctioning is a sterile procedure. Contaminated gloves or catheter must be replaced with sterile ones.

### d. Troubleshoot any problems with the equipment (NBRC code: IIA8) [Difficulty: R]

The three common causes of an equipment failure and explanations of how to fix them are described in the earlier discussion on oropharyngeal suction devices. Remember to completely withdraw the closed airway suctioning catheter from the endotracheal tube into the sheath, or it will partially obstruct the tube.

### 3. Specimen collectors

#### a. Get the necessary equipment (NBRC code: IIA8) [Difficulty: R]

A variety of specimen collectors (commonly called *Lukens traps*) exist. These are packaged as sterile to prevent contamination of the sputum sample with nonpatient organisms. Figs. 13-9 to 13-12 show the key features and functions of several sputum sample collectors. The sputum sample is obtained through a suction catheter or bronchoscope.

The specimen jar has volume markings, and it screws into either a special lid used to suction the specimen or a regular lid for shipment to the laboratory. The special lids used in the systems featured in Figs. 13-9 and 13-10 must be connected to a sterile catheter. Fig. 13-11 shows a system with its own catheter. The vacuum source is provided to these specimen collectors by a length of vacuum tubing, as in the suction catheter systems previously described. Fig. 13-12 shows a DeLee system that is sometimes used in the delivery room. Mouth suction is used to

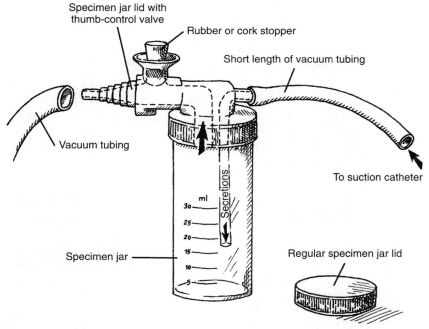

**Fig. 13-9** Features of a sputum specimen collection system with a thumb-control valve.

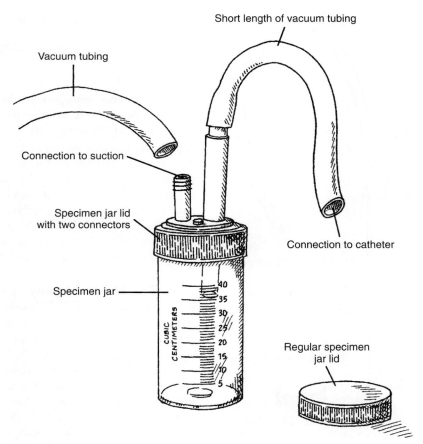

**Fig. 13-10** Features of a sputum specimen collection system without a thumb-control valve.

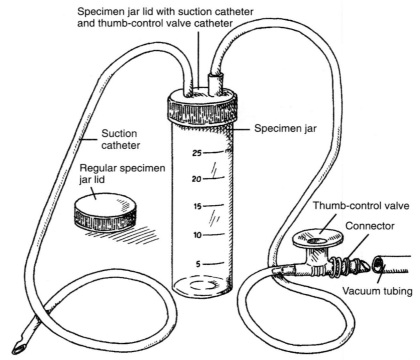

**Fig. 13-11** Features of a sputum specimen collection system with a thumb-control valve built into the catheter.

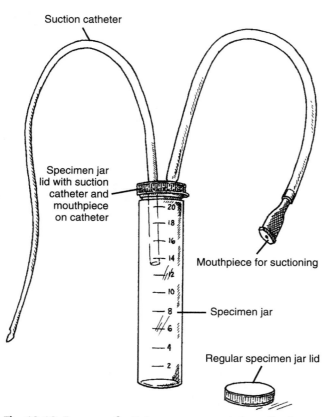

**Fig. 13-12** Features of a DeLee sputum specimen collection system with a mouthpiece through which the practitioner can apply suction.

remove secretions from the newborn. In all of these examples, after the sample has been collected, the special lid is unscrewed and is replaced with the regular specimen jar lid.

### b. Put the equipment together and make sure that it works properly (NBRC code: IIA8) [Difficulty: R]

A properly working specimen collection system provides a vacuum to the tip of the suction catheter when the thumb-control valve or mouthpiece is sealed and vacuum is applied. The vacuum level can be tested by dipping the catheter tip into a container of sterile water or saline solution. The liquid is drawn up the catheter and deposited in the specimen jar. (The water can be emptied out of the jar by simply unscrewing the jar and discarding it.)

### c. Troubleshoot any problems with the equipment (NBRC code: IIA8) [Difficulty: R]

Failure to have a vacuum at the tip of the suction catheter could be caused by any of the previously mentioned possibilities, which can be checked and corrected by the methods listed earlier. An inability to suction secretions has two likely causes. First, the jar is not screwed tightly into the special lid, thus it is drawing in room air. Simply screw it in tightly. Second, the secretion channel is plugged. Discard it and replace it with a new specimen collector.

## MODULE B

### Vacuum regulator systems

**1. Get the necessary vacuum regulator system: vacuum pump, regulator, and collection bottle (NBRC code: IIA20) [Difficulty: R, Ap]**

**2. Put the equipment together and make sure that it works properly (NBRC code: IIA20) [Difficulty: R, Ap]**

Vacuum regulators come preassembled by the manufacturer. The two basic types described here must have components added to make them fully functional.

#### a. Portable vacuum systems

These units are designed to be moved with the patient. They may be mounted on a small platform (Fig. 13-13) or mounted on a wheeled cart. Portable systems generally include an electrically powered vacuum pump with an on/off switch and a collection bottle. Some units have a control valve that can be used for adjusting the level of negative pressure. A negative-pressure gauge is used to determine how much vacuum is being applied. A length of rubber vacuum tubing is used to pass the negative pressure from the pump to the collection bottle. Another length of vacuum tubing is used to pass the vacuum through to the suction catheter. Portable systems are not as powerful as central vacuum systems, and they are not very effective at suctioning large amounts of thick secretions.

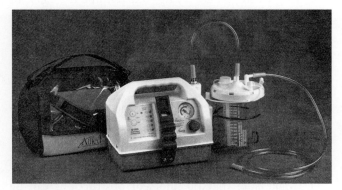

**Fig. 13-13** A portable suction machine. The electrically powered motor, collection bottle and cap, and connecting tubing can be seen. *(Courtesy of Allied Healthcare Products, Inc, St Louis, MO.)*

In general, the following steps are needed to make the units operational:

1. Plug the vacuum pump into a working electrical outlet. Battery-operated units should have fully charged batteries.
2. Place a clean, empty collection bottle into its holder on the cart. The bottle should hold at least 500 mL of fluid.
3. Slip the rubber lid onto the open top of the collection bottle. Both vacuum tubing connectors on the lid must be patent.
4. Slip one end of a short length of vacuum tubing over the connector on the vacuum pump and the other end on one of the tubing connectors on the collection bottle lid.
5. Slip one end of a length of vacuum tubing over the other tubing connector on the collection bottle lid. The vacuum tubing should be no longer than 3 feet. The other end of the vacuum tubing is connected to the suction catheter when needed.
6. Turn on the unit and determine the negative pressure by performing the following:
   a. Pinching closed the long vacuum tubing
   b. Turning on the vacuum pump
   c. Observing the pressure on the negative-pressure gauge
7. If the unit has a fixed vacuum level, the observed negative pressure should match that listed by the manufacturer.
8. If the unit has a variable vacuum level, adjust the vacuum control knob to the desired level.

#### b. Central vacuum systems

Central (wall) vacuum systems are usually available at each patient's bedside in all special care units. Each wall outlet is connected through a hospital-wide piping system to a large electrically powered vacuum pump. Central vacuum systems are capable of generating a negative pressure far greater than that needed in most patient care situations. A regulator is used to reduce the vacuum to the desired clinical level (Fig. 13-14). Either a "quick connect" or diameter index safety system connector is used to attach the regulator to the central vacuum system.

Most regulators include a selector knob that allows the user to turn the vacuum off (Off setting) or to switch between full vacuum (Full setting) and a regulated level of vacuum (Reg setting). The Full setting opens the unit to the maximum level of vacuum available from the central pump. The Reg setting allows the user to adjust the vacuum level through a wide range.

In general, the following steps are needed to make the units operational:

1. Connect the regulator into a working suction outlet.

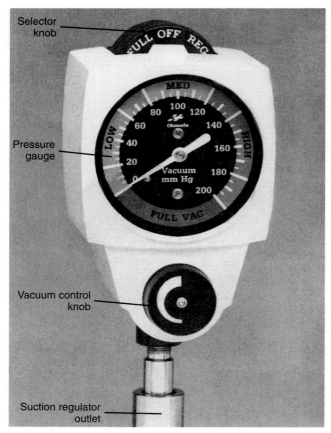

Fig. 13-14 Features of an Ohmeda Medical continuous vacuum regulator with a three-position selector knob. *(Courtesy of Ohmeda Medical, Columbia, MD.)*

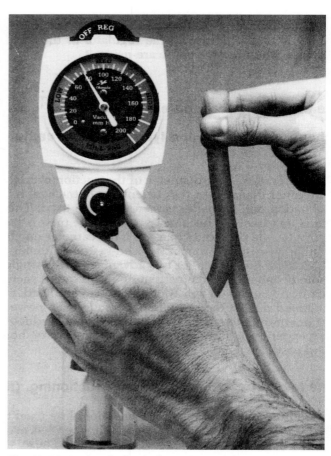

Fig. 13-15 Setting the level of negative pressure on the Ohmeda Medical continuous vacuum regulator by pinching the vacuum tubing and adjusting the vacuum control knob. *(Courtesy of Ohmeda Medical, Columbia, MD.)*

2. Screw a clean, empty collection bottle onto its connector on the regulator. The bottle must hold at least 500 mL of fluid.

3. Slip one end of a length of vacuum tubing over the tubing connector on the collection bottle. The vacuum tubing should be no longer than 3 feet. The other end of the vacuum tubing is connected to the suction catheter when needed.

4. Determine the negative pressure by performing the following:
   a. Pinching closed the vacuum tubing (Fig. 13-15)
   b. Turning the selector knob to Reg
   c. Observing the pressure on the negative-pressure gauge

5. Adjust the vacuum control knob to the desired level. If the secretions are too thick to be drawn up the suction catheter, negative pressure must be increased.

### 3. Troubleshoot any problems with the equipment (NBRC code: IIA20) [Difficulty: R, Ap]

With a *portable* vacuum system, you should check the following when you are trying to determine the cause of a loss of vacuum:

a. Make sure that the vacuum pump is plugged into a working electrical outlet.

b. The vacuum pump must be turned on.

c. Make sure that the vacuum control valve is set at the desired negative pressure.

d. The lid to the collection bottle should be tightly sealed.

e. The vacuum tubing must tightly connect the pump to the collection bottle and the collection bottle to the suction catheter.

f. Make sure that no knots or obstructions can be found in the vacuum tubing or catheter.

g. The collection bottle must not be filled to above its maximum level.

Correct any potential problems. Do not use a portable vacuum system that does not generate the intended negative pressure.

With a *central* vacuum system, check the following when you are trying to determine the cause of a loss of vacuum:

a. Make sure that the regulator is plugged into a working vacuum outlet.
b. Make sure that the vacuum control valve is set at the desired negative pressure.
c. The collection bottle should be tightly screwed onto the suction regulator outlet.
d. The vacuum tubing must tightly connect the collection bottle to the suction catheter.
e. Make sure that no knots or obstructions exist in the vacuum tubing or catheter.
f. The collection bottle must not be filled to above its maximum level.

Correct any potential problems. Do not use a central vacuum system outlet that does not generate the intended negative pressure. Occasionally, less negative pressure than expected occurs when the central vacuum system is being heavily used. No problem exists with the regulator or tubing, and the central vacuum pressure will increase when fewer people are using it.

## MODULE C
### Initiate suctioning procedures to remove tracheal and oral secretions

Tracheal or oral secretions must be actively removed by suctioning whenever the patient cannot clear them out and is at risk for airway obstruction. Suctioning may be needed in patients who are unconscious and who lack swallowing or coughing reflexes, or the patient may be too weak to cough effectively to remove tracheal secretions. The physician often writes a standing order to suction the patient on a regular basis or as needed. However, many institutions have a protocol for suctioning of any patient who is at risk of obstructing his or her airway. For example, the comatose patient who vomits should have the mouth suctioned even though no specific physician's order to do so exists.

Suctioning secretions from a patient's trachea, by any method, places the patient at risk. The following two factors must be understood, identified when they occur, and prevented or corrected.

***Prevent hypoxemia during the suctioning procedure (NBRC code: IIID7) [Difficulty: R, Ap].*** Suctioning the trachea removes air (including $O_2$), as well as secretions, from the lungs. Hypoxemia, however, can be minimized by hyperoxygenation of the patient for 1 to 2 min before suctioning. It is generally recommended that the patient receive 100% $O_2$, if possible. Infants younger than 6 months should be given a fractional concentration of inspired $O_2$ ($F_IO_2$) that is only 10% to 20% greater than base level because of the risk of retinopathy of prematurity.

Check the patient's arterial oxygen ($PaO_2$) results or pulse oximetry ($SpO_2$) value to see whether the patient is hypoxic before you begin the procedure. $SpO_2$ values can also be monitored throughout the suctioning procedure to see how low the saturation drops and when the patient has been resaturated (>90%) after suctioning is performed. The patient's chart should also be checked for any history of cardiac problems. Sudden hypoxemia from suctioning could cause life-threatening arrhythmias such as premature ventricular contractions. Check the patient's pulse rate and rhythm before and after suctioning. If the patient is using a cardiac monitor, it should be watched for rate and rhythm changes related to the suctioning procedure. Tachycardia is frequently seen with hypoxemia. Check the blood pressure of any patient who has suctioning-related arrhythmias. The patient's vital signs should return to normal when oxygenation is restored.

Any modern mechanical ventilator can be set to deliver 100% $O_2$. The most current ventilators have a 100% $O_2$ button designed for just this purpose. Pushing it results in the patient's receiving pure $O_2$ for 1 to 2 min (depending on the manufacturer). Several sigh breaths can also be delivered. A closed airway suction catheter can be used with the ventilator, as has been discussed earlier, to minimize hypoxemia.

A spontaneously breathing patient can have a nonrebreathing mask placed and set to deliver close to 100% $O_2$. If a nonrebreathing mask is not available, turn up the $O_2$ flow or percentage to whatever appliance the patient is using. A spontaneously breathing patient with an endotracheal or tracheostomy tube can have 100% $O_2$ delivered through a Briggs adapter/aerosol T-piece. A manual resuscitation bag can also be used to give the patient several sigh breaths.

All patients must be reoxygenated before another attempt at suctioning is made. Giving 100% $O_2$ after the suctioning episode helps the patient to reoxygenate faster. Giving several sigh breaths also helps reoxygenation to occur faster than does normal tidal volume breathing.

***Vagus/vagal nerve stimulation.*** Vagal nerve endings are found in the hypopharynx and trachea. When these are mechanically stimulated by a suction catheter, any of the following may be seen:

a. The patient may have an induced bronchospasm.
b. The patient may become bradycardic.
c. The patient's blood pressure may drop because of the bradycardia.

Listen to the patient's breath sounds before and after suctioning to detect an increase in wheezing, which shows bronchospasm. Check the patient's heart rate and rhythm by palpation or cardiac monitor to tell whether he or she is becoming bradycardic. Blood pressure can also be measured to check for hypotension.

Further suctioning should be delayed, if possible, until the patient's wheezing and vital signs have returned to normal. The suctioning procedure may need modification that involves not going as deeply and striking the carina, not twisting the catheter, or not suctioning for as long so as to reduce the risk of vagal stimulation. A local anesthetic such as lidocaine (Xylocaine) can be nebulized (with a physician's order) to reduce the local reaction to the catheter.

> ### Exam Hint
>
> **U**nderstand the importance of hyperoxygenating a patient before and after a suctioning procedure. This is usually tested on the examination.

## 1. Perform endotracheal or tracheostomy tube suctioning on the patient (NBRC code: IIIC2) [Difficulty: R, Ap]

The procedure for endotracheal or tracheostomy tube suctioning is the same for both tubes, except that the catheter does not need to be inserted as far into the tracheostomy tube before it hits the carina.

Generally accepted steps in the procedure follow:

a. Check the chart for specific orders, an order to suction as needed, or any special patient considerations.

b. Gather the needed equipment:
1. Suction catheter no larger than one half the ID of the patient's endotracheal or tracheostomy tube
2. Two sterile gloves or one sterile glove and one clean glove (this may be skipped if a closed airway, self-contained system is used)
3. Specimen collector if ordered
4. Vacuum system
5. Sterile water or normal saline in a sterile basin

c. Tell the patient what to expect during the procedure.

d. If possible, place the patient in semi-Fowler's and sniff positions.

e. Give the patient 100% $O_2$ for 1 to 2 min before suctioning and for at least 1 min afterward until the patient is no longer hypoxemic. (The infant who is younger than 6 months can have the $F_IO_2$ increased by 10% to 20%.)

f. Get help if necessary.

g. Wash hands. (This may be skipped if a self-contained system is used or in an emergency.)

h. Using sterile technique, put on the gloves, get the catheter out of its packaging, and connect the vacuum tubing to the catheter.

i. The American Association for Respiratory Care (AARC) clinical practice guidelines (1993) suggest that the vacuum should be set at the lowest possible level that still effectively removes secretions. A number of authors suggest the following ranges for vacuum:
1. Adults: −100 to −120 mm Hg
2. Children: −80 to −100 mm Hg
3. Neonates: −60 to −80 mm Hg

j. Test that the vacuum is reaching the tip of the catheter.

k. Disconnect the ventilator circuit or $O_2$ appliance from the tube (except with a self-contained system).

l. Suction the tube:
1. Without any vacuum, quickly and gently pass the catheter down the tube until an obstruction is felt. Withdraw the catheter 2 cm.
2. In the adult, the entire procedure of disconnection of the $O_2$, suctioning, reconnection of the $O_2$, and normal breathing should take no longer than 10 to 15 sec. In the infant, the entire procedure should take no longer than 10 sec.
3. Withdraw the catheter with a twisting motion while suctioning intermittently. Suction to clear out any secretions. Typically, in the adult, suctioning may be applied for between 5 and 10 sec. In the infant, suctioning may be applied for no longer than 5 sec.
4. Turning the patient's head to the right might help direct the catheter down the left mainstem bronchus. The catheter tends to enter the right mainstem bronchus if the head is in a neutral position or is twisted to the left.

m. Reoxygenate the patient for at least 1 min before suctioning again. Giving 100% $O_2$ (or 10% to 20% more than the base level in the infant) and several sigh breaths help this happen faster.

n. Monitor the patient's vital signs, $O_2$ level, and breath sounds before suctioning again. Suction again, if needed, when the patient is stable.

o. Normal saline solution may be instilled into the tube if the secretions are too thick to be suctioned out easily. The saline solution may help to loosen the secretions. The patient is also likely to cough vigorously. The amount of saline solution to be instilled varies with the size of the patient and the thickness of the secretions. Following are general guidelines for the instillation of normal saline solution:
1. Neonates may be given a few drops to 0.33 mL at a time.
2. Adults may be given 5 to 10 mL at a time, or it may be given in divided doses.
3. A physician's order may be needed to instill saline solution.

| BOX 13-1 | Hazards and Complications of Endotracheal Suctioning |
| --- | --- |

- Cardiac arrest
- Respiratory arrest
- Hypoxemia
- Cardiac arrhythmia
- Bronchospasm
- Increased intracranial pressure
- Hypertension
- Hypotension
- Apnea from interruption of mechanical ventilation
- Pulmonary hemorrhage
- Mechanical trauma to tracheal and bronchial mucosa
- Infection to or from patient and respiratory care practitioner
- Atelectasis

p. Dispose of the catheter and glove by pulling the glove inside-out over the catheter. Self-contained systems may be left in place for up to 24 hr.

q. Rinse the vacuum tubing clear of secretions.

r. Turn off the suction unit.

Refer to Box 13-1 for hazards and complications of endotracheal suctioning.

## 2. Perform nasotracheal suctioning on the patient (NBRC code: IIIC2) [Difficulty: R, Ap]

Generally accepted steps in the procedure follow:

a. Check the chart for specific orders, an order to suction as needed, or any special patient considerations.

b. Gather the needed equipment:
1. Suction catheter no larger than one-half the diameter of the patient's nostril
2. An appropriate size and type of nasopharyngeal airway to minimize nasal mucosal damage
3. Sterile, water-soluble lubricant jelly
4. A sterile 4 × 4-inch gauze pad

c. Tell the patient what to expect during the procedure.

d. If possible, place the patient in semi-Fowler's and sniff positions.

e. Give the patient 100% $O_2$ for 1 to 2 min before suctioning and for at least 1 min afterward until the patient is no longer hypoxemic. (The infant younger than 6 months can have the $F_IO_2$ increased by 10% to 20%.)

f. Get help if necessary.

g. Wash hands. (This may be skipped in an emergency.)

h. Using sterile technique, put on the gloves, get the catheter out of its packaging, apply lubricant jelly to the catheter tip, and connect the vacuum tubing to the catheter.

i. The AARC clinical practice guidelines (1992) suggest that the vacuum should be set at the lowest possible level that still effectively removes secretions. A number of authors suggest the following ranges for vacuum:
1. Adults: −100 to −120 mm Hg
2. Children: −80 to −100 mm Hg
3. Neonates: −60 to −80 mm Hg

j. Test that the vacuum is reaching the tip of the catheter.

k. Remove the $O_2$ appliance from the patient so that the nose may be reached. Directing the end of the $O_2$ tubing or nasal cannula prongs toward the patient's mouth may help to prevent hypoxemia.

l. Suction the trachea:
1. Without any vacuum, advance the catheter into the nasopharyngeal airway. If no nasopharyngeal airway is available, without any vacuum, advance the catheter into the most open nasal passage. The catheter should be advanced parallel to the turbinates to minimize tissue trauma. Never force the catheter. (The most patent nasal passage can be assessed by checking the chart for a history of deviated septum, asking the patient if one side feels more open, or feeling which nostril has greater airflow through it.)
2. Have the cooperative patient stick out his or her tongue. The practitioner or assistant can grasp the uncooperative patient's tongue with a 4 × 4-inch gauze pad or gloved hand.
3. Advance the catheter as the patient inspires. The epiglottis and vocal cords are open at this time, and it is easiest to slip the catheter into the trachea. The cooperative patient should be told to inhale slowly and deeply. Some practitioners find it helpful to disconnect the catheter from the vacuum tubing and listen to the end of the catheter for the sound of air movement. The patient will cough vigorously when the catheter is in the trachea (Fig. 13-16).
4. Advance the catheter until an obstruction is felt. Then, pull the catheter back about 2 cm.
5. Withdraw the catheter with a twisting motion while suctioning intermittently. Suction to clear out any secretions. Typically, in the adult, suctioning may be applied for between 5 and 10 sec. Suctioning in the infant should be applied for no longer than 5 sec. When secretions are cleared, the catheter is pulled out. Practitioners disagree on whether the catheter should be withdrawn or left in place if the patient still

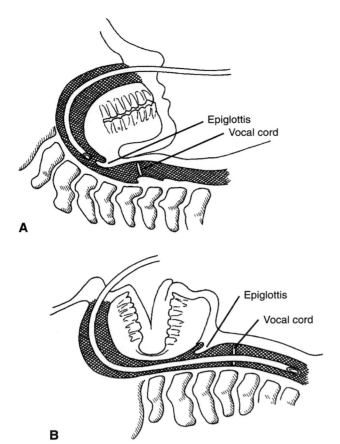

**Fig. 13-16** Cross section through the airway showing nasotracheal suctioning. **A,** Catheter is advanced through the nostril to the level of the vocal cords. **B,** With the head in a sniff position and during an inspiration, the catheter is advanced into the trachea. The patient coughs, and secretions are suctioned.

---

**BOX 13-2  Contraindications and Hazards and Complications of Nasotracheal Suctioning**

**CONTRAINDICATIONS**

*ABSOLUTE*

- Epiglottitis
- Laryngotracheobronchitis (croup)

*RELATIVE*

- Blocked nasal passages
- Nasal bleeding
- Acute facial, neck, or head injury
- Bleeding disorder
- Upper respiratory tract infection
- Irritable airway
- Laryngospasm

**HAZARDS AND COMPLICATIONS**

- Cardiac arrest
- Respiratory arrest
- Hypoxemia
- Cardiac arrhythmia
- Bronchospasm
- Increased intracranial pressure
- Hypertension
- Hypotension
- Pulmonary hemorrhage
- Infection to or from patient and respiratory therapist
- Atelectasis
- Pain
- Catheter misdirected into esophagus
- Gagging or vomiting
- Uncontrolled coughing
- Mechanical trauma: nasal turbinates, perforation of pharynx, nasal bleeding, bleeding of the tracheal and bronchial mucosa

---

has secretions. Some prefer to withdraw the catheter, let the patient rest and reoxygenate, and reinsert the catheter for additional suctioning. Others prefer to leave the catheter in place to minimize tissue trauma from a reinsertion, let the patient rest and reoxygenate, then suction again.

6. The entire procedure usually takes longer than 20 sec, so the $O_2$ tubing must be kept directed toward the patient's mouth.

7. Turning the patient's head to the right might help direct the catheter down the left mainstem bronchus. The catheter will tend to enter the right mainstem bronchus if the head is in a neutral position or is twisted to the left.

m. Reoxygenate the patient for at least 1 min before suctioning again. Giving 100% $O_2$ (or 10% to 20% more than the base level in the infant) helps this happen faster.

n. Monitor the patient's vital signs, $O_2$ level, and breath sounds before suctioning again. Suction again, if needed, when the patient is stable.

o. Normal saline solution may be instilled down the suction catheter by pulling off the vacuum tubing, inserting the tip of the syringe (not needle) into the end of the catheter, covering the thumb-control valve, and squirting the saline solution into the catheter. The other considerations listed earlier would apply here.

p. Dispose of the catheter and glove by pulling the glove inside-out over the catheter.

q. Rinse the vacuum tubing clear of secretions.

r. Turn off the suction unit.

Refer to Box 13-2 for contraindications and hazards and complications of nasotracheal suctioning.

### 3. Perform orotracheal suctioning on the patient (NBRC code: IIIC2) [Difficulty: R, Ap]

Orotracheal suctioning is a more difficult procedure than nasotracheal suctioning and is not performed as often.

Generally accepted steps in the procedure follow:

a. Check the chart for specific orders, an order to suction as needed, or any special patient considerations.

b. Gather the needed equipment:
   1. Suction catheter no larger than one-half the diameter of the patient's nostril. Even though the catheter is going through the mouth, the critical diameter is the trachea. This guideline helps prevent forcing of too large a catheter into the trachea.
   2. The nasopharyngeal airway is not needed.
   3. The sterile, water-soluble lubricant jelly and 4 × 4-inch gauze pad may not be needed if the patient's mouth is moist. Some may always prefer to lubricate the catheter tip.
   4. Use sterile water or normal saline solution and a sterile basin. Pour some water or saline into the basin.

c. Tell the patient what to expect during the procedure.

d. If possible, place the patient in semi-Fowler's and sniff positions.

e. Give the patient 100% $O_2$ for 1 to 2 min before suctioning and for at least 1 min afterward until the patient is no longer hypoxemic. (The infant younger than 6 months can have the $F_IO_2$ increased by 10% to 20%.)

f. Get help if necessary.

g. Wash hands. (This may be skipped in an emergency.)

h. Using sterile technique, put on the gloves, get the catheter out of its packaging, and connect the vacuum tubing to the catheter. Add the following steps if necessary:
   1. With the clean-gloved hand, squeeze some of the lubricant jelly onto the 4 × 4-inch gauze pad.
   2. Lubricate the tip and the first few centimeters of the catheter.

i. The AARC clinical practice guidelines (1992 and 1993) suggest that the vacuum should be set at the lowest possible level that still effectively removes secretions. A number of authors suggest the following ranges for vacuum:
   1. Adults: −100 to −120 mm Hg
   2. Children: −80 to −100 mm Hg
   3. Neonates: −60 to −80 mm Hg

j. Test that the vacuum is reaching the tip of the catheter.

k. Remove the $O_2$ appliance from the patient so that the mouth may be reached. A nasal cannula may be placed on the patient to give supplemental $O_2$. An assistant may be able to direct the end of the $O_2$ tubing toward the patient's mouth to help prevent hypoxemia.

l. Suction the trachea:
   1. Without any vacuum, advance the catheter into the oral pharynx.
   2. Have the cooperative patient stick out his or her tongue. The practitioner or assistant can grasp the uncooperative patient's tongue with a 4 × 4-inch gauze pad or gloved hand.
   3. Advance the catheter as the patient inspires. The epiglottis and vocal cords are open at this time, and it is easiest to slip the catheter into the trachea. The cooperative patient should be told to inhale slowly and deeply. Try to avoid stimulating the patient's gag reflex by not striking the oropharynx with the tip of the catheter. The patient will cough vigorously when the catheter is in the trachea.
   4. Advance the catheter until an obstruction is felt. Then, pull the catheter back about 2 cm.
   5. Withdraw the catheter with a twisting motion while suctioning intermittently. Suction to clear out any secretions. Typically, in the adult, suctioning may be applied for between 5 and 10 sec. Suctioning in the infant may be applied for no longer than 5 sec. When secretions are cleared, the catheter is pulled out. Practitioners disagree on whether the catheter should be withdrawn or left in place if the patient still has secretions. Some prefer to withdraw the catheter, let the patient rest and reoxygenate, and reinsert the catheter for additional suctioning. Others prefer to leave the catheter in place to minimize tissue trauma from a reinsertion, let the patient rest and reoxygenate, then suction again.
   6. The entire procedure usually takes longer than 20 sec, so the $O_2$ tubing must be kept directed toward the patient's mouth.
   7. Turning the patient's head to the right might help direct the catheter down the left mainstem bronchus. The catheter will tend to enter the right mainstem bronchus if the head is in a neutral position or is twisted to the left.

m. Reoxygenate the patient for at least 1 min before suctioning again. Giving 100% $O_2$ (or 10% to 20% more than the base level in the infant) helps this happen faster.

n. Monitor the patient's vital signs, $O_2$ level, and breath sounds before suctioning again. Suction again, if needed, when the patient is stable.

o. Normal saline solution may be instilled down the suction catheter by pulling off the vacuum tubing, inserting the tip of the syringe (not needle) into the end of the catheter, covering the thumb-control valve, and squirting the saline into the catheter. The other considerations listed earlier would apply here.

p. Dispose of the catheter and glove by pulling the glove inside-out over the catheter.
q. Rinse the vacuum tubing clear of secretions.
r. Turn off the suction unit.

## MODULE D
### Respiratory care plan

1. **Analyze the available information to determine the patient's pathophysiologic state** (NBRC code: IIIH1) [Difficulty: R, Ap, An]
2. **Auscultate the patient's breath sounds and interpret any changes** (NBRC code: IIIE11) [Difficulty: R, Ap]
3. **Look for changes in the patient's sputum characteristics** (NBRC code: IIIE5) [Difficulty: R, Ap]

Coarse, intermittent expiratory sounds (crackles or rhonchi) indicate secretions in the airway. Tracheal suctioning should clear these secretions and cause the return of (or at least an improvement in) normal breath sounds. Pneumonia and bronchitis cause chest x-ray film changes that show areas of infiltrate. Right or left lung involvement (or both), individual lobes, and segments with disease can be determined. As the patient's condition improves, the chest x-ray film should show clearing of infiltrates.

4. **Determine the appropriateness of the respiratory care plan and recommend modifications when indicated**
   a. **Make a change in the size and type of suction catheter** (NBRC code: IIIF2g2) [Difficulty: R, Ap]

As has been discussed earlier, the OD of the suction catheter should be no more than half the ID of the patient's endotracheal tube. When secretions are easy to suction, a smaller catheter may be used. The spontaneously breathing patient is less likely to become hypoxic if the tube is less obstructed.

A catheter with a Coudé tip should be used if it needs to be directed into one or the other mainstem bronchus (usually the left). Closed airway catheters, such as those made by Ballard Medical Products, offer two advantages over single-use catheters. First, they are more economical if the patient needs frequent suctioning. Second, patients using mechanical ventilators continue to be ventilated and oxygenated and to have positive end-expiratory pressure maintained during the suctioning episode. Newer catheters that offer intermittent or continuous insufflation of $O_2$ may reduce the hypoxemia that many patients

experience during the suctioning procedure. However, these can be expensive, and their use requires advanced skill.

   b. **Change the level of vacuum used when suctioning** (NBRC code: IIIF2g3) [Difficulty: R, Ap]

In general, the lowest possible vacuum level that adequately removes secretions should be used. As has been mentioned, several authors have listed recommended maximal vacuum levels to be applied to adults, children, and neonates. However, the AARC clinical practice guidelines (1992 and 1993) on suctioning state that the lack of experimental data fails to support these or any other written maximum pressures.

   c. **Instill an irrigating solution into the trachea** (NBRC code: IIIF2g4) [Difficulty: R, Ap]

Sterile normal saline solution (0.9%) is widely instilled into the trachea to dilute and mobilize pulmonary secretions. It should be used whenever secretions are difficult to suction. Also, when secretions are easier to remove, a lower vacuum level can be used. In adults, about 5 to 10 mL can be instilled into the trachea before suctioning. Less is used with children, but no universal guidelines are available. Neonates have been reportedly given a few drops to 0.33 mL.

   d. **Change the frequency of suctioning** (NBRC code: IIIF2g1) [Difficulty: R, Ap]

Secretions obstruct the airways and should be removed, if possible; this usually necessitates more than one suctioning episode. Repeatedly suctioning the patient is not harmful as long as he or she is reoxygenated between suctioning efforts. Watch for any complications (see Boxes 13-1 and 13-2). Also, listen to the patient's breath sounds for crackles or rhonchi, or palpate the chest for secretions between suctioning efforts. Stop suctioning when it is no longer needed.

   e. **Change the duration of the suctioning procedure** (NBRC code: IIIF2g1) [Difficulty: R, Ap]

Suctioning generally takes between 5 and 10 sec; the entire procedure should take between 10 and 15 sec. Some patients may not be able to tolerate this, so be prepared to suction for a shorter period. Suction repeatedly rather than increase the suctioning time.

   f. **Stop the procedure if the patient has an adverse reaction to it** (NBRC code: IIIF1) [Difficulty: R, Ap, An]

As listed in Boxes 13-1 and 13-2, stop the procedure if the patient becomes hypoxic or has tachycardia, bradycardia, arrhythmias, hypotension, or bronchospasm. Bloody secretions indicate possible mucosal damage and justify stopping the procedure. A conscious patient should be able to communicate how he or she feels after secretions have been suctioned. It is hoped that the feeling of dyspnea will improve. Hypoxemia and vagal stimulation can cause unstable vital signs and bronchospasm. Be prepared to stop suctioning, give extra $O_2$, or get help.

### g. Discontinue the procedure based on the patient's response (NBRC code: IIIG1f) [Difficulty: R, Ap]

Hypoxemia, tachycardia, bradycardia, arrhythmias, hypotension, bronchospasm, pneumothorax, or pulmonary hemorrhage that places the patient's life in danger justifies the cancellation of the suctioning order. Once the underlying problem has been corrected and safe suctioning can be performed, the order may be resumed.

---

**Exam Hint**

**P**ast examinations have tested an understanding of the need to alter the suctioning procedure or stop it, as previously discussed.

---

## BIBLIOGRAPHY

American Association for Respiratory Care: Clinical practice guideline: Endotracheal suctioning of mechanically ventilated adults and children with artificial airways, *Respir Care* 38:500, 1993.

American Association for Respiratory Care: Clinical practice guideline: Nasotracheal suctioning, *Respir Care* 37:898, 1992.

Burton GG: Patient assessment procedures. In Barnes TA, editor: *Respiratory care practice*, Chicago, 1988, Mosby.

Caldwell SL, Sullivan KN: Suctioning protocol. In Burton GG, Hodgkin JE, editors: *Respiratory care*, ed 2, Philadelphia, 1984, Lippincott.

Durbin CG: Airway management. In Cairo JM, Pilbeam SP: *Mosby's respiratory care equipment*, ed 7, St. Louis, 2004, Mosby.

Eubanks DH, Bone RC: *Comprehensive respiratory care*, ed 2, St Louis, 1990, Mosby.

Fink JB, Hess DR: Secretion clearance techniques. In Hess DR, MacIntyre NR, Mishoe SC, et al, editors: *Respiratory care principles & practice*, Philadelphia, 2002, WB Saunders.

Guidelines for the prevention of nosocomial infections, *AARTimes* 7:9, September 1983.

Hess DR, Branson RD: Airway and suctioning equipment. In Branson RD, Hess DR, Chatburn RL, editors: *Respiratory care equipment*, ed 2, Philadelphia, 1999, Lippincott Williams & Wilkins.

Lewis RM: Airway care. In Fink JB, Hunt GE, editors: *Clinical practice in respiratory care*, Philadelphia, 1999, Lippincott Williams & Wilkins.

McIntyre D: Airway management. In Wyka KA, Mathews PJ, Clark WF: *Foundations of respiratory care*, Albany, 2002, Delmar.

Pettignano MM, Pettignano R: Airway management. In Barnhart SL, Czervinske MP, editors: *Perinatal and pediatric respiratory care*, Philadelphia, 1995, WB Saunders.

Plevak DJ, Ward JJ: Airway management. In Burton GG, Hodgkin JE, Ward JJ, editors: *Respiratory care*, ed 4, Philadelphia, 1997, Lippincott-Raven.

Rarey KP, Youtsey JW: *Respiratory patient care*, Englewood Cliffs, NJ, 1981, Prentice-Hall.

Roth P: Airway care. In Aloan CA, Hill TV, editors: *Respiratory care of the newborn and child*, ed 2, Philadelphia, 1997, Lippincott.

Scott AA, Koff PB: Airway care and chest physiotherapy. In Koff PB, Eitzmann DV, Neu J, editors: *Neonatal and pediatric respiratory care*, ed 2, St Louis, 1993, Mosby.

Shapiro BA, Harrison RA, Cane RD, et al: *Clinical application of respiratory care*, ed 4, St Louis, 1991, Mosby.

Simmons KF, Scanlan CL: Airway management. In Wilkins RL, Stoller JK, Scanlan CL, editors: *Egan's fundamentals of respiratory care*, ed 8, St Louis, 2003, Mosby.

Wilkins RL: Physical examination of the patient with cardiopulmonary disease. In Wilkins RL, Krider SJ, Sheldon RL, editors: *Clinical assessment in respiratory care*, ed 3, St Louis, 1995, Mosby.

Wilkins RL, Hodgkin JE, Lopez B: *Lung sounds, a practical guide*, St Louis, 1988, Mosby.

Wojciechowski WV: Incentive spirometers, and secretion evacuation devices, and inspiratory muscle training devices. In Barnes TA, editor: *Core textbook of respiratory care practice*, ed 2, St Louis, 1994, Mosby.

## SELF-STUDY QUESTIONS

1. All of the following statements about the use of a Lukens trap are true EXCEPT
   A. A vacuum source is needed
   B. All connections must be tight for it to work properly
   C. Either a suction catheter or a bronchoscope is also needed
   D. It is used to collect a sputum sample from a patient with a strong, productive cough

2. Before a patient with an intubated airway is suctioned for the first time, the chart must be checked for
   I. A history of cardiac disease or arrhythmia
   II. A written order
   III. A history of a strong gag reflex
   IV. Blood gas results or $SpO_2$ results
   V. A history of asthma or bronchospasm
   A. II and III
   B. IV and V
   C. I, II, IV, and V
   D. III and V

3. The properly sized suction catheter should be no larger than what fraction of the ID of a patient's endotracheal tube?
   A. 1/4
   B. 1/2
   C. 2/3
   D. 3/4

4. Placing a suction catheter into your patient's trachea and applying vacuum causes
   I. Transient hypoxemia
   II. Removal of secretions
   III. Stopping of the hypoxic drive because of vagal stimulation
   IV. Removal of air from the lungs
   A. III and IV
   B. III
   C. III and IV
   D. I, II, and IV

5. If your patient has a room air arterial $O_2$ pressure of 65 mm Hg, the most important step to take to prevent hypoxemia during suctioning is to
   A. Give the patient 100% $O_2$ before and after the procedure
   B. Use a large catheter to remove the secretions quickly
   C. Hyperextend the patient's neck and head
   D. Use a small catheter so that the patient can breathe around it

6. The best position for a patient to be placed in before nasotracheal suctioning is
   I. Supine
   II. Trendelenburg
   III. Neck and head hyperextended
   IV. Semi-Fowler's
   A. I and IV
   B. I and III
   C. II and III
   D. III and IV

7. Making sure that a central vacuum system is working properly includes all the following steps EXCEPT
   A. Setting the vacuum control to Full
   B. Screwing a 500-mL collection bottle tightly onto the vacuum connector
   C. Attaching 3 ft of vacuum tubing to the tubing connector on the collection jar
   D. Pinching closed the vacuum tubing when the vacuum is turned on to measure the vacuum level

8. During nasotracheal suctioning, it is important to
   A. Lubricate the catheter in sterile water
   B. Lubricate the catheter tip in a sterile, water-soluble lubricant jelly
   C. Place the catheter in the refrigerator to make it firmer and easier to pass
   D. Lubricate the catheter in sterile normal saline solution

9. You notice that a Yankauer suction catheter you are using is cracked. The best thing to do is to
   A. Continue to use it
   B. Tape over the crack
   C. Put lubricating jelly in the crack to seal it
   D. Replace the catheter

10. You are preparing to suction a patient for a mucus sample when you notice that the vacuum is not reaching the end of the catheter. All of the following are possible causes of this problem EXCEPT
    A. The vacuum is not turned on to the proper level
    B. The vacuum tubing, specimen collector, and catheter system are connected so that they are airtight
    C. The catheter is plugged with foreign matter
    D. The specimen jar is not screwed tightly into the special lid

11. While connecting the suction catheter to the vacuum tubing, you accidentally touch the tip of the catheter with your clean-gloved hand. You would proceed to
    A. Discard the clean glove and start over
    B. Suction the patient
    C. Put a sterile glove over the clean glove and suction the patient
    D. Discard the catheter and start over
12. You are suctioning your patient when the vacuum is lost. You should do all the following EXCEPT
    A. Make sure the vacuum system is working
    B. Make sure a tight connection exists between the suction catheter and the vacuum tubing
    C. Check the catheter to make sure it is not obstructed
    D. Get a larger suction catheter

13. A ventilator-dependent patient required a vacuum pressure of −120 mm Hg to remove her thick secretions. After treatment with a mucolytic drug, her secretions are much easier to remove. What would you recommend?
    A. Reduce her vacuum pressure to −100 mm Hg and monitor the ease of removing her secretions
    B. Maintain the present vacuum level and suction less often
    C. Increase the vacuum level to −140 mm Hg and suction less often
    D. Reduce her vacuum pressure to −60 mm Hg and suction more often

## ANSWER KEY AND RATIONALE

1. **D.** Lukens traps are used only to get a sputum sample from a patient who cannot cough productively.
2. **C.** Suctioning an intubated patient does not stimulate a gag reflex. The other listed items are important to know for the sake of patient safety and legality.
3. **B.** It is commonly accepted that a suction catheter's diameter should not be greater than one-half the ID of the endotracheal tube. This ensures that the patient has room to breathe around the catheter.
4. **D.** Suctioning removes secretions, as intended, as well as air (and its contained $O_2$) from the patient's airways and lungs. This causes a transient drop in the patient's $O_2$ level. Vagal stimulation has no connection to hypoxic drive.
5. **A.** All patients should be preoxygenated before suctioning and given added $O_2$ after suctioning to quickly restore the presuctioning $O_2$ level. $O_2$ at 100% should be given unless a reason exists to give less.
6. **D.** Hyperextending the patient's head and neck helps open the airway so that the catheter can be more easily inserted into the trachea. Placing the patient into semi-Fowler's position helps him or her take a deeper breath as needed.
7. **A.** The Full (maximum) vacuum level is too great to be safely applied to a patient's airway.

8. **B.** Lubricating the tip of the catheter with sterile, water-soluble lubricating jelly helps the catheter slide more easily though the patient's nasal passage. Neither water nor saline is a good lubricant because these drip off of the catheter. A suction catheter should be flexible, not firm.
9. **D.** It is always best to replace a broken or defective piece of equipment.
10. **B.** If the equipment is properly assembled with no air leak, the vacuum should reach the end of the catheter. The other three examples would result in failure of vacuum to reach the end of the catheter.
11. **D.** Suctioning is a *sterile* procedure. A clean-gloved hand is not sterile. The contaminated catheter should be replaced with a sterile one.
12. **D.** A larger suction catheter would not make any difference in restoring vacuum. When the suctioning system is properly working, vacuum should be felt at the end of a catheter of *any* size. Problems with the other listed options could result in loss of vacuum.
13. **A.** It is most reasonable to slightly decrease her vacuum level and find out how easy it is to remove her secretions. Suctioning frequency should not be reduced unless she has fewer secretions. No need exists to increase the vacuum level.

# 14 Intermittent Positive-Pressure Breathing

A review of the most recent Entry Level Examinations has shown an average of 3 questions (2% of the exam) that cover intermittent positive-pressure ventilation.

## MODULE A

**Initiate intermittent positive-pressure (IPPB) breathing therapy to achieve adequate spontaneous ventilation and oxygenation (NBRC code: IIID2a) [Difficulty: R, Ap]**

### 1. Description

The Respiratory Care Committee of the American Thoracic Society published the following definition in its 1980 *Guidelines for the use of intermittent positive-pressure breathing (IPPB)*: "'IPPB treatments' refers to the use of a pressure-limited respirator to deliver a gas with humidity and/or aerosol to a spontaneously breathing patient for periods of time that are generally no greater than 15 to 20 minutes each."

A pressure-limited respirator may be powered by compressed gas or electricity. The patient's tidal volume ($V_T$) should be greater than normal when enhanced by IPPB. This greater-than-normal $V_T$ is caused by the use of positive pressure against the lungs. Pressure is also directed against the airways and, through contact with the airways and lungs, the entire chest. The patient's exhalation is usually passive but can be slowed through modification of the exhalation valve.

Shapiro and associates (1991) list the following as the physiologic effects of IPPB:

#### a. Increased mean airway pressure

By definition of IPPB, the patient is receiving a positive airway pressure instead of generating a negative intrathoracic pressure to create the $V_T$. Most authors recommend that patients with heart disease be monitored closely for the effects of increased mean airway pressure. Decreasing the normal return of venous blood to the heart, thereby decreasing the cardiac output, is possible. Shapiro and associates (1991) recommend an expiratory time that is long enough to allow for normal venous return before the next positive-pressure breath is given. The patient's heart rate and blood pressure can be monitored to ensure that they stay in the normal range.

Pulmonary barotrauma is the second concern raised by the use of positive airway pressure. It is possible for patients with small-airways disease to trap air in the alveoli. This can lead to the rupture of a bleb, thus causing a pneumothorax. Care must be taken with the patient with bullous emphysema to ensure that the $V_T$ is exhaled completely.

#### b. Increased tidal volume

The primary goal of IPPB is to increase the patient's assisted $V_T$ to greater than the spontaneous $V_T$. Indeed, if the spontaneous $V_T$ is greater than the assisted $V_T$, IPPB is not needed for lung expansion.

#### c. Decreased work of breathing

A properly coached passive treatment with the controls set to meet the patient's inspiratory needs causes a decrease in the work of breathing (WOB). This necessitates considerable skill on the part of the practitioner. Sensitivity, inspiratory flow, and peak pressure must be frequently adjusted to minimize the patient's work. The patient must be asked if the control adjustments make it easier or harder for him or her to breathe in. Failure to tailor the breathing treatment to the patient's needs may actually increase the WOB.

#### d. Alteration of the inspiratory:expiratory ratio

Patients with high airway resistance or low lung compliance often change their breathing patterns to reduce the WOB (see Chapter 1). These new breathing patterns may lead to worsening of the patient's condition. Alteration of normal ventilation and perfusion ratios in the lungs may worsen hypoxemia. Properly administered and coached IPPB can be used to adjust the inspiratory:expiratory (I:E) ratio to the benefit of the patient. The patient can be taught how to breathe in a more physiologically normal pattern.

### 2. Indications

The following indications and guidelines are listed in the American Association for Respiratory Care (AARC) clinical practice guidelines (1991 and 2003) on IPPB.

*To treat clinically significant atelectasis when other deep-breathing methods are ineffective.* Patients who are uncooperative, unconscious, or physically incapable of being coached in deep-breathing and coughing techniques or in performance of incentive spirometry (IS) may be helped by IPPB. As has been discussed in Chapter 7, a patient benefits from IPPB rather than IS if he or she cannot generate an inspiratory capacity (IC) greater than 12 mL/kg or a vital capacity (VC) greater than 15 mL/kg, or has a postoperative IC less than 33% of predicted value (1/3 × 50 mL/kg of ideal body weight). An inspiratory pause at the end of the IPPB breath promotes better distribution of the gas to open areas of atelectasis.

The AARC guidelines list the following poor pulmonary function values as supporting the need for IPPB because they suggest that the patient would have an ineffective cough: VC less than 70% of predicted or less than 10 mL/kg, forced expiratory volume in 1 second (FEV$_1$) less than 65% of predicted, or maximum voluntary ventilation (MVV) less than 50% of predicted.

### Exam Hint

It is important to understand the indications for IPPB versus IS in treatment of a patient with atelectasis. This has been questioned on past examinations.

*To more effectively deliver aerosolized medications.* If the patient cannot coordinate his or her breathing pattern to make use of a metered dose inhaler (MDI) or handheld nebulizer, IPPB may be used. Examples of when IPPB would be the better choice include any situation in which the patient is unconscious, uncooperative, or physically incapable. Such patients are physically unable to make effective use of simpler methods of lung inflation (IS) or to take an aerosolized medication (MDI or handheld nebulizer). Included in this classification are the elderly, chronically debilitated patients, those with neuromuscular diseases, and those with kyphoscoliosis. Patients who are fatigued or who have severe hyperinflation may also benefit from IPPB.

*To enhance the patient's cough effort and sputum clearance.* The combination of aerosolized saline (with or without a bronchodilator or mucolytic) and deeper V$_T$s may help the patient to cough more productively. The practitioner must stop the treatment periodically to coach the patient's cough effort.

*To treat impending ventilatory failure as seen by an increased arterial carbon dioxide pressure (PaCO$_2$).* Intubation and mechanical ventilation may be delayed or avoided in the deteriorating patient with chronic obstructive pulmonary disease (COPD). The patient is able to relax and reduce the WOB during a passive IPPB treatment. It may be necessary to give IPPB for 5 to 10 min as often as every 30 to 60 min. Treatment should also be given with the intention of helping the patient's cough and sputum clearance.

The following additional indications are listed in The Respiratory Care Committee of the American Thoracic Society's *Guidelines for the use of intermittent positive-pressure breathing (IPPB)* (1980):

*To help manage the patient with acute pulmonary edema.* IPPB temporarily reduces venous return to the heart. The IPPB procedure does not correct the underlying cardiac problem, which must be treated by other means.

*To induce a sputum sample for culture and sensitivity or other diagnostic studies.* This would be indicated only if simpler methods did not work.

*To deliver medications for special purposes when simpler methods do not work.* This method can be used, for instance, to deliver a local anesthetic such as lidocaine (Xylocaine) before a bronchoscopy procedure.

### 3. Contraindications

*Untreated pneumothorax* is listed by all authors and by the AARC guidelines as an absolute contraindication. Increased intrathoracic pressure converts a simple pneumothorax into a tension pneumothorax. The consequences could be fatal. Once a chest tube has been inserted into the pleural space and a pleural drainage system has been set up, IPPB can be administered. The air leak may increase, but this should not be life threatening.

The AARC guidelines list the following as relative contraindications. Any patient with one of these should be evaluated carefully before a decision about the clinical use of IPPB is made:

a. Active hemoptysis. Coughing up blood indicates that a tear has occurred in the airway or lung tissues. IPPB treatment should be stopped if a large amount of hemoptysis is present. Certainly, massive hemoptysis (greater than 600 mL of blood coughed out in a 16-hr period) contraindicates IPPB
b. Hemodynamic instability
c. Intracranial pressure greater than 15 mm Hg
d. Chest x-ray film that shows a bleb
e. Tracheoesophageal fistula
f. Recent surgery on the esophagus, skull, face, or mouth
g. Untreated, active tuberculosis (hazardous to the practitioner)
h. Nausea, air swallowing, or hiccups (singultation)

### Exam Hint

Past examinations have included questions about the contraindications for IPPB, especially untreated pneumothorax.

### 4. Hazards and precautions

The AARC guidelines list the following hazards and precautions for IPPB therapy:

a. Pneumothorax

b. Barotrauma

c. Increased airway resistance from a bronchospastic reaction to the positive pressure or an adverse reaction to a medication. This can result in alveolar overdistention and air trapping

d. Hyperoxia when 100% $O_2$ is delivered to the patient. Some hypercarbic COPD patients breathing on hypoxic drive may hypoventilate as a result

e. Secretions that may become impacted when inhaled gas is not humidified adequately

f. Nosocomial infection

g. Decreased venous return

h. Increased ventilation-to-perfusion mismatch: This could worsen any hypoxemia

i. Hyperventilation

j. Psychological dependence: This may be seen in the long-term home care patient who does not want to switch to another method of taking inhaled medications

k. Hypocarbia

l. Hemoptysis

m. Gastric distention

n. Air trapping, auto-PEEP, or overdistended alveoli

### 5. Initiation of therapy

#### a. Steps in the basic procedure

1. Check for a complete and proper order that specifies the patient, $O_2$ percentage, frequency of treatment, medication, and any special considerations.

2. Gather the necessary equipment and medications.

3. Set up the equipment outside the patient's room.

4. Introduce yourself, the department, and the purpose of the visit.

5. Confirm the patient's identity.

6. Have the patient sit up in bed or a chair; an obese patient may stand.

7. Interview the patient.

8. Assess the patient's vital signs.

9. Assess the patient's breath sounds.

10. Prepare the IPPB unit for operation with the following guidelines:

    a. If the unit is electric, plug into a working outlet.

    b. If the unit is pneumatic, plug into either a compressed air or $O_2$ outlet as ordered.

    c. Set the following controls:

        i. Set sensitivity at $-1$ cm $H_2O$.

        ii. Set the nebulizer to run on inspiration only.

        iii. Adjust the flow as necessary.

        iv. Set the peak pressure at about 10 to 15 cm $H_2O$.

    d. Test the nebulizer by turning on the machine.

    e. Cover the mouthpiece with a clean tissue to ensure that it cycles off at the preset pressure.

11. Instruct the patient to sip on the mouthpiece like a straw to turn on the machine. Have the patient relax and let the machine fill his or her lungs with air. The patient should hold his or her breath for 2 to 3 sec and exhale slowly.

#### b. Giving a passive treatment

Most authors describe patients who receive a passive treatment. With this treatment, the patient relaxes and lets the machine fill the lungs until the preset pressure is reached. As has been mentioned earlier, the patient is then told to hold his or her breath before exhaling passively. This treatment is given to minimize the patient's WOB. The slowest possible flow rate is used so that any nebulized medication is deposited deeply into the small airways and lungs.

#### c. Giving an active treatment

Several authors advocate giving the patient an active treatment when he or she uses the IPPB machine to get as deep a breath as possible. Welch and associates (1980) have found that the patient's posttreatment IC is greatest when the practitioner (1) uses as high a peak pressure as the patient can tolerate, and (2) coaches the patient to inhale as deeply as possible with the IPPB machine. They and others believe that this is the best way to treat or prevent atelectasis.

### 6. Initial settings on the Bird Mark 7

The older Mark 7 is used as the model respirator of the Bird series. The current Mark 8 has similar features, and other Bird units have slightly different controls and features. Refer to Fig. 14-1 for the following instructions:

a. Adjust the *air-mix* knob to the desired gas mix.

b. Set sensitivity so that the patient has to generate about $-1$ cm $H_2O$ pressure to cycle on the unit. Set the *sensitivity* control (on the left-hand side of the unit when you are facing it) to the reference no. 15 (approximately the 2 o'clock position). Turning the control lever counterclockwise makes the unit more sensitive. Push in the hand timer rod to note that the unit cycles on easily.

c. Flow should be set so that the patient feels comfortable with the inspiratory time. Set the *flow-rate* knob so that the reference no. 15 is at the 12 o'clock position; the *off* sign is at the 8 o'clock position. Turning the *flow-rate* knob counterclockwise increases the flow.

d. Peak pressure should be set at about 10 to 15 cm $H_2O$ pressure. Set the *pressure* control (on the right-hand side of the unit when you are facing it) to reference no. 15 (approximately the 10 o'clock position). Turning the control lever farther clockwise increases the peak pressure. Hold a clean tissue

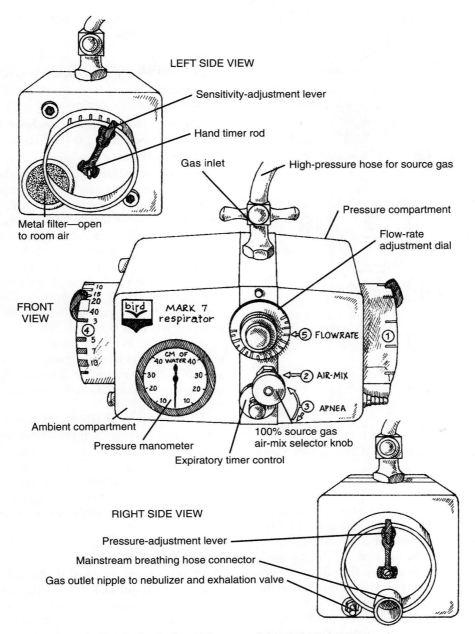

**Fig. 14-1** Controls and features of the Bird Mark 7 IPPB unit.

against the patient's mouthpiece to ensure that the unit cycles off at the desired peak pressure.

### 7. Initial settings on the Bennett PR-2

The PR-2 is used as the model respirator of the Bennett series. (Although the PR-2 is no longer being produced, many are still in clinical use.) Other Bennett units have slightly different controls and features. Refer to Figs. 14-2 and 14-3 for the following instructions:

a. Adjust the *air-dilution* knob to the desired gas mix.

b. Sensitivity should be set so that the patient has to generate about −1 cm $H_2O$ pressure to cycle on the

unit. Turning the control lever counterclockwise makes the unit more sensitive. Push up on the Bennett valve strut to note that the unit cycles on easily.

c. Flow should be set so that the patient feels comfortable with the inspiratory time. The Bennett valve is designed to automatically open and close itself to allow the patient as much flow as desired. Set the *peak flow* control knob as far counterclockwise as possible for its maximal setting. Turning the *peak flow* knob clockwise decreases the patient's peak flow.

Accumulators

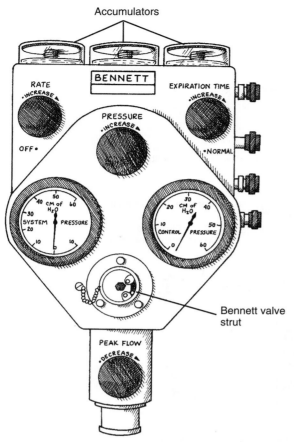

**Fig. 14-2** Front controls and features of the Bennett PR-2 IPPB unit.

d. Peak pressure should be set at about 10 to 15 cm $H_2O$. Dial the *pressure* control clockwise until the *control pressure* gauge shows the desired peak pressure. Hold a clean tissue against the patient's mouthpiece to ensure that when the unit cycles off, the *system pressure* gauge reads the same as the *control pressure* gauge.

e. Turn the *inspiration nebulization* control counterclockwise for medication to be nebulized only during an inspiration. Some practitioners state that the *expiration nebulization* control should be turned on slightly so that the mouthpiece and circuit dead space are filled with medication before the next breath. Others are opposed to this because it wastes medication when the patient stops the treatment.

f. A small leak in the circuit, mouthpiece, or facemask can be overcome with the addition of some additional flow by turning on the *terminal flow* control. It is normally left off. Turn the control counterclockwise to add as much additional flow as necessary to overcome the leak.

Details on the design and control specifications for the various Bird and Bennett models can be found in the manufacturers' literature and in books on respiratory therapy equipment.

## MODULE B

**Adjust intermittent positive-pressure breathing therapy to achieve adequate spontaneous ventilation**

### 1. Change the patient-machine interface (NBRC code: IIIF2a) [Difficulty: R, Ap]

#### a. Mouthpiece

A conscious, cooperative patient can take a treatment with a mouthpiece. He or she must be instructed to place it between the teeth (or gums) and seal the lips around it to prevent leaks. Instruct the patient to sip gently on it to turn on the IPPB machine. As long as the lips are sealed and no other leaks occur, the positive-pressure breath stops when the preset pressure is reached. Noseclips often help to prevent a leak through the nose as the patient is learning how to take the treatment. The noseclips can be removed after the patient has learned how to seal the nasopharynx with the soft palate.

A variety of mouthpieces are available. All share the common features of a raised edge so that the teeth do not slip off and a 22-mm outer diameter (OD) connector end to insert into the IPPB circuit (Fig. 14-4).

#### b. Mouth seal (Bennett seal)

An unconscious, uncooperative, or aged patient who cannot seal his or her lips can be aided by placement of a soft rubber seal around the mouthpiece. The practitioner gently holds the seal around the patient's lips to seal the airway so that the patient can trigger the breath and cycle off the machine (Fig. 14-5). Noseclips are also commonly needed.

#### c. Facemask

The facemask can be used if the mouth seal does not provide an airtight seal. This might occur because of the patient's facial structure or lack of teeth. Mouth trauma, surgery, and lip sores are other reasons to use a facemask.

The mask should be clear and properly sized to fit comfortably over the patient's nose and mouth. The practitioner should be able to get a seal with a minimum amount of hand pressure (Fig. 14-6). The equipment connection opening in the mask has a 22-mm inner diameter (ID) for direct connection to the IPPB circuit. A 22-mm-OD male adapter and a short length of aerosol tubing can be added for flexibility and patient comfort. The clear mask is important so that the practitioner can see whether the patient has vomited or has a large amount of secretions or saliva in his or her mouth. The mask should never be strapped to the patient's face so that the practitioner can attend to another patient.

This is the least effective patient attachment device if the therapeutic goal is to deliver an aerosolized

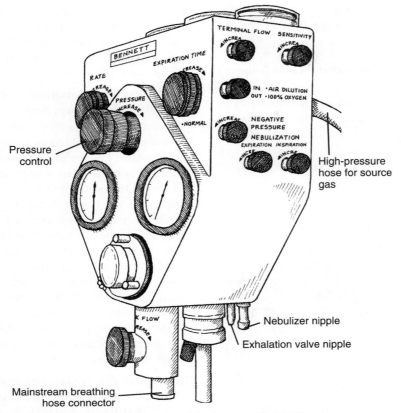

Pressure control

High-pressure hose for source gas

Nebulizer nipple

Exhalation valve nipple

Mainstream breathing hose connector

**Fig. 14-3** Right-side controls and features of the Bennett PR-2 IPPB unit.

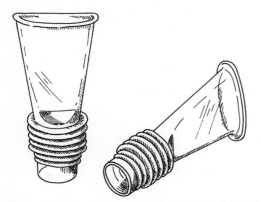

**Fig. 14-4** Universal intermittent positive-pressure breathing mouthpiece with a tapered 22- to 18-mm machine connector.

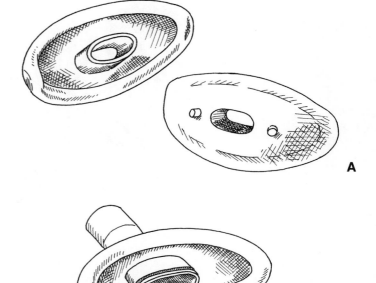

**A**

**B**

**Fig. 14-5  A,** Bennett or mouth flange seal. **B,** Intermittent positive-pressure breathing mouthpiece inserted into the seal.

medication. Much of the medication runs out onto the patient's face or into the nasal passages if he or she is a nose breather.

### d. Tracheostomy/endotracheal tube (elbow) adapter

The elbow adapter connects the patient's tracheostomy or endotracheal tube to the IPPB circuit (or other respiratory care equipment). The IPPB end has a 22-mm-ID connec-

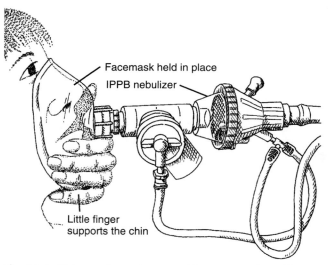

Fig. **14-6** Giving an intermittent positive-pressure breathing (IPPB) treatment with the use of a facemask.

tor. The tracheostomy/endotracheal tube end has a 15-mm-ID connector (Fig. 14-7). If the patient has had the cuff deflated, it must be reinflated to seal the airway. An unsealed cuff results in an air leak, and the gas flow cannot turn off.

### 2. Adjust the sensitivity (NBRC code: IIIF2h1) [Difficulty: R, Ap, An]

The sensitivity of the IPPB unit refers to how much effort or work the patient has to perform to turn on the unit for a breath. Commonly, the sensitivity is set so that the patient has to generate a negative pressure of only about $-1$ cm $H_2O$ to begin an inspiration. This can be verified by looking at the needle deflecting into the negative range on the pressure manometer. Ask the patient whether the machine can be easily turned on to get a breath. The IPPB unit should not be set so sensitively that it self-cycles.

The sensitivity range on the Bird series is $-0.01$ to $-5$ cm $H_2O$. Turning the *sensitivity/starting effort* adjustment lever counterclockwise toward the smaller reference numbers makes the unit more sensitive. The sensitivity range on the Bennett series is $-0.5$ to $-1$ cm $H_2O$. Turning the *sensitivity* control counterclockwise makes the unit easier to turn on.

### 3. Adjust the fractional concentration of inspired oxygen (NBRC code: IIIF2a) [Difficulty: R, Ap]

Both the Bird and Bennett units can be powered by compressed air or $O_2$. The decision as to what $O_2$ percentage

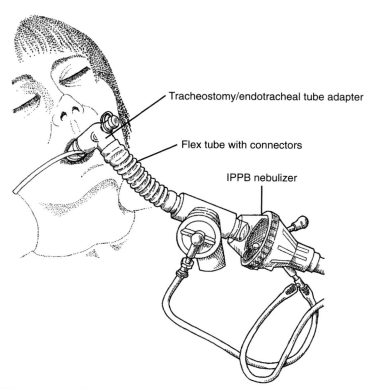

Fig. **14-7** Giving an intermittent positive-pressure breathing (IPPB) treatment with the use of a tracheostomy/endotracheal tube adapter.

to give depends on the patient's condition. The physician may include the $O_2$ percentage in the treatment order. Some departments have $O_2$ protocols in their treatment procedure. Compressed air (21% $O_2$) generally should be used whenever the patient does not need supplemental $O_2$.

Use caution with a patient with COPD who is retaining $CO_2$ and is breathing on hypoxic drive when $O_2$ is used to power the IPPB unit. Many times, compressed air is preferred to power the IPPB unit. The patient may be allowed to keep wearing a nasal cannula with $O_2$ during the treatment so that the blood $O_2$ level remains normal. The lack of availability of piped-in compressed air should not be an excuse for giving a patient a high $O_2$ percentage when it may be harmful. IPPB can be given through a gas-powered unit that is powered by a compressed air cylinder or an electrically powered unit.

Supplemental $O_2$ is given if either unit is powered by $O_2$ and the *air-mix/air-dilution* knob is set to dilute the source gas with room air. This would be appropriate for patients who require supplemental $O_2$ and are not at risk of stopping their spontaneous ventilation. Most practitioners use this method of giving IPPB because piped $O_2$ is usually available in all patients' rooms.

Pure $O_2$ should be given to the severely hypoxemic patient. Examples include acute pulmonary edema, respiratory failure, and CO poisoning. The *air-mix/air-dilution* knob must be set so that only the source gas ($O_2$) is delivered to the patient.

For varying $O_2$ percentages on the Mark 7, note the following guidelines:

a. Pushing the *air-mix* knob into the center body results in pure source gas. This could be either air or $O_2$.
b. Pulling the *air-mix* knob out of the center body results in dilution of the source gas with room air. If $O_2$ is the source gas, room air will dilute the delivered gas to between 60% and 90% (or more) $O_2$.

For varying $O_2$ percentages on the PR-2, note the following guidelines:

a. Pulling the *air-dilution* knob out of the body results in pure source gas. This could be either air or $O_2$.
b. Pushing the *air-dilution* knob into the body results in dilution of the source gas with room air. If $O_2$ is the source gas, room air will dilute the delivered gas to between 40% and 80% $O_2$.
c. Turning on the *terminal flow* control results in the dilution of source gas with room air. This will dilute the final percentage if the source gas is $O_2$.

### 4. Adjust the flow (NBRC code: IIIF2a) [Difficulty: R, Ap]

The patient should initially feel comfortable with the flow rate and the inspiratory time. Ask the patient a simple question, such as, "Is the breath coming too fast or too slow?" He or she can respond with a short answer or even a hand gesture. As treatment progresses, the practitioner may be able to adjust the flow to modify the patient's breathing pattern in an attempt to achieve the therapeutic goal. Consider the following situations:

a. Anxious patients may initially need a fast flow. As they are coached to relax and get used to the treatment, the practitioner should try to reduce the flow.
b. Slower flows cause medications to be deposited more deeply into the lungs, which is important if the patient is having a bronchodilator, mucolytic, or antibiotic nebulized.
c. Faster flows result in the deposition of medications in the upper airways. This is important if the patient is receiving racemic epinephrine for laryngeal edema or lidocaine as a local anesthetic of the upper airway before bronchoscopy.

Turning the *inspiratory time/flow rate* control counterclockwise increases the flow rate on the Bird series. Pulling the *air-mix* knob out from the center body increases the total flow by allowing room air to be entrained along with the source gas. Flow rate in the PR-2 is determined by assessment of the patient's inspiratory effort and evaluation of how open the Bennett valve is. Flow can be decreased somewhat by turning the *peak flow* control clockwise. Flow is not affected by the position of the *air-dilution* knob.

### 5. Adjust the volume, pressure, or both (NBRC code: IIIF2a) [Difficulty: R, AP]

A review of current respiratory care textbooks reveals that all authors agree that the basic goal of IPPB is to increase how deeply the patient inspires. Unfortunately, considerable difference exists about what inspiratory volume is being measured and how much that breath should be increased for therapeutic goals to be achieved. (On a clinical note, it is not practical to measure inhaled tidal volume. So, exhaled tidal volume is measured with a handheld spirometer.) The AARC has released the following statements on the subject of the tidal volume goal during IPPB:

a. The AARC clinical practice guideline (1993) on IPPB states that the $V_T$ delivered during an IPPB-assisted breath should be at least 25% greater than the patient's spontaneous breaths.
b. The AARC clinical practice guideline (1991) on IS states that IPPB is indicated to treat atelectasis rather than IS if (1) the patient's IC is less than 33% of the preoperative value, or (2) the patient's VC is less than 10 mL/kg of ideal body weight.
c. The 2003 revision and update of the 1993 AARC clinical practice guideline on IPPB states that the $V_T$ delivered during an IPPB-assisted breath should be at least 1/3 of the predicted IC ($1/3 \times 50$ mL/kg of ideal body weight).

If the therapeutic goal is to prevent or treat atelectasis, having the patient inspire a deeper than spontaneous $V_T$ breath should help. It seems reasonable to follow the

AARC guidelines both as indications and as clinical goals. They can be used as guidelines if an increased $V_T$ is used as a substitute for the VC. Based on this assumption, an IPPB-delivered $V_T$ goal of at least 10 mL/kg of ideal body weight seems reasonable. Because all of the current IPPB units are pressure-cycled, the only way to increase the inspired volume during a passive treatment is to increase the peak pressure. Coaching the patient during an active treatment results in a larger volume without the need for as great a peak pressure. Decrease the peak pressure if the patient complains of discomfort or cannot hold that much pressure without losing the lip seal.

### 6. Adjust expiratory retard

Expiratory retard is indicated in patients who have small-airways disease and who are air-trapping on exhalation. Over the course of an IPPB treatment, this can lead to an increased functional residual volume (FRC) with the increased risk of pulmonary barotrauma. Adding expiratory retard to the treatment has the same effect as pursed lips breathing. Increased backpressure on the smallest airways keeps them open longer so that the more distal air can be exhaled.

Measurement of exhaled volumes during treatment and monitoring of the patient's responses help the clinician to know how much retard is needed. Too little retard will result in some air trapping and an incompletely exhaled tidal volume. Too much retard will result in an uncomfortably long expiratory time and increased mean intrathoracic pressure. The proper amount of expiratory retard should result in the patient feeling comfortable with the breathing cycle and being able to completely exhale the $V_T$. Listening to the patient's breath sounds is also helpful. If wheezing is present, it will be minimized when the proper amount of retard is added because the backpressure is properly adjusted to minimize the small airway collapse.

Bird makes a retard cap that fits over the exhalation valve port on the permanent circuit. This cap has a series of holes of different sizes through which exhaled gas can pass (Fig. 14-8). Through rotation of the cap progressively from the largest to the smallest opening and evaluation of the patient at each setting, the properly sized opening and appropriate amount of retard can be determined.

Bennett makes a retard exhalation valve that can be substituted for the regular exhalation valve on its permanent circuit (Fig. 14-9). This valve consists of a spring that is attached to a nut and a diaphragm. As the nut is turned counterclockwise, the spring pushes the diaphragm closer to the exhalation valve opening. This causes resistance to exhalation of the $V_T$, and a backpressure is created against the airways. If too much pressure is placed against the exhalation valve opening, the patient will not be able to exhale back to atmospheric pressure. This should not be done without a physician's order.

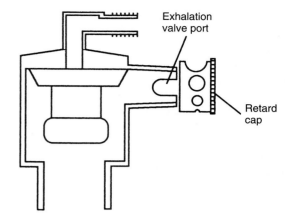

**Fig. 14-8** Bird retard cap that is used to provide adjustable expiratory resistance. *(From McPherson SP, Spearman CP: Respiratory therapy equipment, ed 4, St Louis, 1990, Mosby.)*

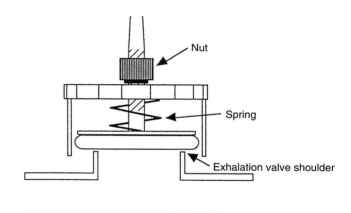

**Fig. 14-9** Bennett retard exhalation valve that is used to provide adjustable expiratory resistance. *(From Cairo JM, Pilbeam SP: Mosby's respiratory care equipment, ed 6, St Louis, 1999, Mosby.)*

Be sure to ask the patient's opinion about the use of expiratory retard. The conscious, cooperative patient can say whether he or she feels as though more air is getting out through the use of the retard, or whether the lungs feel more full because too much retard is being used. Too much retard may make the expiratory time uncomfortably long.

> ### Exam Hint
> Commonly, a question is included that requires the therapist to revise the procedure. Increase the pressure to give a larger tidal volume; decrease the pressure to give a smaller volume. Increase the flow if the patient wants a faster breath.

**7. Stop the treatment if the patient has an adverse reaction to it (NBRC code: IIIF1) [Difficulty: R, Ap, An]**

As has been mentioned, the general treatment length is 15 to 20 min. The patient, particularly one who is aged or debilitated, may not be able to tolerate this period because of fatigue. After rest, treatment may be resumed. Additionally, if the patient is receiving an adrenergic (sympathomimetic) agent, an adverse reaction to the medication can occur. Most commonly, this relates to tachycardia. A common clinical guideline is to stop treatment if the patient's heart rate goes up by 20% or more. If the patient's heart rate slows down in a few minutes, the treatment may be resumed.

## MODULE C

**Intermittent positive-pressure breathing equipment**

**1. Get the proper intermittent positive-pressure breathing circuit for the patient's treatment (NBRC code: IIA11b) [Difficulty: R]**

The two most widely used IPPB machines are the Bird Mark 7/8 (or a variation on it in the series) and the

Bennett PR-2. Both are pneumatically powered and found in most hospitals. Each unit must have a circuit that has been designed specifically for it. Fig. 14-10 shows a permanent (reusable after cleaning) and disposable circuit for a Bennett machine. Fig. 14-11 shows a permanent (reusable after cleaning) and disposable circuit for a Bird machine.

**2. Put the intermittent positive-pressure breathing circuit together, make sure that it works properly, and identify any problems with it (NBRC code: IIA11b) [Difficulty: R]**

See Fig. 14-10 for the Bennett setup and Fig. 14-11 for the Bird setup.

### a. General setup procedures

1. Check for plentiful source gas. Make sure that the $O_2$ or air tank has the proper regulator. Check the pressure in the gas cylinder.
2. Attach the high-pressure hose to the source gas and the IPPB unit at the gas inlet. Make sure that the connections are tight.

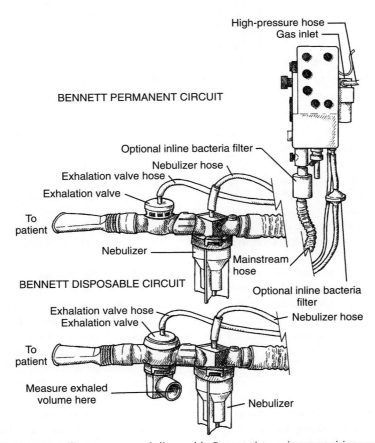

**Fig. 14-10** Features of permanent and disposable Bennett intermittent positive-pressure breathing circuits.

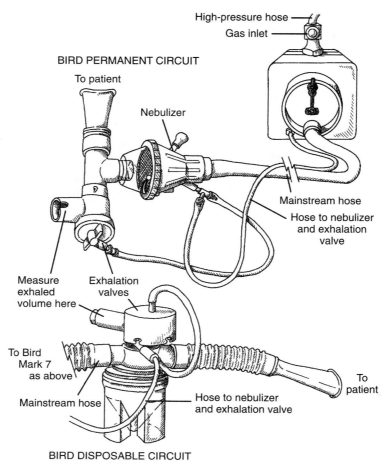

**Fig. 14-11** Features of permanent and disposable Bird intermittent positive-pressure breathing circuits.

3. Bacterial filters are optional. These are inserted between the IPPB unit gas outlets and the mainstream and nebulizer hoses.
4. A cascade-type humidifier is optional. Some practitioners prefer to warm and humidify the mainstream gas before it reaches the patient.
5. Check to see that the IPPB circuit is put together properly and that all of the connections are tight.
6. Set the initial treatment parameters for sensitivity, flow, and peak pressure. Manually cycle on the unit. Cover the mouthpiece to see that the unit cycles off at the preset pressure.
7. Add any medication to the nebulizer. Check to see that the nebulizer is producing a mist.

### b. Bird setup

1. One end of the mainstream (large-bore) hose is connected to the mainstream breathing hose connector on the right side of the unit. The other end is connected to the nebulizer.

2. One end of the nebulizer (small-bore) hose is connected to the small nipple on the right-hand side of the unit. The other end is connected to a T-piece at the nebulizer.
3. A piece of small-bore hose is used to connect one limb of the T-piece with the exhalation valve. Gas flowing through this hose powers both the nebulizer and the exhalation valve.

### c. Bennett setup

1. One end of the mainstream (large-bore) hose is connected to the mainstream breathing hose connector on the underside of the unit. The other end is connected to the nebulizer.
2. One end of the nebulizer (medium-bore) hose is connected to the larger of two nipples on the underside of the unit. The other end is connected to the nebulizer nipple.
3. One end of the exhalation (small-bore) hose is connected to the smaller of two nipples on the underside of the unit. The other end is connected to the exhalation valve nipple.

### 3. Fix any problems with the equipment (NBRC code: IIA11b) [Difficulty: R]

Fixing a problem is possible only after the problem has been identified. The practitioner should be familiar with both permanent and disposable types of Bird and Bennett circuits. Leaks of any sort in the circuit prevent the unit from cycling off so that the patient can exhale. Tighten up any friction fit or screw-type connections to stop the leak. A leak at the source gas connection or high-pressure hose gas-inlet connection results in a rather loud hissing sound. When connections are tightened properly, the hissing and leak stop.

Debris such as mucus or blood plugs the nebulizer capillary tube and prevents the formation of any mist. Disassemble the nebulizer, and rinse it under running water to try to clear the capillary tube. Replace the nebulizer if necessary.

> **Exam Hint**
>
> **P**ast examinations have included questions regarding the reason(s) that an IPPB machine would fail to cycle off. Know how to seal off an air leak around the patient's mouthpiece and how to fix a leak within the circuit such as that resulting from a faulty exhalation valve.

## MODULE D
### Respiratory care plan

### 1. Analyze the available information to determine the patient's pathophysiologic state (NBRC code: IIIH1) [Difficulty: R, Ap, An]

Atelectasis is detected by findings on chest x-ray films and decreased or absent breath sounds over the affected area. Wheezing breath sounds indicate bronchospasm. Pulmonary edema is associated with clear chest x-ray film findings and cardiovascular indicators. Review discussion of these conditions and their findings in Chapters 1 and 5.

### 2. Determine the appropriateness of the respiratory care plan and recommend modifications when indicated

**a. Review the interdisciplinary patient and family care plan (NBRC code: IIIH2b) [Difficulty: R, Ap]**

**b. Review the planned therapy to establish the therapeutic plan (NBRC code: IIIH2a) [Difficulty: R, Ap]**

The patient should be fully cooperative if the full advantages of IPPB are to be attained. It may be counterproductive to try to force an IPPB treatment on a combative or uncooperative patient. A patient with a neuromuscular deficit may need assistance in holding the IPPB circuit or keeping a good mouth seal. A mouth seal or facemask treatment may have to be given. Be prepared to make a recommendation that a patient use IS, positive expiratory pressure therapy, or IPPB for hyperinflation therapy. Also, be prepared to make a recommendation that a patient use an MDI, a small-volume nebulizer, or IPPB for the delivery of an aerosolized medication.

### c. Determine the appropriateness of the prescribed therapy and goals for the patient's pathophysiologic state (NBRC code: IIIH3) [Difficulty: R, Ap, An]

IPPB should be used for hyperinflation therapy only when less expensive options (such as IS) are shown to be impractical. Bedside spirometry should confirm that IPPB is indicated and that the patient's IPPB breath is at least 25% greater than spontaneous. Breath sounds should be heard more clearly at the bases of the lungs. One of the goals of IPPB is to give the patient larger $V_T$s than normal. Additional secretions may be heard in the airways if the larger $V_T$s result in their mobilization. However, if deeper breaths enable the patient to cough more effectively, additional secretions should be coughed out. Wheezing should be diminished if a bronchodilator medication is nebulized to a patient with bronchospasm.

Ask about the patient's feelings toward the treatment, and write them in the chart. Note any significant comments made by the patient. Note the patient's preferred flow and pressure or volume settings.

### d. Recommend changes in the therapeutic plan if supportive data exist (NBRC code: IIIH4) [Difficulty: R, Ap]

### e. Terminate treatment based on the patient's response (NBRC code: IIIG1f) [Difficulty: R, Ap]

If the patient's atelectasis is resolved, IPPB will no longer be needed. Or, a less expensive treatment such as incentive spirometry may be used if the patient can perform it properly. Be prepared to stop treatment if the patient has any of the problems listed in Module A under Contraindications, Hazards, and Precautions. Ttreatment should be canceled if the patient has an untreated pneumothorax or massive hemoptysis. Other serious problems also justify cancellation of the order. Most of these problems are caused by excessive IPPB pressure on the lungs.

Stop treatment if the patient has a pulse change of 20 beats/min or greater. It is most common to see the pulse increase because of a nebulized bronchodilator drug. Decreased venous return to the heart may be demonstrated by increased heart rate or a drop in blood pressure. If these problems happen with each treatment, the physician should be informed, and treatment may need to be terminated.

## BIBLIOGRAPHY

American Association for Respiratory Care: Clinical practice guideline: Incentive spirometry, *Respir Care* 30:1402, 1991.

American Association for Respiratory Care: Clinical practice guideline: Intermittent positive-pressure ventilation—2003 revision & update, *Respir Care* 48:540, 2003.

American Association for Respiratory Care: Clinical practice guideline: Intermittent positive-pressure ventilation, *Respir Care* 38:1189, 1993.

Branson RD, Hess DR, Chatburn RL, editors: *Respiratory care equipment*, ed 2, Philadelphia, 1999, Lippincott Williams & Wilkins.

Cairo JM: Lung expansion devices. In Cairo JM, Pilbeam SP: *Mosby's respiratory care equipment*, ed 7, St. Louis, 2004, Mosby.

Eubanks DH, Bone RC: *Comprehensive respiratory care*, ed 2, St Louis, 1990, Mosby.

Fink JB: Bronchial hygiene and lung expansion. In Fink JB, Hunt GE, editors: *Clinical practice in respiratory care*, Philadelphia, 1999, Lippincott Williams & Wilkins.

Fink JB: Volume expansion therapy. In Burton GG, Hodgkin JE, Ward JJ, editors: *Respiratory care*, ed 4, Philadelphia, 1997, Lippincott.

Fink JB, Hess DR: Secretion clearance techniques. In Hess DR, MacIntyre NR, Mishoe SC: *Respiratory care principles & practices*, Philadelphia, 2002, WB Saunders.

Fluck RJ Jr: Intermittent positive-pressure breathing devices and transport ventilators. In Barnes TA, editor: *Respiratory care practice*, ed 2, St Louis, 1994, Mosby.

McPherson SP, Spearman CB: *Respiratory therapy equipment*, ed 5, St Louis, 1995, Mosby.

Miller WF: Intermittent positive pressure breathing (IPPB). In Kacmarek RM, Stoller JK, editors: *Current respiratory care*, Philadelphia, 1988, BC Decker.

Respiratory Care Committee of the American Thoracic Society: Guidelines for the use of intermittent positive pressure breathing (IPPB), *Respir Care* 25:365, 1980.

Scanlan CL, Wilkins RL, Stoller JK, editors: *Egan's fundamentals of respiratory care*, ed 7, St Louis, 1999, Mosby.

Shapiro BA, Kacmarek RM, Cane RD, et al: *Clinical application of respiratory care*, ed 4, St Louis, 1991, Mosby.

Weizalis CP: Intermittent positive-pressure breathing. In Barnes TA, editor: *Respiratory care practice*, ed 2, St Louis, 1994, Mosby.

Welch MA, Shapiro BJ, Mercurio P, Wagner W, et al: Methods of intermittent positive pressure breathing, *Chest* 78:463, 1980.

White GC: *Equipment theory for respiratory care*, ed 3, Albany, NY, 1999, Delmar.

Wilkins RL: Lung expansion therapy. In Wilkins RL, Stoller CL, Scanlan CL, editors: *Egan's fundamentals of respiratory care*, ed 8, St Louis, 2003, Mosby.

## SELF-STUDY QUESTIONS

1. Your patient complains of difficulty in starting the IPPB treatment. You would adjust which of the following controls?
   - A. Pressure
   - B. Flow
   - C. Sensitivity
   - D. Terminal flow

2. Your patient is having difficulty keeping a tight seal around the mouthpiece. He complains that the breath is too long and takes out the mouthpiece. To help cycle off the PR-2, you would adjust which of the following?
   - A. Pressure
   - B. Flow
   - C. Terminal flow
   - D. Expiratory retard

3. Your patient is going into pulmonary edema. She has rales in both lung fields, has cyanotic lips and nail beds, and is coughing up pink, frothy sputum. What $O_2$ percentage would you recommend for her IPPB treatment?
   - A. 21%
   - B. 40%
   - C. 80%
   - D. 100%

4. All of the following indicate the need for IPPB EXCEPT
   - A. Delivery of medications to a patient who cannot coordinate the use of an MDI or a handheld nebulizer
   - B. Treatment of a comatose patient with atelectasis
   - C. The need for a substitute for IS in a patient with an IC that is 60% of predicted
   - D. Treatment of a cooperative patient with atelectasis

5. You are ordered to give an IPPB treatment to a comatose patient who has lip ulcers. What patient-machine connection would you use?
   - A. Mouthpiece
   - B. Facemask
   - C. Bennett seal with mouthpiece
   - D. Endotracheal tube adapter for intubation

6. The sensitivity control should be set at what level at the start of IPPB treatment?
   - A. 0 cm $H_2O$
   - B. −1 cm $H_2O$
   - C. −3 cm $H_2O$
   - D. −5 cm $H_2O$

7. While coaching an active IPPB treatment, you notice that the needle on the pressure manometer "bounces" around as the pressure increases. To better adjust treatment to the patient's needs, you would do which of the following?
   A. Increase the flow
   B. Decrease the flow
   C. Increase the peak pressure
   D. Decrease the expiratory retard

8. You are giving an IPPB treatment on a Bird Mark 7 unit. To give the patient 100% $O_2$, you push in the air-mix control knob. What effect does this adjustment have on the flow rate to the patient?
   A. Decreases the flow of gas
   B. Increases the flow of gas
   C. No effect
   D. Increases the sensitivity

9. You would stop an IPPB treatment under which of the following conditions?
   I. You suspect that the patient has just developed a pneumothorax
   II. The patient has a difficult time keeping his lips sealed
   III. The patient's wheezing gets worse, and he complains of dyspnea
   IV. The patient coughs up a large amount of blood
   A. I and II
   B. III and IV
   C. II and IV
   D. I, III, and IV

10. A patient with emphysema has been changed from a handheld nebulizer to IPPB for bronchodilator therapy. While evaluating the patient during treatment, you note that her basilar wheezing has increased and her percussion note indicates hyperinflation with lowered hemidiaphragms. What would you recommend?
    A. Decrease the flow
    B. Add expiratory retard
    C. Increase the system pressure
    D. Pull out the air-mix knob

11. You are asked to evaluate a patient for the need for IPPB or IS. She weighs 125 lb. IPPB is indicated if her bedside spirometry values show which of the following?
    I. $V_T$ of 400 mL
    II. IC of 610 mL
    III. IC of 760 mL
    IV. VC of 780 mL
    V. C of 1030 mL
    A. II and IV
    B. I, III, and V
    C. II and V
    D. III and IV

12. A patient who was initially anxious about taking an IPPB treatment and needing a fast breath is now breathing in a more relaxed manner. What adjustment would you make to allow for a longer inspiratory time?
    A. Decrease the peak pressure
    B. Increase the sensitivity
    C. Set the air-mix knob to allow room air to be entrained
    D. Decrease the flow

13. A patient you are evaluating has a spontaneous $V_T$ of 400 mL and has been diagnosed with atelectasis after bowel surgery. IPPB has been ordered. What would you recommend as the minimal volume goal?
    A. 300 mL
    B. 400 mL
    C. 500 mL
    D. 800 mL

14. After 10 min of being given an IPPB treatment, the patient complains of a sharp chest pain. After a few more deep breaths, he says he is short of breath. You notice that his breath sounds are now diminished on the left side. What would you recommend?
    A. Continue the treatment for the next 5 min to finish the ordered time
    B. Decrease the peak pressure and complete the ordered treatment
    C. Discontinue the treatment and notify the physician of the patient's complaints
    D. Monitor the patient closely for the duration of the treatment, and notify the nurse of the patient's complaints

## ANSWER KEY AND RATIONALE

1. **C.** The sensitivity control on all IPPB units determines how much effort (negative pressure) the patient has to generate to trigger a breath.
2. **C.** Terminal flow on a Bennett PR-2 unit is adjusted to attain additional flow at the end on an inspiratory effort. This added flow compensates for a small leak and cycles the unit to exhalation.
3. **D.** Pure $O_2$ is most clearly indicated in a patient with pulmonary edema and signs of hypoxemia. Room air (21% $O_2$) would not be very helpful. Intermediate levels of supplemental $O_2$ (40% or 80%) would be helpful but not as effective as pure $O_2$.
4. **D.** A cooperative patient with atelectasis should first be treated with a less expensive method such as IS. IPPB would be indicated in the other types of patients.
5. **B.** A facemask would allow a treatment to be given without injury to the lip ulcers. A mouthpiece cannot be held by a comatose patient. A Bennett seal would injure the lip ulcers. Intubation is unnecessarily invasive and risky.
6. **B.** A small negative pressure of $-1$ cm $H_2O$ would not make the patient work harder than necessary to turn on the unit. A pressure of 0 cm $H_2O$ would result in the self-cycling of the unit when ambient (room) barometric pressure is reached.
7. **A.** The needle on the pressure manometer bounces when the patient's inspiratory flow is greater than what is leaving the machine. Turn up the inspiratory flow from the unit for a smoother inspiratory effort by the patient.
8. **A.** When the air-mix knob on a Bird unit is pushed in, only pure source gas (100% $O_2$) is given out to the patient. Because no room air is entrained with the source gas, the overall total gas flow is decreased.
9. **D.** Pneumothorax, worsening wheezing and dyspnea, and coughing up of blood indicate a serious patient problem. Treatment should be stopped, the patient evaluated, and help sought.
10. **B.** Adding expiratory retard is the only way to apply backpressure to the patient's airways to attain more complete exhalations.
11. **A.** According to the AARC clinical practice guidelines, these values are less than needed to justify IS rather than IPPB. Review the IC and VC guidelines in this chapter.
12. **D.** Decreasing the inspiratory flow would result in a longer inspiratory time.
13. **C.** It is recommended that an IPPB volume be at least 25% greater than a patient's spontaneous volume.
14. **C.** The patient's signs and symptoms indicate a pneumothorax. Treatment should be stopped, the patient evaluated, and the physician notified.

# 15 Mechanical Ventilation

A review of the most recent Entry Level Examinations has shown an average of 43 questions (31% of the exam) that cover mechanical ventilation. All publicly available versions of the exam feature mechanical ventilation questions that specifically cover the care of adult patients or questions that could apply to adult, neonatal, or pediatric patients. Very few, if any, questions relate exclusively to neonatal or pediatric patients. Chapter 15 is written with the adult patient in mind except when neonatal or pediatric patients are specified.

> ### Exam Hint
>
> **T**he National Board for Respiratory Care (NBRC) is known to ask questions about using and troubleshooting problems with specific ventilators. The scope of this text prevents discussion of all possible mechanical ventilators; such information is available in the manufacturers' literature and in equipment books. All widely accepted ventilators that have been in use for at least 2 years should be reviewed.

## MODULE A
### Review the patient's chart for the following data and recommend and perform the following diagnostic procedures

### 1. Work of breathing

**a. Review the patient's chart for information on work of breathing (NBRC code: IA6c) [Difficulty: R, Ap]**

Work of breathing (WOB) normally refers to how much energy the patient has to expend to inhale. Patients with stiff lungs (low compliance) or high airway resistance (Raw) have an increased WOB. Exhalation is normally passive and requires no work. However, some patients with high Raw may need to work to exhale. Look in the patient's chart for information on signs of increased WOB, such as the patient reporting shortness of breath and tiring easily on exertion.

WOB can be measured in a patient who has been intubated and placed on a modern mechanical ventilator with a microprocessor and graphics software. Fig. 15-1 shows a pressure-volume loop tracing that demonstrates a patient's WOB. WOB is minimized when the ventilator is set to minimize both the negative pressure and the inspiratory flow needed by the patient to trigger a ventilator-assisted breath.

If an intubated and ventilated patient appears to be unsynchronized with the ventilator, his or her WOB should be evaluated. To help assess the problem, ask the conscious patient simple questions about the ease of starting a machine breath or generating fast enough flow. If the ventilator is capable, program it to perform a pressure-volume loop of the patient's WOB. Be prepared to adjust the machine settings (e.g., sensitivity, inspiratory flow) to minimize the patient's workload.

### 2. Ventilator flow, volume, and pressure waveforms

**a. Review the patient's chart for information on ventilator airway graphics (flow, volume, and pressure waveforms) (NBRC code: IA6b) [Difficulty: R, Ap]**

For a patient who has been intubated and placed on a modern mechanical ventilator with a microprocessor and graphics software, ventilator flow, volume, and pressure waveforms can be visualized on the monitor, stored in memory, or printed out. Look for this information and compare it with the patient's current situation.

**b. Perform the procedure to measure ventilator pressure-volume and flow-volume loops (NBRC code: IB7h) [Difficulty: R, Ap]**

Follow the ventilator manufacturer's steps to direct the unit to create pressure-volume and flow-volume loops. The patient must be instructed, according to results of the breathing test, to either actively perform a breathing maneuver or lie passively as the ventilator delivers a breath.

**c. Select ventilator graphics (scales; flow, volume, and pressure waveforms) (NBRC code: IIID3) [Difficulty: R]**

Microprocessor ventilators with a monitor can be configured to show any combination of flow, volume, and pressure waveforms. This information can be used to identify a variety of patient conditions, such as inspiratory flow, expiratory flow, air trapping, ventilator-delivered and

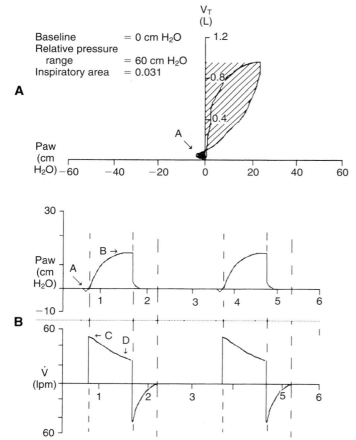

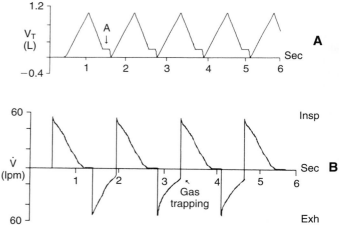

**Fig. 15-2** Two graphic tracings of expiratory air trapping. **A,** Volume vs time. *A* shows that the exhaled tidal volume ($V_T$) tracing does not reach the baseline. The inspiratory $V_T$ is greater than the expiratory $V_T$, which indicates air trapping. **B,** Flow vs time. Inspiratory flow is the tracing above the horizontal baseline of zero flow; expiratory flow is the tracing below the horizontal baseline. The patient's expiratory flow does not return to zero, which indicates air trapping. The higher the flow rate, the greater is the air trapping. Air trapping leads to auto–positive end-expiratory pressure. It can be minimized by increasing the expiratory time, giving an aerosolized bronchodilator to treat bronchospasm, or suctioning any secretions. *(Courtesy of Mallinckrodt, Pleasanton, Calif.)*

**Fig. 15-1** Two graphic tracings of pressure support ventilation. **A,** Pressure-volume loop of a patient triggering a breath. *A,* Amount of work the patient has to provide. The shaded area on the right side of the line indicates how much work was provided by the ventilator. **B,** Airway pressure (Paw) vs time and flow (V̇) in liters per minute (lpm) vs time tracings (seconds). *A,* Where the patient initiated a breath. *B,* Where the ventilator cycled off when the pressure-support level of 15 cm $H_2O$ was reached. *C,* High peak flow at the start of the breath. *D,* How the flow rate decreases as the pressure support level is reached. *(Courtesy of Mallinckrodt, Pleasanton, Calif.)*

**e. Interpret ventilator graphics to identify auto-PEEP** (NBRC code: IB8k) [Difficulty: R, Ap]

Fig. 15-2 demonstrates two ways that air trapping on exhalation can be identified as auto-PEEP (unintended positive end-expiratory pressure). Note in Fig. 15-2, **B,** that the patient's expiratory flow does not reach baseline pressure before another breath is delivered. This proves that air trapping has occurred. The larger the gap between the pressure at the end of expiration and baseline, the greater is the air trapping there.

**3. Airway resistance**

**a. Review the patient's chart for information on airway resistance** (NBRC code: IA6c) [Difficulty: R, Ap]

The airway resistance (Raw) value may have been measured earlier either in the pulmonary function laboratory or on the ventilator. Compare any earlier values with those to be measured. This is important toward attaining an understanding of the patient's trends and assessing an improving or worsening pulmonary condition.

Raw is measured in units of centimeters of water per liter per second (cm $H_2O$/L/sec) at a standard flow rate of 0.5 L/sec (30 L/min). The normal spontaneously

spontaneous tidal volume, and pressure during the breathing cycle. The therapist must be able to identify which data are most important for the clinical situation.

**d. Interpret ventilator pressure-volume and flow-volume loops** (NBRC code: IB8j) [Difficulty: R, Ap]

Many flow, volume, and pressure waveforms have been included in this text for practice. Review Figs. 4-8 and 4-10 for examples of flow-volume loop pulmonary function tests. A pressure-volume loop on a ventilator is shown in Fig. 15-1, **A.** The examples in this chapter include common clinical situations and provide explanations to help with interpretation.

breathing adult's Raw is 0.6 to 2.4 cm $H_2O$/L/sec; the normal 3-kg infant's Raw is 30 cm $H_2O$/L/sec. Do not forget that when this procedure is performed on a patient with an endotracheal tube, the tube adds to the patient's total Raw. The smaller the tube is, the greater is the resistance it offers to gas flowing through it. Alteration of inspiratory flow has an influence on peak pressure measured for the calculation. The lower the flow, the less is the gas turbulence and the lower is the peak pressure. Conversely, a higher flow creates greater turbulence and a higher peak pressure.

The airway resistance calculation is important because it provides valuable information on the patient's pulmonary condition. The Raw value indicates how difficult it is to move the tidal volume ($V_T$) through the patient's airways and whether aerosolized bronchodilator medications are effective.

It is reasonable to recommend a Raw measurement on any patient with an increased airways resistance problem such as chronic obstructive pulmonary disease (COPD), asthma, bronchospasm, or wheezing breath sounds. It is also reasonable to measure Raw before and after a bronchodilator medication is given to determine whether it has provided any benefit.

### b. Determine the patient's airway resistance (NBRC code: IB7g) [Difficulty: R, Ap]

Most microprocessor ventilators offer software for calculating the following values. However, these must be calculated manually for any other situation.

**Procedure for calculating Raw.**

1. Cycle a $V_T$. The patient should be breathing passively; fighting the breath causes an erroneously high peak pressure, and assisting with the breath causes an erroneously low peak pressure.
2. Note the peak airway pressure on the manometer.
3. Briefly prevent the $V_T$ from being exhaled. No air should be moving. Note that the pressure manometer shows a peak pressure and then a static or plateau pressure that is stable as long as the $V_T$ is held in the lungs. Record the plateau pressure.
4. Calculate the flow in liters per second by dividing the flow in liters per minute by 60 sec.
5. Place the peak airway pressure, plateau pressure, and flow into this formula, and solve for Raw:

$$Raw = \frac{peak\ airway\ pressure - plateau\ pressure}{flow\ in\ L/sec}$$

### Exam Hint

The airway resistance calculation has been tested on previous examinations, so review the math.

### EXAMPLE

A mechanically ventilated patient has a peak airway pressure of 30 cm $H_2O$ and a plateau pressure of 20 cm $H_2O$. The peak flow is set at 60 L/min.

Calculate peak flow in liters per second:

$$\frac{60\,L/min}{60\,sec} = 1\,L/sec$$

Calculate Raw:

$$Raw = \frac{30\,cm\,H_2O - 20\,cm\,H_2O}{1\,L/sec} = 10\,cm\,H_2O/L/sec$$

This value is greater than normal for a patient who is breathing spontaneously. However, remember that the patient's airway is intubated, which results in a smaller airway diameter and greater resistance. Some practitioners use the calculated Raw as the basis for setting the pressure support ventilation (PSV) level (discussed later). An increased Raw indicates possible bronchospasm or secretions in the airways. Delivery of an aerosolized bronchodilator or suctioning should result in return of resistance to the original level.

### 4. Determine the patient's plateau pressure (NBRC code: IB7g) [Difficulty: R, Ap]

The plateau pressure on the ventilator is determined for the purpose of evaluating the patient's lung compliance ($C_{LT}$). The change in the patient's lung compliance correlates with changes in the patient's lung condition. The following discussion covers the topics of lung compliance, performance of the lung compliance procedure, and interpretation of the results.

Plateau pressure can be determined in one of two ways. First, have the patient lie passively, and set the ventilator to prevent a delivered tidal volume from being exhaled (inflation hold). Second, have the patient lie passively, and manually cover the end of the expiratory tubing to prevent exhalation of a delivered tidal volume. The breath should be held for about 2 seconds so that the pressure manometer value stabilizes. Record the pressure as the plateau pressure. After plateau pressure has been determined, the patient must exhale completely. It may be necessary to delay the next timed ventilator tidal volume breath so as not to "stack" a new breath when the first has not yet been exhaled. It is recommended that the plateau pressure procedure be repeated to ensure the accuracy of the measured pressure.

### 5. Lung compliance

#### a. Review the patient's chart for information on lung compliance (NBRC code: IA6c) [Difficulty: R, Ap]

The lung and thoracic compliance ($C_{LT}$) value may have been measured earlier either in the pulmonary function laboratory or on the ventilator. Compare any earlier values with those measured later in an attempt to attain a better understanding of the patient's trends toward an improving or worsening pulmonary condition.

Compliance values indicate how easily the $V_T$ can be delivered into the lungs. Static compliance ($C_{st}$) is the measurement of the work needed for the patient to overcome elastic resistance to ventilation, or the measurement of compliance of the lungs and thorax ($C_{LT}$). $C_{st}$ is measured in the unit of milliliters per centimeter of water pressure (mL/cm $H_2O$). The normal adult's $C_{st}$ is 100 mL/cm $H_2O$; the normal 3-kg infant's $C_{st}$ is 5 mL/cm $H_2O$. Dynamic compliance ($C_{dyn}$), sometimes called *dynamic characteristic,* is the measurement of the combination of the $C_{st}$ and the Raw. As has been discussed previously, Raw is the pressure needed to move a $V_T$ through the airways. It is also known as *nonelastic resistance to ventilation.*

$C_{LT}$ should be measured in any patient who has clinical evidence of a significant change in $C_{LT}$. This could result from complications such as acute respiratory distress syndrome (ARDS), pneumonia, pulmonary edema, or pulmonary fibrosis. Compliance can be measured to document the patient's worsening condition and to determine whether compliance is improving with treatment.

### b. Determine the patient's lung compliance (NBRC code: IB7g) [Difficulty: R, Ap]

Most microprocessor ventilators offer software for calculating all of these values. However, these must be calculated manually for any other situation.

***Procedure for calculating the compliance factor.*** Before an actual calculation of the patient's $C_{st}$ and $C_{dyn}$ can be performed, the compliance factor of the breathing circuit should be determined. (In most older ventilators, some of the set $V_T$ never reaches the patient because it is "lost" in the circuit.) To be as accurate as possible in calculating $C_{st}$ and $C_{dyn}$, as well as actual tidal and sigh volumes, this lost volume must be subtracted from the exhaled $V_T$. The term compressed volume is commonly used to describe this lost volume.

1. Remove the patient from the ventilator, and manually ventilate him or her during the remainder of this procedure.
2. Set the pressure limit to as high as possible.
3. Block the breathing circuit at the patient connector.
4. Cycle a $V_T$.
5. Perform either of the following: (a) Note the peak pressure developed in the circuit as the $V_T$ stretches out the circuit, or (b) note the delivered $V_T$ and the pressure limit when the ventilator's peak pressure hits the pressure limit. *Note:* If the patient is on PEEP therapy, subtract the PEEP level from the measured peak pressure to find the true peak pressure.
6. The compliance factor is found by dividing measured $V_T$ by peak pressure.

## EXAMPLE

The patient has a set $V_T$ of 600 mL. With the use of step **5b** just described, the peak pressure is found to be 80 cm $H_2O$, and the measured $V_T$ is found to be 320 mL.

$$\text{Compliance factor} = \frac{320\,\text{mL}}{40\,\text{cm}} = 4\,\text{mL/cm}\,H_2O$$

Compressed volume is found by multiplying the compliance factor by either the peak or the plateau pressure. The compressed volume is then subtracted from the exhaled $V_T$ for determination of the patient's actual $V_T$.

> ### Exam Hint
>
> **E**very previous examination has included questions that require the calculation of $C_{st}$ or $C_{dyn}$. Be able to perform the following calculations.

***Procedure for calculating $C_{st}$.***
1. Determine the compliance factor of the breathing circuit (as previously described).
2. Reattach the patient to the ventilator. Reset all controls to their ordered or preset positions.
3. Cycle a $V_T$. The patient should be breathing passively; fighting the breath causes an erroneously high peak pressure, and assisting with the breath causes an erroneously low peak pressure.
4. Briefly prevent the $V_T$ from being exhaled. No air should be moving. Note that the pressure manometer shows a peak pressure, then a static or plateau pressure that is stable as long as the $V_T$ is held in the lungs. Note the *plateau pressure.*
5. Calculate the $C_{st}$ with this formula:

$$C_{st} = \frac{\text{exhaled }V_T - \text{compressed volume}}{\text{plateau pressure} - \text{PEEP}}$$

where compressed volume = compliance factor × plateau pressure.

***Procedure for calculating $C_{dyn}$.***
1. Determine the compliance factor of the breathing circuit (as previously described).
2. Reattach the patient to the ventilator. Reset all controls to their ordered or preset positions.
3. Cycle a $V_T$. The patient should be breathing passively; fighting the breath causes an erroneously high peak pressure, and assisting with the breath causes an erroneously low peak pressure.
4. Note the *peak pressure* on the manometer. If the pressure at the end of inspiration is less than the peak pressure, the pressure at the end of inspiration should be used in the calculation.

5. Calculate the $C_{dyn}$ with the following formula:

$$C_{dyn} = \frac{\text{exhaled } V_T - \text{compressed volume}}{\text{plateau pressure} - \text{PEEP}}$$

where compressed volume = compliance factor $\times$ peak pressure.

## EXAMPLE

Calculate the $C_{st}$ and the $C_{dyn}$ on a ventilated patient *without PEEP therapy*. The patient has an exhaled $V_T$ of 600 mL. The peak pressure is 30 cm $H_2O$, and the static or plateau pressure is 20 cm $H_2O$. The compliance factor has been determined to be 4 mL/cm $H_2O$. The compressed volume at the plateau pressure is determined to be 80 mL (4 mL/cm compliance factor $\times$ 20 cm). The compressed volume at the peak pressure is determined to be 120 mL (4 mL/cm compliance factor $\times$ 30 cm).

$$C_{st} = \frac{60\,\text{mL} - 80\,\text{mL}}{20\,\text{cm} - 0}$$

$$= \frac{520\,\text{mL}}{20\,\text{cm}}$$

$$= 26\,\text{mL/cm}\,H_2O$$

$$C_{dyn} = \frac{600\,\text{mL} - 120\,\text{mL}}{30\,\text{cm} - 0}$$

$$= \frac{480\,\text{mL}}{30\,\text{cm}}$$

$$= 16\,\text{mL/cm}\,H_2O$$

## EXAMPLE

Calculate the $C_{st}$ and the $C_{dyn}$ on a ventilated patient *with PEEP therapy*. The same patient has an exhaled $V_T$ of 600 mL. Because of refractory hypoxemia, 10 cm of PEEP therapy is started. The peak pressure is now 36 cm $H_2O$, and the static or plateau pressure is now 25 cm $H_2O$. The compliance factor has been determined to be 4 mL/cm $H_2O$. The compressed volume at the plateau pressure is determined to be 60 mL (4 mL/cm compliance factor $\times$ 15 cm [25 cm − 10 cm PEEP]). The compressed volume at the peak pressure is determined to be 104 mL (4 mL/cm compliance factor $\times$ 26 cm [36 cm − 10 cm PEEP]).

$$C_{st} = \frac{60\,\text{mL} - 60\,\text{mL}}{25\,\text{cm} - 10\,\text{cm}}$$

$$= \frac{540\,\text{mL}}{15\,\text{cm}}$$

$$= 36\,\text{mL/cm}\,H_2O$$

$$C_{dyn} = \frac{600\,\text{mL} - 104\,\text{mL}}{36\,\text{cm} - 10\,\text{cm}}$$

$$= \frac{496\,\text{mL}}{26\,\text{cm}}$$

$$= 19\,\text{mL/cm}\,H_2O$$

## 6. Interpret the patient's airway resistance, pulmonary compliance, and plateau pressure values on the ventilator (NBRC code: IB8e) [Difficulty: R, Ap]

### Exam Hint

**E**very previous examination has included questions that deal with interpretation of increasing or decreasing peak pressure, plateau pressure, Raw, or $C_{LT}$. Be able to identify a clinical change, potential causes, and corrective actions.

Any increase in Raw or decrease in $C_{LT}$ increases the patient's WOB. Examples of conditions or situations in which increased Raw occurs include bronchospasm, secretions, mucosal edema, airway tumor, placement of a small endotracheal tube, and biting or kinking of the endotracheal tube. $C_{LT}$ is decreased by pneumonia, pulmonary edema, ARDS, pulmonary fibrosis, atelectasis, consolidation, hemothorax, pleural effusion, air trapping, pneumomediastinum, and pneumothorax. Examples of chest wall and abdominal conditions that lower compliance include various chest wall deformities, circumferential chest or abdominal burns, enlarged liver, pneumoperitoneum, peritonitis, abdominal bleeding, and advanced pregnancy. Correction of the problem should return the patient's ventilator pressure(s) to baseline and normalize the patient's WOB.

Six possible combinations of increasing or decreasing $C_{st}$ and $C_{dyn}$ exist. Each has its own possible causes. Remember that the patient must be passive on the ventilator for the measured values to be accurate. Check two or three breaths for increased accuracy. Let the patient have a normal breath or two between each of the peak and plateau pressure measurement breaths.

### a. Decreased dynamic compliance with stable static compliance

Decreased $C_{dyn}$ with stable $C_{st}$ causes an *increase* in peak pressure with an unchanged plateau pressure (Fig. 15-3). This is caused by an increased Raw (e.g., bronchospasm). Correcting the underlying problem causes the peak pressure to return to the original level.

Note that the inspiratory resistance has doubled from the original 10 to 20 cm $H_2O$ while the plateau pressure has not changed. This confirms that the problem originates in the airway or breathing circuit. The patient's $C_{LT}$ has not changed.

### b. Increased dynamic compliance with stable static compliance

Increased $C_{dyn}$ with stable $C_{st}$ causes a *decrease* in peak pressure with an unchanged plateau pressure (Fig. 15-4).

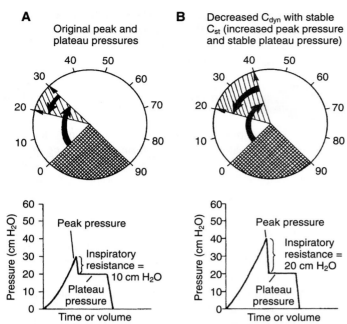

**Fig. 15-3** Decreased dynamic compliance ($C_{dyn}$) with a stable static compliance ($C_{st}$). **A,** Original pressure manometer reading and pressure/volume curve. **B,** Altered pressure manometer reading and pressure/volume curve.

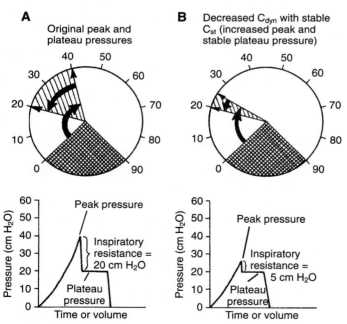

**Fig. 15-4** Increased dynamic compliance ($C_{dyn}$) with a stable static compliance ($C_{st}$). **A,** Original pressure manometer reading and pressure/volume curve. **B,** Altered pressure manometer reading and pressure/volume curve.

This represents an improvement in the patient's Raw from the original condition (e.g., secretions could be diminished, mucus plugs cleared, bronchospasm corrected).

Note that the inspiratory resistance has decreased from the original level of 20 to just 5 cm $H_2O$. This confirms that the patient's Raw has decreased. The patient's $C_{LT}$ has not changed.

### c. False decreased dynamic compliance with true decreased static compliance

False decreased $C_{dyn}$ with true decreased $C_{st}$ causes an *increase* in *both* peak and plateau pressures (Fig. 15-5). This occurs when the patient's $C_{LT}$ worsens. The plateau pressure is elevated and the $C_{st}$ is decreased.

As an artifact of the stiffer lungs, the peak pressure is also elevated and $C_{dyn}$ is decreased. However, the difference between the peak and plateau pressures remains the same. This results in no real increase in the patient's Raw.

### d. True decreased dynamic compliance with true decreased static compliance

True decreased $C_{dyn}$ with true decreased $C_{st}$ causes an *increase* in *both* peak and plateau pressures (Fig. 15-6). This occurs with the combination of a decreased $C_{LT}$ and an increased Raw. Causes of both of these problems were discussed earlier.

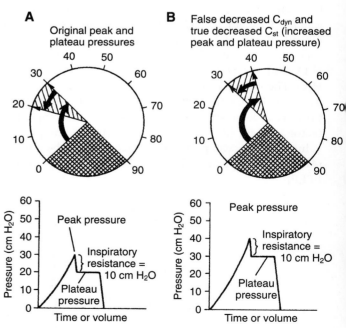

**Fig. 15-5** False decreased dynamic compliance ($C_{dyn}$) with true decreased static compliance ($C_{st}$). **A,** Original pressure manometer reading and pressure/volume curve. **B,** Altered pressure manometer reading and pressure/volume curve.

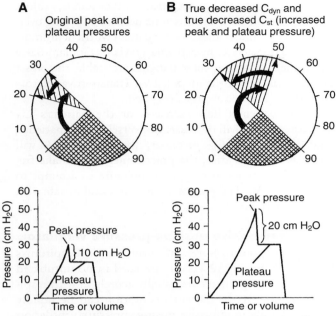

**Fig. 15-6** True decreased dynamic compliance ($C_{dyn}$) with true decreased static compliance ($C_{st}$). **A,** Original pressure manometer reading and pressure/volume curve. **B,** Altered pressure manometer reading and pressure/volume curve.

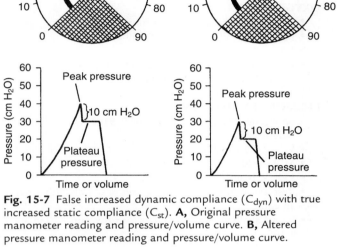

**Fig. 15-7** False increased dynamic compliance ($C_{dyn}$) with true increased static compliance ($C_{st}$). **A,** Original pressure manometer reading and pressure/volume curve. **B,** Altered pressure manometer reading and pressure/volume curve.

### e. False increased dynamic compliance with true increased static compliance

False increased $C_{dyn}$ with true increased $C_{st}$ causes a *decrease* in *both* peak and plateau pressures (Fig. 15-7). This occurs when the patient's $C_{LT}$ improves. The plateau pressure decreases, and as an artifact, the peak pressure also decreases. Notice that the difference between peak and plateau pressures remains the same. This indicates that the patient's Raw is unchanged.

### f. True increased dynamic compliance with true increased static compliance

True increased $C_{dyn}$ with true increased $C_{st}$ causes a *decrease* in *both* peak and plateau pressures (Fig. 15-8). This occurs when both the patient's Raw and $C_{LT}$ improve. Note that the plateau pressure has decreased, thus indicating more compliant lungs. Also, note that the difference between peak and plateau pressures has decreased. This demonstrates that the Raw has also decreased.

Note that a pulmonary embolism should be considered if the patient's condition deteriorates rapidly and no change occurs in the $C_{st}$ or the $C_{dyn}$ value.

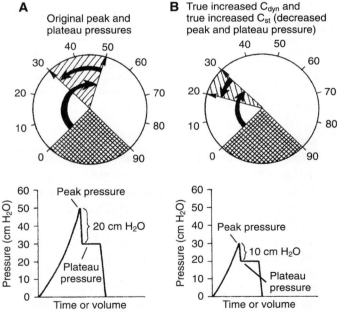

**Fig. 15-8** True increased dynamic compliance ($C_{dyn}$) with true increased static compliance ($C_{st}$). **A,** Original pressure manometer reading and pressure/volume curve. **B,** Altered pressure manometer reading and pressure/volume curve.

---

**BOX 15-1    Indications for Ventilatory Support**

**VENTILATION**
- Apnea
- $PaCO_2 > 55$ torr in a patient who is not ordinarily hypercapneic
- $V_D/V_T$ ratio $> 0.55$–$0.6$ (55%–60%)

**OXYGENATION**
- $PaO_2 < 80$ torr on 50% $O_2$ or more
- $P(A - a)O_2 > 300$–$350$ torr on 100% $O_2$
- Intrapulmonary shunt $> 15\%$–$20\%$
- In a neonate: $PaO_2 < 50$ torr despite maximal CPAP therapy (10 cm $H_2O$) and $> 50\%$ inspired $O_2$

**PULMONARY MECHANICS**
- Spontaneous $V_T < 3$–$4$ mL/lb or $7$–$9$ mL/kg of ideal body weight
- VC $< 10$–$15$ mL/kg
- MIP $< -20$ to $-25$ cm $H_2O$
- $FEV_1 < 10$ mL/kg
- Respiratory rate $< 12$ breaths/min or $> 35$ breaths/min in an adult
- Rapid, shallow breathing index (breaths/min $\div V_T$ in liters) $> 105$

**MISCELLANEOUS**
- Unconscious patient
- Unstable and unacceptable vital signs
- Unstable cardiac rhythm because of hypoxemia or acidosis
- Worsening cardiopulmonary or other major organ system

---

CPAP, continuous positive-airway pressure; $FEV_1$, forced expiratory volume in 1 sec; MIP, maximal inspiratory pressure; $PaCO_2$, arterial $CO_2$ pressure; $PaO_2$, arterial $O_2$ pressure; $P(A - a)O_2$, difference in the partial pressure of $O_2$ in alveolar gas and arterial blood; VC, vital capacity, $V_D/V_T$, dead space/tidal volume.

---

## MODULE B

### Provide mechanical ventilation to adequately oxygenate and ventilate the patient

### 1. Select the appropriate ventilator for the patient (NBRC code: IIA6a) [Difficulty: R, Ap]

A number of physiologic criteria have been compiled to help the clinician determine when a patient is in respiratory or ventilatory failure (Box 15-1). Remember that the patient may not fail each and every criterion; however, the patient will often fail one or more of the criteria in each category. Depending on the patient's condition, one particular type of ventilator may be particularly well suited for the patient. The main classifications of ventilators include pressure cycled, external negative pressure, volume cycled, and high frequency.

### a. Pressure-cycled ventilator

Pressure-cycled ventilators, such as the Bird series or Bennett PR-2, may be acceptable for use with patients who have and are expected to keep normal Raw and $C_{LT}$ values (e.g., a patient who is unconscious because of a drug overdose or who is under anesthesia, a patient with a neuromuscular disease such as myasthenia gravis or Guillain-Barré syndrome). As long as these patients are stable, the preset pressure will deliver the intended $V_T$. Transport ventilators are usually classified as pressure cycled.

If the patient's Raw increases or the patient's $C_{LT}$ decreases, the $V_T$ will decrease. Conversely, if the patient's Raw decreases or $C_{LT}$ increases, the delivered $V_T$ will increase. In either case, the practitioner must make frequent adjustments in the preset pressure to attempt to keep a stable $V_T$. These units are not practical or safe with unstable patients.

### b. Noninvasive positive-pressure ventilator

Noninvasive positive-pressure ventilators (Respironics BiPAP S/T and BiPAP Vision) are used in nonintubated patients. These patients are usually acutely ill with respiratory failure. If the patient's condition can be rapidly improved, only noninvasive positive-pressure ventilation (NPPV) will be necessary. However, if the patient's condition deteriorates, a volume-cycled ventilator will be needed.

### c. Volume-cycled ventilator

A volume-cycled ventilator, such as the Drager Evita 2 Dura, Puritan-Bennett 7200, Bear 1000, and Servo 300A, is indicated when the patient's Raw or $C_{LT}$ is expected to change. These types of units deliver a preset $V_T$ to the patient, at whatever pressure is needed, despite changing patient airway and lung conditions. As a result, volume-cycled ventilators are recommended in most patients who need ventilatory support. In addition, these types of ventilators come with a built-in alarm system for detecting patient problems. Furthermore, they can be used in a variety of modes, can deliver therapeutic PEEP, and can generate greater pressure for delivery of the $V_T$ than can be generated by pressure-cycled or negative-pressure ventilators.

### d. High-frequency ventilator

A high-frequency ventilator is needed when the patient's condition calls for a higher respiratory rate or a smaller $V_T$ than is available on a conventional volume-cycled ventilator. The US Food and Drug Administration has approved these units for use during bronchoscopy and laryngoscopy procedures, in patients with a bronchopleural fistula, and in patients who fail treatment with conventional volume ventilation. Neonatal patients with infant respiratory distress syndrome (RDS) are most frequently ventilated on these types of machines. Current models include the Bunnell Life Pulse High-Frequency Jet Ventilator and the SensorMedics 3100A and 3100B High-Frequency Oscillatory Ventilators.

## 2. Initiate and adjust continuous mechanical ventilation settings (NBRC code: IIID2b) [Difficulty: R, Ap]

Typical ventilator orders include the following:
a. Mode (including control [C], assist/control [A/C], synchronous intermittent mandatory ventilation [SIMV], and pressure support ventilation [PSV])
b. $O_2$ percentage
c. Respiratory rate
d. $V_T$ or minute volume ($\dot{V}_E$)
e. Sigh volume and frequency
f. Special settings (e.g., mechanical dead space, PEEP)

The respiratory therapist is commonly expected to set the following ventilator controls based on department protocol or the patient's condition and response to the ventilator.

### a. Sensitivity

*Sensitivity* describes the amount of work or effort the patient must perform to trigger the ventilator to deliver a $V_T$ breath. With most ventilators, the patient must generate a *negative pressure* to trigger a breath. Pressure sensitivity is usually set at about $-1$ to $-2$ cm $H_2O$ pressure.

Several of the newer ventilators also offer the option of having the patient trigger a ventilator $V_T$ by generating an *inspiratory flow*. The Puritan-Bennett 7200 ventilator is an example of such a ventilator. The term *flow-by* is used to describe this flow sensitivity option on the ventilator. With a ventilator that uses flow sensitivity, the patient triggers a $V_T$ when his or her inspiratory flow is about 2 L/min (33 mL/sec) lower than the set baseline flow through the circuit.

### b. Flow

Flow is adjusted to set the inspiratory time and inspiratory:expiratory (I:E) ratio to meet the patient's needs. Inspiratory flow should be great enough to meet the patient's needs and minimize WOB.

### c. Inspiratory:expiratory ratio

The I:E ratio is adjusted to ensure that the patient can inhale in as physiologically appropriate a manner as possible and can completely exhale the inspired $V_T$. Typically, the initial I:E ratio should be 1:2 or greater. Incomplete exhalation causes air trapping and auto-PEEP (see Fig. 15-2). Eliminate the auto-PEEP by increasing expiratory time, decreasing inspiratory time (higher flow needed), decreasing rate, and/or decreasing tidal volume.

### d. Alarms

Alarm systems are different for each type of ventilator. These are generally set with a safety margin of ±10% from the patient's normal ventilator settings. Variation greater than 10% causes an audible or visual alarm condition. Most ventilators will trigger the alarm if the I:E ratio is 1:1 or less.

### e. Gas temperature

The goal with most patients is to minimize the humidity deficit by giving gas that is humidified and warmed to near body temperature. It is common to see the gas warmed to 31° C to 35° C (90° F to 95° F). This decreases the patient's humidity deficit to a minuscule level and reduces the "rainout" of water vapor that condenses in the ventilator circuit. A temperature probe should be placed in the inspiratory tubing as close to the patient as possible to monitor the inspired gas temperature. This goal can be accomplished with the use of a cascade- or a wick-type humidifier or a heat-moisture exchanger (HME).

### f. Tidal volume for mechanical ventilation

A spontaneously breathing 70-kg (154-lb) adult with normal lungs and metabolism needs a $V_T$ of 7 to 9 mL/kg (3 to 4 mL/lb) of ideal body weight to adequately remove $CO_2$. Splitting the differences, a spontaneous $V_T$ of about 500 mL is considered normal. The Radford nomogram can be used to predict normal spontaneous $V_T$s and rates based on body weight. It can be used to establish an initial $V_T$ for most patients.

Most authors recommend a *set* ventilator $V_T$ of *10 to 15 mL/kg* of ideal body weight. These values are used by the NBRC in most patient situations. For example, the 70-kg (154-lb) adult with normal lungs would need a *set* mechanical ventilator $V_T$ in the following range:

$$10\,\text{mL} \times 70\,\text{kg} = 700\,\text{mL/kg}$$
$$15\,\text{mL} \times 70\,\text{kg} = 1050\,\text{mL/kg}$$

This volume is higher than spontaneous for two reasons. First, some of the set volume is lost to the patient because of gas compression and tubing stretch/compliance (discussed previously). Second, some patients need larger-than-normal $V_T$s because their lungs are not functioning normally. Exceptions include patients with severe chronic restrictive lung disease, those with pneumonectomy, and patients with COPD. The $V_T$ for these patients should be set at about 5 to 10 mL/kg of ideal body weight to avoid excessive ventilating pressure. In addition, giving a patient with COPD a ventilator-delivered $V_T$ in the normal range may cause blowing off of too much $CO_2$, thus causing a respiratory alkalosis.

It is common practice to obtain a set of arterial blood gas (ABG) values after the patient is stable on the ventilator. The $V_T$ can be adjusted within the range depending on whether the patient's arterial $CO_2$ pressure ($PaCO_2$) value is too high or low for the therapeutic goal. The most direct way to change alveolar ventilation is to modify the delivered $V_T$. A larger $V_T$, with everything else the same, results in a lower $PaCO_2$ value. Conversely, a smaller $V_T$, with everything else the same, results in a higher $PaCO_2$ value.

The following formula can be used to help predict the $V_T$ that will produce a desired $PaCO_2$ value:

$$[V_T - (V_{D\,anat} + V_{D\,mech})] \times f \times PaCO_2$$
$$= [V_T' - (V_{D\,anat} + V_{D\,mech})] \times f \times PaCO_2'$$

where

$V_T$ = current $V_T$
$V_{D\,anat}$ = anatomic dead space (calculated at 2.2 mL/kg [1 mL/lb] of ideal body weight)
$V_{D\,mech}$ = added mechanical dead space
$f$ = respiratory (ventilator) rate
$PaCO_2$ = actual patient $PaCO_2$ value
$V_T'$ = *desired* tidal volume
$PaCO_2'$ = *desired* patient $PaCO_2$ value

Note that other, simpler formulas are available for calculating a change in $\dot{V}_E$ or $V_T$. This one is presented because it takes into account a greater number of factors and can be used to calculate a change in $V_T$, rate, or mechanical dead space.

### EXAMPLE

The patient is a 70-kg (154-lb) man who is being ventilated on the control mode (he is apneic). His ventilator settings include a $V_T$ of 1000 mL, rate of 12 times/min, fractional inspired $O_2$ concentration ($F_IO_2$) of 0.3, and no added mechanical dead space. His ABG values are recorded as an arterial $O_2$ pressure ($PaO_2$) of 90 torr, $PaCO_2$ of 30 torr, pH of 7.48, $O_2$ saturation of arterial blood ($SaO_2$) of 95%, and base excess (BE) of 0. The clinical goal is to adjust the patient's $V_T$ as needed to produce a $PaCO_2$ value of 40 torr. A summary follows:

$V_T$ = 1000 mL current tidal volume
$V_{D\,anat}$ = 154 mL of anatomic dead space (calculated at 2.2 mL/kg [1 mL/lb] of ideal body weight)
$V_{D\,mech}$ = no added mechanical dead space
$f$ = 12 times/min for the ventilator rate
$PaCO_2$ = 30 torr actual patient $PaCO_2$ value
$V_T'$ = desired tidal volume
$PaCO_2'$ = 40 torr desired patient $PaCO_2$ value

Placing the data and goal into the formula results in the following:

$$[V_T - (V_{D\,anat} + V_{D\,mech})] \times f \times PaCO_2$$
$$= [V_T' - (V_{D\,anat} + V_{D\,mech})] \times f \times PaCO_2'$$
$$[1000 - (154 + 0)] \times 12 \times 30$$
$$= [V_T' - (154 + 0)] \times 12 \times 40$$
$$[846] \times 12 \times 30 = [V_T' - 154] \times 480$$
$$304{,}560 = 480\,V_T' - 73{,}920$$
$$378{,}480 = 480\,V_T'$$
$$788\,mL = V_T'$$

The solution is to reduce the patient's $V_T$ from 1000 to 788 mL.

---

**Exam Hint**

**E**very available NBRC examination has included several problems that require the examinee to determine an original ventilator $V_T$ or a new $V_T$ to correct for overventilating (low $CO_2$ level) or underventilating (high $CO_2$ level) a patient. Typically, start with a $V_T$ of 10 mL/kg of body weight. Increase or decrease the $V_T$ as needed from this starting point.

---

### g. Rate for mechanical ventilation

Table 1-2 lists the normal resting respiratory frequencies based on age. If the patient is apneic and has a normal temperature and an appropriately set $V_T$, respiratory rates in the indicated ranges will produce a normal $PaCO_2$ level. This must be confirmed by an ABG measurement. If the $V_T$ cannot be changed, adjusting the respiratory rate will modify alveolar ventilation. A higher respiratory rate, with everything else the same, causes a lower $PaCO_2$ level. Conversely, a lower respiratory rate, with everything else the same, results in a higher $PaCO_2$ level.

As has been mentioned, chronically hypercapnic patients must be ventilated with some caution. Giving this type of patient a higher ventilator-delivered rate or larger $V_T$ may result in blowing off of too much $CO_2$, thus causing a respiratory alkalosis. Adult patients with severe chronic restrictive lung disease and those who have had a pneumonectomy may need respiratory rates of 20 to 30/min or greater to meet their $\dot{V}_E$ needs. Their delivered $V_T$ must be smaller than normal because of their lung condition.

Use the same formula for predicting $V_T$ to help predict the *respiratory rate* that will produce a desired $PaCO_2$ value.

### EXAMPLE

Use the same patient parameters listed in the previous section to solve for the new respiratory rate ($f'$). The solution is to reduce the patient's respiratory rate from 12 to 9 breaths/min.

### h. Minute ventilation for mechanical ventilation

The subjects of minute ventilation and alveolar minute ventilation are covered in Chapter 4. Review the calculations as needed. Blood gases must always be evaluated in terms of the $PaCO_2$ level to determine whether the patient's minute ventilation is adequate. A high $CO_2$ level indicates the need for an increase in $V_T$, respiratory rate, or both. A low $CO_2$ indicates the need for decreased $V_T$, respiratory rate, or both. In either case, the key to modifying $CO_2$ level is to modify alveolar ventilation. This is best accomplished by changing the $V_T$ rather than the rate. The following formula can be used to calculate a change in $\dot{V}_E$:

$$\dot{V}_E' = \frac{PaCO_2 \times \dot{V}_E}{PaCO_2'}$$

where

$\dot{V}_E'$ = *desired* minute volume
$\dot{V}_E$ = current minute volume
$PaCO_2$ = current $PaCO_2$ level
$PaCO_2'$ = *desired* $PaCO_2$ level

### EXAMPLE

The patient is the same 70-kg (154-lb) man previously mentioned who is being ventilated on the control mode (he is apneic). His ventilator settings include a $V_T$ of 1000 mL, rate of 12 times/min, $F_IO_2$ of 0.3, and no added mechanical dead space. His ABG values are $PaO_2$ of 90 torr, $PaCO_2$ of 30 torr, pH of 7.48, $SaO_2$ of 95%, and BE of 0. The clinical goal is to adjust the patient's $\dot{V}_E$ as needed to obtain a $PaCO_2$ value of 40 torr. Placing the data and goal into the formula results in the following:

$$\dot{V}_E' = \frac{PaCO_2 \times \dot{V}_E}{PaCO_2'}$$

$$\dot{V}_E = \frac{30 \times 12,000}{40}$$

$$\dot{V}_E = \frac{36,000}{40}$$

$$\dot{V}_E = 9000 \, mL$$

The $PaCO_2$ goal can be accomplished by reducing the $\dot{V}_E$ from 12,000 to 9000 mL. As has been mentioned, this is best done by reducing the $V_T$. Remember that the $V_T$ must be kept at no less than 10 mL/kg of ideal body weight if the development of atelectasis is to be avoided. The respiratory rate may be decreased, if necessary, to obtain this reduced $\dot{V}_E$.

### 3. Perform the following procedures to ensure that the patient is adequately oxygenated

**a. Minimize hypoxemia by positioning the patient properly (NBRC code: IIID6) [Difficulty: R]**

This is discussed in Chapter 6.

**b. Recommend a change in the oxygen percentage (NBRC code: IIIG2c) [Difficulty: R, Ap]**

**c. Administer oxygen, as needed, to prevent hypoxemia (NBRC code: IIID4b) [Difficulty: R, Ap]**

$O_2$ administration and adjustment are discussed in Chapter 6. Briefly, the goal of $O_2$ administration is to keep the $PaO_2$ level of most patients between 60 and 90 torr and the pulse oximetry ($SpO_2$) level greater than 90%. Exceptions include the COPD patient who is breathing on hypoxic drive and the patient who is in a cardiac arrest situation. The following formula can be used to help guide the use of supplemental $O_2$ in most stable patients:

$$\text{Desired } F_IO_2 = \frac{\text{desired } PaO_2 \times \text{current } F_IO_2}{\text{current } PaO_2}$$

### EXAMPLE

A patient has a $PaO_2$ level of 55 torr on 30% $O_2$. The clinical goal is a $PaO_2$ level of 90 torr. What $O_2$ percentage should the patient have?

$$\text{Desired } F_IO_2 = \frac{\text{desired } PaO_2 \times \text{current } F_IO_2}{\text{current } PaO_2}$$

$$\text{Desired } F_IO_2 = \frac{90 \, torr \times 0.3}{55 \, torr}$$

$$\text{Desired } F_IO_2 = \frac{27}{55}$$

$$\text{Desired } F_IO_2 = 0.49 \text{ or } 49\% \, O_2$$

Those patients who have refractory hypoxemia (e.g., ARDS) do not respond with a normal increase in $PaO_2$ level as the $O_2$ percentage is increased. Over the short term, use whatever $O_2$ percentage is needed to achieve the clinical goal. The risk of $O_2$ toxicity increases when the $F_IO_2$ is greater than 0.5 for periods of longer than 48 hr. Always recheck the patient's arterial $O_2$ level after a change has been made in the $F_IO_2$.

Either of the following formulas can be used in the special situation of determining the flows of air and $O_2$ into a "bleed-in" type of intermittent mandatory ventilation (IMV) or continuous positive-airway pressure (CPAP) system for the purpose of obtaining an ordered $F_IO_2$. Either formula can also be used for determining the gas flows, total flow, and $O_2$:air ratio through an air-entrainment (Venturi) mask.

The first formula follows:

$$(L/min\ air \times F_IO_2\ of\ air) + (L/min\ O_2 \times F_IO_2\ pure\ O_2)$$
$$= total\ flow \times unknown\ F_IO_2$$

The second formula follows:

$$F_1C_1 + F_2C_2 = F_TC_T$$

where

$F_1$ = flow of first gas ($O_2$)
$C_1$ = concentration of $O_2$ in the first gas (1.0 for pure $O_2$)
$F_2$ = flow of second gas (air)
$C_2$ = concentration of $O_2$ in the second gas (0.21 for air)
$F_T$ = total flow of both gases
$C_T$ = concentration of $O_2$ in the mix of both gases

Algebraic manipulation enables the practitioner to solve for the unknown.

### EXAMPLE

Determine the oxygen percentage through a "bleed-in" system that has an oxygen flow of 10 L/min and an airflow of 15 L/min. Determine the total flow through the system. Determine the ratio of $O_2$ to air.

$$(L/min\ air \times F_IO_2\ of\ air) + (L/min\ O_2 \times F_IO_2\ pure\ O_2)$$
$$= total\ flow \times unknown\ F_IO_2$$
$$(15 \times 0.21) + (10 \times 1.0) = (15 + 10) \times unknown\ F_IO_2$$
$$(3.15) + (10) = (25) \times unknown\ F_IO_2$$
$$13.15 = 25 \times F_IO_2 \binom{Divide\ both}{sides\ by\ 25.}$$
$$0.526\ or\ 52.6\% = F_IO_2$$
$$Total\ flow = 15 + 10 = 25\ L/min$$
$$Ratio = \frac{10\ L/min\ O_2}{15\ L/min\ air}$$

### d. Adequately oxygenate the patient to prevent accidental hypoxemia before and after suctioning, changing of the ventilator circuit, or other procedures whereby the patient is disconnected from the ventilator (NBRC code: IIID7) [Difficulty: R, Ap]

Ensuring adequate oxygenation during suctioning is discussed in Chapter 13. Briefly, remember to give the adult patient 100% $O_2$ for at least 30 sec before suctioning. Perform the task as quickly and safely as possible. Leave the patient on 100% $O_2$ for at least 1 min after the procedure, or until he or she returns to a stable condition. Children younger than 6 months of age can have the $F_IO_2$ increased by 10% to 20% for the procedure.

It is acceptable to increase an adult's inspired $O_2$ by up to 100% before and after a procedure that requires disconnection from the ventilator. The goal is to prevent hypoxemia. The patient should be manually ventilated with a resuscitation bag, if indicated. Always remember to return the patient to the original $O_2$ percentage when clinically indicated.

### 4. Initiate and adjust modes of ventilation (NBRC code: IIID2b) [Difficulty: R, Ap]

The following modes of ventilation are delivered through most types of electrically powered, volume-cycled ventilators such as the Servo 300A, Puritan-Bennett 7200, Drager Evita 2 Dura, and Bear 1000.

*Control.* Control, the simplest method of providing ventilatory support, is used on an apneic patient. The ventilator is set with a mandatory respiratory rate and $V_T$. The machine is incapable of allowing any patient interaction. For example, the ventilator might be set to deliver a $V_T$ of 700 mL at a rate of 14 times/min. Because of this limitation, it is rarely if ever used in modern medicine except when the patient must be kept sedated or is pharmacologically paralyzed (Fig. 15-9, **A** shows the pressure/time curve).

*Assist/control.* The A/C mode has a set backup respiratory rate but allows the patient to trigger additional machine-delivered breaths. A sensitivity control is adjusted to allow the patient to easily start a breath as needed. All $V_T$s are the same (Fig. 15-9, **B** shows the pressure/time curve).

*Intermittent mandatory ventilation.* IMV has a set backup respiratory rate and $V_T$ for delivery to the patient. In addition, the patient can breathe spontaneously between mandatory breaths as frequently as desired. The patient can also take in as large a spontaneous $V_T$ as needed. The sensitivity control is set so that the patient cannot trigger any extra ventilator $V_T$. For example, the ventilator might be set to deliver a 700 mL $V_T$ 8 times/min. Consider a patient who breathes spontaneously 10 additional times and has an average $V_T$ of 400 mL. The total rate would be counted at 18. The total $\dot{V}_E$ would be the combination of the machine's volume and the patient's volume (Fig. 15-9, **C** shows the pressure/time curve).

*Synchronous intermittent mandatory ventilation.* SIMV is similar to IMV except that the sensitivity control is functional. The patient can trigger a machine-delivered $V_T$ during a preset time interval. The timing of the backup rate is such that the patient can get only as many ventilator breaths as are set. Spontaneous $V_T$s vary with the patient's efforts. The total respiratory rate and total $\dot{V}_E$ would be calculated as previously discussed (Fig. 15-9, **D** shows the pressure/time curve).

*Pressure support ventilation.* PSV is similar to IPPB in that when the patient initiates a ventilator breath, a preset pressure is delivered to the airway. The patient has the flexibility to determine the respiratory rate. The physician orders a PSV level that can either overcome the patient's

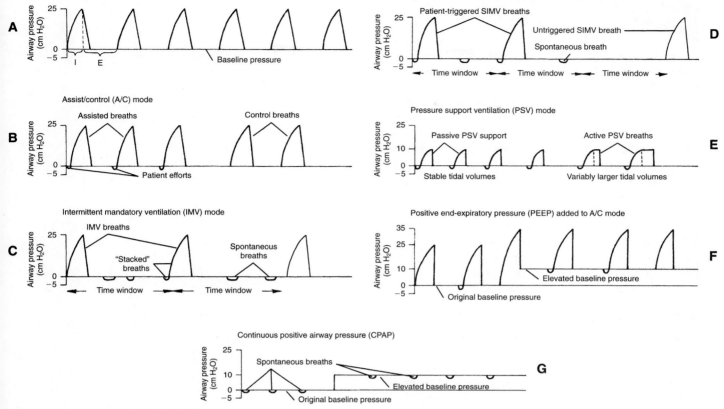

**Fig. 15-9** Pressure-vs-time waveforms for the various modes of mechanical ventilation. **A,** Control (C) mode shows no patient effort and consistent I:E ratios. **B,** Assist/control (A/C) mode shows that the patient's initial effort triggers a machine tidal volume ($V_T$) breath. **C,** Intermittent mandatory ventilation (IMV) mode shows spontaneous $V_T$ breaths occurring between predetermined machine $V_T$ breaths. Note the "stacked" breaths that occur when the patient takes in a breath subsequently supplemented by a machine breath. **D,** Synchronous intermittent mandatory ventilation (SIMV) mode shows that a patient effort within a time window causes the delivery of a machine $V_T$. Any other patient efforts within the time window result in a spontaneous $V_T$. If no patient efforts occur within the time window, a machine $V_T$ will be automatically delivered. **E,** Pressure support ventilation (PSV) mode shows how the patient must initiate all breaths that are then supported to a predetermined airway pressure. Stable $V_T$s will be seen if the patient inhales passively. Variably larger $V_T$s will result if the patient inhales more actively. **F,** Positive end-expiratory pressure (PEEP) therapy can be added to the A/C mode (as shown) or any other mode. The elevated baseline pressure prevents alveolar collapse. The sensitivity control must be set so that the patient is able to trigger a breath without undue effort. **G,** Continuous positive-airway pressure (CPAP) shows that the patient takes spontaneous $V_T$s while exhaling against an elevated baseline pressure.

calculated Raw or deliver a minimum $V_T$, depending on the clinical goal. The $V_T$ will be stable if the patient passively takes the PSV breath, or it will become larger if the patient interacts actively with the delivered pressure (Figs. 15-1 and 15-9, **E** show the pressure/time curve).

***Pressure control ventilation.*** Pressure control ventilation (PCV) involves the delivery of $V_T$ breaths that are pressure limited and time cycled. A ventilator rate can be

set and the patient can trigger additional breaths. Because pressure is limited, the $V_T$s may vary. This needs to be monitored closely in patients with frequently changing $C_{LT}$ and Raw values. As the inspiratory time is increased, it can become longer than the expiratory time and can cause pressure control inverse ratio ventilation (PCIRV). Fig. 15-10 shows volume, flow, and pressure tracings.

### Exam Hint

**N**BRC examinations have included a variety of terms and phrases to describe modes or modifications of modes of ventilation, including the following:
1. Terms related to delivering a set $V_T$: volume ventilation; volume-cycled mechanical ventilation; volume-controlled ventilation; volume-preset ventilation; volume-controlled, flow-limited ventilation; volume-controlled, pressure-limited ventilation; volume-controlled with SIMV, A/C, or control; volume-controlled with continuous-flow IMV circuit added.
2. Terms related to *not* delivering a set $V_T$: pressure-cycled ventilation; pressure control; pressure-controlled, pressure-limited, time-cycled ventilation; pressure-controlled with constant inspiratory time; pressure-limited; any previously mentioned term with inverse ratio.

## 5. Begin and modify positive end-expiratory pressure therapy (NBRC code: IIID2d) [Difficulty: R, Ap]

PEEP is a residual pressure above atmospheric that is maintained at the airway opening at the end of expiration. Fig. 15-9, **F** shows the pressure/time curve. PEEP is administered through a mechanical ventilator and is not a mode by itself. Rather, it is used in conjunction with any of the previously mentioned modes. PEEP is set to prevent the patient from exhaling back to ambient (atmospheric) pressure. The higher the level of PEEP, the more progressively is the patient's functional residual capacity (FRC) increased. The therapeutic goal is to increase the patient's $PaO_2$. A patient most often develops severe hypoxemia because of increased intrapulmonary shunt (perfusion without ventilation). Remember that greater than 5% shunt is abnormal and justifies treatment, such as PEEP or CPAP, to improve ventilation-to-perfusion matching.

PEEP is generally indicated in patients with any bilateral, generalized pulmonary condition in which the FRC is decreased (e.g., generalized atelectasis, pulmonary edema, ARDS, and RDS). All of these patients show a decreased $C_{LT}$ as measured by $C_{st}$. Specific indications for PEEP include the following:
a. Intrapulmonary shunt greater than 15%
b. Refractory hypoxemia ($PaO_2$ less than 60 torr despite an $F_IO_2$ of up to 0.8 to 1.0)
c. An $F_IO_2$ greater than 0.5 for 48 to 72 hr with no indication of a rapidly improving $PaO_2$ (PEEP is added so that the $F_IO_2$ can be lowered to a safer level)

Before PEEP is begun, the patient should be carefully monitored so the baseline condition can be evaluated. These same parameters should be monitored for determi-

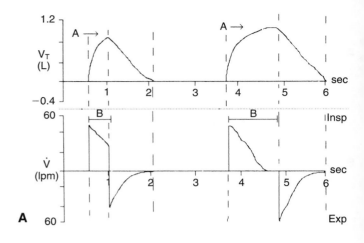

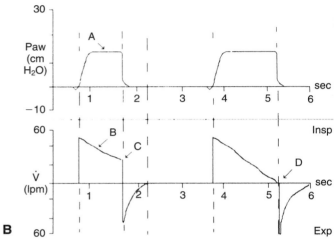

**Fig. 15-10** Two sets of graphic tracings of pressure control ventilation. **A,** Two tracings show tidal volume ($V_T$) vs time and flow ($\dot{V}$) vs time. *A* shows tidal volume; *B* shows inspiratory flow. Note how the $V_T$ increases as the inspiratory time is increased. However, as shown in the lower right tracing, no more volume is delivered as the flow drops to zero. **B,** Two tracings show airway pressure (Paw) vs time and flow vs time. *A* shows the pressure control level being reached with an inspiratory plateau or "square wave" appearance. *B* shows a declining inspiratory flow. *C* shows the final flow when inspiration is time cycled off and exhalation begins. This graphic can be used to help adjust a longer inspiratory time. If pressure control inverse ratio ventilation were being optimally adjusted, the inspiratory time could be increased until inspiratory flow reached zero (indicated by *D*). *(Courtesy of Mallinckrodt, Pleasanton, Calif.)*

nation of the patient's tolerance after each change in the PEEP level. The best or optimal level of PEEP is the level that causes the most efficient delivery of $O_2$ to the tissues (not necessarily the arterial blood). Often, a secondary goal is to reduce the inspired $O_2$ to a safe level. The patient is at risk of $O_2$ toxicity if more than 50% $O_2$ is inhaled for longer than 48 to 72 hr. See Box 15-2 for recommendations on what to monitor during the application of PEEP and how to evaluate the data.

a. Decrease PEEP first if the $PaO_2$ level is greater than 60 torr and the $F_IO_2$ is less than 0.5.
b. Decrease $O_2$ first if the $PaO_2$ level is greater than 60 torr and the $F_IO_2$ is greater than 0.5.

---

## BOX 15-2 Patient Monitoring During Positive End-Expiratory Pressure (PEEP) or Continuous Positive-Airway Pressure (CPAP) Therapy

### GOOD TOLERANCE OF PEEP/CPAP THERAPY
- Increased $PaO_2$ level
- Increased static compliance
- Stable cardiac output as shown by the following:
  ○ Stable heart rate without rhythm disturbances
  ○ Stable blood pressure
  The following can be measured only through a Swan-Ganz/pulmonary artery catheter:
  ○ Stable or increased $P\bar{v}O_2$ (normal is 40 mm Hg)
  ○ Stable cardiac output (adult normal is 4–8 L/min)
  ○ Reduction of elevated pulmonary vascular resistance (normal is 80–240 cynes/seconds/cm$^{-5}$)
  ○ Reduction of elevated intrapulmonary shunt (normal is 5% or less)

### POOR TOLERANCE OF PEEP/CPAP THERAPY
- Increased $PaO_2$ level (this can be deceiving if this is the only information observed)
- Decreased static compliance
- Decreased cardiac output as shown by the following:
  ○ Increased heart rate or rhythm disturbances
  ○ Decreased blood pressure
  The following can be measured only through a Swan-Ganz/pulmonary artery catheter:
  ○ Decreased $P\bar{v}O_2$
  ○ Decreased cardiac output
  ○ Increased pulmonary vascular resistance
  ○ Increased intrapulmonary shunt

---

$PaO_2$, arterial $O_2$ pressure; $P\bar{v}O_2$, mixed venous $O_2$ level.

The application of PEEP does not occur without risks. Hazards of PEEP include the following:

a. Pulmonary barotrauma: pneumothorax, tension pneumothorax, mediastinal emphysema, pulmonary interstitial emphysema in the neonate, subcutaneous emphysema
b. Decreased venous return to the heart (causing a decreased cardiac output): tachycardia, decreased blood pressure, decreased tissue perfusion as measured by a decreased mixed venous $O_2$ ($P\bar{v}O_2$) level, decreased urine output

PEEP therapy is usually begun at levels of 2 to 5 cm $H_2O$. After the patient's response has been determined, an additional 2 to 5 cm $H_2O$ PEEP may be applied. The patient then is reevaluated, and this process goes on until the best or optimal level of PEEP is determined.

As the patient begins to recover, the PEEP level may be reduced in steps of 2 to 5 cm $H_2O$. Again, the patient is evaluated after each change in PEEP level. If the patient's cardiovascular status is normal, the following recommendations can help in decreasing PEEP and $O_2$ levels:

---

### Exam Hint

**K**now to increase PEEP if the patient is hypoxic, is receiving a high $O_2$ percentage, and is hemodynamically stable. Know to decrease PEEP if the patient is well oxygenated and is receiving a moderate $O_2$ percentage, is not hemodynamically stable, or has a PEEP-related complication.

---

## 6. Begin and modify continuous positive-airway pressure (NBRC code: IIID2d) [Difficulty: R, Ap]

Continuous positive airway pressure (CPAP) is a pressure above atmospheric that is maintained at the airway opening throughout the respiratory cycle during spontaneous breathing. Fig. 15-9, **G** shows the pressure/time curve. CPAP is similar to PEEP in purpose and effect. It is different from previously mentioned modes in that the patient receives no ventilator-delivered $V_T$ breaths. The patient must be capable of providing all of the minute ventilation needed for $CO_2$ removal. CPAP can be delivered through some mechanical ventilators when the rate is turned off, or it can be delivered through a free-standing system.

CPAP has the same indications, hazards, and patient evaluation processes as those discussed earlier for PEEP therapy. One possible physiologic benefit of CPAP over PEEP is that reduction in the venous return to the heart is less because the patient breathes spontaneously with CPAP. Therefore, patients treated with CPAP may be able to tolerate higher pressure levels than those tolerated by patients ventilated with PEEP.

CPAP is usually increased and decreased in steps of 2 to 5 cm $H_2O$. As with PEEP, the patient is evaluated before CPAP is begun and again after every change in pressure. See Box 15-2 for recommendations on what to monitor during the application of CPAP and how to evaluate the data.

Before a patient receives CPAP therapy, the practitioner and the physician must be assured that the patient has the ability to breathe adequately to eliminate $CO_2$. CPAP is contraindicated in a patient who is apneic or potentially apneic. (This patient needs to be fully supported on the ventilator.) The patient must have an adequate respiratory rate, $V_T$, and $\dot{V}_E$. Heart rate and blood pressure should be stable. Maximal inspiratory pressure (MIP) and VC values may be acceptable or low. Blood gas analysis typically shows refractory hypoxemia but a normal or low $PaCO_2$ level. This shows that the patient would benefit from an elevated baseline pressure to increase the FRC but is capable of ventilating.

The patient must be carefully monitored for fatigue because the patient is providing all minute ventilation. Signs of fatigue include increasing respiratory rate, decreasing $V_T$ or VC, decreasing MIP, and tachycardia. Blood gas measurement may reveal a stable or decreasing $PaO_2$ value. A rising $PaCO_2$ level is a definite sign of fatigue. The patient may complain of dyspnea. The practitioner can notice that the patient is working harder than normal to breathe, as shown by the increased use of accessory muscles of ventilation and heavy perspiration. When these signs occur, CPAP therapy should be discontinued and mechanical ventilation instituted in a mode that best fits the patient's needs.

---

### Exam Hint

$C$PAP questions often relate to the care of neonatal patients with hypoxemia from increased shunt. Know that CPAP can be used and increased if the patient's $CO_2$ level is normal and hypoxemia is present. In neonates, the upper limit of CPAP is usually 10 cm $H_2O$. Know to switch to mechanical ventilation when this maximal level of CPAP is used and the patient is still hypoxemic.

---

### 7. Begin and modify combinations of ventilatory techniques to adequately oxygenate the patient: synchronous intermittent mandatory ventilation, pressure support ventilation, pressure control ventilation, and positive end-expiratory pressure (NBRC code: IIID2e) [Difficulty: R, Ap]

The current generation of mechanical ventilators offers the physician and practitioner a number of options for how to best tailor ventilatory support to meet the patient's needs. The following should be considered when one is deciding which modes to use and combine.

#### a. Increased work of breathing

Patients who show increased WOB may have a very high Raw, as in status asthmaticus, or may have a very low $C_{LT}$, as in ARDS. Some practitioners believe that the control or A/C mode, when properly applied to a sedated patient, is best for these problems because the patient's breathing efforts are almost eliminated. Other practitioners believe that IMV or SIMV is a physiologically superior mode of ventilation. Recently, PSV has been shown to be beneficial to patients who exert increased efforts at breathing as a result of the high Raw caused by a small-diameter endotracheal tube.

#### b. Hypercapnia

A patient may have hypercapnia (a high $CO_2$ level) because of sedation from a morphine or heroin overdose, or from COPD with worsening of chronic hypercapnia. In either case, the patient becomes progressively more hypoxemic (unless given supplemental $O_2$) as the $CO_2$ level rises. Control and A/C modes are best for setting a minimal $\dot{V}_E$ to determine the maximum $CO_2$ level. As the patient recovers, IMV/SIMV or PSV allows for a gradual reduction in ventilatory support. Box 15-3 lists indications of IMV/SIMV tolerance.

Mandatory minute ventilation (MMV) has also been successful at setting an $\dot{V}_E$ that limits the rise in $CO_2$ as the patient is weaning. MMV is a relatively new variation on the IMV/SIMV mode. With MMV, the patient is assured of a preset $\dot{V}_E$ regardless of his or her spontaneous breathing. It has been proposed as an effective way to ventilate and wean patients who can spontaneously breathe but have an unreliable respiratory drive and unstable $V_T$. Examples include patients who have received narcotic, sedative, anesthetic, or neuromuscular blocking medications. Patient conditions for which MMV would be indicated include encephalopathy and cerebral disorders such as stroke. In addition, MMV may be used during the recovery period for a neuromuscular disease. Ventilators

---

**BOX 15-3    Indications of Intermittent Mandatory Ventilation (IMV)/Synchronous Intermittent Mandatory Ventilation (SIMV) Tolerance**

**GOOD TOLERANCE OF IMV/SIMV THERAPY**
- Stable spontaneous respiratory rate
- Stable heart rate
- Stable spontaneous $V_T$
- Stable VC, MIP or $FEV_1$
- No use or stable use of accessory muscles of ventilation
- Patient indicates he is comfortable
- Stable blood gases

**POOR TOLERANCE OF IMV/SIMV THERAPY**
- Increased spontaneous respiratory rate
- Tachycardia or arrhythmias (e.g., PVCs)
- Drop in the spontaneous $V_T$
- Drop in the VC, MIP, or $FEV_1$
- Beginning or increased use of accessory muscles of ventilation
- Patient complains of dyspnea
- Deterioration of blood gases as seen by falling $PaO_2$ or $SpO_2$ level and a rapidly falling or rising $PaCO_2$ level

$FEV_1$, forced expiratory volume in 1 sec; MIP, maximal inspiratory pressure; $PaCO_2$, arterial $CO_2$ pressure; $PaO_2$, arterial $O_2$ pressure; PVCs, premature ventricular contractions; $SpO_2$, pulse oximetry; VC, vital capacity; $V_T$, tidal volume.

capable of the MMV mode are all controlled by a micro-processor and include the Bear 1000, the Drager E4, and the Hamilton Veolar. The following parameters have been recommended for the initiation of MMV:

1. Set the ventilator $V_T$ according to established guidelines (10 to 15 mL/kg of ideal body weight).
2. Spontaneous breaths may be taken through a demand valve or may be pressure supported.
3. Determine the minimal $\dot{V}_E$ according to the patient's preexisting condition and the clinical goals:
   a. The patient who has been on IMV/SIMV should have the MMV set at 90% of the IMV-delivered $\dot{V}_E$. For example, the patient has an IMV/SIMV rate of 5 breaths/min and a $V_T$ of 800 mL. Therefore, the ventilator is delivering 4 L of $\dot{V}_E$ ($5 \times 800$ mL), and the MMV would be set at 3600 mL (90% of 4 L).
   b. The patient who has been on A/C mode should have the MMV set at 80% of the A/C-delivered $\dot{V}_E$. For example, the patient has an A/C rate of 10 breaths/min and a $V_T$ of 1000 mL. Therefore, the ventilator is delivering 10 L of $\dot{V}_E$ ($10 \times 1000$ mL), and the MMV would be set at 8 L (80% of 10 L).
4. Set the inspired $O_2$ percentage, inspiratory flow, and other values as the patient's clinical condition requires.

Ideally, MMV establishes a minimum safe volume of ventilation. If the patient inhales less than this volume, the ventilator will deliver as many breaths as necessary at the preestablished $V_T$ to make up the difference. Be aware that a patient who is breathing rapidly with a small $V_T$ may move enough gas to exceed the minimal $\dot{V}_E$. Because of this risk, it is important to set a low $V_T$ alarm or a high respiratory rate alarm to give warning. Do not let the programming of a mandatory $\dot{V}_E$ create a false sense of security with these patients.

### c. Hypoxemia

If the problem is the result of a decreased FRC, as in ARDS or atelectasis, the treatment of choice for hypoxemia is CPAP on a free-standing system or PEEP on a conventional volume-cycled ventilator. If the problem results from an increased intrapulmonary shunt, the patient may need PEEP or CPAP, as well as up to 100% $O_2$. Refer to Box 15-2 for patient monitoring during PEEP and CPAP. PCIRV and high-frequency jet ventilation have been used successfully in hypoxemic patients with a pulmonary air leak who have failed conventional volume ventilation.

All of the following were discussed earlier as individual modes of ventilation. When a patient has more than one problem, more than one solution may be needed. Following are discussions about combinations of modes from which to choose.

### d. Pressure control/pressure control inverse ratio ventilation, synchronous intermittent mandatory ventilation, and positive end-expiratory pressure

PCV or, if necessary, PCIRV has been used successfully in patients with low compliance and a pulmonary air leak. With limited peak pressure, less air seems to leak out and tissues are more likely to heal. Therapeutic PEEP is applied to increase the patient's FRC and correct hypoxemia. The SIMV feature is added to let the patient breathe spontaneously if desired and stay more synchronized with the ventilator. With lung healing, the PEEP level is decreased and the inspiratory time is shortened. SIMV with a constant $V_T$ is likely to be used during the weaning phase. Fig. 15-10 shows pressure and flow tracings during PCV.

### e. Intermittent mandatory ventilation/synchronous intermittent mandatory ventilation with pressure support ventilation and positive end-expiratory pressure

IMV/SIMV is used to give the patient a controlled number of deep $V_T$ breaths. The patient can breathe as often as desired between mandatory breaths. The patient's total $\dot{V}_E$ can be determined by adding the IMV/SIMV and the pressure-supported breaths. A maximum acceptable $PaCO_2$ can be established with the proper combination of IMV/SIMV breaths and PSV level. A PSV level greater than 10 cm $H_2O$ may be needed. In addition, the PSV ensures that the Raw of the endotracheal tube is overcome. (Review the Raw calculation from p. 277.) PEEP therapy is applied at the level needed for a clinically safe $PaO_2$ to be achieved at the lowest possible $F_IO_2$. Fig. 15-11, **A** shows the pressure-time curve.

Patients who would benefit from these modes of ventilation have problems with both ventilation and oxygenation. They have the desire to breathe on their own but a very limited ability to do so. All three modes can be independently adjusted to obtain more or less support, as indicated by the patient's clinical condition and blood gas results.

### f. Intermittent mandatory ventilation/synchronous intermittent mandatory ventilation with positive end-expiratory pressure

IMV/SIMV and PEEP therapies are applied as needed to set a baseline $\dot{V}_E$ and FRC. PSV is not needed if the patient is strong enough to overcome the Raw of the endotracheal tube and to breathe with a clinically acceptable $V_T$. Fig. 15-11, **B** shows the pressure-time curve.

### g. Intermittent mandatory ventilation/synchronous intermittent mandatory ventilation with pressure support ventilation

IMV/SIMV and PSV levels are increased or decreased based on the factors discussed earlier. The patient has the

IMV/SIMV with PSV and PEEP

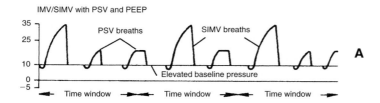

IMV/SIMV with PEEP

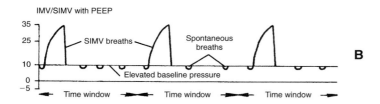

IMV/SIMV with PSV

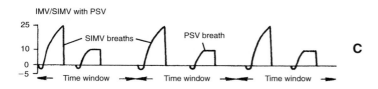

PSV with PEEP

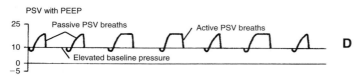

**Fig. 15-11** Modification of combinations of intermittent mandatory ventilation/synchronous intermittent mandatory ventilation (IMV/SIMV), pressure support ventilation (PSV), and positive end-expiratory pressure (PEEP). **A,** IMV/SIMV with PSV and PEEP. **B,** IMV/SIMV with PEEP. **C,** IMV/SIMV with PSV. **D,** PSV with PEEP.

ability to provide some, but not all, of his or her ventilation. The $PaO_2$ is clinically acceptable at an $O_2$ percentage probably no higher than 40%.

A fairly common clinical situation occurs when the recovering patient does well on a gradually decreasing number of IMV/SIMV breaths until he or she can go no lower. The barrier seems to be the Raw of the endotracheal tube. (Review the Raw calculation from p. 277.) The addition of some PSV overcomes that resistance so that the IMV/SIMV level can be further reduced. When the IMV/SIMV frequency is down to 4 breaths/min or less, the patient is providing almost all of his or her $\dot{V}_E$. The decision can then be made to extubate the patient. Fig. 15-11, **C** shows the pressure-time curve.

### h. Pressure support ventilation with positive end-expiratory pressure

PSV and PEEP are applied for reasons previously discussed. This patient has the drive to breathe on his or her own; however, he or she has some limitation in ability to overcome the resistance of the endotracheal tube or to generate a consistently large enough $V_T$. (Review the Raw

calculation from p. 277.) In addition, the patient has a significant oxygenation problem and needs some PEEP therapy. With recovery, both PSV and PEEP can be reduced, either individually or simultaneously, as the patient's strength or oxygenation improves. Fig. 15-11, **D** shows the pressure-time curve.

### 8. Administer prescribed medications (e.g., aerosolized bronchodilators, corticosteroids, saline, mucolytics) to mechanically ventilated patients so that they can be effectively ventilated and airway secretions can be removed (NBRC code: IIIC3 and IIID4a) [Difficulty: R, Ap]

Chapter 9 describes various bronchoactive medications. These can be administered with either a metered-dose inhaler (MDI) or a small-volume nebulizer (SVN). Usually, the nebulizer is placed in line with the inspiratory tubing, at least 18 inches back from the Y, or at the manifold of the circuit. This position prevents the nebulizer from acting as mechanical dead space in the circuit. Inspiratory tubing also acts as a medication reservoir for the next inspiration (Fig. 15-12).

If an MDI is used, a special T-piece medication reservoir must be fitted into the circuit. Activate the dispenser so that the medication is inhaled at the start of the next $V_T$ breath. A sigh volume can deliver the medication even more deeply into the lungs.

An SVN (as shown in Fig. 15-12) must be powered by a high-pressure gas source. Most modern ventilators (e.g., Puritan-Bennett 7200, Bear 1000) are designed to power the nebulizer by diverting part of the $V_T$ through the nebulizer when the nebulizer control is turned on. No change occurs in the patient's $O_2$ percentage, $V_T$, or other ventilator parameters.

Some modern ventilators, such as the Servo 300A, do not have this feature. Medications should be administered with these only by an MDI with a reservoir. Indeed, powering an SVN with an outside flowmeter causes the Servo to report abnormally high volumes. An alarm condition could result, or the ventilator could deliver air at less than preset volumes to compensate for the added flow. In addition, most of the medication would be wasted, and the internal exhalation valve and volume-measuring system would be contaminated.

### 9. Begin and adjust noninvasive positive-pressure ventilation (NBRC code: IIID2c) [Difficulty: R, Ap]

Noninvasive positive pressure ventilation (NPPV) is indicated in stable, unintubated, spontaneously breathing patients who show any of the following clinical situations: elevated $CO_2$ level, hypoxemia despite supplemental $O_2$, chronic ventilatory muscle dysfunction, or sleep apnea from upper airway obstruction. Typically, these patients

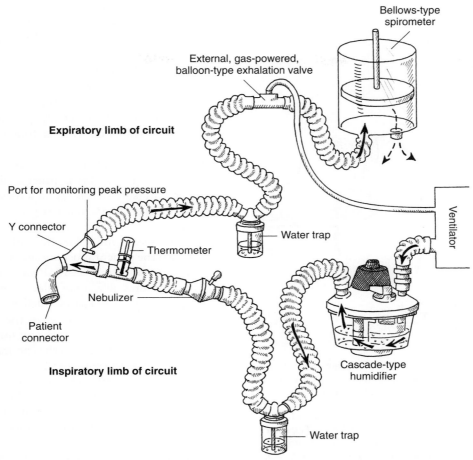

**Fig. 15-12** Continuous mechanical ventilation circuit with external exhalation valve.

are ventilated with the aid of a nasal mask similar to that used to deliver mask CPAP. A full facemask will be needed if the patient leaks through the mouth with a nasal mask. If the patient is critically ill, unstable, needs to be intubated to secure the airway for secretion removal, or needs a high level of therapeutic PEEP to maintain the FRC, he or she should be placed on a standard volume-cycled ventilator.

Patients receiving NPPV are often ventilated with two different levels of positive pressure (bilevel ventilation). The baseline pressure is greater than zero (CPAP or PEEP), and the peak pressure is set to deliver a desired $V_T$ (similar to PSV). Both levels can be independently adjusted. If only the baseline pressure is elevated, the patient receives CPAP. If only the peak pressure is elevated, the patient receives PSV. Respironics has developed two devices for bilevel ventilation for use in the hospital or home for noninvasive mask ventilation: the BiPAP S/T series and the newer BiPAP Vision. The Vision can function as a full ventilatory support system. Supplemental $O_2$ is not available through the BiPAP S/T; however, it can be added through a side port on the nasal mask to meet clinical goals.

The patient must have a properly fitting nasal mask or facemask to receive noninvasive ventilation. These ventilation masks are similar to CPAP masks and are referred to as such in this chapter. CPAP masks come in different sizes for children older than 3 years of age and for adults. Nasal masks are designed to cover only the nose. These allow the patient to eat, drink, speak, and use the mouth as a second airway for breathing in case a malfunction occurs in the CPAP system. The mouth also acts as a pressure-relief route should CPAP pressure become too great. Pressures of up to 10 to 15 cm $H_2O$ can usually be maintained (Fig. 15-13). Usually, the mask is made of a transparent plastic. Facemasks are designed to cover the nose and mouth. They are similar in design to masks used during bag-mask ventilation and are also made of a transparent plastic. The facemask must be used if the patient has persistent mouth breathing and cannot use a nose mask. Pressures greater than 15 cm $H_2O$ can be maintained with a good seal.

All brands and types of CPAP mask have a soft, compliant seal to closely fit the contours of the face. Straps are needed to hold the mask in place. A mask that is too large does not seal and allows gas to leak and pressure to drop.

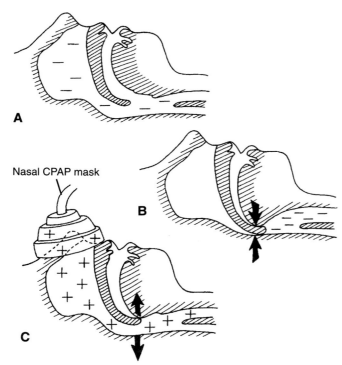

Nasal CPAP mask

**Fig. 15-13** Effect of a nasal continuous positive-airway pressure (CPAP) mask. **A,** Normal upper airway remains patent during sleep. **B,** Abnormal upper airway of a patient with obstructive apnea collapses on inspiration during sleep. **C,** Pressure from a nasal CPAP mask keeps the abnormal upper airway patent during sleep. *(Modified from Scanlan CL: Respiratory failure and the need for ventilatory support. In Scanlan CL, Spearman CB, Sheldon RL, editors: Egan's fundamentals of respiratory care, ed 5, St Louis, 1990, Mosby.)*

The patient may show increased snoring or airway obstruction with periods of apnea. A small or misfitting mask could cause an uneven distribution of pressure on the face, which could lead to abrasions or pressure sores and ulcers on the face.

The BiPAP S/T system can be used for bilevel ventilation or in the CPAP mode. It uses a relatively simple, smooth interior circuit and does not have a humidifier, alarm system, or other attachments seen in a volume-cycled ventilator. A bacteria filter should be inserted between the BiPAP unit and the patient circuit. If a humidifier is desired, it must be a cascade- or wick-type humidifier. An HME cannot be used because it creates too much air flow resistance.

The bilevel settings must be determined at the bedside by asking for the patient's subjective opinion, listening to breath sounds, checking vital signs, and evaluating ABG values. If supplemental $O_2$ is needed, it can be added at a port on the patient's mask, at the humidifier, or at the outlet from the BiPAP unit. Up to 15 L/min can be added without effect on the performance of the BiPAP system. The delivered $O_2$ percentage cannot

be known until after bilevel ventilation settings are determined. The $O_2$ flow should then be gradually increased until the patient's $SpO_2$ value rises to the desired saturation level.

Only the function of the BiPAP S/T system is reviewed in this chapter. The operator can choose among the following five modes of operation:

1. Expiratory positive-airway pressure (EPAP) from 2 to 20 cm $H_2O$. This is functionally similar to CPAP.
2. Inspiratory positive-airway pressure (IPAP) from 2 to 25 cm $H_2O$. This is functionally similar to the peak pressure that is set on a pressure-cycled ventilator. The patient must trigger each IPAP-assisted breath.
3. Spontaneous mode functions like the PSV mode, in which the patient must initiate each assisted breath. The therapist can set IPAP and EPAP levels, a step that ensures delivery of bilevel ventilation.
4. Spontaneous/timed mode delivers between 6 and 30 ventilator breaths/min when the patient's respiratory rate drops to below the set number. Otherwise, it functions similarly to the spontaneous mode and delivers bilevel ventilation.
5. Times mode varies the percentage of each cycle in IPAP from 10% to 90%. This allows the therapist to set an I:E ratio. The first four functions are kept except that the patient cannot trigger an IPAP breath.

With BiPAP units, the difference between IPAP and EPAP is called *pressure boost*; it delivers the $V_T$. It is important to remember that the delivered $V_T$ varies depending on changes in the patient's Raw and $C_{LT}$ values and in machine settings.

---

### Exam Hint

**I**ncreasing the IPAP level will increase the tidal volume; decreasing IPAP will decrease the tidal volume. Increasing the EPAP level will increase the patient's functional residual capacity (FRC) and improve oxygenation. As the patient's oxygenation improves, the EPAP level can be decreased.

---

### MODULE C
### Mechanical ventilation equipment

*Note:* The literature produced by manufacturers and the descriptions used in many standard texts break down the various ventilators into a greater number of categories than are used by the NBRC. To avoid confusion, this text uses the NBRC's more simplified terminology. A *pneumatically powered ventilator* is defined here as one that is powered by compressed gas and that has no electrically powered control system (electrically powered alarm systems may or may not be added). An *electrically powered ventilator* is defined here as one that is electrically powered or controlled. Most volume-cycled ventilators fall into this category. *Microprocessor ventilators* are electrically powered but are controlled by one or more microprocessors (computers). Most current volume-cycled ventilators have microprocessors that control their functions. *Fluidic ventilators* typically make use of electrical circuits with flip-flops to respond to changes in gas flow and pressure through the system. Fluidic ventilators are powered by compressed gas. *Noninvasive positive-pressure ventilators (NPPVs)* are designed for home use or short-term hospital use and are electrically powered and controlled. They have fewer controls and alarms than hospital-based critical care ventilators. A nasal mask or full facemask rather than an endotracheal tube is used to attach the ventilator to the patient.

### 1. Pneumatically powered ventilators

#### a. Get the necessary equipment for the procedure (NBRC code: IIA6a) [Difficulty: R, Ap]

The only commonly used pneumatically powered ventilators are the Bird series and the Bennett PR-2. A control or backup rate can be set on these units in case the patient should become apneic. All other controls and functions are the same as those discussed in Chapter 14. The following equipment is necessary:

1. Bennett PR-2 or Bird ventilator with an air/$O_2$ blender and hoses
2. Bennett or Bird breathing circuit
3. Bacteria filters
4. Proper humidification system: either a passover- or cascade-type humidifier or an HME (discussed later). Sterile, distilled water should be placed in the passover- or cascade-type humidifier
5. One or two water traps for condensation from the circuit
6. Add-on alarm system(s), such as a low-volume bellows spirometer or a low-pressure/disconnection alarm
7. A length of large-bore tubing to connect the exhalation valve to the bellows if a low-volume bellows spirometer alarm is used

#### b. Put the equipment together and make sure that it works properly (NBRC code: IIA6a) [Difficulty: R, Ap]

Refer to figures in Chapter 14 for the IPPB circuits. The ventilator and circuits are similar to those used in IPPB therapy with the following exceptions:

1. Set the ordered $O_2$ percentage on the blender; set the Bird *air-mix* and Bennett *air-dilution* selection controls to obtain pure source gas from the blender.

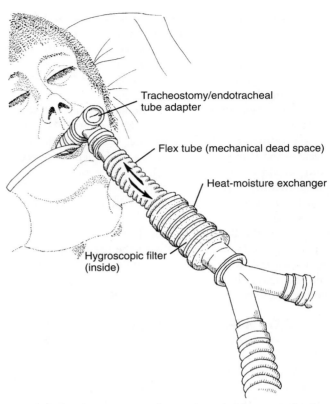

**Fig. 15-14** Heat-moisture exchanger insertion into a patient's breathing circuit. Any extra tubing inserted between the Y and the endotracheal tube acts as mechanical dead space.

Analyze the $F_1O_2$ through a port in the inspiratory limb of the circuit.

2. If a passover- or cascade-type bubble humidifier is used, a short length of large-bore tubing is connected between the outlet of the mainstream inline bacteria filter and the inlet of the humidifier. The inspiratory limb of the circuit is connected to the outlet of the humidifier. If an HME is used, it will be added between the circuit and the tracheostomy/endotracheal tube adapter (Fig. 15-14).
3. A tracheostomy/endotracheal tube adapter must be used to connect the circuit to the patient (see Fig. 15-14).
4. Add at least one disconnection alarm to the circuit. It could be a low-volume spirometer alarm on the expiratory limb or a low-pressure or disconnection alarm added into the inspiratory limb of the circuit with a Briggs adapter/T-adapter.
5. Water traps are placed in the lowest part of the inspiratory and expiratory limbs of the circuit to hold any condensed water vapor.

Fig. 15-12 shows a complete circuit to a volume-cycled ventilator. It is essentially the same circuit as that used on a pressure-cycled ventilator.

*Setting the backup rate for controlled breaths.* For the Bird Mark 7, turn the expiratory timer control counterclockwise to decrease the expiratory time and therefore increase the backup rate. If the expiratory timer control does not trigger a breath, the ventilator is defective and should not be used.

For the Bennett PR-2, turn the *rate* control clockwise from the *off* position to decrease the expiratory time and therefore increase the backup rate. If the unit does not cycle properly into inspiration, the equipment is defective and should not be used. The I:E ratio is preset at 1:1.5 when the unit is time-cycling on and off. Expiratory time can be increased by turning the *expiratory time* control clockwise.

In both the Bennett and Bird units, the backup rate must be timed and adjusted with the use of a stopwatch or wristwatch with a sweep second hand. The I:E ratio may be manually adjusted with the previously mentioned controls and the flow control on the Bird Mark 7.

### c. Troubleshoot any problems with the equipment (NBRC code: IIA6a) [Difficulty: R, Ap]

The Bird and Bennett ventilators previously mentioned send gas through the circuit during an inspiration and do not cycle off until the preset pressure has been reached. Test the tightness of the circuit, backup rate, and delivered $V_T$ by placing a test lung on the patient connection of the circuit. Set the controls to deliver the prescribed order. Be prepared to make final adjustments once either unit has been placed on the patient. The patient's Raw and $C_{LT}$ greatly affect the functioning of both units.

Troubleshooting of problems with these units is discussed in Chapter 14. Make sure that all connections are tight; a greater number of connections are attained by the addition of the humidification system and expiratory limb to the spirometer.

A defective exhalation valve or one in which the small-bore tubing has popped off sends gas through the circuit and not to the patient. If a bellows spirometer is used, it fills during inspiration instead of during expiration, as occurs normally.

### 2. Electrically powered ventilators
### a. Get the necessary equipment for the procedure (NBRC code: IIA6a) [Difficulty: R, Ap]

Most mechanical ventilators are electrically powered or controlled. These primarily function as volume-cycled units, meaning that a preset volume is delivered from the ventilator with each breath regardless of the patient's condition. Each ventilator is unique in its abilities and modes. The scope of this text does not allow discussion of every volume-cycled ventilator, so they are presented in a generic manner. Become familiar with the function of the Servo 300A and other widely used machines.

### b. Put the equipment together and make sure that it works properly (NBRC code: IIA6a) [Difficulty: R, Ap]
### c. Troubleshoot any problems with the equipment (NBRC code: IIA6a) [Difficulty: R, Ap]

The specifics of each ventilator must be learned. The following steps generally should be taken to ensure that the ventilator is functioning properly:

1. Select the proper ventilator for the physician's orders and the patient's needs.
2. Attach the circuit properly, and make sure that all connections are tight (see Fig. 15-12).
3. Select the appropriate humidification device: a passover- or cascade-type bubble humidifier, or HME. Put sterile, distilled water into the passover or cascade-type unit.
4. Preset all physician-ordered parameters and any other settings needed to make the ventilator fully functional.
5. Place a test lung on the circuit at the patient connection.
6. Make sure that the ventilator delivers the preset rate, volume, $O_2$ percentage, and I:E ratio.

A low volume could result from a leak; check all connections, and tighten them as needed. Volume can be measured directly as it leaves the ventilator and at the exhalation valve to help determine the source of the wrong volume. If the unit shows a volume entering the exhalation valve and spirometer instead of the test lung during inspiration, the exhalation valve is broken. All alarms must be working properly. Batteries need to be replaced when discharged.

### 3. Microprocessor ventilators
### a. Get the necessary equipment for the procedure (NBRC code: IIA6a) [Difficulty: R, Ap]

Microprocessor ventilators (e.g., Bennett 7200, Bear 1000, Drager E2 Dura) represent the most advanced generation of mechanical ventilators. These are electrically powered but are controlled by one or more microprocessors (minicomputers). They offer all commonly provided modes of ventilation. In addition, many of these machines offer computer software for measuring bedside spirometry for weaning, WOB, and other parameters that give the clinician much valuable information. Raw, $C_{st}$, and $C_{dyn}$ values can be automatically calculated. Flow, volume, and pressure tracings are graphically displayed on the computer screen. Auto-PEEP can be documented and measured. These units offer the greatest quantity of patient data and the clinical flexibility of all currently available ventilators. The most challenging patients can probably be best cared for on one of these machines.

**b. Put the equipment together and make sure that it works properly** (NBRC code: IIA6a) [Difficulty: R, Ap]

**c. Troubleshoot any problems with the equipment** (NBRC code: IIA6a) [Difficulty: R, Ap]

The previous general discussion about electrically powered ventilators also applies to microprocessor ventilators. An additional advantage of these units is that they self-diagnose most problems and display the problem. If a microprocessor fails, the unit should be removed from the patient. The biomedical department or manufacturer must replace the computer chip.

### 4. Fluidic ventilators

**a. Get the necessary equipment for the procedure** (NBRC code: IIA6a) [Difficulty: R, Ap]

Examples of commonly available fluidic ventilators include the Sechrist IV-100B and the Bio-Med MVP-10. Both are neonatal/pediatric units.

**b. Put the equipment together and make sure that it works properly** (NBRC code: IIA6a) [Difficulty: R, Ap]

Make sure that high-pressure gas hoses between the unit and wall outlets are tightly connected to prevent leaks. The patient circuit and humidification system must be properly installed and operating correctly.

**c. Troubleshoot any problems with the equipment** (NBRC code: IIA6a) [Difficulty: R, Ap]

Typically, fluidic ventilators are pneumatically powered and have fluidic controls. Make sure that the $O_2$ and air sources are up to the required pressure (usually 50 psig). Fluidic controls are very sensitive to any obstruction and to changes in other settings. Make sure that gas inlet and outlet filters are kept clear of obstructions.

### 5. Bilevel/noninvasive positive-pressure ventilators

**a. Get the necessary equipment for the procedure** (NBRC code: IIA2 and IIA6b) [Difficulty: R, Ap]

A bilevel or noninvasive positive-pressure ventilator (NPPV) is intended for an adult patient who is capable of breathing spontaneously. The unit is typically used for a short period with a patient who is having difficulty breathing but who does not need intubation and full ventilatory support. Current ventilators include the Respironics BiPAP S/T series, Respironics BiPAP Vision, Nellcor Puritan-Bennett KnightStar 320, and Healthdyne Quantum PSV.

**b. Put the equipment together and make sure that it works properly** (NBRC code: IIA6b) [Difficulty: R, Ap]

**c. Troubleshoot any problems with the equipment** (NBRC code: IIA6b) [Difficulty: R, Ap]

Follow the manufacturer's guidelines for putting the circuit on the unit and adding a humidification system. In addition, a properly sized nasal mask or full facemask is needed to attach the circuit to the patient. Check carefully for any leakage between the mask and the patient's face.

---

**Exam Hint**

The mask will need to be adjusted or replaced if a leak causes a significant drop in the patient's $V_T$.

---

### 6. Continuous mechanical ventilation and noninvasive ventilation breathing circuits

**a. Get the necessary equipment for the procedure** (NBRC code: IIA11d) [Difficulty: R, Ap]

Either a permanent or a disposable continuous mechanical ventilation (CMV) breathing circuit may be selected based on the type of ventilator on which it must be placed. A circuit with an external exhalation valve must be used with older ventilators, such as the Bennett MA-1 and the Bear 1 and 2. The Puritan-Bennett 7200, Bear 1000, Servo 300A, and other newer ventilators feature internal exhalation valves. If the patient needs to receive aerosolized medications, the circuit should include a nebulizer or should be able to accept one. If not included, the nebulizer or MDI adapter must be added into the inspiratory limb of the circuit.

Also, consider whether an unheated or heated circuit is better to use. Usually, the circuit is unheated. With these, a cascade-type humidifier or HME is used to warm and humidify the inspired gas. However, some practitioners prefer to use a heated circuit in the care of neonates. These circuits have heated wires loosely running through the lumen of the tubing, or they have a wire embedded within the tubing itself. A heated-wire circuit offers finer control over the temperature of the inspired gas and minimizes condensation. Follow the manufacturer's guidelines to make sure that the system can adequately humidify the $\dot{V}_E$ that is being used.

Noninvasive ventilators, such as the Respironics series, have specific circuits designed only for the unit. Traditional ventilator circuits cannot be placed on a noninvasive ventilator.

### b. Put the equipment together and make sure that it works properly (NBRC code: IIA11d) [Difficulty: R, Ap]

Assemble the ventilator circuit with the features needed to manage the patient. Common, but not universal, features of the inspiratory limb of the circuit include a water trap, humidification system, nebulizer, thermometer or temperature probe, pressure monitoring port, and $O_2$ monitoring port. Common, but not universal, features of the expiratory limb of the circuit include an exhalation valve and water trap.

The heated-wire ventilator circuits must be used only with the humidifier with which they are specifically designed to work. The humidifier has a thermostat that regulates warming of the humidifier water and wires heated to the same temperature. Never cover a heated-wire circuit with a patient's sheets or blankets or any other material. Do not rest the circuit on anything such as the bedrail, the patient's body, or medical equipment. These circuits should always be supported on a boom arm or tube tree.

Noninvasive ventilator circuits must be set up as specified for the ventilator. Typically, a heat-moisture exchanger (HME) is added to humidify the patient's tidal volume gas. This is because of the high airway resistance of a wick- or bubble-type humidifier. These ventilators are not powerful enough to provide a stable tidal volume when airway resistance is high.

All circuits use a Y-connector to tie the inspiratory and expiratory limbs together and attach the circuit to the patient. Fig. 15-12 shows a generic ventilator circuit. Make sure that the water level is properly maintained in the humidifier.

### c. Troubleshoot any problems with the continuous ventilation circuit (NBRC code: IIA11d) [Difficulty: R, Ap]

Check the circuit and connections for leaks if the volume returned from the patient is less than what was set or delivered. The set volume should be measured with a handheld spirometer as volume exits the ventilator, at connection points through the circuit, and at the exhalation valve or ventilator spirometer. The volume control or ventilator spirometer may be out of calibration. If the unit shows a volume entering the spirometer instead of the test lung during inspiration, the exhalation valve is broken. Replace a circuit that has a leak or a defective exhalation valve that cannot be fixed. A circuit also needs to be replaced if it is damaged in a way that prevents the patient from being ventilated. This is most commonly seen in circuits with external exhalation valves. If the valve is damaged and cannot close, the circuit needs replacement.

Routine circuit changes are performed for infection control purposes. A circuit that is unclean in appearance (mucus or blood contamination) should be changed. The American Association for Respiratory Care clinical practice guideline on ventilator circuit changes (1994) includes these recommendations:

1. The circuit should be changed every 24 hr if a nebulizer is used for humidification.
2. The circuit may be used for up to 5 days if a cascade- or wick-type humidifier is used for humidification.
3. If an HME is used, it should be changed every 24 hr.

## 7. Ventilator breathing circuits: positive end-expiratory pressure valve assembly

### a. Get the necessary equipment for the procedure (NBRC code: IIA11c) [Difficulty: R, Ap]

A variety of PEEP systems can be added to a ventilator or a CPAP circuit. Consult an equipment book for details of their operation. A number of newer ventilators, such as the Servo 300A and the Puritan-Bennett 7200, have internal exhalation valves and PEEP-generating Venturi systems. No assembly is necessary at the bedside. Failure to generate PEEP indicates that the exhalation valve or the PEEP-generating Venturi system has failed in some manner. Most older ventilators (Bennett MA-1 and Bear 1 and 2) use a balloon-like exhalation valve. A direct relationship exists between the volume of gas kept in the balloon, the pressure and resistance it creates, and the PEEP level generated.

### b. Put the equipment together and make sure that it works properly (NBRC code: IIA11c) [Difficulty: R, Ap]

The key item to be checked with any PEEP-generating system is that the proper level of PEEP is generated and maintained. Once the ordered PEEP level has been set, it should be seen as stable on the pressure manometer throughout the respiratory cycle. The pressure sensitivity control should be set at no greater than $-1$ to $-2$ cm $H_2O$. In this way, the PEEP level is maintained at close to the ordered level, even during an assisted breath. For example, PEEP is set at 10 cm and sensitivity is set at $-1$ cm. Thus, a breath, when triggered by the patient, occurs at 9 cm PEEP.

### c. Troubleshoot any problems with the equipment (NBRC code: IIA11c) [Difficulty: R, Ap]

Malfunctioning internal exhalation valves or PEEP-generating Venturi systems cannot be easily repaired at the bedside. The ventilator needs to be replaced. Balloon-type exhalation valves are prone to the following two problems:

1. The small-bore tube that carries gas from the ventilator to the balloon valve is pulled off. Reconnect the tubing to either the ventilator nipple connection or the exhalation valve nipple connection.

2. The balloon is torn and the gas leaks out. This can be confirmed by disassembling the exhalation valve assembly. Replace the balloon and reassemble the exhalation valve.

Both of the problems just mentioned demonstrate themselves when the inspiratory $V_T$ flows past the patient and directly into the exhaled $V_T$ spirometer. Little or no airway pressure is generated. The patient is poorly ventilated (if at all). This problem must be corrected immediately while the patient is being manually ventilated.

### 8. Continuous positive-airway pressure systems: breathing circuits

#### a. Get the necessary equipment for the procedure (NBRC code: IIA11c) [Difficulty: R, Ap]

Most current-generation ventilators have a built-in CPAP mode. No additional circuitry is needed. After a switch is made to the CPAP mode, the desired level should be set by adjusting the PEEP/CPAP dial, and the reading on the pressure manometer should be watched.

Several manufacturers make CPAP systems for home use in the treatment of patients with obstructive sleep apnea. These CPAP systems typically include an air pump to generate flow to the patient, CPAP generating device, circuit designed to work with the system, patient mask(s), and alarm system.

Free-standing CPAP breathing circuits used in hospitals vary considerably. No manufacturer has developed a system that dominates the marketplace. Each respiratory care department usually develops its own breathing circuit to meet its own needs.

#### b. Put the equipment together and make sure that it works properly (NBRC code: IIA11c) [Difficulty: R, Ap]

Fig. 15-15 shows the typical components used in a CPAP breathing circuit. These components include the following:

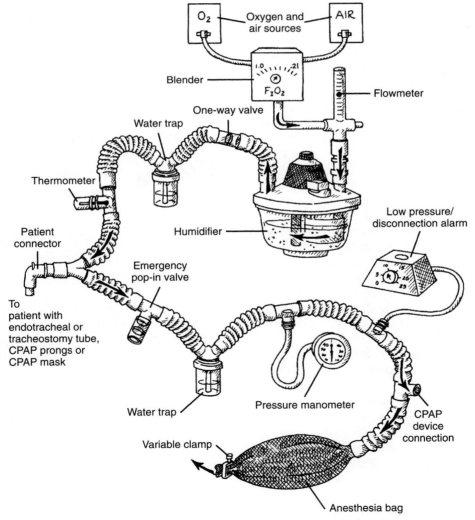

**Fig. 15-15** Patient breathing circuit for continuous positive-airway pressure (CPAP).

1. Air/$O_2$ blender
2. Pediatric or adult flowmeter on the blender
3. Cascade-type bubble humidifier or wick-type humidifier
4. Inspiratory circuit of large-bore/aerosol tubing with the following additions: water trap, one-way valve, and thermometer
5. Y-connector to connect the inspiratory and expiratory limbs of the circuit
6. Patient connector (elbow adapter) to endotracheal/tracheostomy tube, CPAP prongs, or CPAP mask
7. Expiratory circuit of large-bore/aerosol tubing with the following additions: water trap, high-pressure pop-off valve (not shown), pressure manometer for measuring the CPAP level, low-pressure/disconnection audible alarm, anesthesia bag as a reservoir, variable resistance clamp on the tail of the anesthesia bag, Briggs adapters/T-pieces for connecting the various features, emergency pop-in valve in case gas flow is stopped, and CPAP device

The CPAP level is adjusted by means of a variety of devices collectively called *threshold resistors*, which include the following:

1. A column of water with a length of expiratory tubing inserted to the needed depth below the surface.
2. A vertically mounted ball bearing, which creates resistance as gas flows up past it. These ball-bearing resistors come in weights of 2.5, 5, and 10 cm $H_2O$.
3. A spring-loaded resistor (Downs CPAP generator) that is adjusted for application of the desired CPAP level against the airway.
4. A free-standing Venturi PEEP system. Gas from the Venturi jet creates backpressure against the escaping patient $V_T$.

Air exits through each of these devices when they are working properly. All CPAP systems must be adjusted by checking the pressure level on the manometer. Set the low-pressure/disconnection audible alarm to sound at a few centimeters below the CPAP level. For example, if 10 cm $H_2O$ CPAP is ordered, set the alarm to sound if the pressure drops to below 8 cm $H_2O$ of CPAP.

### c. Troubleshoot any problems with the equipment (NBRC code: IIA11c) [Difficulty: R, Ap]

1. Flow through the CPAP breathing circuit must be sufficient to meet the patient's needs. Adjust the flowmeter setting and clamp on the anesthesia bag so that it is somewhat inflated with excess air escaping out past the clamp. With all of these devices, gas escapes through the path of least resistance. All or some may escape through the anesthesia bag, CPAP device, or both. The bag should collapse somewhat during the patient's inspiration and should expand somewhat during expiration. The CPAP level should not drop more than 1 or 2 cm $H_2O$ from baseline during an inspiration.
2. Make sure that the water level is properly maintained in the humidifier. Fill it with sterile, distilled water as needed.
3. A sudden drop in the CPAP level to zero indicates a disconnection at the patient or somewhere in the breathing circuit. Check all connections, and reassemble the break. The patient may need to be manually ventilated while the problem is corrected.
4. If the CPAP level drops more than 2 cm $H_2O$ during an inspiration, the flow is inadequate and should be increased. Flow is also inadequate if the patient shows an increased use of accessory muscles of respiration or complains of increased WOB. Too high a flow is indicated by an inadvertently high level of CPAP or by the patient's complaining of difficulty in exhalation.
5. Water column systems must be frequently monitored because of water loss caused by evaporation. The actual CPAP level is progressively less than desired as the water is gradually lost. This system must regularly have water added to it, or the expiratory tubing must be inserted more deeply to keep the desired CPAP level.
6. The ball-bearing resistor system must be mounted vertically for gravity to keep the desired weight against the circuit. If it falls over and is horizontal, CPAP pressure will be lost.

---

**Exam Hint**

**B**e prepared to troubleshoot problems with a CPAP system that is losing pressure or leaking through a CPAP mask or prongs. If the CPAP pressure is fluctuating with the patient's breathing cycle, the flow may need to be increased.

---

9. **Continuous positive-airway pressure systems: masks**

a. **Get the necessary equipment for the procedure** (NBRC code: IIA2) [Difficulty: R, Ap]

A CPAP mask and breathing circuit are primarily used for patients who have obstructive sleep apnea. CPAP, by means of the mask, forces the soft tissues open to the point that the airway is never obstructed (see Fig. 15-13). The patient is now able to sleep normally and remain oxygenated. The patient should have the CPAP mask, breathing circuit, and proper CPAP level determined by a sleep study in the hospital. The patient can use the system at home once it has been set up properly and he or she has been trained in its use.

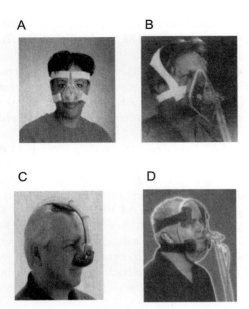

**Fig. 15-16** Types of masks used to deliver continuous positive airway pressure (CPAP) or noninvasive positive pressure ventilation (NPPV). **A,** Nasal mask designed to cover the entire nose. **B,** Full face mask (oronasal mask) designed to cover the nose and mouth. **C,** Nasal pillows that fit into the nostrils. **D,** Total face mask that covers the entire facial area. The key elements for consideration in the decision of which mask should be used are patient fit without leaks and comfort. (**B** From Hill NS: Complications of noninvasive positive pressure ventilation, *Respir Care* 42:432–442, 1997. **A, C,** and **D** from Hess DR, Kacmarek RM: Essentials of mechanical ventilation, ed 2, New York, 2002, McGraw-Hill.)

In recent years, a CPAP mask has been used with a non-invasive mechanical ventilator to temporarily assist the breathing of a patient with respiratory distress. The hope is to support the patient's breathing long enough to treat the underlying problem(s). If this is successful, the patient does not need to be intubated. These patients require careful assessment and monitoring.

The two main categories of CPAP masks are available in different sizes for children older than 3 years of age to adults. See Fig. 15-16 for examples. Nasal mask and nasal pillow systems are designed to cover only the nose. These allow the patient to speak and offer the mouth as a second airway for breathing in case a malfunction occurs in the CPAP system. The mouth also acts as a pressure-relief route if CPAP pressure becomes too great. Pressures of up to 15 cm $H_2O$ can usually be maintained in an adult. Pressures of up to 10 cm $H_2O$ can usually be maintained in a child.

Full face mask and total face mask systems are designed to cover the nose and mouth. These are transparent and similar to the mask used during bag-mask ventilation. The facemask must be used if the patient has persistent mouth breathing and cannot use a nasal mask. With a good seal, pressures of greater than 15 cm $H_2O$ can be maintained.

All types of CPAP mask have a soft, compliant seal that closely fits the contours of the face. This mask must properly fit the patient's face; straps are needed to hold the mask in place.

### b. Put the equipment together and make sure that it works properly (NBRC code: IIA2) [Difficulty: R, Ap]

Several companies manufacture mask CPAP systems for home care. These relatively simple circuits do not have a humidification system or other attachments seen in the hospital. Check the manufacturer's literature for specific directions on the circuit's application to the patient. Any mask CPAP system must be able to generate enough flow to meet the patient's $\dot{V}_E$ and peak flow needs. The CPAP level must be stable throughout the breathing cycle.

### c. Troubleshoot any problems with the equipment (NBRC code: IIA2) [Difficulty: R, Ap]

Too large a mask does not seal and allows gas to leak, which causes decreased CPAP pressure on the manometer. The patient may show increased snoring or airway obstruction with periods of apnea. Too small a mask or a misfitting mask could cause an uneven distribution of pressure on the face, which could lead to abrasions or pressure sores and ulcers on the face.

A sudden drop in CPAP level to zero indicates a disconnection at the patient or somewhere in the breathing circuit. Check all connections and reassemble the break if needed. If the CPAP level drops more than 2 cm $H_2O$ during inspiration, the flow is inadequate and should be increased. Flow is also inadequate if the patient shows an increased use of accessory muscles of respiration or complains of increased WOB. Too high a flow is seen by an inadvertently high level of CPAP or the patient reporting difficulty with exhalation.

### 10. Continuous positive-airway pressure systems: nasopharyngeal tube and nasal prongs

### a. Get the necessary equipment for the procedure (NBRC code: IIA2) [Difficulty: R, Ap]

Nasal CPAP devices are used extensively with neonates. These infants commonly have been born prematurely and have RDS. Their immature lungs lack sufficient surfactant and need CPAP treatment to keep the alveoli open. Often, nasal CPAP meets the patient's needs so that endotracheal intubation and mechanical ventilation can be avoided. Nasal CPAP works with neonates because they are obligate nose breathers.

Nasal CPAP therapy is associated with the hazards of gastric distention and reflux aspiration. These occur when

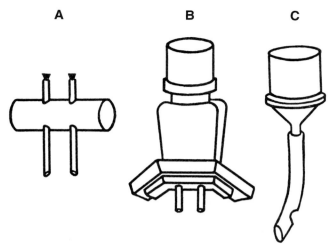

**Fig. 15-17** Nasal continuous positive-airway pressure (CPAP) devices for infants. **A,** Jackson-Reese tubes. **B,** Argyle nasal cannula (prongs). **C,** Endotracheal tube cut shorter for nasopharyngeal insertion (NP tube). *(From Blodgett D: Manual of pediatric respiratory care procedures, Philadelphia, 1982, Lippincott.)*

the airway pressure forces air into the stomach. A gastric tube is usually inserted to vent the air.

### 1. Nasopharyngeal tube

A nasopharyngeal tube is actually an endotracheal tube that has been cut shorter (Fig. 15-17, **C**). Select the largest possible tube that is still easy to insert into the patient. Estimate the needed length by laying the tube along the patient's face and measuring from the ear lobe to the tip of the chin. It is inserted into either naris and is advanced until the tip can be seen behind the uvula. This position can be confirmed by x-ray films of the chest and upper airway. The tube marking for length at the nostril should be recorded.

### 2. Nasal prongs

Nasal prongs come in short and long versions (see Fig. 15-17, **A** and **B**). Both types involve prongs that fit into both nostrils. These prongs are available in different diameters so that the proper size can be found to fit the ID of the infant's nares. Short prongs are inserted 0.5 to 1.0 cm.

### b. Put the equipment together and make sure that it works properly (NBRC code: IIA2) [Difficulty: R, Ap]

All of these patient connection devices fit either into the elbow adapter on the CPAP breathing circuit or directly into the circuit if the Y is removed. All must be secured to the patient in some fashion. A nasopharyngeal tube or long nasal prongs that extend beyond the nose usually need to be taped or tied similar to an endotracheal tube. If the patient is lying quietly, no securing may be needed. Short nasal prongs usually need a securing device because these are easily dislodged from the nostrils.

### c. Troubleshoot any problems with the equipment (NBRC code: IIA2) [Difficulty: R, Ap]

A sudden drop in the CPAP level to zero indicates a disconnection at the patient or somewhere in the breathing circuit. Check all connections, and reassemble the break. The patient may need to be manually ventilated while the problem is corrected.

If the CPAP level drops more than 2 cm $H_2O$ during inspiration, the flow is inadequate and should be increased. Flow is also inadequate if the patient shows an increased use of accessory muscles of respiration or appears to have an increased WOB. Too high a flow is shown by a high level of CPAP or by the appearance of the patient's having difficulty exhaling. A common problem with small-diameter tubes like these is mucus plugging. A plugged tube causes gas to back up and CPAP values to increase, as shown on the manometer. The patient would show distress at the increased WOB. The clinician should suction to clear out the mucus plug, or remove the tube and place a new one.

A pressure of about 10 cm $H_2O$ is usually possible; excessive pressure is vented out of the mouth. Try to prevent the infant from crying because this causes pressure loss.

---

**Exam Hint**

**I**f a newborn infant is receiving 10 cm $H_2O$ CPAP and 50% $O_2$ or more and remains hypoxemic, mechanical ventilation is indicated.

---

### 11. Humidifiers: passover-, cascade-type, bubble, wick

#### a. Get the necessary equipment for the procedure (NBRC code: IIA3) [Difficulty: R, Ap]

#### b. Put the equipment together and make sure that it works properly (NBRC code: IIA3) [Difficulty: R, Ap]

A general discussion of this equipment is presented in Chapter 8. See Figs. 15-12 and 15-15 for setups in ventilator and CPAP breathing circuits, respectively. Both types are capable of providing 100% relative humidity. Passover-type systems are preferred with neonates.

The humidifier's temperature is usually maintained at between 31° C and 35°C. Normally, the temperature should never be greater than 37°C at the patient's airway. (The exception is a hypothermic patient. Inhaled gas that is warmed to a few degrees above normal body temperature speeds up the rewarming process.)

Typically, a temperature probe is added into the inspiratory limb of the circuit near the Y. If a heated-wire circuit is being used with an infant, the temperature probe should be placed outside of the incubator and away from a radiant warmer's direct heat. The humidifier should provide at least 30 mg/L of water vapor.

Ensure that the water level is kept within the recommended range to properly humidify the gas. Avoid being sprayed with any circuit water during disconnections from the patient. It is considered contaminated and should be disposed of similarly to any other contaminated fluid from the patient.

### c. Troubleshoot any problems with the equipment (NBRC code: IIA3) [Difficulty: R, Ap]

A loose connection at the humidifier (or anywhere else in the circuit) causes a loss of volume or pressure to the patient. Check the entire circuit. When the leak is fixed, the volume or pressure is restored. The humidifier should warm to the desired temperature; do not use a humidifier that does not warm properly.

## 12. Humidifiers: heat-moisture exchangers
### a. Get the necessary equipment for the procedure (NBRC code: IIA3) [Difficulty: R, Ap]

A heat-moisture exchanger (HME) is designed to be warmed by the patient's exhaled breath and to absorb water vapor from the gas. The next inspired volume is then humidified by evaporation. The key element in the exchanger is a hygroscopic filter medium. Under ideal conditions, these units can achieve up to 70% to 90% body humidity. They should minimally provide 30 mg/L of water at 30°C. Consider the following when you select an HME:

1. Select a unit with the smallest possible dead space volume. Watch for an increase in the patient's $PaCO_2$ if the HME adds too much dead space or the patient's $V_T$ is too small.
2. Pick the unit that provides the greatest percentage of body humidity. Do not use one that cannot meet the minimal standards described previously.
3. If the patient has had a known pulmonary infection, select an HME that is also a bacteria filter.
4. Should the unit be disposable or reusable? Staffing, infection control, and equipment processing considerations make a difference in the choice of which unit should be used.

### b. Put the equipment together and make sure that it works properly (NBRC code: IIA3) [Difficulty: R, Ap]

Most of these units are preassembled by the manufacturer with nothing to add. A length of large-bore/aerosol tubing or an elbow adapter may need to be attached to make the unit fit onto the Y or endotracheal tube. All come with standard 15- or 22-mm connector ends. Air should flow easily through them with little resistance (see Fig. 15-14).

### c. Troubleshoot any problems with the equipment (NBRC code: IIA3) [Difficulty: R, Ap]

Any disconnections can be easily noticed and reconnected. Replace any unit that has a mucus plug or other debris that obstructs the channel. This might be demonstrated by a sudden rise in the patient's peak airway pressure. Typically, HME units are replaced every 24 hr.

> **Exam Hint**
>
> **A**n HME becomes obstructed when secretions are coughed into it. This will be shown as a rapid increase in peak pressure seen during an inspiration. Remove the obstructed HME. Replace it, or change to a cascade-type humidifier.

## 13. Perform quality control procedures on mechanical ventilators (NBRC code: IIC3) [Difficulty: R]

Follow the manufacturer's guidelines for quality control procedures on a mechanical ventilator. These may include checking for accurate flow, volume delivery, and pressure readings. Microprocessor ventilators usually provide a software package that performs self-diagnostic tests on the unit. Obviously, the ventilator should deliver the set volume, flow, and pressure. Do not use a unit that fails a quality control check.

### MODULE D

**Evaluate and monitor the patient's response to mechanical ventilation**

### 1. Observe the patient for signs of patient-ventilator dyssynchrony (NBRC code: IIIE6) [Difficulty: R, Ap]

Because a patient with an intubated airway cannot speak, simple questions that can be answered with a nod or a shake of the head must be asked. A pad of paper and pencil or picture boards can be used as well.

The issue of a patient's emotional reaction to illness is discussed in Chapter 1. A patient's reaction to the initiation of mechanical ventilation or its prolonged need cannot be predicted. Some patients react with relief and relax when the work of breathing is reduced. Some become angry at the limitations imposed on them; others become depressed. As a result, some patients will try to breathe in faster than is allowed by the inspiratory flow that is set on the ventilator. Note the significant negative pressure on the manometer. If the patient coughs during a breath, the manometer pressure will rapidly swing from negative to positive.

### 2. Measure the tidal volume (NBRC code: IIIE8) [Difficulty: R, Ap]

The patient's exhaled $V_T$ is usually measured and recorded in his or her chart. Many newer ventilators also display an

---

**BOX 15-4  Indications That the Patient Can Probably Be Weaned from the Ventilator**

**OXYGENATION**
- $PaO_2 \geq 80$ torr or $SpO_2 > 90\%$ on $50\%$ $O_2$ or less
- $P(A - a)O_2 < 300$–$350$ torr on $100\%$ $O_2$
- Intrapulmonary shunt of less than 15%

**VENTILATION**
- $PaCO_2 < 55$ torr in a patient who is not ordinarily hypercapnic
- $V_D/V_T$ ratio $< 0.55$–$0.6$ (55%–60%)
- Rapid, shallow breathing index (breaths/minute ÷ tidal volume in liters) $< 105$

**PULMONARY MECHANICS**
- Spontaneous $V_T$ of 3–4 mL/lb or 7–9 mL/kg of ideal body weight
- VC of at least 10–15 mL/kg
- MIP $> -20$ to $-25$ cm $H_2O$
- $FEV_1 > 10$ mL/kg
- Respiratory rate of 12–35 breaths/min (adult)

**MISCELLANEOUS**
- Conscious and cooperative patient who wants to breathe spontaneously
- Stable and acceptable normal blood pressure and temperature
- Stable cardiac rhythm; heart rate should not increase by more than 15%–20%
- Corrected underlying problem that led to ventilatory support
- Normal fluid balance and electrolyte values
- Proper nutritional status

---

$FEV_1$, forced expiratory volume in 1 sec; MIP, maximal inspiratory pressure; $PaO_2$, arterial $O_2$ pressure; $P(A - a)O_2$, difference in the partial pressure of $O_2$ in alveolar gas and arterial blood; $SpO_2$, pulse oximetry; VC, vital capacity; $V_D/V_T$, dead space/tidal volume.

---

inhaled and exhaled $V_T$. Compare the two volumes, if possible. If they do not match closely, check for a leak or other reason for the difference. The patient on an IMV, SIMV, or PSV mode should have both machine-delivered and spontaneous $V_T$s measured and recorded.

The weaning patient needs to have his or her spontaneous $V_T$ measured along with the VC. These and other parameters are used to judge weanability (discussed later; Box 15-4 offers additional information).

### 3. Measure the respiratory rate (NBRC code: IIIE8) [Difficulty: R, Ap]

Count and record the machine-delivered respiratory rate. If the patient is on IMV, SIMV, or PSV, count and record both machine and spontaneous rates. The weaning patient should have his or her spontaneous rate counted and recorded.

**TABLE 15-1  Time Variables in Mechanical Ventilation**

| Term | Symbol | Formula for calculation |
|---|---|---|
| Frequency (rate) | $f$ | Count breaths/min or $\dfrac{60}{t_I + t_E}$ |
| Cycle time | $t_I + t_E$ | Add $t_I + t_E$ or $\dfrac{60}{f}$ |
| Inspiratory time | $t_I$ (I) | $t_I = \dfrac{60}{f} - t_E$ or $t_I = \%t_I \times (t_I + t_E)$ |
| Expiratory time | $t_E$ (E) | $t_E = \dfrac{60}{f} - t_I$ |
| Inspiratory:expiratory ratio | I:E or $t_I/t_E$ | $I:E = \dfrac{t_I}{t_E}$, usually numerator |
| Percent inspiratory time | $\%t_I$ | $\%t_I = \dfrac{t_I}{t_I + t_E} \times 100$ |

From Scanlan CL: Physics and physiology or ventilatory support. In Scanlan CL, Spearman CB, Sheldon RL, editors: *Egan's fundamentals of respiratory care*, ed 5, St Louis, 1990, Mosby.

### 4. Measure the inspiratory:expiratory ratio (NBRC code: IIIE8) [Difficulty: R, Ap]

The I:E ratio should be calculated and recorded. Some newer ventilators display it, whereas others show inspiratory time and expiratory time. The I:E ratio can then be calculated (Table 15-1).

### 5. Measure airway pressures (NBRC code: IIIE8) [Difficulty: R, Ap]

Peak pressure (or $P_{peak}$): The peak pressure reached during the delivery of a $V_T$ is the pressure needed to push the gas through the circuit, the endotracheal tube, and the patient's airways to expand the lungs. The sigh volume necessitates greater pressure because it is a larger volume. These pressures should be recorded regularly whenever the patient and machine are checked. The importance of peak pressure in calculating $C_{dyn}$ is discussed earlier in the chapter.

Plateau pressure (or $P_{plat}$): The plateau pressure occurs when the $V_T$ has been delivered to the lungs and is temporarily held within them. The importance of plateau pressure in calculating $C_{st}$ is discussed earlier in the chapter.

Baseline pressure: The baseline pressure is the pressure measured at the end of exhalation. Normally, it is seen as zero on the ventilator's pressure manometer. (Remember that in this case, "zero" is actually local barometric pressure.) If the patient has therapeutic PEEP or CPAP, the baseline pressure will be greater than zero.

### 6. Monitor mean airway pressure (NBRC code: IIIE8) [Difficulty: R, Ap]

Mean airway pressure is the average pressure over an entire breathing cycle. Most newer ventilators display a mean airway pressure. This pressure results from changes in the patient's peak and baseline pressures plus the I:E ratio.

### 7. Measure the patient's inspired oxygen percentage (NBRC code: IIIE9) [Difficulty: R]

Most ventilators have very accurate $O_2$ delivery systems. However, standard practice requires use of a calibrated, external $O_2$ analyzer. If the patient is receiving IMV with an added flow system, it too should be analyzed. Make sure that the ventilator and the added IMV gas have the same, ordered $O_2$ percentage.

### 8. Test the alarm systems, and adjust them as needed (NBRC code: IIIE8, IIIG3g) [Difficulty: R, Ap]

All alarm systems must function properly, so test all audible and visual alarms. The practitioner should be familiar with the most widely used adult and infant ventilators and their alarm systems. It is common practice to set most alarms at ±10% from the set value. For example,

a. The $V_T$ is 1000 mL. Set the low-volume alarm at 900 mL and the high-volume alarm at 1100 mL.
b. The $\dot{V}_E$ is 10,000 mL. Set the high-volume alarm at 11,000 mL and the low-volume alarm at 9000 mL.
c. The $O_2$ percentage is set at 40%. Set the high-percentage alarm at 45% and the low-percentage alarm at 35%.
d. The low-pressure/disconnection alarm is set to sound if the ventilator-delivered pressure is about 5 cm $H_2O$ below the peak pressure. For example, if the peak pressure has been about 40 cm $H_2O$, the low-pressure/disconnection alarm should be set at 35 cm $H_2O$. If a leak or disconnection occurs, the alarm will sound when the peak pressure does not reach 35 cm $H_2O$. If the patient is on a CPAP system, the low-pressure/disconnection alarm should be set to sound if the pressure drops to about 2 cm $H_2O$ below the set level. For example, if the patient is on 10 cm $H_2O$ CPAP, the alarm should be set to alarm if the pressure drops to less than 8 cm $H_2O$.

Many types of alarms have a timer that can be set to delay the time that the alarm sounds. If the alarm is on a ventilator, this delay should be set at about 3 to 5 sec longer than the cycling time. For example, if the patient has a backup rate of 10 breaths/min, the cycling time between mandatory breaths would be 6 sec. Set the timer to delay the sounding of the alarm for about 10 sec. Thus, if the patient is disconnected from the ventilator and the peak pressure does not reach 35 cm $H_2O$, the alarm will sound in 10 sec. If the patient is on a CPAP system, the timer may be set for no delay or for a short delay. Adjust all alarms to fit the clinical setting and the patient's condition. Some

may need tighter limits, and others may need wider limits, than those just discussed.

### 9. Monitor the cuff pressure to the patient's endotracheal or tracheostomy tube (NBRC code: IIIB5a and IIIE10) [Difficulty: R, Ap]

Monitoring of cuff pressure is presented in Chapter 12; review this if necessary.

### 10. Auscultate the patient's chest and interpret the breath sounds (NBRC code: IIIE11) [Difficulty: R, Ap]

Auscultation of the patient's chest and interpretation of breath sounds are presented in Chapter 1; review this if necessary.

### 11. Interpret arterial blood gas results (NBRC code: IIIE4) [Difficulty: R, Ap]

An arterial blood gas sample should be obtained after every significant change that occurs in the ventilator settings. These include changes in the inspired oxygen percentage, rate, tidal volume, and PEEP level. Interpretation of the ABG results provides vital information for guidance with further ventilator changes.

> **Exam Hint**
>
> Expect to see many arterial blood gas values incorporated into questions about adjusting the ventilator. Hypoxemia should be treated by an increased oxygen percentage or an increased PEEP level. As the patient improves, these can be reduced. If the patient's carbon dioxide level is too high, increase either the rate or the tidal volume. If too much carbon dioxide is blown off, decrease either the rate or the tidal volume.

### MODULE E
**Recommend modifications or independently make modifications in mechanical ventilation based on the patient's response**

### 1. Recommend a change or independently change the type of mechanical ventilator (NBRC code: IIIG3i and IIIF2h9) [Difficulty: R, Ap, An]

Selection of the appropriate type of mechanical ventilator was discussed earlier in this chapter. Briefly, a pressure-cycled unit can be used with a patient without cardiopulmonary disease. Most patients with conditions that cause abnormal Raw or $C_{LT}$ should be placed on electrically powered, volume-cycled units. Microprocessor ventilators offer a greater number of ventilating options and improved monitoring of clinical information; these are the best choice for the most critical patients. Noninvasive ventilation and negative-pressure ventilation are used with patients who do not need intubation and who have some ability to breathe for themselves.

Be prepared to change from one type of ventilator to another as the patient's condition warrants. A malfunctioning ventilator should be replaced with one that is capable of providing the same level of ventilatory support.

## 2. Recommend a change or independently change the ventilator breathing circuit (NBRC code: IIIG3i and IIIF2h9) [Difficulty: R, Ap, An]

Changing of circuits was discussed earlier in this chapter. Briefly, change a circuit that has a leak or is contaminated. Routine changes are performed for infection control purposes.

## 3. Change the type of humidification equipment (NBRC code: IIIF2f2) [Difficulty: R, Ap]

A heat-moisture exchanger (HME) is indicated in the following situations:

a. The patient has few, if any, secretions.
b. The patient will probably be weaned from the ventilator within 96 hr.
c. The patient is being transported on mechanical ventilation.

An HME is contraindicated in the following situations:

a. The patient has thick, bloody, or copious secretions.
b. The patient has a large air leak such that the exhaled volume is less than 70% of the inhaled $V_T$. This causes a relatively dry hygroscopic filter. (Patients with uncuffed equipment or with torn cuffs on their endotracheal tubes or large bronchopleural fistulas would have large $V_T$ leaks.)
c. The patient's temperature is lower than 32°C.
d. The patient's spontaneous $\dot{V}_E$ is greater than 10 L/min.
e. Always remove the HME when nebulized medications are delivered through the circuit.

A cascade-type bubble humidifier is indicated in these situations:

a. The patient has thick or copious secretions. An increase in the amount or thickness of secretions or a change from white to yellow or green justifies the switch to a cascade-type humidifier.
b. The patient will probably require mechanical ventilation for longer than 96 hr.
c. The patient cannot have mechanical dead space added to the breathing circuit. If the patient's (especially a child's) $V_T$ is smaller than the HME's dead space, the HME should not be used. IMV systems typically are set up without mechanical dead space, so an HME should not be used.
d. An HME should not be used with a patient who is receiving very large $V_T$s because the filter's ability to

hold moisture will be exceeded and the patient will breathe in some dry air. Check the manufacturer's literature for the maximal recommended $V_T$.

e. If the patient has a large air leak, as is seen with a deflated cuff or a bronchopleural fistula, an HME should not be used. With a large air leak, more air is inspired than expired and the exchanger cannot fully humidify the inspired $V_T$.

## 4. Enhance oxygenation
### a. Make a recommendation to change the oxygen percentage (NBRC code: IIIG3b) [Difficulty: R, Ap]
### b. Change the oxygen percentage (NBRC code: IIIF2d1) [Difficulty: R, Ap]

As has been discussed earlier, the goal of $O_2$ administration is to keep the $PaO_2$ level of most patients between 60 and 90 torr and the $SpO_2$ level greater than 90%. Exceptions are patients who are breathing on hypoxic drive and who are in a cardiac arrest situation. The patient with COPD who has a chronically low $PaO_2$ level and a chronically high $PaCO_2$ level may be allowed to have a $PaO_2$ value as low as 50 to 55 torr and an $SpO_2$ value as low as 85%. The patient who is extremely hypoxic must be given up to 100% $O_2$. Those patients who have refractory hypoxemia (e.g., ARDS) do not respond with a normal increase in the $PaO_2$ level as the $O_2$ percentage is increased.

## 5. Ventilator graphics
### a. Make a recommendation to change the ventilator settings based on ventilator graphics (NBRC code: IIIG3h) [Difficulty: R, Ap]
### b. Change the ventilator settings based on ventilator graphics (NBRC code: IIIF2h8) [Difficulty: R, Ap, An]

See the discussion on pages 276 and 310.

## 6. Tidal volume
### a. Make a recommendation to change the tidal volume (NBRC code: IIIG3c) [Difficulty: R, Ap]
### b. Change the tidal volume (NBRC code: IIIF2h3) [Difficulty: R, Ap, An]

The specific $V_T$ to be selected was discussed earlier in this chapter. Conditions in which the $V_T$ should be increased include atelectasis, consolidation, and situations in which the present $V_T$ is at the small end of the normal range and the patient has an elevated $CO_2$ level. The NBRC uses the upper level for a set $V_T$ in an adult of 15 mL/kg of ideal body weight. Conditions in which the $V_T$ should be decreased include air trapping, hyperinflated lungs as seen on the chest x-ray film by wide intercostal margins or flattened hemidiaphragms, and situations in which the present $V_T$ is at the large end of the normal range and the patient has a decreased $CO_2$ level. The NBRC uses the lower level for a set $V_T$ in an adult of 10 mL/kg of ideal body weight.

An additional consideration is whether to give the patient a sigh breath, which represents a volume larger than the normal $V_T$. People normally sigh every few minutes. This serves the purpose of opening up atelectatic alveoli and reorienting the surfactant in the alveoli so that they are stable. A sigh breath is usually given only to a patient in the assist/control (A/C) mode.

Most patients who are being ventilated in the A/C mode receive a ventilator sigh volume just as they do a $V_T$. A sigh volume is typically 1.5 to 2 times the $V_T$ if the $V_T$ is in the low to middle range of normal. If the patient has a problem of atelectasis or consolidation, a larger sigh volume may be indicated. The patient may not need a sigh volume if the set $V_T$ is at the 15-mL/kg upper limit. A patient with bullous emphysema, pneumothorax, or cardiac status that is sensitive to high peak pressures may be contraindicated for a sigh volume. The patient with air trapping of the $V_T$ should have a smaller (possibly no) sigh volume. Compare the inspired and expired volumes to ensure that no air trapping exists. Most current ventilators allow the clinician to tailor the sigh frequency to best meet the patient's clinical needs. The sigh frequency should be increased in patients with atelectasis or consolidation. The sigh frequency may need to be decreased or eliminated in patients who are air-trapping the $V_T$ or sigh volume. Sighs are usually not given when the patient is in the IMV/SIMV mode.

### 7. Respiratory rate
   **a. Make a recommendation to change the respiratory rate (NBRC code: IIIG3c) [Difficulty: R, Ap]**
   **b. Change the respiratory rate (NBRC code: IIIF2h3) [Difficulty: R, Ap, An]**

Respiratory rate selection has been discussed earlier in this section. Increase the backup rate on the ventilator if the patient has an elevated $CO_2$ level and the $V_T$ is at the high end of the normal range. Decrease the backup rate on the ventilator if the patient has a decreased $CO_2$ level and the $V_T$ is at the low end of the normal range.

### 8. Make a recommendation to change inspiratory effort (sensitivity) to improve patient synchrony (NBRC code: IIIG3a) [Difficulty: R, Ap]

Sensitivity has been discussed earlier in this chapter. If the patient seems to be working too hard to trigger a ventilator breath, make a recommendation to increase the sensitivity. Be careful to avoid making the ventilator so sensitive that it self-cycles.

### 9. Monitor and adjust the alarm settings (NBRC code: IIIF2h7) [Difficulty: R, Ap]

Alarm settings have been discussed earlier in this chapter. Be prepared to adjust the alarm settings based on the patient's clinical situation.

### 10. Make a recommendation to change the mechanical dead space (NBRC code: IIIG3j) [Difficulty: R]

Mechanical dead space is added to make the patient rebreathe gas from his or her anatomic dead space for the purpose of increasing the patient's $PaCO_2$ level. This high-$CO_2$ gas is then inhaled back to the alveolar level, which increases the patient's $PaCO_2$ level. Mechanical dead space is created by inserting a length of large-bore/aerosol tubing into the breathing circuit between the Y and the patient's endotracheal or tracheostomy tube (see Fig. 15-14). The more dead space tubing is used, the greater the amount of $CO_2$ that is retained. It is important to realize that this same rebreathed volume of gas is lower in $O_2$ because of its diffusion into the patient's pulmonary circulation. If a large amount of mechanical dead space is added, the $F_1O_2$ will need to be increased to keep the ordered level. Measure the $O_2$ percentage between the dead space and the endotracheal or tracheostomy tube adapter.

Mechanical dead space is used only in the control and A/C modes; it should not be used in IMV/SIMV, PSV, or CPAP modes. The following formula can be used to predict what amount of *mechanical dead space* ($Vd_{mech}$) produces a desired $PaCO_2$ level:

$$[(V_T - V_{D\,anat}) - V_{D\,mech}] \times f \times PaCO_2$$
$$= [(V_T - V_{D\,anat}) - V_{D\,mech}'] \times f \times PaCO_2'$$

### EXAMPLE

Use the same patient conditions listed earlier when a change in $V_T$ was calculated. The solution to this problem is to increase the patient's mechanical dead space from zero to 212 mL.

### 11. Mode of ventilation
   **a. Make a recommendation to change the mode of ventilation to improve patient synchrony (NBRC code: IIIG3a) [Difficulty: R, Ap]**
   **b. Change the mode of ventilation to improve patient synchrony (NBRC code: IIIF2h1) [Difficulty: R, Ap, An]**

Changing the mode of ventilation was discussed earlier in this chapter. Be prepared to change the mode as the patient's condition varies. A patient who is apneic can be placed on the assist/control mode. A patient with an acceptable spontaneous tidal volume can be placed on the synchronous intermittent mandatory ventilation mode. Pressure support can be added to any mode to reduce the patient's work of breathing.

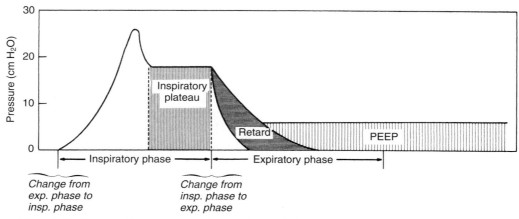

**Fig. 15-18** Pressure-time waveform showing how exhalation can be modified. An inspiratory plateau (inflation hold) is seen when the tidal volume is held within the lungs for a certain period. With expiratory retard, the gas is more slowly exhaled than during a passive breath. These two modifications of exhalation may or may not be combined with PEEP. *(From Kirby RR, Smith RA, Desautels DA: Mechanical ventilation. In Burton GG, Hodgkin JE, editors: Respiratory care: a guide to clinical practice, ed 2, Philadelphia, 1984, Lippincott.)*

## 12. Positive end-expiratory pressure (PEEP) therapy

**a. Make a recommendation to change the level of PEEP to improve oxygenation (NBRC code: IIIG3b) [Difficulty: R, Ap]**

**b. Change the level of PEEP to improve oxygenation (NBRC code: IIIF2h2) [Difficulty: R, Ap, An]**

PEEP therapy has been discussed earlier in this chapter. Remember that therapeutic PEEP is indicated for situations in which the patient has bilaterally small lungs with a reduced FRC. This causes hypoxemia. The proper level of PEEP restores the FRC and improves oxygenation. Watch for adverse effects of barotrauma or decreased cardiac output from too much pressure. The patient should be carefully monitored with blood gas analysis and vital sign checks before PEEP is started and after each change is made.

## 13. Continuous positive-airway pressure therapy (CPAP)

**a. Make a recommendation to change the level of CPAP to improve oxygenation (NBRC code: IIIG3b) [Difficulty: R, Ap]**

**b. Change the level of continuous CPAP to improve oxygenation (NBRC code: IIIF2h2) [Difficulty: R, Ap, An]**

CPAP therapy has been discussed earlier. Briefly, all of the considerations for PEEP apply to CPAP except that the patient must be able to breathe adequately to maintain a normal $CO_2$ level.

## 14. Inspiratory hold/plateau pressure

**a. Initiate and adjust inspiratory hold (NBRC code: IIID2e) [Difficulty: R, Ap]**

**b. Recommend a change in the ventilator to reduce the inspiratory plateau pressure (NBRC code: IIIG3k2) [Difficulty: R, Ap]**

Inspiratory hold (also known as *inflation hold*) is a technique whereby the patient is temporarily prevented from exhaling the ventilator-delivered $V_T$. Fig. 15-18 shows the pressure/time waveform. The pressure found during the inspiratory hold period is called the *inspiratory plateau*. Inspiratory hold is added therapeutically to improve the distribution of the $V_T$. Patients with ARDS and pulmonary edema can benefit from this. Oxygenation should improve in direct proportion to the duration of the inspiratory plateau. The duration of the inspiratory plateau is measured in different ways, depending on the ventilator. For example, with the Bear 1000 and the Puritan-Bennett 7200, it can be added in steps of 0.1 sec up to several seconds total. With the Servo 900C, it can be added as a variable percentage of the total duration of the breathing cycle. The inspiratory plateau must be reduced as the patient's ventilation and $C_{LT}$ improve. Patients with normal ventilation and compliance should receive no inspiratory plateau.

Notice that the use of an inspiratory plateau increases the inspiratory phase of the breathing cycle, which causes a shorter expiratory time if the rate is kept the same (or the rate must be reduced to keep the same I : E ratio). Again, as has been discussed earlier, make sure that the $V_T$ is completely exhaled. The patient's condition should be monitored closely to enable determination of whether the level of inspiratory plateau is appropriate.

Nontherapeutic inspiratory plateau is added temporarily to allow determination of the plateau pressure on the ventilator. This is considered to be the pressure needed to deliver the $V_T$. With this information, the patient's effective $C_{st}$ can be calculated. Its calculation and interpretation have been discussed earlier in this chapter. An inspiratory plateau of 1.0 sec is usually long enough to enable determination of the plateau pressure. Remember to turn off the inspiratory plateau afterward.

Expiratory retard is also shown in the Fig. 15-18 pressure/time waveform. Some ventilators have a control that adjusts both inspiratory hold and expiratory retard. So, care must be taken when a change is made in either. As has been discussed in Chapter 14, expiratory retard is indicated in any patient who is air-trapping and is not exhaling completely. It functions similarly to pursed-lip breathing in the spontaneously breathing patient. Backpressure prevents collapse of the smallest airways. Expiratory retard may be indicated in a patient with asthma, emphysema, or bronchitis. It is important with these types of patients that the inspiratory and expiratory $V_T$ values be measured. Air trapping is confirmed by an expiratory volume that is less than the inspiratory volume. When you are listening to the patient's breath sounds, you will note that no pause occurs at the end of exhalation before the next inspiration is started. In extreme cases, the pressure manometer does not return to the baseline level. These patients should be checked for the presence and level of auto-PEEP. The proper level of expiratory retard is determined by trial and error. The following parameters should be monitored so that the proper amount can be determined:

a. The inspiratory and expiratory $V_T$s should be the same.
b. The patient's breath sounds should reveal that wheezing is absent or minimal and that a silent pause occurs at the end of exhalation before the next $V_T$ is delivered.
c. Auto-PEEP should not occur.
d. The patient should subjectively feel that he or she has exhaled completely before the next breath is given.

The patient must be monitored frequently when expiratory retard is being used. As the patient is treated with bronchodilating medications, the bronchospasm should diminish. Expiratory retard should not be necessary when airway resistance has returned to normal.

15. **Pressure support level**
    a. **Recommend a change in the pressure support level (NBRC code: IIIG3e) [Difficulty: R, Ap]**
    b. **Change the pressure support level (NBRC code: IIIF2h5) [Difficulty: R, Ap, An]**

When the PSV level is adjusted for delivery of a $V_T$, this is called maximum PSV ($PSV_{max}$). Clinical guidelines for $PSV_{max}$ include the following:

1. Use enough pressure to deliver a $V_T$ of 10 to 12 mL/kg of ideal body weight.
2. The patient should not have to assist the ventilator at a rate greater than 20 times/min to achieve acceptable ABG values.

$PSV_{max}$ has been used in patients with resolving acute respiratory failure. Usually, these patients have been maintained on the A/C mode for several days to minimize their WOB while they are undergoing treatment for their condition. $PSV_{max}$ is considered ideal for reconditioning of the diaphragm and other respiratory muscles. Reconditioning occurs when the assist or "trigger" pressure for the breath is kept as low as possible ($-1$ to $-2$ cm $H_2O$ pressure) and the $V_T$ is kept large. This pattern results in a low respiratory muscle workload. As the patient continues to improve, the PSV level is reduced. The patient's $V_T$ is stable as long as the patient passively takes in the PSV-supported breath; the $V_T$ can be larger if the patient interacts actively with the delivered pressure. See Fig. 15-1 for a pressure/flow curve and Fig. 15-9, **E** for a pressure/time curve.

The PSV level has also been used to overcome the Raw caused by the patient's endotracheal tube. (See the example calculated earlier in the chapter.) Too small an endotracheal tube may prevent some patients from successfully weaning by means of the IMV/SIMV mode. The addition of enough PSV to overcome the additional WOB caused by the tube enables the patient to wean successfully and the airway to be extubated.

The PSV level is reduced, as tolerated, when the patient's $C_{LT}$ or Raw improves. As both return to normal, the only barrier to extubation is the resistance offered by the endotracheal tube. Some practitioners advocate extubation when the PSV level is 10 cm $H_2O$ or less, which is probably the pressure level needed to overcome the tube's resistance. Thus, the patient should tolerate extubation with no increase in the WOB.

16. **Pressure control ventilation level**
    a. **Recommend a change in the pressure control level (NBRC code: IIIG3e) [Difficulty: R, Ap]**
    b. **Change the pressure control level (NBRC code: IIIF2h5) [Difficulty: R, Ap, An]**

Pressure control ventilation (PCV) involves the delivery of $V_T$ breaths that are pressure limited and time cycled. It has been advocated for patients with bilateral low-compliance conditions (e.g., ARDS).

The PCV level is set as low as possible so that an adequate $V_T$ can be achieved for gas exchange. The exhaled volume must be monitored continuously because the $V_T$ will decrease if the patient's $C_{LT}$ or Raw worsens. If either or both improve, the $V_T$ will increase. The patient with a pulmonary air leak loses variable amounts of $V_T$ from the chest tube, depending on changes in compliance and resistance. An ABG sample must be evaluated with a change in the PCV level or $V_T$. The PCV mode is well tolerated by many patients because of the freedom they have to set the rate, the inspiratory flow through the demand valve, and the $\dot{V}_E$. PCV may also be combined with SIMV and PSV as the clinical situation indicates. Following are some suggestions for initial PCV settings:

a. Set the PEEP to the same level that is used on the constant-volume ventilator to maintain the patient's FRC.
b. Set the PCV level at the patient's static lung compliance pressure. Be prepared to increase this pressure. The clinical goal is to give a $V_T$ close to that delivered previously.
c. Set the rate so it is the same as before.
d. Set the inspired $O_2$ so it is the same as before. Some may prefer to set it at 100% until blood gas results show that it can be lowered.
e. Set the inspiratory time under pressure control so that the I:E ratio is the same as before.

Check the patient's vital signs for tolerance, and get an ABG sample in about 15 min. If the Raw or $C_{LT}$ worsens, the PCV level must be increased to maintain or increase the $V_T$. Obviously, as the patient's Raw and $C_{LT}$ improve (or pulmonary air leak decreases), the PCV level must be decreased to maintain the desired $V_T$.

## 17. Inspiratory-to-expiratory (I:E) ratio
   **a. Recommend a change in the I:E ratio settings** (NBRC code: IIIG3d) [Difficulty: R, Ap]
   **b. Change the I:E ratio settings** (NBRC code: IIIF2h4, IIIF2h2) [Difficulty: R, Ap, An]

A general discussion of I:E ratio was presented earlier. An increase in expiratory time to eliminate auto-PEEP is discussed in the next section. This discussion will focus on the need to increase inspiratory time. This is done to improve oxygenation by holding the tidal volume in the lungs for longer than normal. When the inspiratory time is longer than the expiratory time (e.g., 2:1), the patient is said to have an *inverse I:E ratio* and an *inverse ratio ventilation* (IRV). This technique has been used successfully in low lung compliance adult patients who do not respond to PCV. Increased inspiratory time and

decreased expiratory time should be used in any condition in which the patient has a small time constant of ventilation ($T_C$). ($T_C = C_{LT} \times$ Raw.) This would be observed clinically as a normal Raw but a low $C_{LT}$ in such conditions as ARDS, pulmonary edema, pneumonia, or an enlarged abdomen. Increasing the inspiratory time to create an inverse I:E ratio keeps the alveoli inflated longer to provide additional time for $O_2$ to diffuse, to prevent atelectasis, and to maintain the FRC. Typically, patients who are considered for IRV are already being ventilated in the pressure control mode. Therefore, the merging of the two modes is called *pressure-control inverse ratio ventilation (PCIRV)*. The following have been recommended as initial PCIRV settings:

a. If the patient is being switched from volume-cycled ventilation to PCIRV, set the PCV level at the patient's static lung compliance pressure. However, if the patient was already on PCV at a higher pressure, keep this higher pressure.
b. Set the $O_2$ at 100%.
c. Keep the current respiratory rate.
d. Keep the I:E ratio at 1:1 for now.
e. PEEP should be removed if it is currently less than 8 cm $H_2O$. Cut the PEEP level in half if it is currently greater than 8 cm $H_2O$. As the I:E ratio is made inverse, air trapping increases the patient's FRC.

Draw a set of ABGs after 15 min on PCIRV and check the patient's vital signs. Monitor the exhaled $V_T$ for a decrease. If the ventilator gives a real-time graph of pressure, volume, and flow, these should be monitored for air trapping (auto-PEEP). See Fig. 15-2 for an auto-PEEP flow/time tracing.

If the initial set of blood gases on PCIRV does not show adequate oxygenation, the inspiratory time will have to be increased. The inspiratory time must be progressively increased and expiratory time decreased if the patient's $C_{LT}$ worsens. It is also possible to alternate between a 2- and 3-cm $H_2O$ increase in the PCV level with small increases in the inspiratory time. Blood gases must be analyzed with each increase in inspiratory time, decrease in expiratory time, or increase in PCV. Once an acceptable $PaO_2$ has been established, it is usually not necessary to make further increases in the inspiratory time if the patient's pulmonary condition does not worsen. Look for an increase in $PaCO_2$ or end-tidal $CO_2$ as a sign of inadequate $V_T$. It may be necessary to increase the PCV level to increase the $V_T$. Also, monitor the patient's vital signs and cardiac output, if possible, to look for a decrease in cardiac output. PCIRV ratios as inverse as 3:1 or 4:1 have been reported. When this happens, the pressure volume curve takes on a characteristic "square wave" shape, as shown in Fig. 15-10, **B**. The I:E ratio must be returned to normal as the patient's $C_{LT}$ improves by a gradual decrease in the inspiratory time or increase in the expiratory time. The patient's blood gas results should be evaluated at each step to ensure that oxygenation is maintained at a safe level.

## 18. Recommend a modification in the ventilator settings to eliminate auto-PEEP (NBRC code: IIIG3k1) [Difficulty: R, Ap]

If a patient has auto-PEEP (see Fig. 15-2), every attempt should be made to determine why the patient is air-trapping. Although the basic problem is an expiratory time that is too short for full exhalation of the tidal volume, a more specific reason should be found. Then, a solution can be found. Following are possible reasons for air trapping and auto-PEEP and solutions:

| Problem | Solution(s) |
|---|---|
| a. Bronchospasm causing slow expiratory flow | Administer a bronchodilator medication. Increase expiratory time. Add expiratory retard. |
| b. Secretions causing slow expiratory flow | Suction the patient's airway. |
| c. Large tidal volume that is not fully exhaled | Reduce the tidal volume. Increase the expiratory time. |

Not every possible solution can be used. The patient's situation must be considered. For example, increasing the expiratory time will reduce the inspiratory time if the same rate is to be kept. Increasing the expiratory time and keeping the same inspiratory time will reduce the patient's respiratory rate. This will reduce the minute volume, causing an increase in the patient's carbon dioxide level. Additionally, reducing the tidal volume will reduce the minute volume and will elevate the patient's carbon dioxide level.

## 19. Noninvasive positive-pressure ventilation
### a. Recommend a change in noninvasive positive-pressure ventilation (NBRC code: IIIG3f) [Difficulty: R, Ap]
### b. Change the level of noninvasive positive-pressure ventilation (NBRC code: IIIF2h6) [Difficulty: R, Ap, An]

NPPV was discussed earlier in this chapter. Briefly, if the patient's $V_T$ needs to be increased, the level of positive pressure must be increased. Lowering the level of positive pressure decreases the $V_T$. Blood gases and vital signs should always be monitored after any change is made.

## 20. Monitor the mean airway pressure to determine the patient's response to respiratory care (NBRC code: IIIE8) [Difficulty: R, Ap]

Paw is the average pressure over an entire breathing cycle. Many current neonatal and adult ventilators are able to calculate the value (Fig. 15-19). Paw is influenced by the

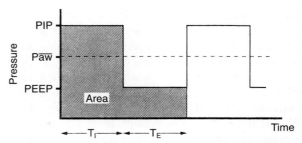

**Fig. 15-19** Pressure-time tracing showing where mean airway pressure (Paw) would be found. PEEP, positive end-expiratory pressure; PIP, peak inspiratory pressure; $T_E$, expiratory time; $T_I$, inspiratory time. *(From Chatburn RL: Principles and practice of neonatal and pediatric mechanical ventilation, Respir Care 36:569, 1991.)*

patient's $C_{LT}$, Raw, and ventilator settings. If a volume-cycled ventilator is being used, a decrease in compliance or an increase in resistance will result in an increase in Paw. It takes greater pressure to deliver the $V_T$; a higher peak pressure is observed. Conversely, if the patient's compliance increases or resistance decreases, the Paw will decrease. The patient must be further evaluated when a change in Paw is noticed because the new pressure, by itself, does not show whether a change in compliance and/or resistance has occurred. Any treatments that improve $C_{LT}$ and reduce Raw would be shown by a reduced airway pressure. Both $C_{dyn}$ and $C_{st}$ (discussed earlier) must be calculated when one is trying to determine how the patient's condition has changed.

## 21. Recommend the use of sedatives or muscle relaxants (paralyzing agents) as needed (NBRC code: IIIG1b) [Difficulty: R, Ap]

An adult who is attempting to inhale or exhale out of sequence with the ventilator is considered to be "bucking" or "fighting" the ventilator. This problem is most commonly seen in the control and A/C modes. If the asynchrony between the patient's efforts and the ventilator is too great, an increased risk of hypoxemia, air trapping, and pneumothorax exists. Carefully evaluate the patient to determine whether he or she is breathing rapidly because of pain, anxiety, or improper adjustment of the ventilator. Make sure that the settings (e.g., inspiratory flow, respiratory rate, pressure limit) are correctly set for the patient's condition. Sedation or paralysis should be considered only after all other causes of asynchrony have been ruled out. The following patient conditions must be considered before a medication choice is made for controlling the patient's breathing efforts:

Is the patient in pain? If so, an opiate analgesic such as morphine sulfate is commonly administered intravenously for fast onset. Morphine has the additional effects of reducing anxiety and inducing sleep. Because all opiates are central nervous system depressants, make sure that the ventilator alarm systems are functioning properly in case the patient becomes disconnected.

Is the patient agitated? Asynchrony with the ventilator for no known physical reason can often be attributed to anxiety or fear. Benzodiazepines, including diazepam (Valium) and midazolam (Versed), are the drugs of choice for treatment of agitation. They have a sedating effect within minutes when given intravenously.

Does the patient need to be paralyzed? If total muscular relaxation along with apnea is necessary, a skeletal muscle–paralyzing agent should be used. Usually, a short-term, depolarizing neuromuscular blocker such as succinylcholine (Anectine) is used during a difficult intubation. A single intravenous dose paralyzes a combative patient for about 10 min. For paralysis during mechanical ventilation, one of the following long-term, nondepolarizing neuromuscular-blocking agents is commonly used: pancuronium (Pavulon), atracurium (Tracrium), and vecuronium (Norcuron). These are given intravenously and cause paralysis that lasts for 2 to 4 hr.

Remember that these paralyzing agents have no effect on the patient's ability to feel pain or fear of what is happening. Pain medications such as morphine must be given as necessary. A sedating agent such as Valium is always given to counteract the emotional stress of being awake but unable to move.

## 22. Wean the patient from the ventilator
### a. Recommend procedures for weaning the patient (NBRC code: IIIG1d) [Difficulty: R, Ap]

Indications that the patient can tolerate weaning should include some, if not all, of the criteria listed in Box 15-4. The patient need not pass each and every criterion. However, the more the patient can attain, the more likely he or she is to successfully wean. Individual physicians and practitioners may favor some of these conditions over others and may include other factors not listed.

Some patients do not wean successfully even though objective criteria indicate that they should. Conversely, some patients wean successfully even when objective criteria indicate otherwise. Keep in mind that each patient must be evaluated individually. Look at the objective criteria and assess how the patient actually performs during weaning.

### b. Initiate and modify weaning procedures (NBRC code: IIID5) [Difficulty: R, Ap, An]
### c. Make changes in the weaning procedures (NBRC code: IIIF2i) [Difficulty: R, Ap, An]

Each of the five methods presented in Fig. 15-20 has its advocates and a body of clinical evidence showing it as a

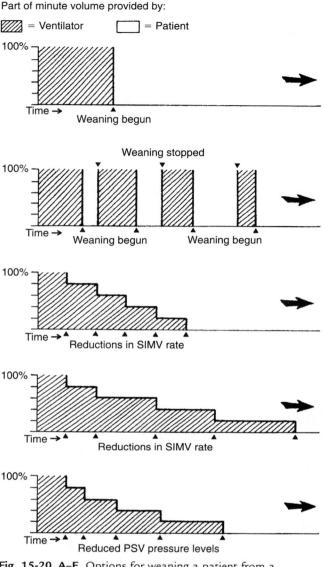

**Fig. 15-20 A–E,** Options for weaning a patient from a mechanical ventilator. See the text for discussion. PSV, pressure support ventilation; SIMV, synchronous intermittent mechanical ventilation.

valid weaning technique. The practitioner must evaluate the patient before recommending any particular weaning method and during the weaning trial to determine if the method chosen is meeting the patient's needs. The practitioner needs to be prepared to discontinue weaning if the patient is failing and must be ready to try another weaning approach to help ensure success.

### 1. Ventilator discontinuance

Ventilator discontinuance (also called a T-piece trial) is widely used with patients who have been ventilated for a short period and are now fully prepared to breathe on their own (see Fig. 15-20, **A**). When the patient is stable, awake, and alert and meets the criteria listed in Box 15-4, he or she can be prepared for weaning. The patient should be instructed about the weaning, should be suctioned, and should be put in Fowler's or semi-Fowler's position, if possible. The ventilator circuit is disconnected, and an aerosol and $O_2$ mix is breathed in through a T-piece (Briggs adapter). The $O_2$ percentage should be the same as originally inspired or up to 10% higher, depending on the patient's $PaO_2$ level on the ventilator.

Ventilator discontinuance and weaning begin at the same moment. The ventilator goes from providing 100% of the $\dot{V}_E$ for the patient to providing none of it. The patient should be watched continuously because he or she is now breathing totally independently. Vital signs and respiratory mechanics should be measured every 5 to 10 min throughout the procedure. If the patient is stable, an ABG sample should be taken after about 20 min, or $SpO_2$ and end-tidal $CO_2$ can be monitored. If the blood gas results are acceptable and the patient appears stable, weaning is continued, or the patient can be extubated. In a stable patient, a T-piece wean should not be needed for longer than 1 to 2 hours before extubation. Several clinical studies have shown that about 75% of the patients who tolerate ventilator discontinuance can be extubated.

When the patient deteriorates, ventilator therapy should be reestablished. After a rest period, intermittent ventilator discontinuance or another mode of weaning might be tried, as follows.

### 2. Intermittent ventilator discontinuance

This method is used after ventilator discontinuance proves unsuccessful. The patient is started on a schedule of intermittent weaning periods and rest periods on the ventilator (see Fig. 15-20, **B**). The method shown has a cycle of lengthening weaning periods and shortening rest periods. This would go on until the patient has been weaning for an extended period, as has been discussed earlier. Another method involves a cycle of set rest periods (commonly ½ to 1 hr) and lengthening weaning periods as the patient becomes stronger. Again, blood gas values should be monitored after about 20 min of weaning. The weaning period can be extended as long as the patient is stable or until extubation.

### 3. Regular steps in synchronous intermittent mandatory ventilation weaning

Regular steps involve one of two SIMV weaning methods. As has been discussed earlier, IMV/SIMV was originally developed as a ventilating mode and has since become a widely used weaning mode. It allows the patient to achieve a more gradual transition toward providing all of the WOB. SIMV seems to work especially well in weaning patients who have been ventilator dependent for an extended period. By gradually taking over more of the

WOB, the patient reconditions respiratory muscles that may have atrophied through lack of use. The patient is also gaining confidence that complete weaning will occur. An additional benefit is that all ventilator alarm systems are functional, and the patient does not need to be directly watched as closely as in the two previously mentioned weaning methods.

This particular SIMV weaning pattern can be applied to a patient who is stable and is making rapid progress (see Fig. 15-20, **C**). The weaning pattern might involve an IMV rate reduction in increments of about 2/min on a set time schedule. About 20 min after the SIMV rate has been reduced, blood gas values should be monitored. The patient's respiratory mechanics are monitored closely. It is important that the patient's spontaneous $\dot{V}_E$ be calculated (rate × $V_T$). This should be approximately the same volume as that subtracted from the ventilator-delivered $\dot{V}_E$. The process continues as long as the patient tolerates each decrease in SIMV rate. The stable, strong patient can be rather quickly weaned down to an SIMV rate of 2 to 4 times/min. The decision is often made at this point to use a T-piece, as has been discussed earlier, or to extubate the airway.

### 4. Irregular steps in synchronous intermittent mandatory ventilation weaning

This method is applied when the regular SIMV method is less than successful. Often, the patient starts out on a cycle of regular reductions in SIMV rate until a point is reached at which the patient has a setback and cannot tolerate any further reductions. The rate may be kept at that level for an extended period until the patient is ready for a further decrease (see Fig. 15-20, **D**). Further drops in the IMV rate proceed as the patient tolerates them. No attempt is made to set up a regular pattern of rate reduction.

It may be necessary to increase the rate to higher previous levels if the patient has a serious setback. One possible reason why rates are unable to go any lower is resistance to breathing through the demand valve and breathing circuit. A trial on a T-piece (which offers no resistance) may be the final step in weaning. The patient would likely fail this if resistance should occur from the endotracheal tube. The PSV weaning method should then be tried on the patient.

### 5. Weaning by pressure support ventilation

The PSV mode is available on most modern electrically powered and microprocessor ventilators and can be used as the newest weaning method (see Fig. 15-20, **E**). When it is used as a weaning method, the PSV level is gradually reduced. Decreases in PSV in steps of 2 to 5 cm $H_2O$ are commonly made. The patient has to gradually increase the WOB to inspire a $V_T$. Blood gas values and respiratory mechanics should be evaluated after each drop in PSV level. A modest PSV level of 2 to 5 cm $H_2O$ is maintained to overcome any resistance of the endotracheal tube. If the patient does well during an extended trial of minimal PSV, extubation is performed, unless the endotracheal tube is needed for other reasons. Recent research has demonstrated that most patients who fail a T-piece trial and need prolonged ventilatory support can be eventually weaned with pressure support ventilation that is used to overcome the airway resistance of the endotracheal tube.

The criteria listed in Box 15-4 can be used in the evaluation of any patient who is being weaned by any of these methods. General signs that the patient is not tolerating weaning include anxiety, agitation, a large increase or decrease in respiratory rate, angina, tachycardia, increase in PVCs or other serious arrhythmias, bradycardia, hypertension, hypotension, cyanosis, hypoxemia, and hypercarbia with acidemia. The patient probably will not exhibit all of these signs; some tend to be seen together because they relate to the patient's WOB. Others appear to give conflicting signals of success or failure. The practitioner is responsible for evaluating the patient's condition to determine whether weaning should be continued or ventilatory support resumed.

---

### Exam Hint

**E**xpect to see several questions that relate to evaluating a patient's ability to wean. This will include such information as initial bedside spirometry, arterial blood gas results, and vital signs. If a patient is able to wean, expect to make recommendations on which method(s) to use. Lastly, expect to see questions related to evaluating a patient who is weaning. You will evaluate current bedside spirometry, arterial blood gas results, and vital signs and will make a decision to continue weaning, change the weaning procedure, or put the patient back on the ventilator.

---

### 23. Make a recommendation to extubate the patient (NBRC code: IIIG1e) [Difficulty: R, Ap, An]

Extubation can usually be safely accomplished when the patient has met the criteria listed in Box 15-4, has demonstrated the ability to breathe effectively for a clinically significant time as measured by the listed criteria, has acceptable blood gas results, is alert enough to protect his or her airway, and can effectively cough out any secretions. Some patients need the endotracheal tube even though

they no longer need ventilatory support. The tube provides a suctioning route if the patient is unable to cough out large amounts of secretions. The tube also protects the airway from the risk of aspiration in a comatose patient who may vomit. See Chapter 12 for an explanation of the extubation procedure.

---

### Exam Hint

**E**xpect to see at least one question that relates to evaluating a weaning patient and recommending extubation if the patient is meeting weaning and extubation criteria, or the resumption of mechanical ventilation if the patient has failed weaning and extubation criteria.

---

## MODULE F
### Respiratory care plan

### 1. Analyze the available information to determine the patient's pathophysiologic state (NBRC code: IIIH1) [Difficulty: R, Ap, An]

Remember to get an ABG after every ventilator change that could result in a different $PaO_2$ ($SpO_2$ or transcutaneous $O_2$ may be substituted) or $PaCO_2$ (end-tidal $CO_2$ or transcutaneous $CO_2$ may be substituted). Mixed venous blood gas values should also be obtained when possible.

Physical responses to mechanical ventilation, as measured by vital signs, can vary considerably. A patient who is anxious, angry, or in pain will often have an increase in heart rate and blood pressure. A patient who is relaxed, who has reduced WOB, and whose blood gas values are now normal shows a return to normal vital signs. Watch carefully for the patient whose drop in blood pressure coincides with a tachycardia. This patient may be having decreased venous return to the heart resulting from increased intrathoracic pressure.

Patients with ventilation/perfusion mismatching or shunting may not show an increase in the $PaO_2$ despite a high percentage of inspired oxygen. This finding demonstrates refractory hypoxemia. In these cases, PEEP is applied with the goal of increasing the patient's functional residual capacity (FRC) to improve oxygenation. As has been mentioned, tachycardia and hypotension can result from too much PEEP. A pulmonary artery catheter (Swan-Ganz catheter) is often placed into these patients to monitor the patient's cardiac output (CO). Remember that a normal adult's cardiac output is 4 to 8 L/min. Too much PEEP will result in a drop in cardiac output. The PEEP level should be decreased to promote venous return to the heart and increase cardiac output.

2. **Determine the appropriateness of the prescribed therapy and goals for the patient's pathophysiologic state** (NBRC code: IIIH3) [Difficulty: R, Ap, An]
3. **Recommend changes in the therapeutic plan if supportive data exist** (NBRC code: IIIH4) [Difficulty: Ap, An]
4. **Stop the treatment or procedure if the patient has an adverse reaction to it** (NBRC code: IIIF1) [Difficulty: R, Ap, An]
5. **Discontinue treatment based on the patient's response** (NBRC code: IIIG1f) [Difficulty: R, Ap]

Be prepared to make recommendations on changing ventilator parameters based on the patient's condition, blood gas values, chest x-ray films, breath sounds, and vital signs. This information can be found in this chapter and throughout this text.

## BIBLIOGRAPHY

Aloan CA, Hill TV, editors: *Respiratory care of the newborn and child,* ed 2, Philadelphia, 1997, Lippincott-Raven.

American Association for Respiratory Care: Clinical practice guideline: Humidification during mechanical ventilation, *Respir Care* 37:887, 1992.

American Association for Respiratory Care: Clinical practice guideline: Patient-ventilator system checks, *Respir Care* 37:882, 1992.

American Association for Respiratory Care: Clinical practice guideline: Endotracheal suctioning of mechanically ventilated adults and children with artificial airways, *Respir Care* 38:500, 1993.

American Association for Respiratory Care: Clinical practice guideline: Application of continuous positive airway pressure in neonates via nasal prongs or nasopharyngeal tube, *Respir Care* 39:817, 1994.

American Association for Respiratory Care: Clinical practice guideline: Neonatal time-triggered, pressure-limited, time-cycled mechanical ventilation, *Respir Care* 39:808, 1994.

American Association for Respiratory Care: Clinical practice guideline: Ventilator circuit changes, *Respir Care* 39:797, 1994.

American Association for Respiratory Care: Clinical practice guideline: Long-term invasive mechanical ventilation in the home, *Respir Care* 40:1313, 1995.

American Association for Respiratory Care: Clinical practice guideline: capnography/capnometry during mechanical ventilation, *Respir Care* 40:1321, 1995.

American Association for Respiratory Care: Clinical practice guideline: Removal of the endotracheal tube, *Respir Care* 44:85, 1999.

American Association for Respiratory Care: Clinical practice guideline: Selection of device, administration of bronchodilator, and evaluation of responses to therapy in mechanically ventilated patients, *Respir Care* 44:105, 1999.

American Association for Respiratory Care: Consensus statement on the essentials of mechanical ventilation, *Respir Care* 37:1000, 1992.

American Association for Respiratory Care: Clinical practice guideline: In-hospital transport of the mechanically ventilated patient—2002 revision & update, *Respir Care* 47:721-723, 2002.

American Association for Respiratory Care: Evidence-based clinical practice guidelines: Care of the ventilator circuit and its relation to ventilator-associated pneumonia, *Respir Care* 48:869-879, 2003.

Banner MJ, Lampotang S: Clinical use of inspiratory and expiratory waveforms. In Kacmarek RM, Stoller JK, editors: *Current respiratory care,* Philadelphia, 1988, BC Decker.

Barnes TA, editor: *Core textbook of respiratory care practice,* ed 2, St Louis, 1994, Mosby.

Bone RC: Pressure-volume measurements in detection of bronchospasm and mucous plugging in acute respiratory failure, *Respir Care* 21:620, 1976.

Boysen PG, McGough E: Pressure-control and pressure-support ventilation: Flow patterns, inspiratory time, and gas distribution, *Respir Care* 33:620, 1988.

Branson RD, Campbell RS, Davis K Jr, et al: Altering flowrate during maximum pressure support ventilation (PSV$_{max}$): Effects on cardiorespiratory function, *Respir Care* 35:1056, 1990.

Branson RD, Chatburn RL: Technical description and classification of modes of ventilator operation, *Respir Care* 37:1026, 1992.

Branson RD, Hess DR, Chatburn RL, editors: *Respiratory care equipment,* ed 2, Philadelphia, 1999, Lippincott Williams & Wilkins.

Branson RD, Hurst JM: Laboratory evaluation of moisture output of seven airway heat and moisture exchangers, *Respir Care* 32:741, 1987.

Burton GC, Hodgkin JE, Ward JJ, editors: *Respiratory care: A guide to clinical practice,* ed 4, Philadelphia, 1997, Lippincott-Raven.

Cairo JM, Pilbeam SP: *Mosby's respiratory care equipment,* ed 7, St Louis, 2004, Mosby.

Campbell RS, Davis BR: Pressure-controlled versus volume-controlled ventilation: Does it matter? *Respir Care* 47:416-426, 2002.

Chang DW: *Clinical application of mechanical ventilation,* ed 2, Albany, NY, 2001, Delmar.

Chatburn RL: A new system for understanding mechanical ventilation, *Respir Care* 36:1123, 1991.

Chatburn RL: Classification of mechanical ventilators, *Respir Care* 37:1009, 1992.

Dantzker DR, MacIntyre NR, Bakow ED, editors: *Comprehensive respiratory care,* Philadelphia, 1995, WB Saunders.

Drinker PA, McKhann CF III: Landmark perspective: The iron lung: First practical means of respiratory support, *JAMA* 256:1476, 1986.

Epstein SK: Extubation, *Respir Care* 47:483-495, 2002.

Epstein SK: Weaning from mechanical ventilation, *Respir Care* 47:454-468, 2002.

Evidence-based guidelines for weaning and discontinuing ventilator support. *Respir Care* 47:69-90, 2002.

Felix WR Jr, MacDonnell KF, Jacobs L: Resuscitation from drowning in cold water, *N Engl J Med* 304:843, 1981.

Fink JB, Hunt GE, editors: *Clinical practice in respiratory care,* Philadelphia, 1999, Lippincott-Raven.

Fink JB, Tobin MJ, Dhand R: Bronchodilator therapy in mechanically ventilated patients, *Respir Care* 44:53, 1999.

Greer K: Hypothermia: A quiet killer, *Adv Respir Ther,* Jan 15, 1990.

Gregg BL: Invasive mechanical ventilation. In Wyka KA, Mathews PJ, Clark WF, editors: *Foundations of respiratory care,* Albany, 2002, Delmar.

Gurevitch MJ: Selection of the inspiratory:expiratory ratio. In Kacmarek RM, Stoller JK, editors: *Current respiratory care,* Philadelphia, 1988, BC Decker.

Hess DR: Mechanical ventilation of the adult patient: Initiation, management, and weaning. In Burton GG, Hodgkin JE, Ward JJ, editors: *Respiratory care: A guide to clinical practice,* ed 4, Philadelphia, 1997, Lippincott-Raven.

Hess DR, Branson RD: Mechanical ventilation. In Hess DR, MacIntyre NR, Mishoe SC, et al, editors: *Respiratory care principles & practice,* Philadelphia, 2002, WB Saunders.

Hess DR, Kacmarek RM: *Essentials of mechanical ventilation,* ed 2, New York, 2002, McGraw-Hill.

Hess DR, McCurdy S, Simmons M: Compression volume in adult ventilator circuits: A comparison of five disposable circuits and a nondisposable circuit, *Respir Care* 36:1113, 1991.

Hill NS: Clinical application of body ventilators, *Chest* 90:897, 1986.

Hill NS, Eveloff SE, Carlisle CC, Goff SG: Efficacy of nocturnal nasal ventilation in patients with restrictive thoracic disease, *Am Rev Respir Dis* 145:365, 1992.

Hirsch C, Kacmarek RM, Stanek K: Work of breathing during CPAP and PSV imposed by the new generation mechanical ventilators: A lung model study, *Respir Care* 36:815, 1991.

International consensus conferences in intensive care medicine: Ventilator-associated lung injury in ARDS, *Am J Respir Crit Care Med* 160:2118-2124, 1999.

Kacmarek RM: The role of pressure support ventilation in reducing work of breathing, *Respir Care* 33:99, 1988.

Kacmarek RM, Foley K, Cheever P: Determination of ventilatory reserve in mechanically ventilated patients: A comparison of techniques, *Respir Care* 36:1085, 1991.

Kacmarek RM, Hess D: Pressure-controlled inverse-ratio ventilation: Panacea or auto-PEEP? *Respir Care* 35:945, 1990.

Kirby RR: Modes of mechanical ventilation. In Kacmarek RM, Stoller JK, editors: *Current respiratory care,* Philadelphia, 1988, BC Decker.

Kuhlen R, Rossaint R: The role of spontaneous breathing during mechanical ventilation, *Respir Care* 47:296-307, 2002.

MacIntyre NR: Pressure support: Inspiratory assist. In Kacmarek RM, Stoller JK, editors: *Current respiratory care,* Philadelphia, 1988, BC Decker.

MacIntyre NR: Setting the frequency-tidal volume pattern, *Respir Care* 47:266-278, 2002.

MacIntyre NR: Weaning from mechanical ventilatory support: Volume-assisting intermittent breaths versus pressure-supporting every breath, *Respir Care* 33:121, 1988.

MacIntyre NR, Branson RD: *Mechanical ventilation,* Philadelphia, 2001, WB Saunders.

Martz KV, Joiner JW, Rodger MS: *Management of the patient-ventilator system: A team approach,* ed 2, St Louis, 1984, Mosby.

Pennock BE, Kaplan PD, Carlin BW, et al: Pressure support ventilation with a simplified ventilatory support system administered with a nasal mask in patients with respiratory failure, *Chest* 100:1371, 1991.

Pierson DJ: Indications for mechanical ventilation in adults with acute respiratory failure, *Respir Care* 47:249-265, 2002.

Pilbeam SP: *Mechanical ventilation: Physiological and clinical applications,* ed 3, St Louis, 1998, Mosby.

Quan SF, Parides GC, Knoper SR: Mandatory minute volume (MVV) ventilation: An overview, *Respir Care* 35:898, 1990.

Radford EP Jr: Ventilation standards for use in artificial respiration, *J Appl Phys* 7:451, 1955.

Respironics: Guidelines for invasive applications with BiPAP systems, Monroeville, Penn.

Respironics: Product literature on the suggested protocol for initiation of the BiPAP S/T or BiPAP S/T-D Ventilatory Support System, Monroeville, Penn.

Saura P, Blanch L: How to set positive end-expiratory pressure, *Respir Care* 47:279-295, 2002.

Scanlan CL, Wilkins RL, Stoller JK, editors: *Egan's fundamentals of respiratory care,* ed 8, St Louis, 2003, Mosby.

Shapiro BA, Kacmarek RM, Cane RD, et al, editors: *Clinical application of respiratory care,* ed 4, St Louis, 1991, Mosby.

Shelledy DC, Mikles SP: Newer modes of mechanical ventilation. I. Pressure support, *Respir Management* July/Aug 14-20, 1988.

Shelledy DC, Mikles SP: Newer modes of mechanical ventilation, II. Mandatory minute volume ventilation, *Respir Management* July/Aug 21, 1988.

Stoller JK: Establishing clinical unweanability, *Respir Care* 36:186, 1991.

Strumpf DA, Carlisle CC, Millman RP, et al: An evaluation of the Respironics BiPAP Bi-Level CPAP device for delivery of assisted ventilation, *Respir Care* 35:415, 1990.

Tobin MJ: Monitoring of pressure, flow, and volume during mechanical ventilation, *Respir Care* 37:1081, 1992.

Tobin MJ, Lodato RF: PEEP, auto-PEEP, and waterfalls, *Chest* 96:449, 1989.

Waldhorn RE: Nocturnal nasal intermittent positive pressure ventilation with bi-level positive airway pressure (BiPAP) in respiratory failure, *Chest* 101:516, 1992.

Waugh JB, Deshpande VM, Harwood RJ: *Rapid interpretation of ventilator waveforms,* Upper Saddle River, NJ, 1999, Prentice-Hall.

Whitaker K: *Comprehensive perinatal & pediatric respiratory care,* ed 2, Albany, NY, 1997, Delmar.

White GC: *Equipment theory for respiratory care,* ed 4, Albany, NY, 2005, Delmar.

Wright J, Gong H: "Auto-PEEP": Incidence, magnitude, and contributing factors, *Heart Lung* 19:352, 1990.

## SELF-STUDY QUESTIONS

1. A 40-year-old patient is brought to the emergency room after being in an automobile accident. She has broken ribs on her right side and a right-sided pneumothorax. Which of the following ventilators would you recommend for her?
   A. PR-2
   B. Bird Mark 7
   C. Servo 300A
   D. Bird Mark 14

2. Your patient needs to be placed on a ventilator. His body weight is 86 kg (190 lb). The most appropriate uncorrected ventilator $V_T$ would be
   A. 800 mL
   B. 860 mL
   C. 1350 mL
   D. 500 mL

3. Two patients are brought into the emergency room simultaneously. One has taken an accidental overdose of sleeping pills and has respiratory center depression. The other has pneumonia and bronchitis and is coughing up large amounts of thick, yellow secretions. The airways of both are intubated, and they will undergo mechanical ventilation. You have available only a Bird Mark 7 and a Puritan-Bennett 7200. Which would you recommend for the patient who has taken the overdose of sleeping pills?
   A. Bird Mark 7
   B. Puritan-Bennett 7200
   C. Either is acceptable for either patient.
   D. Neither is acceptable.

4. Which of the following parameters indicate that weaning should be successful?
   I. Spontaneous $V_T$ of 7 mL/kg of ideal body weight
   II. $V_D/V_T$ ratio of 0.4
   III. Intrapulmonary shunt of 10%
   IV. VC of 9 mL/kg of ideal body weight
   V. MIP of −15 cm $H_2O$
   A. I and II
   B. III, IV, and V
   C. I, II, and III
   D. II, III, and IV

5. The physician asks your opinion on which weaning method would be most successful in the patient with the weaning parameters listed in Question 4. The patient is on the A/C mode with a ventilator $V_T$ of 800 mL and a backup rate of 12 times/min. Her spontaneous $V_T$ is 400 mL. You would recommend which of the following methods?
   A. T-piece and extubation in 30 min
   B. Intermittent ventilator discontinuance
   C. SIMV weaning
   D. PCV

6. Your patient with a $V_T$ of 4 mL/kg of ideal body weight has the desire to breathe spontaneously. Because of facial trauma from an automobile accident, she has an endotracheal tube that is smaller than the ideal size. She also suffered lung contusions in the crash. Her $PaO_2$ level is 63 torr on 55% $O_2$. What ventilator mode would you recommend for her?
   A. PSV with PEEP
   B. CPAP
   C. SIMV with PSV and PEEP
   D. SIMV with PSV

7. Your patient is recovering from ARDS and is receiving 10 cm $H_2O$ CPAP and 40% $O_2$. In evaluating the patient after 1 hr, you notice the following: His $SpO_2$ has dropped from 95% to 90%, his respiratory rate has increased from 14 to 23 breaths/min, and he is complaining of tiredness. You would recommend which of the following?
   A. Continue for another hour and reevaluate
   B. Raise the CPAP level to 13 cm $H_2O$ because the $SpO_2$ value has decreased
   C. Decrease the CPAP level to 7 cm $H_2O$ because the patient is becoming tired at the present level
   D. Initiate SIMV with 10 cm PEEP

8. Your patient has an HME in place for humidification purposes. You notice that the peak pressure has increased by 10 cm $H_2O$ in the past hour. The nurse reported to you that the patient's secretions were difficult to suction the last time because they were rather thick. You would recommend which of the following?
   A. Switch the HME to a cool passover-type humidifier
   B. Switch to a heated cascade-type humidifier
   C. Have the nurse instill a few milliliters of normal saline solution before suctioning
   D. Turn up the temperature on the HME

9. Your ventilated patient with ARDS has the following blood gas values on 40% $O_2$: $PaO_2$ 75 torr, $PaCO_2$ 35 torr, and pH 7.43. She is on the A/C mode with a backup rate of 10 breaths/min and is assisting at a rate of 18 breaths/min. Her peak airway pressure is 65 cm $H_2O$, and her plateau pressure is 45 cm $H_2O$. She has developed a pneumothorax caused by the ventilating pressures. What would you suggest?
   A. Switch her to the PCV mode
   B. Switch her to the SIMV mode
   C. Switch her to the CPAP mode
   D. Sedate her so that she does not assist

10. The sensitivity control should be set at what level when the patient is being ventilated on the A/C mode?
    A. 0 cm $H_2O$
    B. $-1$ to $-2$ cm $H_2O$
    C. $-5$ cm $H_2O$
    D. 1 to 2 cm $H_2O$

11. In preparing for a mode change from A/C to SIMV, the following must be done:
    I. Turn the sensitivity control off
    II. Inform the patient of the change in ventilator function
    III. Turn off the ventilator's sigh control
    IV. Add 5 cm $H_2O$ of therapeutic PEEP to reduce the WOB
    V. Remove any mechanical dead space from the patient's breathing circuit
    A. I, III, and IV
    B. III and IV
    C. II, IV, and V
    D. II, III, and V

12. Which of the following indicate that the patient is not tolerating PEEP?
    I. Increased $C_{st}$
    II. Decreased $C_{st}$
    III. Increased intrapulmonary shunt
    IV. Stable heart rate
    V. Decreasing blood pressure
    A. I, III, and V
    B. II and III
    C. III and IV
    D. II, III, and V

Use the following information for questions 13 and 14: Your ventilated patient has an exhaled $V_T$ of 800 mL. Because of refractory hypoxemia, 8 cm of PEEP therapy is started. The peak pressure is 40 cm $H_2O$ and the static or plateau pressure is 30 cm $H_2O$. The compliance factor has been determined to be 3 mL/cm $H_2O$.

13. Calculate the $C_{st}$ for this patient.
    A. 22 mL/cm $H_2O$
    B. 32 mL/cm $H_2O$
    C. 27 mL/cm $H_2O$
    D. 17 mL/cm $H_2O$

14. Calculate the $C_{dyn}$ for this patient.
    A. 32 mL/cm $H_2O$
    B. 20 mL/cm $H_2O$
    C. 25 mL/cm $H_2O$
    D. 21 mL/cm $H_2O$

15. Your patient is being ventilated by a volume-cycled ventilator with an external exhalation valve. The nurse calls you to evaluate the patient because the alarm is going off. When you arrive, you notice that the patient's chest is barely moving during a control breath, the peak pressure does not rise above 3 cm $H_2O$, and the exhaled $V_T$ spirometer shows the set $V_T$ when the control breath is delivered. The most likely cause of these findings is
    A. The machine is self-cycling
    B. The inspiratory and expiratory limbs of the circuit are reversed at the cascade humidifier
    C. The tubing to the exhalation valve is disconnected
    D. The spirometer is out of calibration

16. Expiratory retard would be indicated in a patient with
    A. Pulmonary edema
    B. Air trapping on exhalation
    C. Pleural effusion
    D. Pneumothorax

17. All of the following parameters indicate the need for intubation and mechanical ventilation EXCEPT
    A. VC of less than 15 mL/kg of ideal body weight
    B. MIP of less than $-25$ cm $H_2O$
    C. $P(A - a)O_2$ on 100% $O_2$ of 40 torr
    D. $V_D/V_T$ of 0.7

18. Your polio patient is being ventilated with a BiPAP system and has an IPAP level of 15 cm water and an EPAP level of 5 cm water. She complains of being short of breath. You check her $V_T$ and find that it has dropped. How should the tidal volume be restored?
    A. Lower the IPAP level
    B. Lower the EPAP level
    C. Raise the IPAP level
    D. Raise the EPAP level

19. You are working with a patient with obstructive sleep apnea who is receiving bilevel NPPV through a nasal mask. During a sleep period, you notice that he is snoring. You would recommend the following ventilator adjustment:
    A. Increase the respiratory rate
    B. Increase the upper pressure level
    C. Increase the lower pressure level
    D. Loosen the nasal mask so that it is not as tight on the patient's face

20. You are working with an 80-kg (176-lb) patient who is apneic after suffering a stroke. He is being ventilated with the A/C mode and has the following settings:

    | | |
    |---|---|
    | $\dot{V}_E$ | 8 L |
    | Rate | 10/min |
    | I:E ratio | 1:3 |
    | Inspired $O_2$ | 40% |
    | Mechanical dead space | 200 mL |

    The ABG results show the following:

    | | |
    |---|---|
    | $PaO_2$ | 90 torr |
    | $PaCO_2$ | 50 torr |
    | pH | 7.30 |
    | $HCO_3^-$ | 24 mEq/L |

    Which of the following would you recommend?
    A. Decrease the mechanical dead space
    B. Decrease the patient's $\dot{V}_E$
    C. Change the I:E ratio to 1:2
    D. Add 5 cm $H_2O$ PEEP

21. Factors causing an increased peak pressure without a change in static pressure include the following:
    I. Retained secretions
    II. Pleural effusion
    III. Bronchospasm
    IV. Pulmonary edema
    A. II and IV
    B. I and II
    C. I and III
    D. III and IV

22. Which of the following will have the greatest impact on the mean airway pressure?
    A. Increasing the inspiratory flow
    B. Adding 5 cm $H_2O$ PEEP
    C. Adding 0.5 sec of inflation hold
    D. Increasing the inspiratory time by 0.25 sec

## ANSWER KEY AND RATIONALE

1. **C.** The Servo 300A is the only volume-cycled ventilator among those listed. It delivers a set $V_T$ despite changes in the patient's pulmonary condition. The other ventilators are pressure cycled and cannot ensure a consistent $V_T$.

2. **B.** The minimal-set $V_T$ for a ventilated patient is 10 mL/kg. This would result in a set patient $V_T$ of 860 mL (10 mL × 86 kg).

3. **A.** The patient with the drug overdose should be easily ventilated on a pressure-cycled ventilator such as the Bird Mark 7. The Puritan-Bennett 7200 is a volume-cycled ventilator and should be reserved for the patient with serious pulmonary problems.

4. **C.** The listed patient parameters are close to normal. The other two items are not normal and do not indicate successful weaning. Review Box 15-4.

5. **C.** SIMV would be the safest weaning method for this patient with an acceptable $V_T$ but inadequate VC or MIP. The ventilator will still provide intermittent deep breaths and alarms for safety. T-piece weaning offers no alarms, and the patient is not ready for extubation. PCV is not a weaning method.

6. **C.** SIMV offers intermittent deep breaths while allowing the patient to breathe spontaneously. PSV helps to overcome the Raw caused by the small endotracheal tube. PEEP is needed to maintain her FRC and oxygenation.

7. **D.** SIMV decreases the patient's WOB by providing a set number of large $V_T$ breaths. The patient can breathe between machine breaths as he wishes. Keep the same PEEP/CPAP level to maintain his FRC and oxygenation. Decreasing the CPAP causes a lower FRC and less oxygenation. Raising the CPAP level may increase FRC and oxygenation but does not help the patient's fatigue and WOB.

8. **B.** A heated cascade-type humidifier will do the best job of providing 100% relative humidity to the patient. Neither instilling a few milliliters of saline nor switching to a cool passover-type humidifier would do a good a job of adding moisture to the patient's secretions. HME devices can be heated only by the patient's warm exhaled gas.

9. **A.** The PCV mode will allow the therapist and physician to lower her peak pressure. She should be able to ventilate without further injury to her lung(s). SIMV will still deliver the set $V_T$s with high pressures. CPAP will not ventilate the patient at all. Sedation will not lower the high delivered ventilator pressures.

10. **B.** The sensitivity control should be set so that the patient has to begin an inhalation and generate a slightly negative pressure. A pressure of 0 cm $H_2O$ or in the positive range will result in self-cycling of the ventilator to inspiration.

11. **D.** The patient should be told of any significant change in the ventilator unless a clinically based reason exists not to do so. Sigh breaths are not used with SIMV because the mandatory breaths should be large enough to serve as a sigh. Mechanical dead space should be removed because it could result in $CO_2$ retention during the patient's spontaneous breaths.

12. **D.** Too much PEEP will overstretch the lungs and result in decreased compliance. The overstretched lung areas compress their pulmonary capillaries, which causes blood to be diverted to other lung areas. This is likely to increase shunting. If the level of PEEP is too great, the lungs will compress the heart. This will reduce venous return to the heart. As a result, the cardiac output will drop, as will the blood pressure.

13. **B.** $C_{st}$ is caluulated as follows:

$$C_{st} = \frac{\text{exhaled } V_T - \text{compressed volume}}{\text{plateau pressure} - PEEP}$$

$$\text{Compressed volume} = \frac{\text{compliance factor} \times \text{plateau pressure}}{(3\,mL/cm\,H_2O \times 30\,cm\,H_2O)}$$

$$= \frac{800\,mL - 90\,mL}{30 - 8}$$

$$= \frac{710\,mL}{22}$$

$$C_{st} = 32\,mL/cm\,H_2O$$

14. **D.** $C_{dyn}$ is calculated as follows:

$$C_{dyn} = \frac{\text{exhaled } V_T - \text{compressed volume}}{\text{peak pressure} - PEEP}$$

$$\text{Compressed volume} = \frac{\text{compliance factor} \times \text{peak pressure}}{(3\,mL/cm\,H_2O \times 40\,cm\,H_2O)}$$

$$= \frac{800\,mL - 120\,mL}{40 - 8}$$

$$= \frac{680\,mL}{32}$$

$$C_{dyn} = 21\,mL/cm\,H_2O$$

15. **C.** Disconnecting the tubing to the external exhalation valve will cause it to fail, which causes the machine $V_T$ to bypass the patient. A self-cycling ventilator would deliver the $V_T$ to the patient. If the inspiratory and expiratory limbs of the circuit were reversed, no volume would be delivered and the peak pressure alarm would sound. Even if the spirometer were out of calibration, the $V_T$ would be delivered to the patient, and pressure would build in the system.

16. **B.** Expiratory retard is indicated in a condition with air trapping on exhalation, such as asthma. The other three conditions do not interfere with exhalation.

17. **C.** The patient's oxygenation is normal. The other three parameters are not normal. Review Box 15-1.

18. **C.** Increasing the IPAP (inspiratory positive airway pressure) level will lead to an increased tidal volume. If the IPAP level is decreased, the tidal volume will also decrease. The EPAP (expiratory positive airway pressure) level is similar to CPAP or PEEP in its effect on the patient's functional residual capacity (FRC). Therefore, EPAP is adjusted only to change FRC to affect the patient's oxygenation.

19. **C.** Increasing the lower pressure level will increase the CPAP pressure to open the patient's throat soft tissues and stop the snoring. A rate change will not affect the ventilator pressures. Increasing the upper pressure level will increase the $V_T$; it will not affect the lower pressure to stop the snoring. A facemask would be indicated if the patient did not tolerate the nasal mask or had a significant leak out of his mouth. He does not have these problems.

20. **A.** Decreasing the mechanical dead space will decrease the patient's $CO_2$ level. Decreasing the $\dot{V}_E$ will increase the $CO_2$ level. Neither changing the I:E ratio nor adding PEEP has any effect on $CO_2$ elimination.

21. **C.** Retained secretions and bronchospasm are Raw problems and cause only the peak pressure to increase. The other two conditions decrease $C_{LT}$ and make the plateau pressure increase. The peak pressure increases as a result.

22. **B.** PEEP elevates the patient's baseline pressure and raises the P$\overline{aw}$ by the same amount. Although the other three options would increase the P$\overline{aw}$, they would not have as much impact as the PEEP.

# 16 | Home Care and Pulmonary Rehabilitation

A review of the most recent Entry Level Examinations has shown an average of 3 questions (2% of the exam) that cover home care and pulmonary rehabilitation.

## MODULE A

### Interview the patient

**1. What is the patient's social history? (NBRC code: IB4c) [Difficulty: R, Ap]**

The patient's family and social life is an important consideration in discharge planning with the patient and family. Whether the patient is an adult or a child, his or her home life should be understood. Probably no one knows more about the patient or cares more about his or her well-being than the immediate family. Very close friends can assist the family or even replace a nonexistent one.

The following questions can be asked of an adult patient and family:

a. "Is your spouse able to help you at home?"
b. "Do you have other family members who can help you at home?"
c. "Are there neighbors or family friends who can help you at home?"
d. "Do you belong to any clubs or a church? Can you get to them?"
e. "Do you have a garden, a pet, or any hobbies at your home?"
f. "Have you smoked? If yes, for how long? How many packs of cigarettes a day?"
g. "Have you used illegal drugs? What have you used? For how long?"

The following questions can be asked of the family of a minor child:

a. "Do both parents live at home? If not, with whom does the child live? Do both parents care for the child?"
b. "Are there any siblings who can help in caring for the child?"
c. "Do you have other family members who can help you care for the child at home?"
d. "Are there neighbors or family friends who can help you care for the child at home?"
e. "Does the child belong to any clubs or a church? Can you get the child to them? Can they help you care for the child at home?"
f. "Can you get the child to and from school?"

The answers to these types of questions may lead to other questions about the patient's family and social life. Consider the patient's disease or condition and the answers that are given to determine a discharge plan that minimizes any disturbances in family life.

**2. How much exercise can the patient tolerate, and how active is the patient on a daily basis? (NBRC code: IB4b) [Difficulty: R, Ap]**

The following subject areas and questions can help the therapist to further determine the patient's exercise tolerance and activities of daily living:

#### a. Personal grooming

1. "Do you get short of breath when dressing?"
2. "What is the most difficult part of dressing?"
3. "Are you able to wash your hair regularly?"
4. (For men) "Are you able to shave regularly?"
5. "Does using extra $O_2$ help you to do these things without getting as short of breath?"

#### b. In-home activities

1. "Can you go up and down stairs without getting short of breath?"
2. "Can you walk through your home without getting short of breath?"
3. "Can you cook and prepare nutritious meals?"
4. "Does using extra $O_2$ help you do these things without getting as short of breath?"

#### c. Out-of-home activities

1. "Can you go shopping without getting short of breath?"
2. "What clubs, church, and so forth do you attend regularly?"
3. "Can you do yard or garden work?"
4. "Do you have a pet dog that you walk through the neighborhood?"

5. "Does using extra $O_2$ help you do these things without getting as short of breath?"

The patient with chronic and severe cardiopulmonary disease may speak of a very restricted and limited lifestyle. Extra $O_2$ may have only limited benefit. The patient with chronic, but moderate, cardiopulmonary disease can live a somewhat limited but full lifestyle. Extra $O_2$ may help greatly at times when the patient becomes short of breath. The otherwise healthy patient with an acute cardiopulmonary disease should tell of a previously full and enjoyable lifestyle. Extra $O_2$ may be needed now, but it is hoped that it will not be needed upon recovery.

### 3. What are the patient's learning needs?
(NBRC code: IB5) [Difficulty: R]

It is very important to determine what the patient understands about his or her cardiopulmonary condition and the care that has been ordered to help with it. If the patient is found to need additional teaching in some area, it should be incorporated into the respiratory care plan.

### MODULE B
**Home respiratory care services**

### 1. Instruct the patient and family to ensure safety and infection control (NBRC code: IIIK4) [Difficulty: R, Ap]

Home care equipment is essentially the same as that found in any hospital. The same types of equipment problems can occur in the patient's home as in the hospital. Teach the patient and family about the equipment so that they can correct minor concerns and direct major concerns to the home care therapist.

Evaluate the following aspects of the patient's home environment:

a. Does the patient live alone or have a spouse or companion to help provide care? Make sure that telephone numbers for relatives, helpful neighbors, the patient's physician, ambulance service, local hospital, pharmacy, and any other support services are posted by each telephone.

b. Make sure that all respiratory care equipment is cleaned (Chapter 2 has suggestions on methods of disinfection) and functioning properly.

c. Check that home $O_2$ systems are working properly. If the patient has an $O_2$ concentrator, make sure that the filters are cleaned and that the alarms are set and working. Make sure that an $O_2$ cylinder, a regulator, and an $O_2$ delivery system are working properly as a backup system if the $O_2$ concentrator fails.

d. Have the patient centrally locate all necessary items for daily living. The patient should avoid unnecessary stair climbing. It might be recommended that the patient convert the living room, if it is located near the kitchen and bathroom, into a bedroom.

Clothing can be modified with Velcro fasteners, snaps, or zippers if the patient cannot use buttons easily. Shoes can be more easily put on with a long-handled shoehorn. Avoid shoes with laces. A long-handled comb or brush makes grooming easier.

e. The kitchen should be modified so that all commonly used equipment is on the counter. Everyday dishes, utensils, and foods should be placed so that they can be easily reached in cabinets and drawers within an arm's reach. The patient should not have to bend over, stoop down, or climb onto a footstool to retrieve anything.

f. It may be necessary to have handholds added to the walls by the toilet and shower or tub for extra security. A shower chair can be added so that the patient can sit while bathing. A handheld showerhead might make bathing easier.

g. Check the home for airborne irritants. Smoking by the patient or anyone else in the home must be stopped. The patient should avoid contact with other forms of indoor pollution, such as aerosol sprays, paints, varnishes, and dust. A high-efficiency particulate air (HEPA) filtration system is best for removing indoor airborne pollutants and irritants. Indoor kerosene-fueled space heaters should not be used because of their release of carbon monoxide.

h. The patient should avoid contact with any known allergens, people who smoke, or substances to which he or she has a bad reaction.

> ### Exam Hint
>
> **P**ast examinations have included questions on the maintenance of $O_2$ concentrators for low-flow oxygen in the home and the use of backup sources of $O_2$ when an $O_2$ concentrator fails. In addition, questions have been asked about how to deal with a home care patient whose nasal cannula has no flow. Telephone instructions include having the patient place the cannula under water to check for bubbling, tightening all tubing connections, confirming that gas is flowing from the $O_2$ concentrator, cleaning its filters, replacing a defective cannula, and switching to an $O_2$ cylinder if the concentrator has malfunctioned.

### MODULE C
**Respiratory care plan**

### 1. Analyze the available information to determine the patient's pathophysiologic state (NBRC code: IIIH1) [Difficulty: R, Ap, An]

The respiratory therapist should have a solid understanding of the pathophysiology of commonly found cardiopulmonary and cardiovascular conditions. These include, but are not limited to, asthma, emphysema, chronic bronchitis, pneumonia, pulmonary fibrosis, cystic fibrosis, right and left heart failure, stroke, and neuromuscular disease. The scope of this text prevents a full discussion of these conditions; the reader is referred to the many excellent pathology textbooks that are available.

In addition, review the information presented in Chapters 1, 3, 4, and 5. These chapters discuss bedside patient assessment, blood gas interpretation, pulmonary function testing, and hemodynamic monitoring that the NBRC has determined to be testable on the entry level examination. Be prepared to evaluate areas such as vital signs, breath sounds, blood gas values, pulmonary function results, and cardiac study results to determine the patient's condition.

## 2. Counsel the patient and family about the importance of smoking cessation (NBRC code: IIIA6, IIIK3) [Difficulty: R, Ap, An]

Absolute proof exists that smoking causes emphysema, chronic bronchitis, lung cancer, and heart disease. These conditions occur in the smoker and in the nonsmoking spouse and children. Asthmatic patients often find that their bronchospasm is worsened when they inhale tobacco smoke. Obviously, any patient with a smoking-related cardiopulmonary disease and the patient's family members must cease smoking. Continued exposure to tobacco smoke will harm the patient.

Because the nicotine found in tobacco is highly addictive, many patients find that they cannot stop smoking without suffering withdrawal symptoms. To aid in stopping smoking, it is often helpful to meet with other people who are also trying to stop. This group support helps the patient feel less alone in his or her efforts to stop smoking. The patient's physician also needs to be involved in this process.

If the patient has been unable to stop smoking because of withdrawal symptoms, he or she is likely addicted to nicotine. A nicotine replacement system that allows gradual withdrawal can aid greatly in smoking cessation. Although no smoking cessation plan works in every case, the highest percentage of patients are able to stop smoking using a combination of psychological support and gradual reduction in nicotine.

Several well-established nicotine replacement and reduction systems currently exist. All are available without prescription. The Commit lozenge is held in the mouth to release a controlled amount of nicotine. Nicotine polacrilex (Nicorette) is a gum that is chewed by the patient to release a dose of nicotine. The Nicotrol Inhaler allows the user to inhale nicotine through a device shaped like a cigarette. Nicotine transdermal patches are another nicotine reduction system. Prostep, Nicoderm, and Habitrol are three brands of patch that, when placed onto the skin, allow a set amount of nicotine to be absorbed. With these systems, the patient starts with a relatively high dose of the drug and, over a period of weeks, goes through a series of patches with less and less nicotine. It is critical that the patient not smoke while using any of these systems. Patients who continue to smoke run the risk of a nicotine overdose, which increases the risk for myocardial infarction.

A third option is taking bupropion HCl (Zyban). It was originally found to help patients who were suffering from depression; it acts to alter the brain's chemistry so that nicotine cravings are reduced. A physician must prescribe this drug.

## 3. Determine the appropriateness of the prescribed respiratory care plan and recommend modifications when indicated

### a. Review the interdisciplinary patient and family care plan (NBRC code: IIIH2b) [Difficulty: R, Ap]

### b. Review the planned therapy to establish the therapeutic plan (NBRC code: IIIH2a) [Difficulty: R, Ap]

Determination of the patient's ideal therapeutic goals is best done with a team approach. The patient's physician, nurse, and respiratory therapist should work together. The first consideration should be the patient's diagnosis. Then, it should be determined whether the patient's condition is permanent, improving, or worsening. Objective information such as arterial blood gas results, pulmonary function testing results, chest x-ray film findings, sputum production, and vital signs must be evaluated. The patient cannot be expected to do more than he or she is physically capable of doing. The therapist must also evaluate the patient's mental state. Is he or she emotionally ready to go home and be taught about self-care or start a rehabilitation program? The therapeutic goals for each patient must be individualized. If the patient is not physically or emotionally ready to take care of himself or herself, the family or a paid care provider is needed. Following are common therapeutic goals:

a. The primary goal is to improve the patient's functional ability as much as possible. This can best be determined by finding out what the patient wants to be able to do in his or her life. From this, a list of attainable short- and long-term goals can be developed. One of the primary short-term goals should be that the patient feels better. He or she should be able to control or reduce any symptoms. Make sure that the patient's goals are realistic and can be reached. The family needs to be involved with any major decision making. Often, it is helpful to break a large goal down into several smaller tasks. In this way, the patient and family receive frequent positive feedback.

b. Improve the patient's self-image. This should follow when the first goal is reached.

c. Enhance the patient's ability to exercise. How this is approached may depend on the level of the patient's disability. In general, the worse the patient's lung disease, the less able the patient is to increase his or her exercise level.

d. Decrease the frequency and length of any hospitalizations.

e. Prolong the patient's life through the proper use of $O_2$ and other respiratory care modalities.

Respiratory care protocols may be used at home and in the hospital. An $O_2$ therapy protocol can be implemented that uses the patient's pulse oximetry ($SpO_2$) values to adjust the $O_2$ percentage or flow up or down. For example, keep the patient's $SpO_2$ at less than 95% but greater than 85%. A second protocol could involve the use of inhaled sympathomimetic bronchodilators based on the patient's peak flow results.

## c. Determine the appropriateness of the prescribed therapy and goals for the patient's pathophysiologic state (NBRC code: IIIH3) [Difficulty: R, Ap, An]

The patient's physical condition must be evaluated before a home care or rehabilitation program is designed. Besides the primary diagnosis, the patient may have other conditions that further limit his or her ability to safely participate. If the patient is too ill or too limited in ability, he or she should not be placed into a home care or rehabilitation program.

Although the patient's physical condition is the most important thing to be evaluated from a safety point of view, other aspects of his or her life must also be explored. These include a nutritional review, a psychosocial assessment, and a vocational evaluation. Because these areas are beyond the scope of practice of most respiratory therapists, other experts must be called in by the physician.

A rehabilitation program is an individually structured sequence of events that is designed to safely increase the patient's exercise tolerance. In 1942, the Council of Rehabilitation defined rehabilitation as "the restoration of the individual to the fullest medical, mental, emotional, social, and vocational potential of which he/she is capable" (Hodgkin, 1993). In 1974, The American College of Chest Physicians' Committee on Pulmonary Rehabilitation adopted the following: "Pulmonary rehabilitation may be defined as an art of medical practice wherein an individually tailored, multidisciplinary program is formulated which through accurate diagnosis, therapy, emotional support, and education, stabilizes or reverses both the physio- and psychopathology of pulmonary diseases and attempts to return the patient to the *highest possible functional capacity* (italics added) allowed by his pulmonary handicap and overall life situation" (Petty, 1975).

It further states: "In the broadest sense, pulmonary rehabilitation means providing good, comprehensive respiratory care for patients with pulmonary disease."

## d. Recommend changes in the therapeutic plan if supportive data exist (NBRC code: IIIH4) [Difficulty: R, Ap]

Be prepared to evaluate the patient's condition and make suggestions for changing goals and methods. The therapist must have a thorough understanding of the patient's condition and individual goals to evaluate the progress. Objectively consider the patient's physical, emotional, and social condition. The therapist must also listen to the patient's subjective opinion about his or her situation. Be prepared to make recommendations to the patient and attending physician for modifying the goals according to the patient's changing condition.

The following signs indicate that the patient is stable or making progress:

1. The patient subjectively feels that he or she is doing as well as can be expected. The patient is motivated to try new things.
2. Symptoms are reduced or at least under control.
3. Cardiopulmonary function tests and blood gases show improvement. Even a slowing in the patient's formerly rapid rate of decline is a good sign.
4. The patient reports an increase in the distance that can be walked at his or her own pace.
5. The patient reports an increase in the 6- or 12-min walking distance.

The following indicate that the patient's health is deteriorating:

1. He or she subjectively feels worse. The patient is afraid to try new things.
2. Symptoms are worse. The patient feels dyspnea at less exertion than before.
3. The sputum has changed. It could be thick and harder to cough out or could have changed color to yellow or green. The patient may be coughing out more than before or less if the sputum cannot be brought up.
4. Cardiopulmonary function tests and blood gases are worse. The patient may need increased $O_2$, more aerosolized bronchodilator, or other cardiopulmonary medications.
5. The patient cannot walk or perform as much work as before without worsening of symptoms.

### Exam Hint

Increased walking distance is an indication that the patient's pulmonary rehabilitation program is succeeding.

**e. Explain therapy and goals in understandable terms** (NBRC code: IIIK1) [Difficulty: R, Ap]

**f. Conduct patient education and disease management programs** (NBRC code: IIIK2) [Difficulty: R, Ap]

Effective teaching methods include the following:

1. Speak at the patient's and family's levels of understanding. Medical language usually reserved for peer discussions is not typically understood by people without a medical background. However, use of overly simple explanations can be insulting to someone who is intelligent or well educated. In either case, the important information does not get across as intended. Give the patient written instructions as needed.

2. Frequently ask the patient and family whether they have any questions, then answer them.

3. Have the patient and family repeat in their own words what they were just told to ensure understanding.

4. Have the patient and family demonstrate all procedures and techniques.

5. Reteach anything that is misunderstood.

6. Retest the patient and family as needed.

7. Document in the patient's chart what has been taught.

The therapist should be able to implement a patient's disease management program. In addition, the therapist should monitor the patient's compliance with the program. For example, is the patient faithfully following the smoking cessation program or has he or she "cheated"? Is the patient following the asthma control program by monitoring his or her peak flow and adjusting inhaled medications according to the physician's order?

## BIBLIOGRAPHY

American Association for Respiratory Care: Clinical practice guideline: Oxygen therapy in the home or extended care facility, *Respir Care* 37:918, 1992.

American Association for Respiratory Care: Clinical practice guideline: Discharge planning for the respiratory care patient, *Respir Care* 40:1308, 1995.

American Association for Respiratory Care: Clinical practice guideline: Long-term invasive mechanical ventilation in the home, *Respir Care* 40:1313, 1995.

American Association for Respiratory Care: Clinical practice guideline: Providing patient and caregiver training, *Respir Care* 41:658, 1996.

American Association for Respiratory Care: Clinical practice guideline: Suctioning of the patient in the home, *Respir Care* 44:99, 1999.

Bell CW, Blodgett D, Goike C, et al: *Home care and rehabilitation in respiratory medicine*, Philadelphia, 1984, JB Lippincott.

Belman MJ, Wasserman K: Exercise training and testing in patients with chronic obstructive pulmonary disease, *Basics Respir Dis* 10, 1981.

Branson RD, Hess DR, Chatburn RL: *Respiratory care equipment*, ed 2, Philadelphia, 1999, Lippincott Williams & Wilkins.

Cairo JM, Pilbeam SP: *Mosby's respiratory care equipment*, ed 7, St Louis, 2004, Mosby.

Christopher KL: At-home administration of oxygen. In Kacmarek RM, Stoller JK, editors: *Current respiratory care*, Toronto, 1988, BC Decker.

Connors G, Hilling L, editors: *American Association of Cardiovascular and Pulmonary Rehabilitation: Guidelines for pulmonary rehabilitation programs*, Champaign, Ill, 1993, Human Kinetics.

Des Jardins T, Burton GG: *Clinical manifestations and assessment of respiratory disease*, ed 4, St Louis, 2002, Mosby.

Dunlevy CL: Patient education and health promotion. In Scanlan CL, Wilkins RL, Stoller JK, editors: *Egan's fundamentals of respiratory care*, ed 7, St Louis, 1999, Mosby.

Edge RS: Infection control. In Barnes TA, editor: *Respiratory care practice*, Chicago, 1988, Mosby.

Eubanks DH, Bone RC: *Comprehensive respiratory care*, ed 2, St Louis, 1990, Mosby.

Farzan S, Farzan D: *A concise handbook of respiratory disease*, ed 4, Stamford, Conn, 1997, Appleton & Lange.

Gilmartin M: Transition from the intensive care unit to home: Patient selection and discharge planning, *Respir Care* 39:456, 1994.

Gourley DA: Respiratory home care. In Wyka KA, Mathews PJ, Clark WF, editors: *Foundations of respiratory care*, Albany, 2002, Delmar.

Heuer AJ, Scanlan CL: Respiratory care in alternative settings. In Wilkins RL, Stoller JK, Scanlan CL, editors: *Egan's fundamentals of respiratory care*, ed 8, St Louis, 2003, Mosby.

Hodgkin JE: Home care and pulmonary rehabilitation. In Kacmarek RM, Stoller JK, editors: *Current respiratory care*, Toronto, 1988, BC Decker.

Hodgkin JE et al: *Pulmonary rehabilitation*, ed 2, Philadelphia, 1993, Lippincott.

Hodgkin JE, Connors GA: Pulmonary rehabilitation. In Burton GG, Hodgkin JE, Ward JJ, editors: *Respiratory care: A guide to clinical practice*, ed 4, Philadelphia, 1997, JB Lippincott.

Holden DA, Stelmach KD, Curtis PS, et al: The impact of a rehabilitation program on functional status of patients with chronic lung disease, *Respir Care* 35:332, 1990.

Kwiatkowski CA, Tougher-Decker R, O'Sullivan-Maillet J: Nutritional aspects of health and disease. In Scanlan CL, Wilkins RL, Stoller JK, editors: *Egan's fundamentals of respiratory care*, ed 7, St Louis, 1999, Mosby.

Lewis ML, Hagarty EM, Lawlor B: Home respiratory care. In Fink JB, Hunt GE, editors: *Clinical practice in respiratory care*, 1999, Lippincott Williams & Wilkins.

Lucas J, Golish JA, Sleeper G, et al: *Home respiratory care*, Norwalk, Conn, 1988, Appleton & Lange.

MacIntyre NR: Pulmonary rehabilitation. In Hess DR, MacIntyre NR, Mishoe SC, et al, editors: *Respiratory care principles & practice*, Philadelphia, 2002, WB Saunders.

May DF: *Rehabilitation and continuity of care in pulmonary disease*, St Louis, 1991, Mosby.

McInturff SL, O'Donohue WJ Jr: Respiratory care in the home and alternate sites. In Burton GG, Hodgkin JE, Ward JJ, editors: *Respiratory care: A guide to clinical practice*, ed 4, Philadelphia, 1997, JB Lippincott.

Mulligan SC, Masterson JG, Devane JG, et al: Clinical and pharmacokinetic properties of a transdermal nicotine patch, *Clin Pharmacol Ther* 47:331, 1990.

Nett LM: The physician's role in smoking cessation, *Chest Suppl* 97:28s, 1990.

Petty TL: Pulmonary rehabilitation, Basics of respiratory disease (journal), New York, 1975, American Thoracic Society.

Petty TL: Pulmonary rehabilitation: Better living with new technology, *Respir Care* 30:98, 1985.

Petty TL, Nett LM: *Enjoying life with emphysema*, Philadelphia, 1987, Lea & Febiger.

Pulmonary rehabilitation: Official American Thoracic Society statement, *Am Rev Respir Dis* 124:663, 1981.

Rennard SI, Daughton D: Transdermal nicotine for smoking cessation, *Respir Care* 38:290, 1993.

Scanlan CL, Heuer A, Wyka KA: Respiratory care in alternate sites. In Scanlan CL, Wilkins RL, Stoller JK, editors: *Egan's fundamentals of respiratory care*, ed 7, St Louis, 1999, Mosby.

Sobush D, Dunning M, McDonald K: Exercise prescription components for respiratory muscle training: Past, present, and future, *Respir Care* 30:34, 1985.

Taylor C, Lillis C, LeMond P: *Fundamentals of nursing: The art and science of nursing care*, ed 2, Philadelphia, 1993, JB Lippincott.

White GC: *Equipment theory for respiratory care*, ed 3, Albany, NY, 1999, Delmar.

Wilkins RL, Dexter JR: *Respiratory disease: A case study approach to patient care*, ed 2, Philadelphia, 1998, FA Davis.

Wyka KA: Cardiopulmonary rehabilitation. In Wilkins RL, Stoller JK, Scanlan CL, editors: *Egan's fundamentals of respiratory care*, ed 8, St Louis, 2003, Mosby.

Wyka KA: Pulmonary rehabilitation. In Wyka KA, Mathews PJ, Clark WF, editors: *Foundations of respiratory care*, Albany, 2002, Delmar.

## SELF-STUDY QUESTIONS

1. After instructing a home care patient on the use of her small-volume nebulizer, you want to be sure that she understands how to fill and clean it. How could you confirm this?
   - I. Have the patient demonstrate use of the nebulizer to you
   - II. Have the patient's boyfriend demonstrate use of the nebulizer to you
   - III. Have the patient answer your questions about the nebulizer
   - IV. Have the patient tell you how the equipment is set up and cleaned
   - A. I, III, and IV
   - B. I and II
   - C. III and IV
   - D. II, III, and IV

2. Your patient with chronic obstructive pulmonary disease (COPD) had been coughing out about 20 mL/day of white mucus until 3 days ago. Since then, she has been coughing out only 5 mL. She tells you that the mucus is more difficult to cough out and that she is getting more short of breath. What is the most likely cause of these recent changes?
   - A. Her lung disease is improving
   - B. She is overhydrated
   - C. She has an infection or mucus plugging
   - D. Treatments have decreased the amount of mucus she is producing

3. A home care patient tells you that she cannot feel any $O_2$ coming to her nasal cannula from the $O_2$ concentrator. You would do all of the following EXCEPT
   - A. Refill the humidifier bottle with sterile water
   - B. Place the cannula prongs under water to see if any gas is bubbling out
   - C. Tighten all the equipment connections
   - D. Switch the patient over to her tank of $O_2$

4. On surveying a patient's home, you notice that four steps lead to the front door. The patient's bedroom is upstairs, and his wife smokes about one pack of cigarettes a day. You would recommend all the following EXCEPT
   - A. The patient's wife should stop smoking
   - B. The patient should use a cane when climbing stairs
   - C. The patient's bedroom should be moved downstairs
   - D. A ramp should be added to facilitate entering through the front door

5. When first visiting a home care patient's house, the therapist should evaluate all of the following to attempt to eliminate risks associated with the patient's performance of daily activities:
    I. Bathroom facilities, including an assessment of ease of getting into and out of the shower or bathtub
    II. Television and remote control for operation
    III. Kitchen facilities, including all cooking and eating utensils placed within arm's reach
    IV. Properly cleaned HEPA filtration system
    A. I
    B. I, II, III, and IV
    C. III and IV
    D. I and III

6. In attempts to determine the daily exercise tolerance of a male COPD patient, all of the following questions might be asked EXCEPT
    A. How far can you walk your pet dog around the yard?
    B. Are you able to shave every day?
    C. Is your wife or a relative able to drive you to the grocery store?
    D. How many flights of stairs can you climb before you have to stop?

7. The main goal of a pulmonary rehabilitation program should be to
    A. Reduce the amount of sputum coughed out every day
    B. Return the patient to his or her highest possible level of functioning
    C. Reduce the amount of supplemental $O_2$ needed
    D. Increase the patient's appetite to achieve weight gain

8. Your patient and her husband are both smokers. She is about to be discharged after treatment for bronchitis. Which of the following would you recommend?
    I. She should stop smoking
    II. She should see her physician to get help to stop smoking
    III. Her husband should stop smoking
    IV. She should switch to her husband's brand of cigarettes to reduce the conflict between them
    A. I and II
    B. III
    C. I, II, and III
    D. I, II, III, and IV

## ANSWER KEY AND RATIONALE

1. **A.** The best way to be sure that the patient really understands the purpose of the equipment is to ask her questions about it and have her describe its function. Any misunderstandings then can be clarified. In addition, the patient should show that she has the necessary dexterity to make the equipment operate.

2. **C.** The patient's complaint of decreased mucus clearance, greater difficulty coughing out secretions, and increased shortness of breath all indicate a worsening secretion problem.

3. **A.** The level of water in the humidifier does not affect the ability of $O_2$ to flow through the $O_2$ delivery system. Tightening of all connections and placement of the cannula prongs under water reveal whether gas is flowing through the prongs. If no gas is flowing out from the $O_2$ concentrator, the nasal cannula should be switched over to the $O_2$ tank.

4. **B.** A cane should not be used without a documented need. The patient's life situation can improve if his spouse stops smoking and he minimizes climbing of stairs.

5. **D.** Many injuries occur in the bathroom and kitchen when weak patients fall while climbing into showers or tubs or onto chairs to reach high objects.

6. **C.** A patient's exercise tolerance is not evaluated by finding out if a relative can drive the patient somewhere. Exercise tolerance can be assessed by finding out the patient's ease or difficulty in performing specific tasks.

7. **B.** Restoring the patient to his or her highest possible functional capacity is the main goal of a rehabilitation program. All other goals are secondary to this.

8. **C.** The patient and her husband must both stop smoking. If she is the only one to quit, she will continue to inhale second-hand smoke from her husband. Her physician should be involved in her care to offer medical support and recommend group support.

# 17 Special Procedures

A review of the most recent Entry Level Examinations has shown an average of 3 questions (2% of the exam) that cover special procedures.

## MODULE A

### Assist the physician with procedures

### 1. Cardioversion (NBRC code: IIIJ2) [Difficulty: R, Ap]

Cardioversion (or *countershock*) refers to deliberate sending of a direct current electrical shock through the patient's heart. Its purpose is to suppress an abnormal heartbeat so that the normal pacemaker at the sinoatrial (SA) node takes over. This is accomplished if a great enough electrical current is sent through the chest wall to cause depolarization of a critical mass of myocardial cells. After this, the SA node should take over as the pacemaker, provided that the heart muscle is oxygenated and is not too acidotic.

Synchronized cardioversion is similar in some ways to defibrillation (see Chapter 11). An electrical shock is sent by two paddles through the heart to suppress paroxysmal atrial tachycardia, atrial flutter, atrial fibrillation, and hemodynamically stable ventricular tachycardia so that the SA node takes over. Its major difference from defibrillation is that the electrical shock is administered automatically by the defibrillator after an R wave has been recognized by the electrocardiograph (ECG) monitor. The ECG electrodes must be in place and the best lead (often lead II) selected for a clear, strong, upright R wave to be shown. The defibrillator unit is set for synchronized cardioversion. The physician holds the paddles on the patient's right anterior and left lateral chest wall. When the discharge buttons are pushed on the paddles, the shock is sent after the next R wave has been identified by the ECG monitor. Box 17-1 shows the sequence of increasingly powerful countershocks that can be given.

Cardioversion is not considered to be an emergency; however, it is performed as quickly as possible so that the patient does not stay in the abnormal rhythm any longer than necessary. Synchronized cardioversion is performed only if medical treatment with antiarrhythmia drugs or carotid artery massage has no effect. Because these patients are usually conscious, they should be sedated with diazepam (Valium), midazolam (Versed), or a similar medication. Patients who are hypotensive or already unconscious should not be sedated.

The respiratory therapist's role in cardioversion involves the following:

a. Making sure that the ECG electrodes are properly positioned for either monitoring or diagnosing the rhythm, as the physician requires
b. Making sure that the ECG machine and monitor are working properly
c. Making sure that the selected ECG lead can provide a strong R wave; usually, the R wave is upright in lead II
d. Charging the defibrillator to the power level ordered by the physician
e. Adding the electrode cream to the electrode paddles to decrease the skin's resistance to electricity
f. Being prepared to keep a patent airway, manually ventilate the patient, or begin chest compressions, if necessary

### 2. Bronchoscopy (NBRC code: IIIJ1) [Difficulty: R, Ap]

Bronchoscopy involves looking directly into the patient's tracheobronchial airways. The physician can perform a number of diagnostic and therapeutic tasks under direct vision. (Box 17-2 lists uses, limitations, and risks of bronchoscopy.)

The rigid bronchoscope is a straight, hollow, stainless steel tube (Fig. 17-1). It has a distal light source so that the airway can be seen and a side port for providing $O_2$ or mechanical ventilation to the patient. The right and left mainstem bronchi can be observed by passing a mirror through the main channel. A hook or net can be passed through the main channel into the trachea or either bronchus to remove a foreign body. A rigid bronchoscope is preferred for the treatment of massive hemoptysis or for removal of a foreign body.

Flexible fiberoptic bronchoscopy (FFB) is a small-diameter flexible tube with two sets of fiberoptic bundles that shine light into the airway and allow viewing of the airway. It has gained wide popularity because it is well tolerated by the patient and allows for clear visualization and collection of specimens from small bronchi (Figs. 17-2 and 17-3). The adult bronchoscopy tube is about 5 to 6 mm in outer diameter (OD), and the pediatric tube is about 3 mm in OD. Small diameter and an ability to guide the catheter allow the operator to

---

### BOX 17-1   Wattage Used in Synchronous Cardioversion and Defibrillation

**SYNCHRONIZED CARDIOVERSION OF AN INFANT**
- 0.5-1.0 joules (watt-seconds)/kg
- Stepwise increases in energy should be used if the initial shock fails to convert the rhythm

**SYNCHRONIZED CARDIOVERSION OF AN ADULT**
*ATRIAL FLUTTER AND PAROXYSMAL ATRIAL TACHYCARDIA*
- 50 joules
- Stepwise increases in energy should be used if the initial shock fails to convert the rhythm

*ATRIAL FIBRILLATION*
- 100 joules
- Stepwise increases in energy should be used if the initial shock fails to convert the rhythm

*VENTRICULAR TACHYCARDIA WITH A REGULAR FORM AND RATE WITH OR WITHOUT A PULSE*
- 100 joules
- Stepwise increases in energy should be used if the initial shock fails to convert the rhythm

*VENTRICULAR TACHYCARDIA WITH AN IRREGULAR FORM AND RATE*
- 200 joules
- Stepwise increases in energy should be used if the initial shock fails to convert the rhythm

**DEFIBRILLATION**
*INFANT*
- 2 joules/kg
- 4 joules/kg for second and succeeding attempts

*ADULT*
- 200 joules on first attempt
- 200-300 joules on second attempt
- Up to 360 joules on third and succeeding attempts

---

### BOX 17-2   Uses, Limitations, and Risks of Bronchoscopy

**RIGID BRONCHOSCOPY**
*DIAGNOSTIC USE*
- Biopsy of tumors within the main airway

*THERAPEUTIC USES*
- Treatment of massive hemoptysis by cold-saline lavage, or placement of a Fogarty catheter to occlude the airway
- Removal of foreign bodies in infants and small children
- Aspiration of inspissated secretions and mucus plugs

*LIMITATIONS*
- Cannot be used for observing or treating problems beyond the left or right mainstem bronchus
- Cannot be used with patients with disease or trauma of the cervical spine who cannot hyperextend the neck
- Cannot be used with patients with disease or trauma of the jaw who cannot open the mouth widely enough to pass the tube

**FIBEROPTIC BRONCHOSCOPY**
*DIAGNOSTIC USES*
- Search for the origin of a positive sputum cytology
- Evaluate lung lesions and perform transbronchial biopsy of lung tissue (should be done only under fluoroscopic control)
- Stage lung cancer preoperatively
- Investigate unexplained hemoptysis, unexplained cough, localized wheeze, or stridor
- Search for the cause of unexplained paralysis of a vocal cord or hemidiaphragm
- Search for the cause of superior vena cava syndrome, chylothorax, or unexplained pleural effusion
- Assess airway patency, and investigate suspected bronchial tear or other injury after thoracic trauma
- Investigate a suspected tracheoesophageal fistula
- Investigate problems related to an endotracheal tube, such as tracheal damage, airway obstruction, or tube placement
- Obtain mucus for identification of pathogens
- Investigate suspected injury as a result of inhaled superheated gas and smoke from an enclosed fire
- Investigate suspected injury as a result of the aspiration of gastric contents
- Perform bronchoalveolar lavage

*THERAPEUTIC USES*
- Remove secretions or mucus plugs that cannot be cleared by other methods
- Remove small foreign bodies
- Remove abnormal endobronchial tissue or foreign material by forceps or laser techniques

**INCREASED RISKS RELATED TO RIGID OR FIBEROPTIC BRONCHOSCOPY**
- Recent myocardial infarction or unstable angina
- Unstable cardiac arrhythmia
- Partial tracheal obstruction
- Unstable bronchial asthma
- Severe hypoxemia
- Hypercarbia
- Pulmonary hypertension (risk of hemorrhage after biopsy)
- Bleeding disorder (risk of hemorrhage after biopsy)
- Lung abscess (airway could be flooded with purulent material)
- Pulmonary infection from contaminated equipment
- Pneumothorax from transbronchial biopsy
- Respiratory failure requiring mechanical ventilation of the patient

look into the bronchus to view each lung segment (segmental bronchi). The fiberoptic bronchoscope is preferred over the rigid one when the patient is being mechanically ventilated or has disease or trauma to the skull, jaw, or cervical spine. As is shown in Fig. 17-2, a photo connection allows the assistant to either take still photographs of pulmonary anatomy or videotape the entire procedure.

A limitation of the pediatric unit is that no channel outlet exists for suctioning purposes because of its small size. If a patient has an obstructing bronchial tumor, a special laser fiberoptic bronchoscope is used to burn away part of it. This enables the patient to breathe more easily but is not a cure for the cancer.

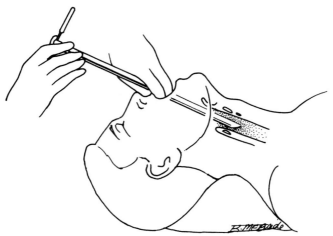

**Fig. 17-1** Rigid tube bronchoscope being inserted into a patient's trachea. Note how the head and neck must be hyperextended. *(From Scanlan CL, Simmons KF: Airway management. In Scanlan CL, Wilkins RL, Stoller JK, editors: Egan's fundamentals of respiratory care, ed 7, St Louis, 1999, Mosby.)*

Typical duties of the respiratory therapist during bronchoscopy include the following:

1. Inform the patient of the procedure and have him or her sign the medical release form.
2. Have a sedative (e.g., Versed, Valium) administered if needed.
3. Nebulize a topical anesthetic (e.g., 4% Xylocaine) to the airway.
4. Check the fiberoptic unit for proper function: working light source, working thumb control to flexible tip, adjustable focus on eyepiece, patency of the suction/biopsy channel.
5. Check the functioning of the biopsy brush and forceps.
6. Set up and monitor the patient's ECG.
7. Monitor the patient's vital signs.
8. Place and monitor the pulse oximeter on the patient.
9. Administer $O_2$ through a nasal catheter or the suction/biopsy channel on the unit.
10. Collect all suctioned or other specimens for culture and sensitivity.
11. Perform biopsies and brushings for cytology.
12. Operate any photographic equipment.
13. If the patient is being mechanically ventilated during fiberoptic bronchoscopy, perform the following:
    a. Place a bronchoscopy adapter between the endotracheal tube and the Y of the circuit. This keeps a seal around the bronchoscopy tube to minimize any drop in tidal volume ($V_T$).
    b. Watch for an increase in peak pressure because of the increased resistance caused by the bronchoscopy tube.
    c. Be prepared to make adjustments in inspired $O_2$, rate, flow, and $V_T$.

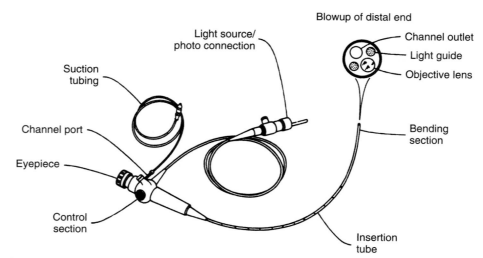

**Fig. 17-2** Flexible fiberoptic bronchoscope with its components and special features. *(From Scanlan CL, Simmons KF: Airway management. In Scanlan CL, Wilkins RL, Stoller JK, editors: Egan's fundamentals of respiratory care, ed 7, St Louis, 1999, Mosby.)*

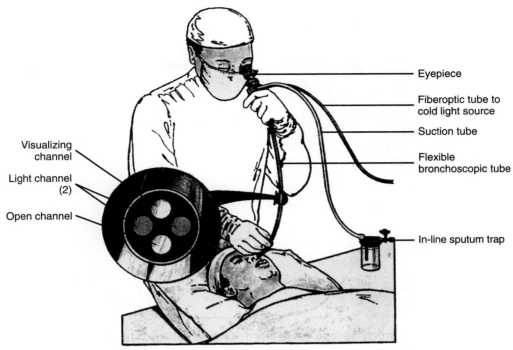

**Fig. 17-3** A flexible fiberoptic bronchoscopy being performed on a patient. *(From Williams SF, Thompson JM: Respiratory disorders, St Louis, 1990, Mosby.)*

d. Be prepared to switch from conventional volume ventilation to high-frequency jet ventilation, if needed.
14. Tend to the patient's comfort.
15. Disinfect equipment between patients.

### 3. Pleural drainage systems

#### a. Select a pleural drainage system (NBRC code: IIA20) [Difficulty: R, Ap]

*Thoracentesis* refers to the surgical puncture and drainage of the thoracic cavity. A chest tube (or *tube thoracostomy*) may be inserted into either one or both pleural spaces around the lungs (Fig. 17-4), the mediastinal space, or the pericardial space around the heart. This procedure is indicated when air or fluid in any of these spaces interferes with normal lung or heart function. Box 17-3 lists the indications for insertion of a chest tube.

> **Exam Hint**
>
> **M**ost past examinations have included a question that relates to identifying a patient who has a tension pneumothorax and needs to have a pleural chest tube inserted.

Modern drainage systems consist of either three or four chambers or sections designed to regulate the vacuum

---

**BOX 17-3   Indications for the Insertion of a Chest Tube**

**PLEURAL SPACE** (see Fig. 17-4, *D*)
- Tension pneumothorax
- Greater than a 10%-20% simple pneumothorax
- Hemothorax
- Empyema
- Pleural effusion
- Chylothorax

**MEDIASTINAL SPACE**
- Free air
- Free blood or other fluid

**PERICARDIAL SPACE**
- Cardiac tamponade
- Pneumopericardium

---

level, hold any drained fluids, prevent any outside air from entering the patient's thorax, and act as a pressure-relief valve in case the vacuum regulator should fail. Argyle and Pleurovac are two well-known manufacturers. Systems for draining the pleural space are discussed here; the principles are the same for draining mediastinal and pericardial spaces.

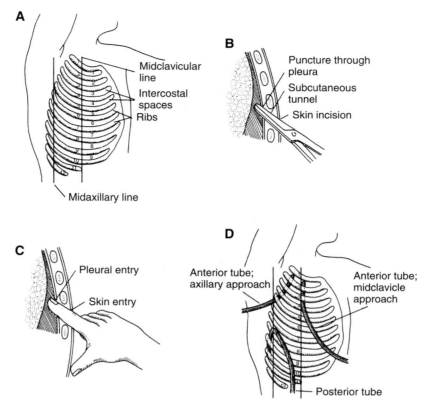

**Fig. 17-4** Technique for inserting a pleural chest tube. **A,** Anatomic landmarks. **B,** Dissecting through the tissues with a hemostat. **C,** Using a finger to widen the opening and ensure that the lung has not been punctured. **D,** Proper tube placement. Air is removed by a tube placed toward the apex of the lung. Fluid is removed by a tube placed toward the posterior base of the lung. *(Modified from Anderson HL, Bartlett RH: Respiratory care of the surgical patient. In Burton GG, Hodgkin JE, Ward JJ, editors: Respiratory care: a guide to clinical practice, ed 3, Philadelphia, 1991, JB Lippincott.)*

### b. Put a pleural drainage system together and make sure that it works properly (NBRC code: IIA20) [Difficulty: R, Ap]

Refer to Fig. 17-5 for an illustration of the assembly and operation of the three-chamber drainage system. The four-chamber drainage system is shown in Fig. 17-6 and is discussed concurrently.

*Vacuum level.* The operation of the central (wall) vacuum systems is discussed in Chapter 13. A partial vacuum setting of −15 to −20 cm $H_2O$ pressure to the pleural space is common practice.

*Suction control.* The suction control chamber is dry when the unit is unpacked. Follow the manufacturer's instructions for adding the correct amount of water to it. The proper water level, which is generally 15 to 20 cm high, causes whatever level of vacuum that is being applied to the patient's pleural space.

Room air drawn into the opening on top and bubbling through the water column is normal. This corresponds to chamber C in Fig. 17-6. Constant air bubbling causes the water level to gradually drop as the result of evaporation. Water will have to be added occasionally.

*Water seal.* The water seal chamber, which corresponds to chamber B in Fig. 17-6, is a safety feature. It is dry when unpacked. Follow the manufacturer's directions regarding the amount of water to be added. Typically the water seal tube should have about 2 cm of water in it for any patient air to bubble through. As indicated by the arrows (chamber B in Fig. 17-6), the tube is designed to permit air to leave the patient's chest cavity. (Air also can be seen bubbling through when fluid enters the drainage collection chamber and displaces some of its air.) However, room air cannot be drawn "backward" through the water so that it enters the chest if the vacuum fails or is disconnected.

The water seal chamber must be checked regularly for detection of any air that may be bubbling through from the patient's chest. If this is happening, the patient has an active air leak. If the chest tube has been placed into the pleural space, the air bubbling indicates that the patient has an unhealed pneumothorax or bronchopleural fistula. If the chest tube has been placed into the mediastinum or pericardium, bubbling indicates that air is leaking through a tear in the lung structures adjacent to these areas. Cessation of the air leak indicates that the tissues have healed over the tear.

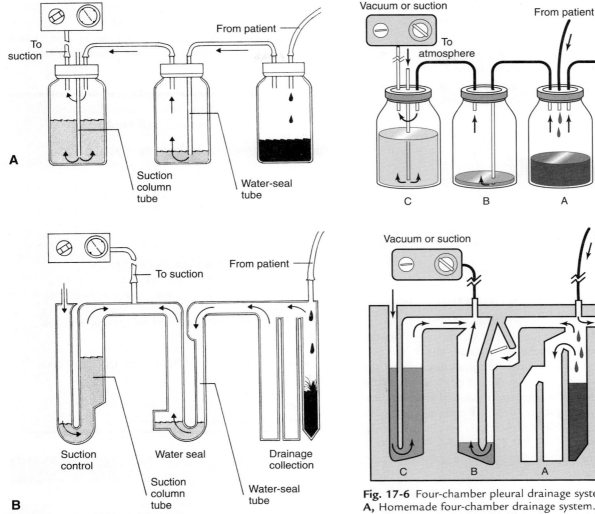

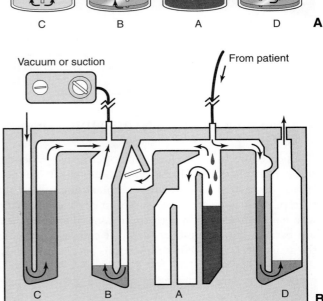

**Fig. 17-5** Three-chamber pleural drainage systems.
**A,** Homemade three-chamber drainage system. The depth at which the suction column tube is placed under water determines the level of vacuum that should be applied against the patient's pleural space. **B,** Schematic drawing of a modern manufactured three-chamber drainage system. *(From Shapiro BA, Kacmarek RM, Cane RD, et al: Clinical application of respiratory care, ed 4, St Louis, 1991, Mosby.)*

**Fig. 17-6** Four-chamber pleural drainage systems.
**A,** Homemade four-chamber drainage system. The depth at which the suction column tube in chamber C is placed under water determines the level of vacuum that will be applied against the patient's pleural space. **B,** Schematic drawing of a modern manufactured four-chamber drainage system. Chamber D acts to vent high-pressure air should the vacuum be turned off or malfunction *(Modified from Pilbeam SP, Deshpande VM: Chest tubes and pleural drainage, Curr Rev Respir Ther 5:151, 1983.)*

***Drainage collection.*** The drainage collection chamber, which corresponds to chamber A in Fig. 17-6, is designed to hold any fluid that is removed from the pleural space. It is divided into several sections that are marked off for volume measurement. The volume that has accumulated in the chamber should be recorded each hour. A sudden, significant increase in the amount of drainage should be called to the physician's attention. This is especially important if the patient is losing blood. Note the color of the drainage. Blood would obviously be red, chyle would be white, pus from an empyema would be yellow or green, and pleural effusion fluid would be a straw-yellow color.

The whole drainage system must be replaced when the drainage collection chamber becomes filled.

***Pressure-relief valve on the four-chamber system.*** This additional chamber, a safety feature, is seen on four-chamber systems such as those shown in Fig. 17-6. Its purpose is to act as an escape route for any gas that may be leaking from the patient if the vacuum system is accidentally turned off or disconnected. Without the relief valve, air pressure from a pneumothorax could increase to a dangerous level. Instead, air and pressure are released. In three-chamber systems, the pressure has to build up to the point that water in the suction control chamber "geysers" out before the pressure is relieved.

### c. Troubleshoot any problems with the pleural drainage system (NBRC code: IIA20) [Difficulty: R, Ap]

A number of problems can occur with chest drainage systems. The practitioner must understand how the systems are designed and must know how to recognize and correct the situation. Table 17-1 shows examples of problems and ways to correct them.

---

#### Exam Hint

**R**emember that a pleural drainage system is operating properly when air leaking from a pneumothorax is seen bubbling through the water seal. Most examinations have included a question that concerns this.

---

### 4. Intubation (NBRC code: IIIJ3) [Difficulty: R, Ap]

The procedure by which a therapist performs oral endotracheal intubation is discussed in Chapter 12. The following discussion is limited to an explanation of how the therapist can assist an anesthesiologist or other physician who has been trained in performing a nasal endotracheal intubation. The respiratory therapist commonly acts as the assistant. Box 17-4 lists indications and contraindications, and Box 17-5 lists complications of nasal endotracheal intubation. Two different procedures for passing an endotracheal tube by the nasal route can be used: blind nasotracheal intubation and direct vision nasotracheal intubation.

---

#### BOX 17-4 Indications and Contraindications for Nasal Endotracheal Intubation

**GENERAL INDICATIONS FOR ENDOTRACHEAL INTUBATION**
- Provide a secure, patent airway
- Provide a route for mechanical ventilation
- Prevent aspiration of stomach or mouth contents
- Provide a route for suctioning the lungs
- General anesthesia

**INDICATIONS FOR NASAL INTUBATION**
- Patient has a cervical spine abnormality or injury
- Use of muscle relaxants may cause complete loss of the airway
- Limited movement of the cervical spine or mandible
- Lower facial injury or surgery

**CONTRAINDICATIONS FOR NASAL INTUBATION**
- Basilar skull fracture
- Nasal tumors
- Deviated nasal septum
- Severe coagulation disorder

---

#### TABLE 17-1 Troubleshooting Problems with Chest Drainage Systems

| PROBLEM | CORRECTIVE ACTION |
| --- | --- |
| Drainage system is cracked open, or drainage tubing is disconnected from the drainage system | If the patient has a leaking pneumothorax: Leave the tube open to room air so the pleural air can be vented out. As quickly as possible, place the distal end of tubing into a glass of water to create a water seal. If the patient does not have a leaking pneumothorax, clamp the distal end of the tube to prevent room air from being drawn into the pleural space. In either case, attach the tube to a new drainage system as soon as possible. |
| No bubbling through the suction control chamber | Increase the vacuum pressure. Correct any leak in the system |
| Water is spouting out of the suction control chamber (3-bottle system) | Turn on the vacuum. Remove obstruction inside the tubing between vacuum and drainage system |
| Air leak through the water seal chamber | Check the patient for a pneumothorax; report a new air leak to the physician. Check for a leaking seal between the drainage tube and the patient's chest. Check for a hole in the drainage tube, a loose connection between the tube and the drainage system, or a fenestration in the tubing that has pulled out of the chest wall |
| Fluid has filled a dependent loop in the tubing | Drape the tubing so that there are no loops or kinks |
| No change in drainage | Check for loops or kinks in tube. Milk the tube to remove any clots. Take no action if drainage has ceased |
| Drainage collection chamber is full | Prepare another unit, clamp the tube while making the exchange, and unclamp the tube after the new unit is functioning |

---

### BOX 17-5    Complications of Nasal Endotracheal Intubation

**GENERAL COMPLICATIONS**
- Reflex laryngospasm
- Perforation of the esophagus or pharynx
- Esophageal intubation
- Bronchial intubation
- Reflex bradycardia
- Tachycardia or other arrhythmias from hypoxemia
- Hypotension
- Bronchospasm
- Aspiration of tooth, blood, gastric contents, or laryngoscope bulb
- Laceration of pharynx or larynx
- Nosocomial infection
- Vocal cord injury
- Laryngeal or tracheal injury from the tube or excessive cuff pressure
- Mucosal bleeding
- Trauma to the larynx during an attempted blind intubation
- Sinusitis

**COMPLICATIONS AFTER EXTUBATION**
- Reflex laryngospasm
- Aspiration of stomach contents or oral secretions
- Sore throat
- Hoarseness
- Laryngeal edema (postintubation croup)

---

***Blind nasotracheal intubation.*** Be prepared to assist in blind nasotracheal intubation by positioning the patient properly, providing supplemental O$_2$ or manual ventilation to the patient, and getting and preparing the endotracheal tube or other equipment. A stylet is not indicated. Often, the physician orders that the patient should be prepared by having 1% phenylephrine sprayed into the nares. This medication vasoconstricts the blood vessels; it dilates the nasal passages to make intubation easier and reduce the risk of bleeding. Often, 4% Xylocaine is sprayed into the nares for its local anesthetic effect. The distal end of the endotracheal tube is usually covered with sterile Xylocaine ointment.

This procedure is performed without the aid of a laryngoscope to visualize the patient's anatomy and expose the trachea. The general procedure is to place the patient in the sniff position, advance the tube to the oropharynx, and then advance it only on inspiration. Changing the patient's head position, feeling for air movement through the tube, applying pressure over the larynx, or pulling on the tongue may be needed to help guide the tube into the trachea. In addition, several different devices can aid in this intubation. For example, a *fiberoptic bronchoscope* can

be placed through the tube and guided into the patient's trachea. The tube is then advanced and the bronchoscope removed.

***Direct vision nasotracheal intubation.*** The respiratory therapist assists with direct vision nasotracheal intubation and prepares the patient and the endotracheal tube, as with blind endotracheal intubation. This procedure is different from the previous procedure in that intubation equipment is used to visualize the patient's anatomy and to see the glottis. Prepare a laryngoscope handle, a straight or curved blade (depending on the physician's choice), and a Magill forceps.

The lubricated tube is advanced to the oropharynx. The laryngoscope blade is then placed into the mouth and is used to expose the glottis. The Magill forceps is then placed into the mouth to grasp the endotracheal tube and guide it into the trachea (Fig. 17-7). Care must be taken to avoid placing the pincers over the cuff and possibly tearing it.

With either method, the tube must be properly positioned so that the cuff is within the trachea beyond the vocal cords (Fig. 17-8). The cuff is then inflated, its pressure adjusted to a safe level, the tube secured in place by tape, and an x-ray film taken of the chest and neck.

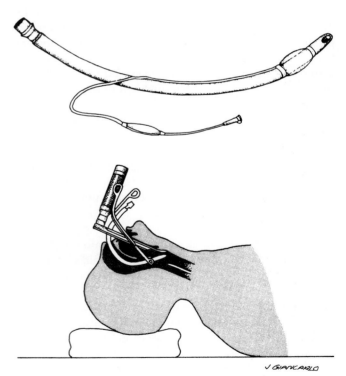

**Fig. 17-7** Direct vision nasotracheal intubation. Note that the Magill forceps and the laryngoscope and blade are used. The Magill forceps is used to grasp the tip of the endotracheal tube and pull it anteriorly into the trachea. *(From Shapiro BA, Harrison RA, Cane RD: Clinical application of respiratory care, ed 4, St Louis, 1991, Mosby.)*

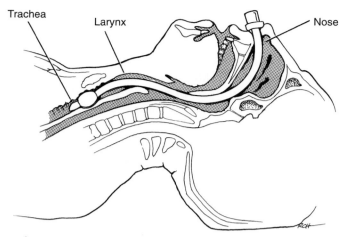

**Fig. 17-8** A properly placed nasotracheal tube. *(From Shapiro BA, Harrison RA, Cane RD: Clinical application of respiratory care, ed 4, St Louis, 1991, Mosby.)*

## MODULE B

### Sleep-disordered breathing

### 1. Overnight pulse oximetry

#### a. Perform overnight pulse oximetry (NBRC code: IB7j) [Difficulty: R, Ap]

A sleep apnea study (cardiopulmonary sleep study or polysomnography) is performed to determine whether the patient has sleep-disordered breathing. Furthermore, it can help to determine the type of disorder and to monitor the patient's response to treatment. Box 17-6 lists the indications for a polysomnography sleep study. The following procedures are usually performed before the sleep study is done:

1. A history of the problem from both the patient's and the bed partner's viewpoints
2. Physical examination, including neck, upper airway, blood pressure, heart rate, and respiratory rate and pattern
3. Arterial blood gas (ABG) or pulse oximetry
4. Hemoglobin
5. Thyroid function
6. Chest and upper airway x-ray examinations; may include a computed axial tomographic scan of the upper airway if obstructive sleep apnea is suspected
7. ECG

The following physiologic parameters are usually measured during a polysomnography sleep study:

1. Pulse oximetry for $O_2$ saturation. An ear or bridge nose oximetry probe is recommended. Finger oximetry is not recommended because the unit may fall off during patient movement
2. Sleep stages through an electroencephalographic (EEG) recording of brain wave activity and an electrooculographic (EOG) recording of eye movements

---

**BOX 17-6   Indications for a Polysomnography Sleep Study**

- Patient with COPD whose awake $PaO_2 > 55$ torr but who has pulmonary hypertension, right heart failure (cor pulmonale), or polycythemia
- Patient whose awake $PaO_2 < 55$ torr without continuous supplemental $O_2$ and who needs to have the proper $O_2$ flow rate set for sleeping at night. Overnight sleep ear oximetry should be performed
- Patient with restrictive ventilatory impairment as a result of chest wall or neuromuscular disturbances who also has chronic hypoventilation, polycythemia, pulmonary hypertension, disturbed sleep, morning headaches, or daytime somnolence and fatigue
- Patient with awake $PaCO_2 > 45$ torr who also has polycythemia, pulmonary hypertension, disturbed sleep, morning headaches, or daytime somnolence or fatigue
- Patient with snoring, obesity, and other symptoms that indicate a disturbed sleep pattern
- Patient with excessive daytime sleepiness or sleep maintenance insomnia
- Patient with nocturnal cyclic bradytachyarrhythmias, atrioventricular conduction abnormalities while asleep, or increased abnormal ventricular beats compared with those when awake

*COPD, Chronic obstructive pulmonary disease; $PaCO_2$, arterial $CO_2$ pressure; $PaO_2$, arterial $O_2$ pressure.*

---

3. Inspiratory and expiratory airflow by nasal thermistor, pneumotachograph, or end-tidal $CO_2$ analyzer
4. Inspiratory and expiratory effort by respiratory inductive plethysmography (Some may prefer to have the patient swallow a transducer to allow measurement of esophageal pressure changes.)
5. Body position related to normal and abnormal breathing patterns
6. Periodic arm and leg movements
7. ECG for monitoring heart rate and arrhythmias

Because of the cost involved in a polysomnography study, overnight pulse oximetry (OPO) has been studied as a less expensive way to determine desaturation from sleep apnea. OPO can be performed in the patient's home or in the hospital setting. The respiratory therapist may be responsible for preparing the patient and setting up the equipment and supplies. Each hospital or physician may have a prescribed procedure. The general steps are listed here:

1. Inform the patient of the procedure, and have him or her sign the medical release form.
2. Attach the pulse oximeter, ECG leads, and other monitoring equipment to the patient.
3. Calibrate the equipment, and make sure it is working properly.

4. Record the patient's parameters during the course of a 6-hr or longer sleep period. The patient may also be recorded on videotape and audiotape during the sleep period.

5. Make any needed adjustments in the patient's respiratory care equipment.

6. Dispose of any used supplies after the procedure has been completed.

7. Tend to the patient's comfort.

### b. Interpret the results of overnight pulse oximetry (NBRC code: IB8g) [Difficulty: R, Ap]

Apnea is the cessation of breathing for 10 sec or longer. Sleep apnea is diagnosed when a patient experiences at least 30 apneic periods during 6 hr of sleep. Numerous studies have shown that overnight pulse oximetry can be used to screen patients with moderate to severe sleep apnea. These patients had at least 10 apnea episodes per hour during which their $SpO_2$ values dropped at least 4% and <90%. In cases in which the overnight pulse oximetry results were difficult to interpret, polysomnography was called for.

During polysomnography, the EEG tracing should confirm that apneic periods occur during both of the major sleep stages. The first stage is called *non–rapid eye movement* (non-REM) sleep and starts soon after the person loses consciousness. The second stage is called *rapid eye movement* (REM) sleep and follows after the non-REM stage. Normally, people cycle through both stages about every 1 to 1 ½ hours during the night. This normal cycle of sleep is important for both mental and physical health. People with disturbed sleep do not dream as they should and are not physically rested when they awaken. Whether the patient is evaluated by overnight pulse oximetry or polysomnography, the results should lead to one of the following classifications for sleep apnea.

***Obstructive sleep apnea.*** Obstructive sleep apnea results when the patient's upper airway is obstructed despite continued breathing efforts (Figs. 17-9 and 17-10). Patients with this problem often exhibit the following symptoms: loud snoring (reported by the bed partner), morning headache, excessive daytime sleepiness, depression or other personality changes, decreased intellectual ability, sexual dysfunction, bed-wetting (nocturnal enuresis), or abnormal limb movements during sleep.

Obstructive sleep apnea is associated with the following: middle-aged males, obesity, short neck, hypothyroidism, testosterone administration, myotonic dystrophy, temporomandibular joint disease, narrowed upper airway from excessive pharyngeal tissue, enlarged tongue (macroglossia), enlarged tonsils or adenoids, deviated nasal septum, recessed jaw (micrognathia), goiter, laryngeal stenosis or web, and pharyngeal neoplasm. Management of patients with obstructive sleep apnea may include any of the following:

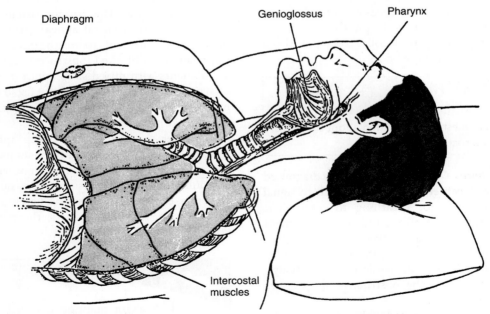

**Fig. 17-9** Obstructive sleep apnea. These patients often obstruct when lying supine, and the genioglossus muscle of the tongue fails to oppose the negative force on the airway during inspiration. *(From Des Jardins TL: Clinical manifestations of respiratory disease, ed 2, Chicago, 1990, Mosby.)*

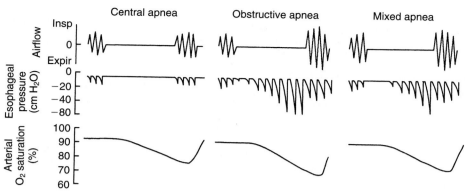

**Fig. 17-10** Typical patterns of airflow, esophageal pressure (or respiratory inductive plethysmography) showing respiratory effort, and arterial $O_2$ desaturation produced by central, obstructive, and mixed sleep apnea. Central apnea shows a lack of respiratory effort, which causes no airflow. Obstructive apnea shows a continued respiratory effort but no airflow because of the airway obstruction. Mixed apnea starts out with an initial lack of respiratory effort (central apnea). Later, breathing efforts are made but no airflow occurs because of the airway obstruction (obstructive apnea). Arterial desaturation results from all three types of apnea. When the desaturation becomes great enough and the $CO_2$ level high enough, the patient (it is hoped) awakens enough to breathe again. *(From Des Jardins TL: Clinical manifestations and assessment of respiratory disease, ed 2, Chicago, 1990, Mosby.)*

1. Weight reduction
2. Sleeping on either side or the abdomen; do not sleep in the supine position
3. Continuous positive airway pressure (CPAP) mask or BiPAP mask
4. Surgery to open the airway: Mandibular advancement, palatopharyngoplasty, or tracheostomy
5. Protriptyline (Triptil, Vivactil) to decrease REM sleep (when most obstructive episodes occur)
6. Have the patient wear a tongue-retaining device to prevent it from obstructing the pharynx
7. Have the patient wear a neck collar to keep the head and neck aligned with the body

> **Exam Hint**
>
> **O**ften, a question is included about the use of CPAP to treat obstructive sleep apnea.

**Central sleep apnea.** Central sleep apnea is diagnosed when the respiratory center of the medulla fails to signal the respiratory muscles for breathing to occur. The patient makes no respiratory effort, and no air movement occurs (see Fig. 17-10). Patients with this problem often exhibit normal weight, mild snoring, insomnia, and lesser levels of daytime sleepiness, depression, or sexual dysfunction than are seen in the obstructive sleep apnea patient.

Central sleep apnea is associated with primary alveolar (idiopathic) hypoventilation (Ondine's curse), muscular dystrophy, bilateral cervical cordotomy, bulbar poliomyelitis, encephalitis, brain stem infarction or neoplasm, spinal surgery, or hypothyroidism. Management of patients with central sleep apnea may include the following:

1. Negative pressure ventilation for sleeping
2. Intubation or tracheostomy and positive-pressure ventilation if the patient has acute ventilatory failure
3. Phrenic nerve pacemaker

**Mixed sleep apnea.** Mixed sleep apnea is diagnosed when the patient shows evidence of both central and obstructive apnea. The patient usually first stops all breathing efforts (central apnea). After some time, the patient makes attempts to breathe but cannot because the upper airway is blocked (obstructive apnea) (see Fig. 17-10). Patients with mixed sleep apnea may show a variety of symptoms and traits (see those listed earlier). Clinical management may include any of the treatments mentioned that prove to be effective.

Whatever the cause of the sleep apnea, it must be treated. If apnea is left to continue its pathologic course, the patient may develop a number of other problems, such as pulmonary hypertension, cor pulmonale, polycythemia, cardiac arrhythmia, and even unexplained nocturnal death. At the very least, the patient's personal, family, and social life will suffer.

> **Exam Hint**
>
> **U**sually, a question is asked about how to identify a patient who has obstructive sleep apnea. The key is to recognize that the patient will not be moving any air despite breathing efforts.

## 2. Apnea monitoring
### a. Perform apnea monitoring (NBRC code: IB7i) [Difficulty: R]

Apnea monitoring is indicated in an infant with documented periods of apnea of prematurity because of an immature central nervous system. This condition is most commonly seen in infants of less than 35 weeks' gestational age. The usual monitoring guidelines include apneic periods that last longer than 20 sec and are associated with bradycardia with a heart rate of less than 100 beats/min. See Box 17-7 for guidelines on starting and stopping home apnea monitoring.

---

**BOX 17-7   Guidelines for Starting and Stopping Home Apnea Monitoring**

**INDICATIONS FOR STARTING HOME APNEA MONITORING**
- Infant has had one or more apparent life-threatening apnea events
- Infant is preterm and symptomatic of apnea
- Infant is a sibling of two or more victims of sudden infant death syndrome
- Infant has central nervous system–based hypoventilation

**INDICATIONS FOR STOPPING HOME APNEA MONITORING**
- Two to three months have passed without a significant number of alarms
- Two to three months have passed without an apnea episode
- Infant can tolerate stress of illnesses (e.g., nasopharyngitis) or immunizations (e.g., diphtheria-tetanus-pertussis [DPT]) without apnea episodes

---

The following are desirable features of a home apnea monitor: (1) Ability to store and display events for later analysis, (2) identification of breathing patterns and apnea periods, (3) identification of heart rate patterns, (4) estimation of $V_T$, and (5) identification of hypoxemia by pulse oximetry. Setting up a home apnea monitor involves placing the electrodes properly on the infant's chest, turning on the monitor, and setting the proper high and low limits for the alarms.

Apnea monitors use impedance pneumography to determine breathing and heart rates. Impedance pneumography measures changes in electrical resistance between two electrodes in relationship with a patient's breathing and heartbeats. For best results, the infant's chest should be washed with mild soap and water and dried before the electrodes are placed. This creates optimal electrical conduction between the electrodes. Do not use baby oils, lotions, or powders over the electrode sites. Two electrodes are typically placed where the greatest amount of movement occurs during breathing, usually on the infant's upper chest between the nipples and the armpits (Fig. 17-11). With older infants, the electrodes might have to be placed on the sides over the lower ribs. Occasionally, one electrode is placed on the chest and the other on the infant's abdomen. The monitor sends out a small, constant electrical current, which results in a voltage across the two electrodes on the infant's chest. As the infant breathes and the chest wall expands and contracts, a change in voltage occurs. This fluctuation is measured and interpreted as inhalation and exhalation. Similarly, smaller voltage changes are measured with each heartbeat, and these are measured and interpreted as the heart rate. Attach the lead wires to the electrodes. These connect to the patient cable that is then connected to the monitor.

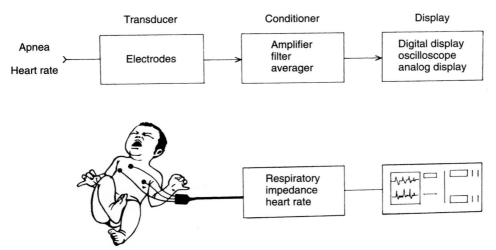

**Fig. 17-11** Block diagram for impedance apnea and heart rate monitor. *(From Lough MD: Newborn respiratory care procedures. In Lough MD, Williams TJ, Rawson JE, editors: Newborn respiratory care, Chicago, 1979, Mosby.)*

Occasionally, static electricity causes some interference with the signal. A third chest electrode is then added to act as a ground wire.

The monitor should be plugged into a working electrical outlet and turned on. Set the unit to charge the internal battery so that it can be made portable for later use. Ensure that the infant's respiratory and heart rates are being sensed and displayed. If pulse oximetry (SpO$_2$) is a feature on the unit, the probe should be properly placed on the infant, and an SpO$_2$ value should be displayed. Set the high and low alarm values according to the physician's orders or established protocols. For example,

1. Set the apnea alarm to trigger after 20 sec.
2. Set the low heart rate alarm to trigger if the heart rate is less than 100 beats/min.
3. If available, set the SpO$_2$ alarm to trigger if the SpO$_2$ drops below 90%.
4. If available, set the high heart rate alarm to trigger if the heart rate is greater than 150 beats/min.

Multiple alarms provide a greater margin of patient safety. They also indicate what physiologically deteriorates first in the infant. These backup alarm systems are important because the apnea monitor senses chest wall movement, not air movement. The infant can have an upper airway obstruction and continue to make breathing attempts; when this occurs, the apnea monitor would not alarm because the chest wall is moving. The bradycardia or desaturation alarms would signal that the infant is in trouble. It is critically important that the parent(s) know about the infant's medical condition. They must understand how the monitor functions and what to do if the alarms sound.

### b. Interpret apnea monitoring results (NBRC code: IB8f) [Difficulty: R, Ap]

Alarm situations fall into two basic categories: patient alarms and equipment alarms. *Patient alarms* mean that the infant is apneic, has a heart rate below or above an acceptable level, or is desaturated. One, any two, or all three alarms could be triggered. An audible or visual alarm flash indicates the problem(s), and the recording device keeps track of the events. Parents should be instructed to first care for the infant; then, when the infant is back to normal, they should reset the alarms.

Three types of *equipment alarms* exist: electrode or lead problem, low battery, and monitor failure. The unit should have different visual and audible alarms for equipment failure so that the family does not mistakenly think that the infant is in trouble. An electrode or lead problem alarm usually occurs because the electrode comes off of the infant, or the lead disconnects. The family should be taught how to fix these types of problems. A low-battery alarm indicates that not much time is left for the monitor to function on battery power. The family should be instructed to plug the monitor into a functioning

electrical outlet and set the unit to recharge the battery. A monitor failure alarm indicates a serious internal problem with the monitor. It is not functioning properly and should not be used. The family should be instructed to continuously observe the infant and call the home care company for a replacement monitor.

Apnea monitors in current use record and store these alarm situations. The information can usually be downloaded into a computer for a visual display of breathing and heart rate patterns, equipment problems, and the dates and times of their occurrences. The therapist or physician should review all these data to determine what types of problems the patient was having.

## MODULE C
### Respiratory care plan

### 1. Analyze the available information to determine the patient's pathophysiologic state (NBRC code: IIIH1) [Difficulty: R, Ap, An]

Some discussion on pathophysiology was presented with each of the procedures just described. Further reading is recommended as needed.

### 2. Recommend changes in the therapeutic plan if supportive data exist (NBRC code: IIIH4) [Difficulty: R, Ap]

Review the discussion on each of the procedures just described. Use other chapters in this text as well, if needed.

### 3. Stop the procedure if the patient has an adverse reaction to it (NBRC code: IIIF1) [Difficulty: R, Ap, An]

Review Box 17-2 for bronchoscopy risks and Boxes 17-4 and 17-5 for contraindications and complications of nasal endotracheal intubation.

### BIBLIOGRAPHY

American Association for Respiratory Care: Clinical practice guideline: Fiberoptic bronchoscopy assisting, *Respir Care* 38:1173, 1993.

American Association for Respiratory Care: Clinical practice guideline: Management of airway emergencies, *Respir Care* 40:749, 1995.

American Association for Respiratory Care: Clinical practice guideline: Polysomnography, *Respir Care* 40:1236, 1995.

Arand DL, Bonnet MH: Sleep-disordered breathing. In Burton GC, Hodgkin JE, Ward JJ, editors: *Respiratory care: A guide to clinical practice*, ed 4, Philadelphia, 1997, Lippincott-Raven.

Barnes TA, editor: *Core textbook of respiratory care practice*, ed 2, St Louis, 1994, Mosby.

Branson RD, Hess DR, Chatburn RL, editors: *Respiratory care equipment*, ed 2, Philadelphia, 1999, Lippincott Williams & Wilkins.

Brutinel WM, Cortese DA: Fiberoptic bronchoscopy. In Burton GC, Hodgkin JE, Ward JJ, editors: *Respiratory care: A guide to clinical practice,* ed 4, Philadelphia, 1997, Lippincott-Raven.

Cairo JM: Sleep diagnostics. In Cairo JM, Pilbeam SP, editors: *Mosby's respiratory care equipment,* ed 7, St Louis, 2004, Mosby.

Cairo JM: Assessment of physiologic function. In Cairo JM, Pilbeam SP, editors: *Mosby's respiratory care equipment,* ed 6, St Louis, 1999, Mosby.

Chadha TS, Schneider AW, Tobin MJ, et al: Noninvasive monitoring of breathing patterns during wakefulness and sleep, *Respir Ther* 27, May/June, 1985.

Chavis AD, Grum CM: Fiberoptic bronchoscopy with mechanical ventilation, *Choices Respir Management* 21:4, 1991.

Chavis AD, Grum CM: Pulmonary procedures during mechanical ventilation, *Choices Respir Management* 21:29, 1991.

Chediak AD: Pathogenesis of obstructive sleep apnea, *Respir Care* 43:265, 1998.

Coppolo DP, Brienza LT, Pratt DS, et al: A role for the respiratory therapist in flexible fiberoptic bronchoscopy, *Respir Care* 30:323, 1985.

Decker MJ, Smith BL, Strohl KP: Center-based vs. patient-based diagnosis and therapy of sleep-related respiratory disorders and role of the respiratory care practitioner, *Respir Care* 39:390, 1994.

Deshpande VM, Pilbeam SP, Dixon RJ: *A comprehensive review in respiratory care,* East Norwalk, Conn, 1988, Appleton & Lange.

Des Jardins T: *Clinical manifestations of respiratory disease,* ed 4, St Louis, 2000, Mosby.

Downey R III, Dexter JR: Assessment of sleep and breathing. In Wilkins RL, Krider SJ, Sheldon RL, editors: *Clinical assessment in respiratory care,* ed 3, St Louis, 1995, Mosby.

Epstein LJ, Dorlac GR: Cost-effectiveness analysis of nocturnal oximetry as a method of screening for sleep apnea-hypopnea syndrome, *Chest* 113:97, 1998.

Erickson RA: Chest drainage, I, *Nursing89* 19:37, 1989.

Erickson RA: Chest drainage, II, *Nursing89* 19:47, 1989.

Eubanks DH, Bone RC: *Comprehensive respiratory care: A learning system,* ed 2, St Louis, 1990, Mosby.

Garay SM: Therapeutic options for obstructive sleep apnea, *Respir Management* 17:11, 1987.

Guidelines for fiberoptic bronchoscopy, *ATS News* 12:14, 1986.

Homedco, *Home infant monitoring guidelines,* Fountain View, Calif.

Howard TP: Foreign body extraction by means of combined rigid and flexible bronchoscopy: A case report, *Respir Care* 33:786, 1988.

Indications and standards for cardiopulmonary sleep studies, *Am Rev Respir Dis* 139:559, 1989.

Johnson MD: Noninvasive monitoring. In Aloan CA, Hill TV, editors: *Respiratory care of the newborn and child,* ed 2, Philadelphia, 1997, Lippincott-Raven.

Kendall Hospital Products, Curity thoracentesis tray, package insert, Boston, Mass.

Khoury JB, Radtke RA: Sleep assessment. In Hess DR, MacIntyre NR, Mishoe SC, et al, editors: *Respiratory care principles & practices,* Philadelphia, 2002, WB Saunders.

Kilkenny LA, Fernandes KS, Strollo PJ Jr: Disorders of sleep. In Wilkins RL, Stroller JK, Scanlan CL, editors: *Egan's fundamentals of respiratory care,* ed 8, St Louis, 2003, Mosby.

Lewis CA, Eaton TE, Fergusson W, et al: Home overnight pulse oximetry in patients with COPD: More than one recording may be needed, *Chest* 123:1127, 2003.

Lough MD: Newborn respiratory care procedures. In Lough MD, Williams TJ, Rawson JE, editors: *Newborn respiratory care,* Chicago, 1979, Mosby.

Madama VC: *Pulmonary function testing and cardiopulmonary stress testing,* ed 2, Albany, NY, 1998, Delmar.

Mathewson HS: Drug therapy for obstructive sleep apnea, *Respir Care* 31:717, 1986.

Mims BC: You *can* manage chest tubes confidently, *RN* 48:39, 1985.

Mishoe SC: The diagnosis and treatment of sleep apnea syndrome, *Respir Care* 32:183, 1987.

Netzer N, Eliasson AH, Netzer C, Kristo DA: Overnight pulse oximetry for sleep-disordered breathing in adults. *Chest* 2001.

Peters RM: Chest trauma. In Moser KM, Spragg RG, editors: *Respiratory emergencies,* ed 2, St Louis, 1982, Mosby.

Phillips BA: Clinical diagnosis of sleep apnea, *Respir Care* 43:288, 1998.

Phillipson EA: Breathing disorders during sleep, *Basics Respir Dis* 7:1, 1979.

Plevak DJ, Ward JJ: Airway management. In Burton GC, Hodgkin JE, Ward JJ, editors: *Respiratory care: A guide to clinical practice,* ed 4, Philadelphia, 1997, Lippincott-Raven.

Podnos SD, Chappell TR: Hemoptysis: A clinical update, *Respir Care* 30:977, 1985.

Poe RH, Israel RH: Flexible fiberoptic bronchoscopy in 1998, *Respir Care* 43:811, 1998.

Rapaport DM: Techniques for administering nasal CPAP, *Respir Management* 17:17, 1987.

Ruppel G: *Manual of pulmonary function testing,* ed 6, St Louis, 1994, Mosby.

Sachs S: Fiberoptic bronchoscopy. In Hess DR, MacIntyre NR, Mishoe SC, et al, editors: *Respiratory care principles & practices.* Philadelphia, 2002, WB Saunders.

Shapiro BA, Kacmarek RM, Cane RD, et al: *Clinical application of respiratory care,* ed 4, St Louis, 1991, Mosby.

Smalling T, Valente J: Examining laser surgery, *J Respir Care Pract* 11:93, 1998.

Strollo PJ Jr, Fernandes KS: Disorders of sleep. In Scanlan CL, Wilkins RL, Stoller JK, editors: *Egan's fundamentals of respiratory care,* ed 7, St Louis, 1999, Mosby.

Whitaker K: *Comprehensive perinatal & pediatric respiratory care,* ed 2, Albany, NY, 1997, Delmar.

Williams SF, Thompson JM: Respiratory disorders, St Louis, 1990, Mosby.

## SELF-STUDY QUESTIONS

1. Home apnea monitoring on an infant can usually be stopped when all of the following conditions exist EXCEPT
   A. The infant has gone 30 days without an apnea episode
   B. The infant has had a DPT immunization without any consequences
   C. Three months have passed without any alarms sounding
   D. Two months has passed without an apnea episode

2. Your patient is being mechanically ventilated when the nurse calls you to evaluate the patient's condition. You discover that her breath sounds are absent over the left lung field, the left-sided percussion note is hyperresonant, and peak airway pressures have increased from 40 to 65 cm $H_2O$. What would you recommend?
   A. Place a pleural chest tube into the right side
   B. Increase the $V_T$ to better inflate the atelectatic left lung
   C. Change the mode to synchronous intermittent mechanical ventilation from assist/control
   D. Place a pleural chest tube into the left side

3. You notice that air is bubbling through the water seal of the patient's pleural drainage system when she coughs. This tells you that
   A. The vacuum has to be increased
   B. Air is still leaking through a tear in the lung
   C. The proper level of vacuum has been set
   D. There is a leak in the system

4. After a sleep study has been performed, your patient is given a diagnosis of obstructive sleep apnea. His physician asks for your advice on the best method of management. You would recommend that
   A. The patient should use nasal CPAP when sleeping
   B. The patient should sleep with an oropharyngeal airway to keep the tongue forward in the mouth
   C. The patient should always sleep on his back
   D. A tracheostomy should be performed, and the patient should be placed on a volume-cycled ventilator to sleep.

5. An adult patient with obstructive sleep apnea and frequent pulse oximetry desaturations is fitted with a nasal CPAP system. A pressure of 7 cm water is set. After the CPAP system is set up, the patient's $SpO_2$ value stays above 90%. How should the results be interpreted?
   A. The CPAP system has corrected the patient's problem
   B. Greater CPAP pressure is needed
   C. Improved gas flow is needed through the CPAP system
   D. The delivered oxygen percentage should be increased

6. Your mechanically ventilated patient is going to have a flexible fiberoptic bronchoscopy performed. Of what kinds of considerations must you be aware?
   I. The $V_T$ must be monitored for a leak
   II. The inspiratory flow resistance will increase
   III. The inspiratory pressure will decrease
   IV. The inspiratory pressure will increase
   A. I and II
   B. III
   C. II and III
   D. I, II, and IV

7. During the transport of your patient, the chest tube drainage system is pulled off of the drainage tubing and cracked open. Your best response is to
   A. Clamp the tube near the patient's chest at once
   B. Hold the distal end of the tubing a few centimeters below the surface of a bottle of sterile water or saline
   C. Leave the tube open to the atmosphere
   D. Have the patient perform the Valsalva maneuver until a new system can be set up

8. When preparing to assist the physician with the cardioversion of a patient, you must check the following:
   I. A strong R wave should be seen on the ECG monitor
   II. The charge level should be set as ordered
   III. The electric paddles should be kept clean for the best possible conduction
   IV. Ensure that the ECG electrodes are attached properly
   A. I and III
   B. I, II, and IV
   C. III and IV
   D. I, II, III, and IV

9. A 28-year-old patient has aspirated a tooth that was knocked out during a sporting event. The chest x-ray film shows the tooth to be lodged in the right mainstem bronchus; the neck x-ray film is normal. What would you recommend as the best way to quickly remove the tooth?
   A. Flexible fiberoptic bronchoscopy
   B. Positive expiratory pressure breathing
   C. Rigid tube bronchoscopy
   D. Postural drainage therapy

10. A patient is referred for a sleep study. The attending physician wants to know which parameters are measured during the study. You would measure all of the following EXCEPT
   A. $SpO_2$
   B. ECG
   C. Inspiratory and expiratory breathing efforts
   D. ABG values

## ANSWER KEY AND RATIONALE

1. **A.** Current guidelines indicate that apnea monitoring can be stopped if an infant has gone at least 2 months without an apnea episode. The other items are all indications to stop monitoring. Review Box 17-7.

2. **D.** The physical signs indicate that the patient has a left-sided pneumothorax; a pleural chest tube is indicated. Do not place a tube into the right pleural space. Increasing the $V_T$ or changing the mode would not correct the problem.

3. **B.** An air leak through the water seal when the patient coughs indicates that the air is coming from the patient's lung. If a leak exists in the system, air will bubble through the water seal at all times. The vacuum level has no impact on the air leak from the patient.

4. **A.** Nasal CPAP would be indicated for the management of a patient with obstructive sleep apnea. An oropharyngeal airway would be indicated only in an obtunded patient with an obstructed upper airway. For many patients, sleeping on the back worsens the obstruction. A tracheostomy and mechanical ventilation may be indicated in a patient with central sleep apnea if all other efforts have failed.

5. **A.** A normal $SpO_2$ value indicates that the CPAP system at 7 cm water pressure has corrected the patient's problem. There is no need to raise the CPAP level because the patient's pulse oximetry value is normal. There is no indication of inadequate flow through the CPAP system. There is no need to raise the delivered oxygen percentage because the saturation is within the normal range.

6. **D.** Performing a bronchoscopy on a ventilated patient necessitates the use of a special bronchoscopy adapter between the endotracheal tube and the circuit. The bronchoscope is placed through the adapter, which may result in a $V_T$ leak. In addition, the bronchoscope partially obstructs the endotracheal tube, which increases resistance and causes inspiratory pressure to increase.

7. **B.** The easiest way to seal the chest tube but allow air leaking from the patient to escape is to place the distal end of the tube under water. Clamping the tube does not allow any pleural air to escape. Leaving the tube open allows pleural air to escape but also allows room air to enter the pleural space. The Valsalva maneuver would require breath-holding by the patient for an extended time and is not practical.

8. **B.** Cardioversion requires a strong R wave on the ECG monitor, a proper electrical charge level, and proper placement of the ECG leads. The electrode paddles should be well covered with a conducting jelly to maximize the flow of current into the patient without a burn.

9. **C.** Rigid tube bronchoscopy is preferred in the removal of a large foreign body from a large airway. FFB may be used with a small foreign body or one that is in a smaller airway. PEP and PDT are not likely to dislodge a large foreign body such as a tooth. PDT with percussion may dislodge a foreign body.

10. **D.** ABGs are not monitored during a sleep study because it is an invasive procedure and the patient would wake up as the blood sample is drawn. The other items are routinely monitored during a sleep study.

# Detailed Content Outline for the Entry Level CRT Examination

| | **Items** | | | |
|---|---|---|---|---|
| | **Cognitive Levels** | | | |
| | Recall | Application | Analysis | Totals |

## Detailed Content Outline for the Entry Level CRT Examination

Open cells show an examination could include items from indicated cognitive levels.
Shaded cells prevent appearance of items on examinations.

| | Recall | Application | Analysis | Totals |
|---|---|---|---|---|
| **I. PATIENT DATA EVALUATION** | 7 | 18 | 0 | 25 |
| **A. Review Existing Data in the Patient Record Including** | 2 | 4 | 0 | 6 |
| 1. Patient history [e.g., present illness, admission notes, respiratory care orders, progress notes, diagnoses, DNR status] | | | | |
| 2. Physical examination relative to the cardiopulmonary system [e.g., vital signs, physical findings] | | | | |
| 3. Pulmonary function results | | | | |
| 4. Blood gas results | | | | |
| 5. Imaging studies [e.g., radiographic, CT, MRI, PET, $\dot{V}/\dot{Q}$ scan, angiogram] | | | | |
| 6. Monitoring data | | | | |
|   a. pulmonary mechanics [e.g., maximum inspiratory pressure, vital capacity] | | | | |
|   b. respiratory monitoring [e.g., rate, tidal volume, minute volume, I:E, inspiratory and expiratory pressures; airway graphics] | | | | |
|   c. pulmonary compliance, airways resistance, work of breathing | | | | |
|   d. noninvasive monitoring [e.g., $V_D/V_T$, capnography, pulse oximetry, transcutaneous $O_2/CO_2$] | | | | |
| **B. Collect and Evaluate Additional Pertinent Clinical Information** | 5 | 14 | 0 | 19 |
| 1. Assess patient's overall cardiopulmonary status by **inspection** to determine | | | | |
|   a. general appearance [e.g., muscle wasting, venous distention, peripheral edema, diaphoresis, clubbing, cyanosis, capillary refill, chest configuration, evidence of diaphragmatic movement, breathing pattern, accessory muscle activity, asymmetrical chest movement, intercostal and/or sternal retractions, nasal flaring] | | | | |
|   b. cough, amount and character of sputum | | | | |
| 2. Assess patient's overall cardiopulmonary status by **palpation** to determine | | | | |
|   a. heart rate, rhythm, and force | | | | |
|   b. asymmetrical chest movements, tactile fremitus, crepitus, tenderness, secretions in the airway, tracheal deviation | | | | |
| 3. Assess patient's overall cardiopulmonary status by **auscultation** to determine presence of | | | | |
|   a. breath sounds [e.g., normal, abnormal] | | | | |
|   b. heart sounds and rhythms [e.g., normal, abnormal] | | | | |
|   c. blood pressure | | | | |
| 4. Interview patient to determine | | | | |
|   a. level of consciousness/sedation, orientation to time, place and person, emotional state, ability to cooperate, level of pain | | | | |
|   b. presence of dyspnea and/or orthopnea, work of breathing, sputum production, exercise tolerance and activities of daily living | | | | |
|   c. social history [e.g., smoking, substance abuse] | | | | |
|   d. advance directives [e.g., DNR status] | | | | |

| | | Items | | |
|---|---|---|---|---|
| **Detailed Content Outline for the Entry Level CRT Examination** | | **Cognitive Levels** | | |
| | Recall | Application | Analysis | Totals |
| Open cells show an examination could include items from indicated cognitive levels. Shaded cells prevent appearance of items on examinations. | | | | |
| 5. Assess patient's learning needs | ░ | | ░ | |
| 6. Review chest radiograph to determine | ░ | | | |
|    a. position of endotracheal or tracheostomy tube | | | ░ | |
|    b. presence of or change in pneumothorax or subcutaneous emphysema, other extrapulmonary air, consolidation and/or atelectasis, pulmonary infiltrates | | | ░ | |
|    c. presence and position of foreign bodies | | | ░ | |
|    d. position of or change in hemidiaphragms, hyperinflation, pleural fluid, pulmonary edema, mediastinal shift, patency and size of major airways | | | ░ | |
| 7. Perform procedures including | ░ | ░ | | |
|    a. 12-lead ECG | | ░ | | |
|    b. pulse oximetry, capnography | | | | |
|    c. tidal volume, minute volume, peak flow, vital capacity | | | | |
|    d. bedside spirometry [e.g., FVC, $FEV_1$] | | | | |
|    e. arterial sampling—percutaneous or line | | | | |
|    f. blood gas/hemoximetry analysis | | | | |
|    g. lung mechanics [e.g., MIP, MEP, pulmonary compliance, plateau pressure, airways resistance] | | | | |
|    h. ventilator pressure-volume and flow-volume loops | | | | |
|    i. apnea monitoring | | ░ | | |
|    j. overnight pulse oximetry | | | | |
|    k. tracheal tube cuff pressure and/or volume | | ░ | | |
|    l. tracheal intubation | | | | |
|    m. pulmonary function laboratory studies [e.g., flows, volumes, diffusion studies, pre- and post-bronchodilator] | | | | |
| 8. Interpret procedure results including | ░ | | | |
|    a. pulse oximetry, capnography | | | | |
|    b. tidal volume, minute volume, peak flow, vital capacity | | | | |
|    c. bedside spirometry [e.g., FVC, $FEV_1$] | | | | |
|    d. blood gas/hemoximetry analysis | | | | |
|    e. lung mechanics [e.g., MIP, MEP, pulmonary compliance, plateau pressure, airways resistance] | | | | |
|    f. apnea monitoring | | | | |
|    g. overnight pulse oximetry | | | | |
|    h. tracheal tube cuff pressure and/or volume | | | | |
|    i. pulmonary function laboratory studies [e.g., flows, volumes, diffusion studies, pre- and post-bronchodilator] | | | | |
|    j. ventilator pressure-volume and flow-volume loops | | | | |
|    k. auto-PEEP | | | | |
| 9. Recommend blood gas analysis, pulse oximetry, transcutaneous $O_2/CO_2$ monitoring to obtain additional data | | | ░ | |

# Detailed Content Outline for the Entry Level CRT Examination

Open cells show an examination could include items from indicated cognitive levels.
Shaded cells prevent appearance of items on examinations.

| | Items | | | |
| --- | --- | --- | --- | --- |
| | Cognitive Levels | | | |
| | Recall | Application | Analysis | Totals |
| **II. EQUIPMENT APPLICATION AND CLEANLINESS** | 13 | 17 | 0 | 30 |
| **A. Select, Assemble, Use, and Troubleshoot Equipment Including** | 10 | 15 | 0 | 25 |
| 1. Oxygen administration devices | ▓ | | ▓ | ▓ |
|   a. low-flow devices [e.g., nasal cannula] | | | ▓ | ▓ |
|   b. high-flow devices [e.g., air entrainment mask] | | | ▓ | ▓ |
| 2. CPAP devices—mask, nasal, or bi-level | | | ▓ | ▓ |
| 3. Humidifiers [e.g., bubble, passover, cascade, wick, heat moisture exchanger] | | ▓ | ▓ | ▓ |
| 4. Pneumatic aerosol generator (nebulizer) | | ▓ | ▓ | ▓ |
| 5. Resuscitation devices [e.g., manual resuscitator (bag-valve), mouth-to-valve mask resuscitator] | | | ▓ | ▓ |
| 6. Ventilators | ▓ | ▓ | ▓ | ▓ |
|   a. pneumatic, electric, fluidic, microprocessor | | | ▓ | ▓ |
|   b. noninvasive positive pressure | | | ▓ | ▓ |
| 7. Artificial airways | ▓ | ▓ | ▓ | ▓ |
|   a. oro- and nasopharyngeal airways | | | ▓ | ▓ |
|   b. endotracheal tubes | | | ▓ | ▓ |
|   c. tracheostomy tubes and buttons | | | ▓ | ▓ |
|   d. intubation equipment [e.g., laryngoscope and blades, fiberoptic devices, exhaled $CO_2$ detection devices] | | | ▓ | ▓ |
| 8. Suctioning devices [e.g., suction catheters, specimen collectors, oropharyngeal suction devices] | | ▓ | ▓ | ▓ |
| 9. Gas cylinders, regulators, reducing valves, connectors and flowmeters, air/oxygen blenders | | ▓ | ▓ | ▓ |
| 10. Point-of-care blood gas analyzers | | | ▓ | ▓ |
| 11. Patient breathing circuits | ▓ | ▓ | ▓ | ▓ |
|   a. continuous mechanical ventilation | | ▓ | ▓ | ▓ |
|   b. IPPB | | ▓ | ▓ | ▓ |
|   c. CPAP, PEEP valve assembly | | | ▓ | ▓ |
|   d. non-invasive ventilation | | ▓ | ▓ | ▓ |
| 12. Aerosol (mist) tents | | ▓ | ▓ | ▓ |
| 13. Incentive breathing devices | | ▓ | ▓ | ▓ |
| 14. Percussors and vibrators | | ▓ | ▓ | ▓ |
| 15. Positive expiratory pressure (PEP) devices | | | ▓ | ▓ |
| 16. Vibratory PEP [e.g., Flutter®] mucous clearance devices | | ▓ | ▓ | ▓ |
| 17. Manometers [e.g., water, mercury, and aneroid] | | ▓ | ▓ | ▓ |
| 18. Respirometers [e.g., flow-sensing devices (pneumotachometer)] | | | ▓ | ▓ |
| 19. ECG machines (12-lead) | | ▓ | ▓ | ▓ |
| 20. Vacuum systems [e.g., pumps, regulators, collection bottles, pleural drainage devices] | | | ▓ | ▓ |
| 21. Oximetry monitoring devices [e.g., pulse oximeter, transcutaneous] | ▓ | | ▓ | ▓ |
| 22. Metered dose inhalers (MDI), MDI spacers | | ▓ | ▓ | ▓ |
| 23. Dry powder inhalers | | ▓ | ▓ | ▓ |

| | Items | | | |
|---|---|---|---|---|
| **Detailed Content Outline for the Entry Level CRT Examination** | **Cognitive Levels** | | | |
| | Recall | Application | Analysis | Totals |
| Open cells show an examination could include items from indicated cognitive levels. Shaded cells prevent appearance of items on examinations. | | | | |
| 24. Spirometry screening equipment for bedside | | | | |
| 25. Troubleshoot speaking tubes and valves | | | | |
| **B. Ensure Infection Control** | **2** | **0** | **0** | **2** |
| 1. Assure selected equipment cleanliness [e.g., select or determine appropriate agent and technique for disinfection and/or sterilization, perform procedures for disinfection and/or sterilization, monitor effectiveness of sterilization procedures] | | | | |
| 2. Assure proper handling of biohazardous materials | | | | |
| **C. Perform Quality Control Procedures For** | **1** | **2** | **0** | **3** |
| 1. Blood gas analyzers, co-oximeters, and sampling devices | | | | |
| 2. Oxygen analyzers | | | | |
| 3. Mechanical ventilators | | | | |
| 4. Gas metering devices [e.g., flowmeter] | | | | |
| **III. THERAPEUTIC PROCEDURE INITIATION AND MODIFICATION** | **15** | **38** | **32** | **85** |
| **A. Maintain Records and Communicate Information** | **1** | **4** | **2** | **7** |
| 1. Record therapy and results using conventional terminology as required in the health care setting and/or by regulatory agencies | | | | |
| a. specify therapy administered, date, time, frequency of therapy, medication, and ventilatory data | | | | |
| b. note and interpret patient's response to therapy including | | | | |
| 1) effects of therapy, adverse reactions, patient's subjective and attitudinal response to therapy | | | | |
| 2) auscultatory findings, cough and sputum production and characteristics | | | | |
| 3) vital signs [e.g., heart rate, respiratory rate, blood pressure, body temperature, pain level] | | | | |
| 4) pulse oximetry, heart rhythm, capnography | | | | |
| c. verify computations and note erroneous data | | | | |
| 2. Communicate information | | | | |
| a. regarding patient's clinical status to appropriate members of the health care team | | | | |
| b. relevant to coordinating patient care and discharge planning [e.g., scheduling, avoiding conflicts, sequencing of therapies] | | | | |
| 3. Apply computer technology to | | | | |
| a. document patient management | | | | |
| b. monitor workload assignments | | | | |
| 4. Communicate results of therapy and alter therapy per protocol(s) | | | | |
| 5. Explain planned therapy and goals to patient in understandable terms to achieve optimal therapeutic outcome | | | | |
| 6. Counsel patient and family concerning smoking cessation and disease management education | | | | |

# Detailed Content Outline for the Entry Level CRT Examination

Open cells show an examination could include items from indicated cognitive levels.
Shaded cells prevent appearance of items on examinations.

| | Items | | | |
|---|---|---|---|---|
| | **Cognitive Levels** | | | |
| | Recall | Application | Analysis | Totals |
| **B. Maintain a Patent Airway Including the Care of Artificial Airways** | 1 | 2 | 2 | 5 |
| 1. Properly position patient | | | | |
| 2. Insert oro- and nasopharyngeal airways | | | | |
| 3. Identify tube placement by available means | | | | |
| 4. Change tracheostomy tubes | | | | |
| 5. Maintain | | | | |
|    a. proper cuff inflation | | | | |
|    b. adequate humidification | | | | |
| 6. Perform extubation procedure | | | | |
| **C. Remove Bronchopulmonary Secretions** | 1 | 2 | 0 | 3 |
| 1. Perform | | | | |
|    a. postural drainage and percussion and/or vibration | | | | |
|    b. nasotracheal suctioning | | | | |
|    c. oropharyngeal suctioning | | | | |
| 2. Suction artificial airways | | | | |
| 3. Administer aerosol therapy, administer prescribed agents [e.g., bronchodilators, corticosteroids, saline, mucolytics] | | | | |
| 4. Instruct and encourage bronchopulmonary hygiene techniques | | | | |
| **D. Achieve Adequate Respiratory Support** | 1 | 4 | 2 | 7 |
| 1. Instruct in | | | | |
|    a. proper breathing technique, encourage deep breathing, instruct and monitor techniques of incentive spirometry | | | | |
|    b. inspiratory muscle training techniques | | | | |
| 2. Initiate and adjust | | | | |
|    a. IPPB therapy | | | | |
|    b. continuous mechanical ventilation settings | | | | |
|    c. noninvasive ventilation | | | | |
|    d. elevated baseline pressure [e.g., CPAP, PEEP] | | | | |
|    e. combinations of ventilatory techniques [e.g., SIMV, PEEP, PS, PCV, IRV, inspiratory hold] | | | | |
| 3. Select ventilator graphics [e.g., waveforms, scales] | | | | |
| 4. Administer | | | | |
|    a. aerosolized drugs [e.g., bronchodilators, corticosteroids, mucolytics] | | | | |
|    b. oxygen—on or off a ventilator | | | | |
| 5. Initiate and modify weaning procedures | | | | |
| 6. Position patient to minimize hypoxemia | | | | |

| | Items | | | |
|---|---|---|---|---|
| **Detailed Content Outline for the Entry Level CRT Examination** | **Cognitive Levels** | | | |
| | Recall | Application | Analysis | Totals |
| Open cells show an examination could include items from indicated cognitive levels. Shaded cells prevent appearance of items on examinations. | | | | |
| 7. Prevent procedure-associated hypoxemia [e.g., oxygenate before and after suctioning and equipment changes] | | | ▓ | ▓ |
| 8. Adhere to infection control policies and procedures [e.g., Standard Precautions] | | ▓ | | |
| **E. Evaluate and Monitor Patient's Objective and Subjective Responses to Respiratory Care** | **4** | **5** | **0** | **9** |
| 1. Recommend and review chest radiograph | | | ▓ | |
| 2. Obtain a blood gas sample | ▓ | | ▓ | |
| a. by puncture | | | ▓ | |
| b. from an arterial or pulmonary artery catheter | | | ▓ | |
| 3. Perform | ▓ | | ▓ | |
| a. pulse oximetry | | | ▓ | |
| b. blood gas and co-oximetry analyses | | | ▓ | |
| c. capnography | | | ▓ | |
| 4. Interpret blood gas and co-oximetry results | | | ▓ | |
| 5. Observe changes in sputum characteristics | | | ▓ | |
| 6. Observe for signs of patient-ventilator dysynchrony | | | ▓ | |
| 7. Perform spirometry, determine vital capacity, measure pulmonary compliance and airways resistance, interpret airway graphics, measure peak flow | | | ▓ | |
| 8. Monitor mean airway pressure, adjust and check alarm systems, measure tidal volume, respiratory rate, airway pressures, I:E, and maximum inspiratory pressure | | | ▓ | |
| 9. Measure $F_IO_2$ and/or liter flow | | ▓ | | |
| 10. Monitor endotracheal or tracheostomy tube cuff pressure | | | ▓ | |
| 11. Auscultate chest and interpret changes in breath sounds | | | ▓ | |
| **F. INDEPENDENTLY MODIFY Therapeutic Procedures Based on the Patient's Response** | **2** | **4** | **19** | **25** |
| 1. Terminate treatment based on patient's response to therapy | | | | ▓ |
| 2. Modify treatment techniques including | ▓ | | | |
| a. IPPB [e.g., volume, flow, pressure, $F_IO_2$, mouthpiece/mask] | | | ▓ | |
| b. Incentive breathing devices | ▓ | | | |
| c. aerosol therapy | ▓ | | ▓ | |
| 1) modify patient breathing patterns | | | ▓ | |
| 2) change type of equipment, change aerosol output | | | ▓ | |
| 3) change dilution of medication, adjust temperature of the aerosol | | | ▓ | |
| d. oxygen therapy | ▓ | | ▓ | |
| 1) change mode of administration, adjust flow, and $F_IO_2$ | | | ▓ | ▓ |
| 2) set up or change an $O_2$ blender | | ▓ | ▓ | ▓ |

# Detailed Content Outline for the Entry Level CRT Examination

Open cells show an examination could include items from indicated cognitive levels.
Shaded cells prevent appearance of items on examinations.

| | Recall | Application | Analysis | Totals |
|---|---|---|---|---|
| e. bronchial hygiene therapy [e.g., alter patient position and duration of treatment and techniques; coordinate sequence of therapies such as chest percussion, postural drainage, and PEP therapy] | | | ▓ | ▓ |
| f. management of artificial airways | ▓ | ▓ | ▓ | ▓ |
| 1) reposition or change endotracheal or tracheostomy tube | | | | ▓ |
| 2) change type of humidification equipment | | | ▓ | ▓ |
| 3) initiate suctioning | | | ▓ | ▓ |
| 4) inflate and/or deflate the cuff | | | ▓ | ▓ |
| 5) perform tracheostomy care | | | ▓ | ▓ |
| g. suctioning | ▓ | ▓ | ▓ | ▓ |
| 1) alter frequency and duration of suctioning | | | ▓ | ▓ |
| 2) change size and type of catheter | | | ▓ | ▓ |
| 3) alter negative pressure | | | ▓ | ▓ |
| 4) instill irrigating solutions | | | ▓ | ▓ |
| h. mechanical ventilation | ▓ | ▓ | ▓ | ▓ |
| 1) improve patient synchrony [e.g., sensitivity, mode] | | | | ▓ |
| 2) enhance oxygenation [e.g., $F_IO_2$, PEEP/CPAP level, inspiratory time] | | | | ▓ |
| 3) improve alveolar ventilation [e.g., tidal volume, rate] | | | | ▓ |
| 4) adjust I:E settings | | | | ▓ |
| 5) modify ventilator techniques [e.g., pressure support, pressure control] | | | | ▓ |
| 6) adjust noninvasive positive pressure ventilation | | | | ▓ |
| 7) monitor and adjust alarm settings | | | ▓ | ▓ |
| 8) adjust ventilator settings based on ventilator graphics | | | | ▓ |
| 9) change type of ventilator, change patient breathing circuitry | | | | ▓ |
| i. procedures for weaning from mechanical ventilation | | | ▓ | ▓ |
| **G. RECOMMEND Modifications in the Respiratory Care Plan Based on the Patient's Response** | 1 | 9 | 2 | 12 |
| 1. Recommend | ▓ | ▓ | ▓ | ▓ |
| a. institution of bronchopulmonary hygiene procedures | | | ▓ | ▓ |
| b. sedation and/or use of muscle relaxant(s) | | | ▓ | ▓ |
| c. insertion or change of artificial airway [e.g., endotracheal tube, LMA, tracheostomy] | | | ▓ | ▓ |
| d. procedures for weaning from mechanical ventilation | | | ▓ | ▓ |
| e. extubation | | | | ▓ |
| f. discontinuing treatment based on patient response | | | ▓ | ▓ |

# Detailed Content Outline for the Entry Level CRT Examination

Open cells show an examination could include items from indicated cognitive levels.
Shaded cells prevent appearance of items on examinations.

| | Recall | Application | Analysis | Totals |
|---|---|---|---|---|
| 2. Recommend changes in | | | | |
|   a. patient position | | | | |
|   b. aerosol drug dosage or concentration | | | | |
|   c. $F_IO_2$ and oxygen flow | | | | |
| 3. Recommend changes in mechanical ventilation to | | | | |
|   a. improve patient synchrony [e.g., sensitivity, mode] | | | | |
|   b. enhance oxygenation [e.g., $F_IO_2$, PEEP/CPAP level, inspiratory time] | | | | |
|   c. improve alveolar ventilation [e.g., tidal volume, rate] | | | | |
|   d. adjust I:E settings | | | | |
|   e. modify ventilator techniques [e.g., pressure support, pressure control] | | | | |
|   f. adjust noninvasive positive pressure ventilation | | | | |
|   g. monitor and adjust alarm settings | | | | |
|   h. adjust ventilator settings based on ventilator graphics | | | | |
|   i. change type of ventilator, change patient breathing circuitry | | | | |
|   j. alter mechanical dead space | | | | |
|   k. modify ventilator settings to | | | | |
|     1) eliminate auto-PEEP | | | | |
|     2) reduce plateau pressure | | | | |
| 4. Recommend use of pharmacologic interventions including | | | | |
|   a. bronchodilators [e.g., adrenergics, anticholinergics, theophyllines] | | | | |
|   b. antiinflammatory drugs [e.g., leukotriene modifiers, corticosteroids, NSAID, cromolyn sodium] | | | | |
|   c. mucolytics/proteolytics [e.g., acetylcysteine, RhDNAse] | | | | |
|   d. sedatives | | | | |
|   e. diuretics | | | | |
| **H. Determine the Appropriateness of the Prescribed Respiratory Care Plan and Recommend Modifications When Indicated** | 1 | 3 | 5 | 9 |
| 1. Analyze available data to determine pathophysiological state | | | | |
| 2. Review | | | | |
|   a. planned therapy to establish therapeutic plan | | | | |
|   b. interdisciplinary patient and family plan | | | | |
| 3. Determine appropriateness of prescribed therapy and goals for identified pathophysiological state | | | | |
| 4. Recommend changes in therapeutic plan when indicated based on data | | | | |
| 5. Perform respiratory care quality assurance | | | | |

| | Items | | | |
|---|---|---|---|---|
| **Detailed Content Outline for the Entry Level CRT Examination** | **Cognitive Levels** | | | |
| | Recall | Application | Analysis | Totals |
| Open cells show an examination could include items from indicated cognitive levels. Shaded cells prevent appearance of items on examinations. | | | | |
| 6. Develop outcomes of | | | | |
|    a. quality improvement programs | | | | |
|    b. respiratory care protocols | | | | |
| 7. Monitor outcomes of | | | | |
|    a. quality improvement programs | | | | |
|    b. respiratory care protocols | | | | |
| 8. Apply respiratory care protocols | | | | |
| **I. Initiate, Conduct, or Modify Respiratory Care Techniques in an Emergency Setting** | 1 | 3 | 0 | 4 |
|   1. Treat cardiopulmonary collapse according to | | | | |
|    a. BCLS | | | | |
|    b. ACLS | | | | |
|    c. Pediatric Advanced Life Support (PALS) | | | | |
|    d. Neonatal Resuscitation Program (NRP) | | | | |
|   2. Participate in | | | | |
|    a. intra-hospital patient transport | | | | |
|    b. disaster management | | | | |
| **J. Act as an Assistant to the Physician Performing Special Procedures Including** | 1 | 1 | 0 | 2 |
|   1. Bronchoscopy | | | | |
|   2. Cardioversion | | | | |
|   3. Intubation | | | | |
| **K. Initiate and Conduct Pulmonary Rehabilitation and Home Care Within the Prescription** | 1 | 1 | 0 | 2 |
|   1. Explain planned therapy and goals to patient in understandable terms to achieve optimal therapeutic outcome | | | | |
|   2. Educate patient and family in disease management | | | | |
|   3. Counsel patient and family concerning smoking cessation | | | | |
|   4. Instruct patient and family to assure safety and infection control | | | | |
| **TOTALS** | 35 | 73 | 32 | 140 |

# Index